CLINICAL NEUROSURGERY

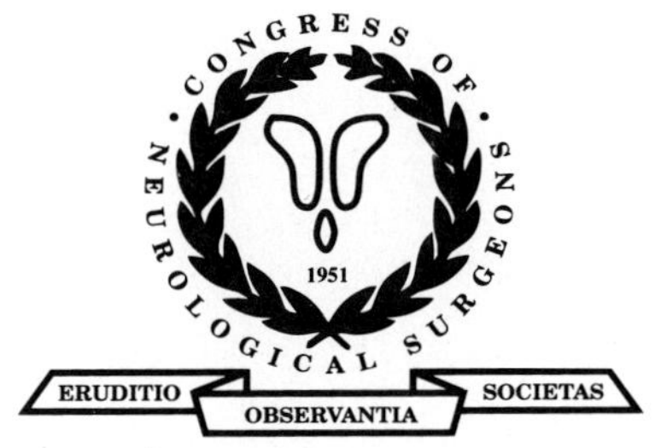

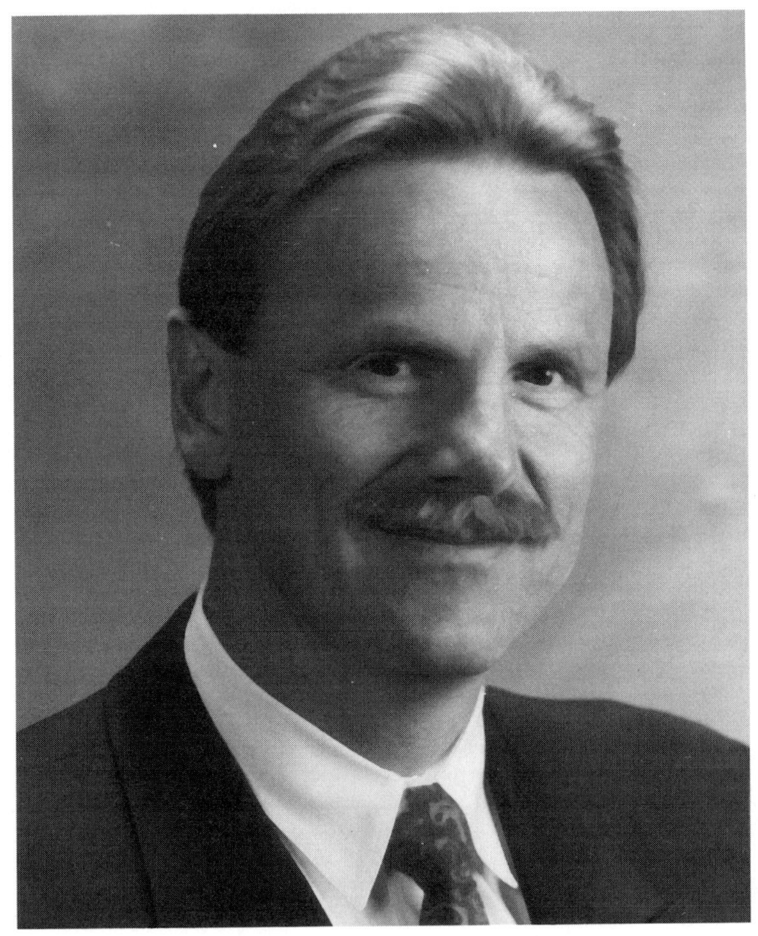

ROBERT F. SPETZLER, M.D.

CLINICAL NEUROSURGERY

Proceedings

OF THE
CONGRESS OF NEUROLOGICAL SURGEONS

Chicago, Illinois
1994

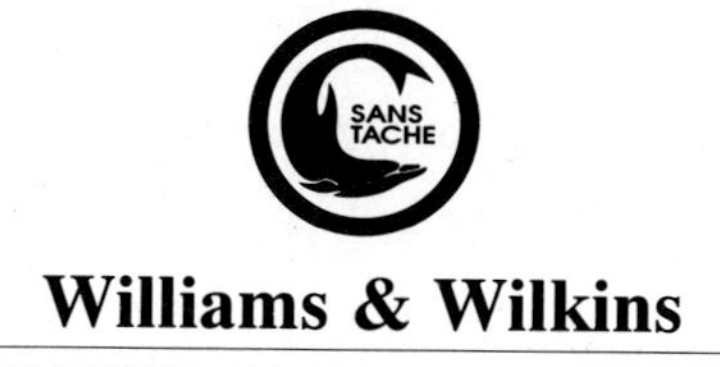

Williams & Wilkins

BALTIMORE • PHILADELPHIA • HONG KONG
LONDON • MUNICH • SYDNEY • TOKYO

A WAVERLY COMPANY

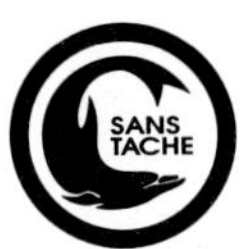

Copyright © 1995
THE CONGRESS OF NEUROLOGICAL SURGEONS

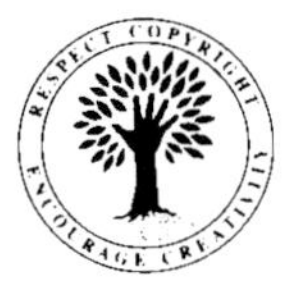

Accurate indications, adverse reactions, and dosage schedules for drugs are provided in this book, but it is possible that they may change. The reader is urged to review the package information data of the manufacturers of the medications mentioned.

ISBN 0-683-02039-0

Printed in the United States of America
(ISBN 0-683-02039-0)

95 96 97 98
1 2 3 4 5 6 7 8 9 10

Reprints of Chapters may be purchased from Williams & Wilkins in quantities of 100 or more. Contact Trudy Rutherford, telephone: (800) 882-0483 or 410-361-8036.

Preface

The 44th Annual Meeting of the Congress of Neurological Surgeons was held in Chicago, Illinois at McCormick Place from October 1–6, 1994. Volume 42 of *Clinical Neurosurgery* represents the official compendium of the platform presentations at that meeting. The meeting was organized and executed by a large number of Congress volunteers led by the Annual Meeting Chairman, H. Hunt Batjer and the General Scientific Program Chairman, Marc R. Mayberg. The McCormick Place facilities were enormous and readily accommodated the record number of neurosurgeons who enrolled for this meeting.

This scientific program was keynoted by the selection of Dr. Robert Spetzler as the honored guest of the Congress. Doctor Spetzler's invited presentations on resection of anterior skull base lesions and on giant aneurysms are included as Chapters 7 and 16 of this volume. As is the custom at the Congress meeting, the general scientific sessions were organized into four broad themes under the direction of the President, Dr. Richard Roski. The first general scientific session was Emerging Health Care Issues in 1994. It should be noted that two of these presentations (those of Doctors Desmarais and Smits) were transcribed from the meeting tapes and edited by the editorial board of *Clinical Neurosurgery*. The flavor of these manuscripts may vary somewhat from the usual submitted form. The remaining general scientific sessions were: Controversies on Skull Base Surgery; Controversies in the Management of Cerebrovascular Malformations; and The Management of Low-Grade Gliomas. Sections I, II, III, and IV of this volume thus reflect the organization of the general scientific sessions at the Congress meeting.

Doctor Roski's eloquent and thoughtful Presidential Address, "The Winds of Change" is presented as Chapter 1. It reflects his broad experience with managed care and socioeconomic issues in neurosurgery; his leadership on this issue is evident.

Notwithstanding the logistical difficulties on opening day engendered by the Chicago Bears game at Soldier Field, the general consensus was that the 44th Annual Meeting of the Congress was a tremendous scientific and social success. The Annual Meeting Committees are to be congratulated on their diligent efforts in presenting an elegant program. From the standpoint of *Clinical Neurosurgery,* I would like to express my gratitude to the eight associate editors all of whom have been called upon to edit specific manuscripts within their section of this volume. Their willingness to perform this task for the 3-year term is greatly appreciated. I would also like to express my gratitude to Carole Pippin and Trudy Rutherford at Williams & Wilkins for all their efforts and for ensuring the timely publication of *Clinical Neurosurgery,* and to my secretary at The University of Iowa, Kathy Escher, who quietly and efficiently handles the vast amount of work that is required from the standpoint of this office to streamline the editorial process. My thanks are also due to Dr. Mark Hadley who volunteered to organize the IRIS response data presented in the final chapter of this book.

CHRISTOPHER M. LOFTUS, M.D., F.A.C.S.
Editor-in-Chief

Editorial Board

ISSAM A. AWAD
KEITH L. BLACK
ROBERT J. DEMPSEY
JAMES T. GOODRICH
M. SEAN GRADY
FREDRIC B. MEYER
JEFFREY J. OLSON
VINCENT C. TRAYNELIS

Editors-in-Chief
Clinical Neurosurgery

Volume	Date	Editor-in-Chief
1	1953	Raymond K. Thompson, M.D.
2	1954	Raymond K. Thompson, M.D. & Ira J. Jackson, M.D.
3	1955	Raymond K. Thompson, M.D. & Ira J. Jackson, M.D.
4	1956	Ira J. Jackson, M.D.
5	1957	Robert G. Fisher, M.D.
6	1958	Robert G. Fisher, M.D.
7	1959	Robert G. Fisher, M.D.
8	1960	William H. Mosberg, Jr., M.D.
9	1961	William H. Mosberg, Jr., M.D.
10	1962	William H. Mosberg, Jr., M.D.
11	1963	John Shillito, Jr., M.D. & William H. Mosberg, Jr., M.D.
12	1964	John Shillito, Jr., M.D.
13	1965	John Shillito, Jr., M.D.
14	1966	Robert G. Ojemann, M.D. & John Shillito, Jr., M.D.
15	1967	Robert G. Ojemann, M.D.
16	1968	Robert G. Ojemann, M.D.
17	1969	Robert G. Ojemann, M.D.
18	1970	George T. Tindall, M.D.
19	1971	George T. Tindall, M.D.
20	1972	Robert H. Wilkins, M.D.
21	1973	Robert H. Wilkins, M.D.
22	1974	Robert H. Wilkins, M.D.
23	1975	Ellis B. Keener, M.D.
24	1976	Ellis B. Keener, M.D.
25	1977	Ellis B. Keener, M.D.
26	1978	Peter W. Carmel, M.D.
27	1979	Peter W. Carmel, M.D.
28	1980	Peter W. Carmel, M.D.
29	1981	Martin H. Weiss, M.D.
30	1982	Martin H. Weiss, M.D.
31	1983	Martin H. Weiss, M.D.
32	1984	John R. Little, M.D.
33	1985	John R. Little, M.D.
34	1986	John R. Little, M.D.
35	1987	Peter McL. Black, M.D., Ph.D.
36	1988	Peter McL. Black, M.D., Ph.D.
37	1989	Peter McL. Black, M.D., Ph.D.
38	1990	Warren R. Selman, M.D.
39	1991	Warren R. Selman, M.D.
40	1992	Warren R. Selman, M.D.
41	1993	Christopher M. Loftus, M.D.
42	1994	Christopher M. Loftus, M.D.

Honored Guests

1952—Professor Herbert Olivecrona, Stockhom, Sweden
1953—Sir Geoffrey Jefferson, Manchester, England
1954—Dr. Kenneth G. McKenzie, Toronto, Canada
1955—Dr. Carl W. Rand, Los Angeles, California
1956—Dr. Wilder G. Penfield, Montreal, Canada
1957—Dr. Francis C. Grant, Philadelphia, Pennsylvania
1958—Dr. A. Earl Walker, Baltimore, Maryland
1959—Dr. William J. German, New Haven, Connecticut
1960—Dr. Paul C. Bucy, Chicago, Illinois
1961—Professor Eduard A. V. Busch, Copenhagen, Denmark
1962—Dr. Bronson S. Ray, New York, New York
1963—Dr. James L. Poppen, Boston, Massachusetts
1964—Dr. Edgar A. Kahn, Ann Arbor, Michigan
1965—Dr. James C. White, Boston, Massachusetts
1966—Dr. Hugo A. Krayenbühl, Zurich, Switzerland
1967—Dr. W. James Gardner, Cleveland, Ohio
1968—Professor Norman M. Dott, Edinburgh, Scotland
1969—Dr. Wallace B. Hamby, Cleveland, Ohio
1970—Dr. Barnes Woodhall, Durham, North Carolina
1971—Dr. Elisha S. Gurdjian, Detroit, Michigan
1972—Dr. Francis Murphey, Memphis, Tennessee
1973—Dr. Henry G. Schwartz, St. Louis, Missouri
1974—Dr. Guy L. Odom, Durham, North Carolina
1975—Dr. William A. Sweet, Boston, Massachusetts
1976—Dr. Lyle A. French, Minneapolis, Minnesota
1977—Dr. Richard C. Schneider, Ann Arbor, Michigan
1978—Dr. Charles G. Drake, London, Ontario, Canada
1979—Dr. Frank H. Mayfield, Cincinnati, Ohio
1980—Dr. Eben Alexander, Jr., Winston-Salem, North Carolina
1981—Dr. J. Garber Galbraith, Birmingham, Alabama
1982—Dr. Keiji Sano, Tokyo, Japan
1983—Dr. C. Miller Fisher, Boston, Massachusetts
1984—Dr. Hugo V. Rizzoli, Washington, D.C.
      Dr. Walter E. Dandy (posthumously), Baltimore, Maryland
1985—Dr. Sidney Goldring, St. Louis, Missouri
1986—Dr. M. Gazi Yasargil, Zurich, Switzerland
1987—Dr. Thomas W. Langfitt, Philadelphia, Pennsylvania

1988—Professor Lindsay Symon, London, England
1989—Dr. Thoralf M. Sundt, Jr., Rochester, Minnesota
1990—Dr. Charles Byron Wilson, San Francisco, California
1991—Dr. Bennett M. Stein, New York, New York
1992—Dr. Robert G. Ojemann, Boston, Massachusetts
1993—Dr. Albert L. Rhoton, Jr., Gainesville, Florida
1994—Dr. Robert F. Spetzler, Phoenix, Arizona

Officers of the Congress
of
Neurological Surgeons
1994

RICHARD A. ROSKI, M.D.
President

RALPH G. DACEY, JR.
President-Elect

STEPHEN J. HAINES, M.D.   DANIEL L. BARROW, M.D.
Vice-President   *Secretary*

WILLIAM A. FRIEDMAN, M.D.
Treasurer

EXECUTIVE COMMITTEE

ISSAM AWAD
ROY P. BAKER
H. HUNT BATJER
MARK H. CAMEL
STEVEN L. GIANNOTTA
RAJ K. NARAYAN
STEPHEN M. PAPADOPOULOS

STANLEY PELOFSKY
RICHARD G. PERRIN
SHIGEAKI KOBAYASHI
MARC R. MAYBERG
LINDA L. STERNAU
JOSEPH ZABRAMSKI
GREG ZORMAN

Contributors

CARGILL ALLEYNE, M.D., Department of Neurosurgery, The Emory Clinic, Atlanta, Georgia (Chapter 15)

OSSAMA AL-MEFTY, M.D., Department of Neurosurgery, University of Arkansas Medical Center, Little Rock, Arkansas (Chapter 11)

DANIEL L. BARROW, M.D., Department of Neurosurgery, The Emory Clinic, Atlanta, Georgia (Chapter 15)

STEPHEN P. BEALS, M.D., Barrow Neurological Institute, Phoenix, Arizona (Chapter 6)

GHASSAN BEJJANI, M.D., Department of Neurological Surgery, The George Washington University Medical Center, Washington, D.C. (Chapter 13)

MITCHEL S. BERGER, M.D., F.A.C.S., Department of Neurological Surgery, University of Washington, Seattle, Washington (Chapter 26)

ALFRED P. BOWLES, M.D., Department of Neurological Surgery, University of Mississippi Medical Center, Jackson, Mississippi (Chapter 11)

J. GREGORY CAIRNCROSS, M.D., Departments of Clinical Neurological Sciences and Oncology, University of Western Ontario and London Regional Cancer Centre, London, Ontario, Canada (Chapter 24)

PAUL J. CAMARATA, M.D., Department of Neurosurgery, University of Minnesota, Minneapolis, Minnesota (Chapter 21)

TAMERLA D. CHAVIS, M.D., School of Medicine and Biomedical Sciences, State University of New York at Buffalo, Buffalo, New York (Chapter 17)

E. ANTONIO CHIOCCA, M.D., PH.D., Department of Surgery and Molecular Neurogenetics Unit, Massachusetts General Hospital, Boston, Massachusetts (Chapter 22)

HENRY DESMARAIS, M.D., M.P.A., Health Policy Alternatives, Washington, DC (Chapter 2)

PAUL A. EBERT, M.D., F.A.C.S., American College of Surgeons, Chicago, Illinois (Chapter 5)

WINK S. FISHER III, M.D., Division of Neurosurgery, University of Alabama at Birmingham, Birmingham, Alabama (Chapter 18)

JOHN C. FLICKINGER, M.D., Department of Neurological Surgery and Radiation Oncology, University of Pittsburgh Medical Center, Pittsburgh, Pennsylvania (Chapter 8)

ITZHAK FRIED, M.D., PH.D., Division of Neurosurgery, School of Medicine, Center for the Health Sciences, Los Angeles, California (Chapter 27)

WILLIAM A. FRIEDMAN, M.D., Department of Neurosurgery, University of Florida, Gainesville, Florida (Chapter 20)

MARY DUFFY FRONCKOWIAK, PH.D., School of Medicine and Biomedical Sciences, State University of New York at Buffalo, Buffalo, New York (Chapter 17)

TAKANORI FUKUSHIMA, M.D., D.M.SC., Center for Skull Base Surgery, Alleghany Neuroscience Institute, Pittsburgh, Pennsylvania (Chapter 9)

KEVIN J. GIBBONS, M.D., School of Medicine and Biomedical Sciences, State University of New York at Buffalo, Buffalo, New York (Chapter 17)

MURAT GUNEL, M.D., Section of Neurosurgery, Yale University School of Medicine, New Haven, Connecticut (Chapter 31)

LEE R. GUTERMAN, PH.D., M.D., School of Medicine and Biomedical Sciences, State University of New York at Buffalo, Buffalo, New York (Chapter 17)

MARK N. HADLEY, M.D., Department of Neurological Surgery, University of Alabama, Birmingham, Alabama (Chapter 32)

MARK G. HAMILTON, M.D.C.M., Alberta Children's Hospital, Alberta, Canada (Chapter 6)

GRIFFITH R. HARSH IV, M.D., Massachusetts General Hospital, Boston, Massachusetts (Chapter 7)

ROBERTO C. HEROS, M.D., Department of Neurosurgery, University of Minnesota, Minneapolis, Minnesota (Chapter 21)

L. NELSON HOPKINS, M.D., School of Medicine and Biomedical Sciences, State University of New York at Buffalo, Buffalo, New York (Chapter 17)

EDWARD F. JOGANIC, M.D., Barrow Neurological Institute, Phoenix, Arizona (Chapter 6)

HIDEFUMI JOKURA, M.D., Department of Neurosurgery, Tohoku University School of Medicine, Sendai, Japan (Chapter 19)

PATRICK J. KELLY, M.D., F.A.C.S., Department of Neurological Surgery, New York University Medical Center, New York, New York (Chapter 25)

HIROYUKI KINOUCHI, M.D., PH.D., Department of Neurosurgery, Tohoku University School of Medicine, Sendai, Japan (Chapter 19)

DOUGLAS KONDZIOLKA, M.D., M.SC., FRCS(C), Departments of Neurological Surgery and Radiation Oncology, University of Pittsburgh, Pittsburgh, Pennsylvania (Chapters 8 and 28)

EDWARD R. LAWS, JR., M.D., F.A.C.S., Department of Neurosurgery, University of Virginia Health Science Center, Charlottesville, Virginia (Chapter 29)

MICHAEL T. LAWTON, M.D., Barrow Neurological Institute, Phoenix, Arizona (Chapters 6 and 16)

L. DADE LUNSFORD, M.D., F.A.C.S., Department of Neurological Surgery, Radiology and Radiation Oncology, University of Pittsburgh Medical Center, Pittsburgh, Pennsylvania (Chapters 8 and 28)

LEONARD I. MALIS, M.D., F.A.C.S., Department of Neurosurgery, The Mount Sinai School of Medicine, New York, New York (Chapter 14)

KAZUO MIZOI, M.D., Department of Neurosurgery, Tohoku University School of Medicine, Sendai, Japan (Chapter 19)

AAGE R. MØLLER, , PH.D., Department of Neurological Surgery, Presbyterian-University Hospital, Pittsburgh, Pennsylvania (Chapter 12)

PETER NORA, M.D., Department of Neurological Surgery, The George Washington University Medical Center, Washington, DC (Chapter 13)

ERIC S. NUSSBAUM, M.D., Department of Neurosurgery, University of Minnesota, Minneapolis, Minnesota (Chapter 21)

ROBERT G. OJEMANN, M.D., Massachusetts General Hospital, Boston Massachusetts (Chapter 7)

JOSEPH M. PIEPMEIER, M.D., F.A.C.S., Section of Neurosurgery, Yale University School of Medicine, New Haven, Connecticut (Chapter 31)

MICHAEL D. PRADOS, M.D., Department of Neurological Surgery, and Brain Tumor Research Center, University of California, San Francisco, California (Chapter 23)

RICHARD A. ROSKI, M.D., F.A.C.S., Quad City Neurological Associates, PA., Davenport, Iowa (Chapter 1)

DAVID SEGAL, M.D., Department of Neurosurgery, The Mount Sinai Medical Center, New York, New York (Chapter 10)

LALIGAM N. SEKHAR, M.D., F.A.C.S., Department of Neurological Surgery, The George Washington University Medical Center, Washington, DC (Chapter 13)

CHANDRANATH SEN, M.D., Department of Neurosurgery, The Mount Sinai Medical Center, New York, New York (Chapter 10)

EDWARD G. SHAW, M.D., Division of Radiation Oncology, Mayo Clinic, Rochester, Minnesota (Chapter 30)

HELEN L. SMITS, Health Care Financing Administration, Washington, DC (Chapter 4)

SALVADOR SOMAZA, M.D., Department of Neurological Surgery, Radiology and Radiation Oncology, University of Pittsburgh Medical Center, Pittsburgh, Pennsylvania (Chapter 28)

ROBERT F. SPETZLER, M.D., Barrow Neurological Institute, Phoenix, Arizona (Chapters 6 and 16)

SCOTT C. STANDARD, M.D., School of Medicine and Biomedical Sciences, State University of New York at Buffalo, Buffalo, New York (Chapter 17)

AKIRA TAKAHASHI, M.D., Department of Neurosurgery, Tohoku University School of Medicine, Sendai, Japan (Chapter 19)

ALLAN F. THORNTON, M.D., Massachusetts General Hospital, Boston, Massachusetts (Chapter 7)

PEDRO L. VERA, PH.D., Department of Neurological Surgery, The George Washington University Medical Center, Washington, DC (Chapter 13)

DAVID E. VOGEL, M.S., David E. Vogel and Associates, Phoenix, Arizona (Chapter 3)

CHARLES B. WILSON, M.D., Department of Neurological Surgery, and Brain Tumor Research Center, University of California, San Francisco, California (Chapter 23)

THOMAS C. WITT, M.D., Department of Neurological Surgery, University of Pittsburgh Medical Center, Pittsburgh, Pennsylvania (Chapter 8)

TAKASHI YOSHIMOTO, M.D., Department of Neurosurgery, Tohoku University School of Medicine, Sendai, Japan (Chapter 19)

Biography of Robert F. Spetzler, M.D.

Robert F. Spetzler attended Knox College in Galesburg, Illinois, from 1963 to 1966 and graduated *cum laude* with a Bachelor's of Science degree in Biology and Chemistry. Before graduating, he spent a year at the Free University of Berlin on a scholarship. In 1967, he entered medical school at Northwestern University, where he obtained his M.D. in 1971 and completed his internship in 1972.

In 1972 Dr. Spetzler moved to the University of California at San Francisco, where he trained as a resident under Charles B. Wilson, MD, Professor and Chairman of the Department of Neurosurgery. It was there, under the expert tutelage of Dr. Wilson, that his interest in neurovascular surgery developed. His commitment to academic neurosurgery also was established at this time. Before finishing his residency, he had already published 15 articles in refereed journals, on 8 of which he was first author; had helped edit two books; and had made almost 20 presentations at national and international meetings. During the last year of his residency, he was awarded a Trauma Fellowship from the National Institutes of Health (NIH). He also received the Annual Resident Award at the 27th Annual Meeting of the Congress of Neurological Surgeons.

After completing his residency in 1977, Dr. Spetzler joined the Department of Neurosurgery at Case Western Reserve University School of Medicine in Cleveland, Ohio, as an Assistant Professor. In 1980 he received his first major grant from NIH, developing a baboon model of stroke that has since been particularly generative for testing new therapeutic treatments for stroke and cerebral ischemia. In 1981, he was promoted to Associate Professor, holding that appointment until 1983. His commitment to clinical research during that period was rewarded with about 40 articles published in refereed journals and 16 book chapters.

In 1983 Dr. Spetzler was recruited by Dr. John R. Green to assume the J. N. Harber Chair of Neurological Surgery at the Barrow Neurological Institute (BNI) in Phoenix, Arizona. Two years later when Dr. Green retired, Dr. Spetzler assumed the position of Director of the Institute. Under Dr. Spetzler's leadership, the BNI has grown from primarily a regional center to an internationally recognized center of excellence that attracts both visiting health care professionals and patient referrals from around the world. The residency program has become one of the most highly sought after programs because of the diversity of clinical experience and the emphasis on developing independent research projects.

Just a few of Dr. Spetzler's contributions have been the development of theories on normal perfusion pressure break-through and how the size of arteriovenous malformations (AVMs) is related to their rupture; the development of a heuristic grading system for AVMs; advances in the surgical treatment of complex cerebrovascular lesions based on hypothermia, barbiturates, and cardiac arrest; and the development of innovative surgical approaches for skull base surgery. In the last decade this work has been reflected in 100 articles published in refereed journals; 83 book chapters either published or in press; the establishment of the official journal of the BNI, the *BNI Quarterly;* and several books and neurosurgical atlases.

These accomplishments underscore the reasons Dr. Spetzler has been chosen as the Honored Guest of the Congress of Neurological Surgeons—the youngest member ever to receive this coveted honor.

Bibliography of Robert F. Spetzler, M.D.

BOOKS

KOOS WT, BOCK FW, SPETZLER RF: *Clinical Microsurgery.* Stuttgart, Georg Thieme Verlag, 1976.

SCHMIEDEK P, GRATZL O, SPETZLER RF: *Microsurgery for Stroke.* New York, Springer-Verlag, 1977.

KOOS WT, SPETZLER RF, LANG J (eds) (with contributions from Pendl G, Perneczky A): Color Atlas of Microneurosurgery. Stuttgart, Georg Thieme, 1986.

SPETZLER RF, CARTER LP, SELMAN, WR, *et al.* (eds): *Cerebral Revascularization for Stroke.* New York, Thieme-Stratton, 1985.

KOOS WT, SPETZLER RF, LANG J (eds) (with contributions from Pendl G. Perneczky A): *Color Atlas of Tumors.* Stuttgart, Georg Thieme Verlag, 1993, ed 2.

KOOS WT, SPETZLER RF, LANG J (eds) (with contributions from Pendl G, Perneczky A): *Color Atlas of Microneurosurgery.* Stuttgart, Georg Thieme Verlag, 1993, ed 2.

SPETZLER RF, KOOS WT, LANG J (eds) (with contributions from Perneczky A, Richling B, Zabramski JM: *Color Atlas of Cerebrovascular Tumors,* Stuttgart, Georg Thieme Verlag, in press, 1995.

CARTER LP, SPETZLER RF, HAMILTON MG (eds): *Neurovascular Surgery,* New York, McGraw Hill, 1995.

REFEREED JOURNALS

Manuscripts in Press (3)

GOLFINOS JG, DICKMAN CA, SONNTAG VKH, ZABRAMSKI JM, SPETZLER RF: Repair of vertebral artery injury during anterior cervical decompression. **Spine** 19(22):2552–2556, 1995.

Manuscripts Submitted in 1994 (19)

ANSON JA, SPETZLER RF: Characteristics and surgical treatment of dolichoectatic and fusiform aneurysms. **J Neurosurg,** submitted for publication, 1994–95.

APOSTOLIDES PJ, JOHNSON PC, SPETZLER RF: Ectomesenchymal hamartoma (benign "ectomesenchymoma") of the eighth nerve. **J Neurosurg,** submitted for publication, 1994–95.

BALDWIN HZ, SPETZLER RF, WASCHER TM, DASPIT CP: The far-lateral-combined supra- and infratentorial approach: Clinical experience. **Acta Neurochir,** in press, 1995.

GREENE KA, MARCIANO FF, JACOBOWITZ R, JOHNSON BA, SPETZLER RF, HARRINGTON TR: Impact of traumatic subarachnoid hemorrhage on outcome in non-penetrating head injury. A proposed CT grading scale. **J Neurosurg,** in press, 1995.

GOLFINOS JG, FITZPATRICK BC, SMITH LR, SPETZLER RF: Clinical use of a frameless stereotactic arm: Results of 325 cases. **J Neurosurg,** in press, 1995.

GREENE KA, KARAHALIOS DG, MARCIANO FF, DICKMAN CA, SPETZLER RF: Glossopharyngeal neuralgia associated with vascular compression and choroid plexus papilloma. **Br J Neurosurg,** in press, 1995.

GREENE KA, MARCIANO FF, DICKMAN CA, COONS SW, JOHNSON PC, BAILES JE, SPETZLER RF: Anterior communicating artery aneurysm paraparesis syndrome: Clinical manifestations and pathological correlates. **Neurology,** in press, 45:, 1995.

HERMAN JM, SPETZLER RF, BEDERSON JB, KURBAT JM, ZABRAMSKI JM: Genesis of a dural arteriovenous malformation (AVM): A rat model. **J Neurosurg,** in press, 1995.

KRAUS G, HERMAN JM, LEE KS, SPETZLER RF, FREY JL: Middle cerebral artery endarterectomy: Experience with two cases. **Surg Neurol,** in press, 1995.

LAWTON MT, HAMILTON MG, SPETZLER RF: Multimodality treatment of deep arteriovenous malformations: Thalamus, basal ganglia, and brain stem. Neurosurgery, in press, 1995.

PORTER RW, LAWTON MT, HAMILTON MG, SPETZLER RF: Concurrent rupture of basilar artery aneurysm and thrombosis of high grade internal carotid artery stenosis: Case report. **Neurosurgery,** submitted for publication, 1994–95.

SMITH KA, SPETZLER RF: Supratentorial-infraoccipital approach for posteromedial temporal lobe lesions. **J Neurosurg,** in press.

ZABRAMSKI JM, SPETZLER RF, BALDWIN HZ, FRAM EK: A new primate model of reversible focal cerebral ischemia: Description and characterization. **Stroke,** submitted for publication, 1994–95.

Manuscripts Published in 1994 (7)

BALDWIN HZ, MILLER CG, VAN LOVEREN HR, KELLER JT, DASPIT CP, SPETZLER RF: The far lateral/combined supra- and infratentorial approach: A human cadaveric prosection model for routes of access to the petroclival region and ventral brain stem. **J Neurosurg** 81: 60–68, 1994.

GREENE KA, MARCIANO FF, HAMILTON MG, HERMAN JM, REKATE HL, SPETZLER RF: Cardiopulmonary bypass, hypothermic circulatory arrest, and barbiturate cerebral protection for the treatment of giant vertebrobasilar aneurysms in children. **Pediatr Neurosurg** 21:124–133, 1994.

HAMILTON MG, SPETZLER RF: The prospective application of a grading system for arteriovenous malformations. **Neurosurgery** 34(1):2–7, 1994.

KHAYATA MH, SPETZLER RF, MOOY JJA, HERMAN JM, REKATE HL: Combined surgical and endovascular treatment of giant vertebral artery aneurysm in a child: Case report. **J Neurosurg** 81:304–307, 1994.

McCORMICK PW, McCORMICK J, ZABRAMSKI JM, SPETZLER RF: Hemodynamics of subarachnoid hemorrhage arrest. **J Neurosurg** 80: 710–715, 1994.

SMITH KA, KRAUS GE, JOHNSON BA, SPETZLER RF: Giant posterior communicating artery aneurysm presenting a third ventricular mass with obstructive hydrocephalus. **J Neurosurg** 81:299–303, 1994.

ZABRAMSKI JM, WASCHER TM, SPETZLER RF, JOHNSON B, GOLFINOS J, DRAYER BP, BROWN B, BROWN G: The natural history of familial cavernous malformations: Results of an ongoing study. **J Neurosurg** 80:422–432, 1994.

Manuscripts Published in 1993 (15)

ANSON JA, HEISERMAN JE, DRAYER BP, SPETZLER RF: Surgical decisions based on magnetic resonance angiography of the carotid arteries. **Neurosurgery** 32(3):335–343, 1993.

ANSON JA, SPETZLER RF: Endarterectomy of the intradural vertebral artery via the far lateral approach. **Neurosurgery** 33(5):804–811, 1993.

ANSON JA, SPETZLER RF: Surgical resection of intramedullary spinal cord cavernous malformations. **J Neurosurg** 78(3):446–451, 1993.

DEAN BL, FLOM RA, WALLACE RC, KHAYATA MH, OBUCHOWSKI NA, HODAK JA, ZABRAMSKI JM, SPETZLER RF: Efficacy of endovascular treatment of meningiomas: Evaluation with matched samples. **AJNR** 15:1675–1680, 1994.

FRITSCHI JA, REULEN H-J, SPETZLER RF, ZABRAMSKI JM: Cavernous malformations of the brain stem. A review of 139 cases. **Acta Neurochir** (Wien) 130:35–46, 1994.

DICKMAN CA, PAPADOPOULOS SM, SONNTAG VKH, SPETZLER RF, REKATE HL, DRABIER J: Traumatic occipitoatlantal dislocations. **J Spinal Disord** 6(4):300–313, 1993.

EGEMEN N, TURKER RK, SANLIDILEK U, ZORLUTUNA A, BILGIC S,

BASKAYA M, UNLU A, CAGLAR S, SPETZLER RF, MCCORMICK JM: The effect of intrathecal sodium nitroprusside on severe chronic vasospasm. **Neurol Res** 15:310–315, 1993.

FITZPATRICK BC, SPETZLER RF, BALLARD JL, ZIMMERMAN RS: Cervical-to-petrous internal carotid artery bypass: Technical procedure. **J Neurosurg** 79(1):138–141, 1993.

GREENE KA, ANSON JA, MARTINEZ JA, SPETZLER RF, JOHNSON PC: Multicystic metastatic carcinoid to brain: Case report. **J Neurooncol** 17:15–20, 1993.

GREENE KA, ANSON JA, SPETZLER RF: Giant serpentine middle cerebral artery aneurysm treated by extracranial-intracranial bypass: Case report. **J Neurosurg** 78(6):974–978, 1993.

HERMAN JM, SPETZLER RF: An evaluation of the Superlux 300 illumination system. **Neurosurgery** 32(6):1048, 1993.

KHAYATA M, SONNTAG VKH, SPETZLER RF: The intraoperative applications of the Diasonics 9400 mobile neuroimaging system. **Neurosurgery** 32(5):869–870, 1993.

KHAYATA ME, ZABRAMSKI JM, JOHNSON PC, FLOM R: False aneurysm associated with rupture of an arteriovenous malformation—Implications for treatment: Case report. **Neurosurgery** 33(4):753–756, 1993.

MCCORMICK JM, MCCORMICK PW, ZABRAMSKI JM, SPETZLER RF: Intracranial pressure reduction by a central alpha-2 adrenoreceptor agonist following subarachnoid hemorrhage. **Neurosurgery** 32(6): 974–979, 1993.

MCCORMICK PW, SPETZLER RF, JOHNSON PC, DRAYER BP: Cerebellar hemorrhage associated with capillary telangiectasia and venous angioma: A case report. **Surg Neurol** 39(6):451–457, 1993.

SPETZLER RF, HERMAN JM, BEALS S, JOGANIC E, MILLIGAN J: Preservation of olfaction in anterior craniofacial approaches. **J Neurosurg** 79(1):48–51, 1993.

WASCHER TM, SPETZLER RF, ZABRAMSKI JM: Improved transdural exposure and temporary occlusion of the petrous internal carotid artery for cavernous sinus surgery: Technical note. **J Neurosurg** 78(5):834–837, 1993.

Manuscripts Published in 1992 (7)

BEDERSON JB, SPETZLER RF: Anastomosis of the anterior temporal artery to a secondary trunk of the middle cerebral artery for treatment of a giant M1 segment aneurysm. Case report. **J Neurosurg** 76(5):863–866, 1992.

BEDERSON JB, ZABRAMSKI JM, SPETZLER RF: Treatment of fusiform intracranial aneurysms by circumferential wrapping and clip-reinforcement: Technical note. **J Neurosurg** 77(3):478–480, 1992.

HERMAN JM, HAMILTON M, SPETZLER RF: Skull base neurosurgery. **Crit Rev Neurosurg** 2:257–265, 1992.

HERMAN JM, REKATE HL, SPETZLER RF: Pediatric intracranial aneurysms: Simple and complex cases. **Pediatr Neurosurg** 17(2): 66–73, 1991–92.

MCCORMICK PW, SPETZLER RF, BAILES JE, ZABRAMSKI JM, PREY JL: Thromboendarterectomy of the symptomatic occluded internal carotid artery. **J Neurosurg** 76(5):752–758, 1992.

SPETZLER RF, DASPIT CP, PAPPAS CTE: The combined supra- and infratentorial approach for lesions of the petrous and clival regions: Experience with 46 cases. **J Neurosurg** 76:588–599, 1992.

SPETZLER RF, HARGRAVES RW, MCCORMICK PW, ZABRAMSKI JM, FLOM RA, ZIMMERMAN RS: Relationship of perfusion pressure and size to risk of hemorrhage from arteriovenous malformations. **J Neurosurg** 76(6):918–923, 1992.

Manuscripts Published in 1991 (10)

CARTER LP, GRAHM T, BAILES JE, BICHARD W, SPETZLER RF: Continuous postoperative monitoring of cortical blood flow and intracranial pressure. **Surg Neurol** 35(1):36–39, 1991.

CULICCHIA F, SPETZLER RF, FLOM RA: Failure of transluminal angioplasty in the treatment of myointimal hyperplasia of the internal carotid artery: Case report. **Neurosurgery** 28(1):148–151, 1991.

DASPIT CP, SPETZLER RF, PAPPAS CT: Combined approach for lesions involving the cerebellopontine angle and skull base: Experience with 20 cases—Preliminary report. **Otolaryngol Head Neck Surg** 105(6):788–796, 1991.

PAPADOPOULOS SM, DICKMAN CA, SONNTAG VKH, REKATE HL, SPETZLER RF: Traumatic atlantooccipital dislocation with survival. **Neurosurgery** 28(4):574–579, 1991.

RIGAMONTI D, JOHNSON PC, SPETZLER RF, HADLEY MN, DRAYER BP: Cavernous malformations and capillary telangiectasia: A spectrum within a single pathological entity. **Neurosurgery** 28(1):60–64, 1991.

ROSENBAUM D, ZABRAMSKI J, FREY J, YATSU F, MARLER J, SPETZLER R, GROTTO J: Early treatment of ischemic stroke with a calcium antagonist. **Stroke** 22:437–441, 1991.

SPETZLER RF, DASPIT CP, PAPPAS CTE: Combined approach for lesions involving the cerebellopontine angle and skull base: Experience with 30 cases. **Skull Base Surg** 1(4):226–234, 1991.

WILLIAMS FC JR, ZABRAMSKI JM, SPETZLER RF, REKATE HL: Anterolateral transthoracic transvertebral resection of an intramedullary spinal arteriovenous malformation: Case report. **J Neurosurg** 74(6):1004–1008, 1991.

Zabramski JM, Spetzler RF, Lee KS, Papadopoulos SM, Bovill E, Zimmerman RS, Bederson JB: Phase I trial of tissue plasminogen activator for the prevention of vasospasm in patients with aneurysmal subarachnoid hemorrhage. **J Neurosurg** 75(2):189–196, 1991.

Zimmerman RS, Spetzler RF, Lee KS, Zabramski JM, Hargraves RW: Cavernous malformations of the brain stem. **J Neurosurg** 75:32–39, 1991.

Manuscripts Published in 1990 (13)

Bailes JE, Spetzler RF, Hadley MN, Baldwin HZ: Management morbidity and mortality of poor-grade aneurysm patients. **J Neurosurg** 72:559–566, 1990.

Benes V, Zabramski JM, Boston M, Puca A, Spetzler RF: Effect of intra-arterial tissue plasminogen activator and urokinase on autologous arterial emboli in the cerebral circulation of rabbits. (Corrected; published erratum appears in **Stroke** Feb:22(2):285, 1991.) **Stroke** 21:1594–1599, 1990.

Dickman CA, Shedd SA, Spetzler RF, Shetter AG, Sonntag VKH: Spinal epidural hematomas associated with epidural anesthesia: Complications of systemic heparinization in patients receiving peripheral vascular thrombolytic therapy. **Anesthesiology** 72:947–950, 1990.

Grahm TW, Williams FC Jr, Harrington T, Spetzler RF: Civilian gunshot wounds to the head: A prospective study. **Neurosurgery** 27(5)696–700, 1990.

Lee, KS, Spetzler RF: Spinal cord cavernous malformation in a patient with familial intracranial cavernous malformations. **Neurosurgery** 26(5):877–880, 1990.

Lee KS, Liu SS, Spetzler RF, Rekate HL: Intracranial mycotic aneurysm in an infant: Report of a case. **Neurosurgery** 26:129–133, 1990.

Liu SS, Williams KD, Drayer BP, Spetzler RF, Sonntag VKH: Synovial cysts of the lumbosacral spine: Diagnosis by imaging. **ARJ** 154(1):163–166,1990.

Martin NA, King WA, Wilson CB, Nutik S, Garter LP, Spetzler RF: Management of dural arteriovenous malformations of the anterior cranial fossa. **J Neurosurg** 72:692–697, 1990.

Puca A, Spetzler RF, Zabramski JM: Hydrostatic dilatation of autologous vein grafts: A technical note. **Neurosurgery** 26(6):1071–1072, 1990.

RIGAMONTI D, SPETZLER RF, MEDINA M, RIGAMONTI K, GECKLE DS, PAPPAS CT: Cerebral venous malformations. **J Neurosurg** 73(4): 560–564, 1990.

RIGAMONTI D, PAPPAS CTE, SPETZLER RF, JOHNSON PC: Extracerebral cavernous angiomas of the middle fossa. **Neurosurgery** 27:306–310, 1990.

SPETZLER RF, FUKISHIMA T, MARTIN N, ZABRAMSKI JM: Petrous carotid-to-intradural carotid saphenous vein graft for intracavernous giant aneurysm, tumor, and occlusive cerebrovascular disease. **J Neurosurg** 73(4):496–501, 1990.

SPETZLER RF, LEE KS: Reconstruction of the temporalis muscle for the pterional craniotomy: Technical note. **J Neurosurg** 73(4):636–637, 1990.

Manuscripts Published in 1989 (7)

BALDWIN H, HADLEY MN, PITTMAN H, SPETZLER RF, DROVER BP: Gadolinium-DTPA enhancement of a recurrent intramedullary ependymoma: A case report. **Surg Neurol** 31:220–223, 1989.

DASPIT CP, SPETZLER RF: Synovial chondromatosis of the temporomandibular joint with intracranial extension: Case report. **J Neurosurg** 70:121–123, 1989.

HADLEY MN, ZABRAMSKI JM, SPETZLER RF, RIGAMONTI D, FIFIELD MS, JOHNSON PC: The efficacy of intravenous nimodipine in the treatment of focal cerebral ischemia in a primate model. **Neurosurgery** 25(1)63–70, 1989.

HADLEY MN, SPETZLER RF, SONNTAG VKH: The transoral approach to the superior cervical spine. A review of 53 cases of extradural cervicomedullary compression. **J Neurosurg** 71:16–23, 1989.

LIU SS, WILLIAMS KD, DRAYER BP, SPETZLER RF, SONNTAG VKH: Synovial cysts of the lumbosacral spine: Diagnosis by MR imaging. **AJNR** 10:1239–1242, 1989.

SPETZLER RF, HADLEY MN: Protection against cerebral ischemia: The role of barbiturates. **Cerebrovasc Brain Metab Rev** 1:212–229, 1989.

SPETZLER RF, ZABRAMSKI JM, FLOM RA: Management of juvenile spinal AVMs by embolization and operative excision. **J Neurosurg** 70:628–632, 1989.

Manuscripts Published in 1988 (12)

BOJANOWSKI WM, RIGAMONTI D, SPETZLER RF, FLOM R: Angiographic demonstration of the meningeal branch of the posterior cerebral artery. **AJNR** 9(4):808, 1988.

BOJANOWSKI WM, SPETZLER RF, CARTER LP: Reconstruction of the MCA bifurcation after excision of a giant aneurysm: A technical note. **J Neurosurg** 60:974–977, 1988.

HADLEY MN, MARTIN NA, SPETZLER RF, SONNTAG VKH, JOHNSON PC: Comparative transoral dural closure techniques: A canine model. **Neurosurgery** 22(2):392–397, 1988.

HADLEY MN, SPETZLER RF, MARTIN NA, JOHNSON PC: Middle cerebral artery aneurysm due to *Nocardia asteroides*. Case report of aneurysm excision and extracranial-intracranial bypass. **Neurosurgery** 22(5):923–928, 1988.

MARANO SR, JOHNSON PC, SPETZLER RF: Recurrent Lhermitte-Duclos disease in a child. **J Neurosurg** 69(10):599–603, 1988.

RIGAMONTI D, SPETZLER RF, DRAYER BP, BOJANOWSKI WM, HODAK J, RIGAMONTI KH, PLENGE K, POWERS M, REKATE H: Appearance of venous malformations on magnetic resonance imaging. **J Neurosurg** 69:535–539, 1988.

RIGAMONTI D, HADLEY MN, DRAYER BP, JOHNSON PC, HOENIG-RIGA-MONTI K, KNIGHT JT, SPETZLER RF: Cerebral cavernous malformations: Incidence and familial occurrence. **N Engl J Med** 319:343–347, 1988.

RIGAMONTI D, SPETZLER RF: The association of venous and cavernous malformations. Report of four cases and discussion of the pathophysiological, diagnostic, and therapeutic implications. **Acta Neurochir (Wien)** 92:100–105, 1988.

RIGAMONTI D, REKATE H, PITTMAN H, SPETZLER RF: Cavernous malformations (angiomas) in children. **J Pediatr Neurosci** 4(1):55–59, 1988.

SPETZLER RF, HADLEY MN, RIGAMONTI D, CARTER LP, RAUDZENS PA, SHEDD SA, WILKINSON E: Aneurysms of the basilar artery treated with circulatory arrest, hypothermia, and barbiturate cerebral protection. **J Neurosurg** 68(6):868–879, 1988.

SPETZLER RF, HADLEY MN, SONNTAG VKH: The transoral approach to the anterior superior cervical spine. A review of 29 cases. **Acta Neurochir** 43:69–74, 1988.

SPETZLER RF, ZABRAMSKI JM: Surgical management of large AVMs. **Acta Neurochir (Suppl)** 42:93–97, 1988.

Manuscripts Published in 1987 (10)

AWAD IA, SPETZLER RF, HODAK JA, AWAD CA, WILLIAMS F JR, CAREY R: Incidental lesions noted on magnetic resonance imaging of the brain—prevalence and clinical significance in various age groups. **Neurosurgery** 20(2):222–227, 1987.

AWAD IA, CARTER LP, SPETZLER RF, MEDINA M, WILLIAMS F: Clinical vasospasm after subarachnoid hemorrhage: Response to hypervolemic hemodilution and arterial hypertension. **Stroke** 18(2):365–372, 1987.

HADLEY, MN, MARTIN NA, SPETZLER, RF, JOHNSON PC: Multiple intracranial aneurysms due to *Coccidioides immitis:* Case report. **J Neurosurg** 66:453–456, 1987.

HADLEY MN, SPETZLER RF, FIFIELD MS, BICHARD WD, HODAK JA: The effect of nimodipine on intracranial pressure: Volume-pressure studies in a primate model. **J Neurosurg** 66:387–393, 1987.

HOPKINS LN, MARTIN NA, HADLEY MN, SPETZLER RF, BUDNY J, CARTER LP: Vertebrobasilar insufficiency. Part II: Microsurgical treatment of intracranial vertebrobasilar disease. **J Neurosurg** 66(5)662–674, 1987.

NEHLS DG, TODD MM, SPETZLER RF, DRUMMOND JC, THOMPSON RA, JOHNSON PC: A comparison of the cerebral protective effects of isoflurane and barbiturates during temporary focal ischemia in primates. **Anesthesiology** 66:453–464, 1987.

RIGAMONTI D, DRAYER BP, JOHNSON PC, HADLEY MN, ZABRAMSKI J, SPETZLER RF: The MRI appearance of cavernous malformations (angiomas). **Neurosurgery** 67:518–524, 1987.

RIGAMONTI D, SPETZLER RF, SHETTER A, DRAYER BP: Magnetic resonance imaging and trigeminal schwannoma. **Surg Neurol** 28:67–70 1987.

SPETZLER RF, MARTIN NA, CARTER LP, FLOM RA, RAUDZENS RA, WILKINSON E: Surgical management of large AVM's by staged embolization and operative excision. **J Neurosurg** 67:17–28, 1987.

SPETZLER RF, HADLEY MN, MARTIN NA, HOPKINS LN, CARTER LP, BUDNY J: Vertebrobasilar insufficiency. Part I: Microsurgical treatment of extracranial vertebrobasilar disease. **J Neurosurg** 66(5): 648–661, 1987.

Manuscripts Published in 1986 (10)

AWAD IA, SPETZLER RF: Extracranial-intracranial bypass surgery: A critical analysis in light of the International Cooperative Study. **Neurosurgery** 19(4):655–664, 1986.

AWAD IA, SPETZLER RF, HODAK JA, AWAD CA, CAREY R: Incidental subcortical lesions identified on magnetic resonance imaging in the elderly. I. Correlation with age and cerebrovascular risk factors. **Stroke** 17(6):1084–1089, 1986.

AWAD IA, JOHNSON PC, SPETZLER RF, HODAK JA: Incidental subcortical lesions identified on magnetic resonance imaging in the elderly.

II. Postmortem pathological correlations. **Stroke** 17(6):1090–1097, 1986.

BLAZIER CJ, HADLEY MN, SPETZLER RF: The transoral surgical approach to craniovertebral pathology. **J Neurosci Nurs** 18(2):57–62, 1986.

MARANO SR, BROOKS RA, SPETZLER RF, REKATE HL: Giant congenital cellular blue nevus of the scalp of a newborn with an underlying skull defect and invasion of the dura mater. **Neurosurgery** 18(1): 85–89, 1986.

MARTIN NA, HADLEY MN, SPETZLER RF, CARTER LP: Management of asymptomatic carotid atherosclerosis. **Neurosurgery** 18(4):505–513, 1986.

SPETZLER RF, MARTIN NA: A proposed grading system for arteriovenous malformation. **J Neurosurg** 65(4):476–483, 1986.

SPETZLER RF, MARTIN NA, HADLEY MN, THOMPSON RA, WILKINSON E, RAUDZENS PA: Microsurgical endarterectomy under barbiturate protection: A prospective study. **J Neurosurg** 65:63–73, 1986.

ZABRAMSKI JM, SPETZLER RF, BONSTELLE C: Chronic cerebral vasospasm: Effect of volume and timing of hemorrhage in a canine model. **Neurosurgery** 18(1):1–6, 1986.

ZABRAMSKI J, SPETZLER RF, BONSTELLE C: Chronic cerebral vasospasm: Effect of calcium antagonists. **Neurosurgery** 18(2):129–135, 1986.

Manuscripts Published in 1985 (10)

ARCHIBALD JE, DRAZKOWSKI JP, WILKINSON E, SPETZLER RF: Human variance to high dose thiopental therapy as determined by EEG/CSA monitoring. **Am J EEG Technol** 25:225–239, 1985.

CARTWRIGHT MJ, NEHLS DG, CARRION CA, SPETZLER RF: Synovial cyst of a cervical facet joint: Case report. **Neurosurgery** 16(6):850–852, 1985.

HADLEY MN, GRAHM TW, DASPIT CP, SPETZLER RF: Otolaryngologic manifestations of posterior fossa arachnoid cysts. **Laryngoscope** 95:678–681, 1985.

HADLEY MN, SPETZLER RF, MASFERRER R, MARTIN NA, CARTER LP: Occipital artery to extradural vertebral artery bypass procedure: Case report. **J Neurosurg** 63:622–625, 1985.

NEHLS DG, FLOM RA, CARTER LP, SPETZLER RF: Multiple intracranial aneurysms: Determining the site of rupture. **J Neurosurg** 63:342–348, 1985.

NEHLS DG, MARANO SR, SPETZLER RF: Transcallosal approach to the contralateral ventricle: Technical note. **J Neurosurg** 62:304–306, 1985.

NEHLS DG, MARANO SR, SPETZLER RF: Positional intermittent occlusion of the internal carotid artery: Case report. **J Neurosurg** 62:435–437, 1985.

SPETZLER RF, CARTER LP: Revascularization and aneurysm surgery: Current status. **Neurosurgery** 16(1):111–116, 1985.

SPETZLER RF, ZABRAMSKI JM, KAUFMAN B: Clinical role of magnetic resonance imaging in the neurosurgical patient. **Neurosurgery** 16(4):511–524, 1985.

ZABRAMSKI JM, SPETZLER RF, KAUFMAN B: Magnetic resonance imaging: Comparative study of radiofrequency pulse techniques in the evaluation of focal ischemia. **Neurosurgery** 16(4):502–510, 1985.

Manuscripts Published in 1984 (9)

CARTER LP, CROWELL RM, SONNTAG VKH, SPETZLER RF: Cortical blood flow during extracranial-intracranial bypass surgery. **Stroke** 15(5):836–839, 1984.

LOCKHART C, SELMAN WR, RODZIEWICZ G, SPETZLER RF: Percutaneous insertion of peritoneal shunt catheters with use of the Veress needle: Technical note. **J Neurosurg** 60:444–446, 1984.

MARANO SR, SONNTAG VKH, SPETZLER RF: Planum sphenoidale meningioma mimicking pituitary apoplexy: A case report. **Neurosurgery** 15(6):859–862, 1984.

RODZIEWICZ GS, KAUFMAN B, SPETZLER RF: Diagnosis of sacral perineural cysts by nuclear magnetic resonance. **Surg Neurol** 22:50–52, 1984.

SELMAN WR, SPETZLER RF: New lumboperitoneal shunt catheter. **Surg Neurol** 21:58–60, 1984.

SPETZLER RF: Neurosurgeon of the Year: Charles B. Wilson. **Surg Neurol** 21:1–2, 1984.

SPETZLER RF, SELMAN WR, CARTER LP: Elective EC-IC bypass for unclippable intracranial aneurysms. **Neurol Res** 6:64–68, 1984.

ZABRAMSKI JM, SPETZLER RF: Intraoperative barbiturate therapy during temporary vessel occlusion. **J Chron Dis Ther Res** 138–148, 1984.

ZABRAMSKI JM, SPETZLER RF, SELMAN WR, ROESSMANN UR, HERSHEY LA, CRUMRINE RC, MACKO R: Naloxone therapy during focal cerebral ischemia evaluation in a primate model. **Stroke** 15(4):621–627, 1984.

Manuscripts Published in 1983 (5)

SELMAN WR, CRUMRINE R, ZABRAMSKI JM, MACKO R, ANTON AH, SPETZLER RF: Brain barbiturate concentration in focal cerebral ischemia. *J Cereb Blood Flow Metab* 3(Suppl 1):S361–S364, 1983.

SPETZLER RF, ZABRAMSKI JM, KAUFMAN B, YEUNG H: NMR imaging: Preliminary laboratory and clinical evaluation of focal cerebral ischemia. **J Cereb Blood Flow Metab** 3(Suppl 1):S87–S88, 1983.

SPETZLER RF, ZABRAMSKI JM, KAUFMAN B, YEUNG HN: Acute NMR changes during MCA occlusion: A preliminary study in primates. **Stroke** 14(4):185–191, 1983.

SPETZLER RF, ROSKI RA, ZABRAMSKI J: Middle cerebral artery perfusion pressure in cerebrovascular occlusive disease. **Stroke** 14(4):552–555, 1983.

STRICKLAND RD, GOLDBERG JS, LAZARUS HM, SPETZLER RF: Phenytoin-induced agranulocytosis after treatment for a gunshot wound to the face. **Oral Surg** 56(5):500–501, 1983.

Manuscripts Published in 1982 (7)

HOPKINS LN, BUDNY JL, SPETZLER RF: Revascularization of the rostral brain stem. **Neurosurgery** 10(3):364–369, 1982.

MAPSTONE T, SPETZLER RF: Vertebrobasilar insufficiency secondary to vertebral artery occlusion from a fibrous band: Case report. **J Neurosurg** 56(4):581–583, 1982.

ROSKI RA, SPETZLER RF, HOPKINS LN: Occipital artery to posterior inferior cerebellar artery bypass for vertebrobasilar ischemia. **Neurosurgery** 10(1):44–49, 1982.

ROSKI RA, HORWITZ SJ, SPETZLER RF: Atypical trigeminal neuralgia in a 6-year-old boy. Case Report. **J Neurosurg** 56:424–425, 1982.

SELMAN WR, SPETZLER RF, ROSKI RA, ROESSMANN U, CRUMRINE R, MACKO R: Barbiturate coma in focal cerebral ischemia. Relationship of protection to timing of therapy. **J Neurosurg** 56:685–690, 1982.

SPETZLER RF, ROSKI RA, SELMAN WR: The microscope in anterior cervical spine surgery. **Clin Orthop** 168:17–23, 1982.

SPETZLER RF, SELMAN WR, ROSKI RA, BONSTELLE C: Cerebral revascularization during barbiturate coma in primates and humans. **Surg Neurol** 17(2):111–115, 1982.

Manuscripts Published in 1981 (12)

CUNAT JS, MODIC MT, BONSTELLE CT, SPETZLER RF: The radiographic anatomy of surgical extracranial-intracranial anastomoses. **Radiology** 140:115–121, 1981.

KOPANIKY D, SPETZLER RF, BONSTELLE C: Severe otorrhagia resulting from a ruptured aneurysm of the extracranial internal carotid artery. **Surg Neurol** 15(2):141–143, 1981.

RHODES RS, SPETZLER RF, ROSKI RA: Improved neurologic function after cerebrovascular accident with extracranial-intracranial arterial bypass. **Surgery** 90:433–438, 1981.

ROSKI RA, ROESSMANN U, SPETZLER RF, KAUFMAN B, NULSEN FE: Clinical and pathological study of dysplastic gangliocytoma. **J Neurosurg** 55:318–321, 1981.

ROSKI RA, SPETZLER RF, NULSEN FE: Late complications of carotid ligation in the treatment of intracranial aneurysms. **J Neurosurg** 54:583–587, 1981.

ROSKI RA, GARDNER JH, SPETZLER RF: Intrachiasmatic arteriovenous malformation. Case report. **J Neurosurg** 54:540–541, 1981.

SELMAN WR, SPETZLER RF, ROESSMANN UR, ROSENBLATT JI, CRUMRINE RC: Barbiturate-induced coma therapy for focal cerebral ischemia. Effect after temporary and permanent MCA occlusion. **J Neurosurg** 55:220–226, 1981.

SELMAN WR, SPETZLER RF, JACKSON D, ROSKI RA, CRUMRINE RC: Regional cerebral blood flow following middle cerebral artery occlusion and barbiturate therapy in baboons. **J Cereb Blood Flow Metab** 1(Suppl 1):S214–S215, 1981.

SELMAN WR, SPETZLER RF, ROSKI RA: Barbiturate resuscitation from focal cerebral ischemia—A review. **Resuscitation** 9:189–196, 1981.

SELMAN WR, SPETZLER RF, ANTON AH, CRUMRINE RC: Management of prolonged therapeutic barbiturate coma. **Surg Neurol** 15(1):9–10, 1981.

SELMAN WR, SPETZLER RF, BROWN R: The use of intraoperative fluoroscopy and spinal cord monitoring for transoral microsurgical odontoid resection. **Clin Orthop** 154:51–56, 1981.

SPETZLER RF, IVERSEN AA: Malleable microsurgical suction device: Technical note. **J Neurosurg** 54:704–705, 1981.

Manuscripts Published in 1980 (12)

GRUNDY BL, SPETZLER RF: Subdural pneumocephalus resulting from drainage of cerebrospinal fluid during craniotomy. **Anesthesiology** 52(3):269–271, 1980.

SELMAN WR, SPETZLER RF: Therapeutics for focal cerebral ischemia. **Neurosurgery** 6(4):446–452, 1980.

SELMAN WR, SPETZLER RF, WILSON CB, GROLLMUS JW: Percutaneous lumboperitoneal shunt: Review of 130 cases. **Neurosurgery** 6(3):255–257, 1980.

SPETZLER RF, ROSKI RA, RHODES RS, MODIC MT: The "bonnet bypass." Case report. **J Neurosurg** 53:707–709, 1980.

Spetzler RF, Modic M, Bonstelle C: Spontaneous opening of large occipital-vertebral artery anastomosis during embolization: Case report. **J. Neurosurg** 53:849–850, 1980.

Spetzler RF, Rhodes RS, Roski RA, Likavec MJ: Subclavian to middle cerebral artery saphenous vein bypass graft. **J Neurosurg** 53: 465–469, 1980.

Spetzler RF, Roski RA, Kopaniky DR: Alternative superficial temporal artery to middle cerebral artery revascularization procedure. **Neurosurgery** 7(5):484–487, 1980.

Spetzler RF, Spetzler H: Holographic interferometry applied to the study of the human skull. **J Neurosurg** 52:825–828, 1980.

Spetzler RF, Selman WR: New design for an implantable vessel occluder. **Surg Neurol** 13(4):317–319, 1980.

Spetzler RF, Roski RA, Schuster H, Takaoka Y: The role of EC-IC in the treatment of giant intracranial aneurysms. **Neurol Res** 2(3–4):345–359, 1980.

Spetzler RF, Schuster H, Roski RA: Elective extracranial-intracranial arterial bypass in the treatment of inoperable giant aneurysms of the internal carotid artery. **J Neurosurg** 53:22–27, 1980.

Spetzler RF, Selman WR, Weinstein P, Townsend J, Mehdorn M, Telles D, Crumrine RC, Macko R: Chronic reversible cerebral ischemia: Evaluation of a new baboon model. **Neurosurgery** 7(3): 257–261, 1980.

Manuscripts Published in 1979 (9)

Miller CF II, Spetzler RF, Kopaniky DJ: Middle meningeal to middle cerebral arterial bypass for cerebral revascularization. Case report. **J Neurosurg** 50:802–804, 1979.

Owen MP, Brown RH, Spetzler RF, Nash CL Jr, Brodkey JS, Nulsen FE: Excision of intramedullary arteriovenous malformation using intraoperative spinal cord monitoring. **Surg Neurol** 12(4):271–276, 1979.

Roski RA, Roessmann U, Spetzler RF, Kaufman B: Vermian hematoma in a four-year-old child. **Surg Neurol** 11(3):173–174, 1979.

Selman W, Spetzler RF: Neurophysiological monitoring of barbiturate induced coma. **Acta Neurol Scand** 60(Suppl 72):74–75, 1979.

Spetzler RF, Selman WR, Nash CL Jr, Brown RH: Transoral microsurgical odontoid resection and spinal cord monitoring. **Spine** 4(6):506–510, 1979.

Spetzler RF, Myers MD, Bell M: Microsurgery in stroke management. **AORN J** 30(5):885–890, 1979.

SPETZLER RF, OWEN MP: Extracranial-intracranial arterial bypass to a single branch of the middle cerebral artery in the management of a traumatic aneurysm. **Neurosurgery** 4(4):334–337, 1979.

SPETZLER RF, NORMAN D, SELMAN WR, KAUFMAN B, WILSON CB: Computerized tomographic diagnosis: Pitfalls for neurosurgeons. **Neurosurgery** 5(2):231–236, 1979.

SPETZLER RF: Extracranial-intracranial arterial anastomoses for cerebrovascular disease. **Surg Neurol** 11(3):157–161, 1979.

Manuscripts Published in 1978 (3)

HOFF JT, SPETZLER RF, WINESTOCK D: Head injury and early signs of tentorial herniation. A management dilemma. **West J Med** 128: 112–116, 1978.

ROSKI R, SPETZLER RF, OWEN M, CHANDAR K, SHOLL JG, NULSEN FE: Reversal of seven-year old visual field defect with extracranial-intracranial arterial anastomosis. **Surg Neurol** 10(4):267–268, 1978.

SPETZLER RF, WILSON CB: Management of recurrent CSF rhinorrhea of the middle and posterior fossa. **J Neurosurg** 49:393–397, 1978.

Manuscripts Published in 1977 (5)

HOFF JT, PITTS LH, SPETZLER RF, WILSON CB: Barbiturates for protection from cerebral ischemia in aneurysm surgery. **Acta Neurol Scand** 56(Suppl 64):158–159, 1977.

SPETZLER RF, WEINSTEIN PR, CHATER N, WILSON CB: Cisternoatrial, ventriculocisternal, and other cisternal shunts simplified. A percutaneous technique. **J Neurosurg** 47:299–302, 1977.

SPETZLER RF, SCHMIEDEK P, GRATZL O: Summary of the Third International Symposium on Microneurosurgical Anastomoses for Cerebral Ischemia. **Stroke** 8(1):16–19, 1977

SPETZLER RF, WILSON CB, SCHULTE R: Simplified percutaneous lumboperitoneal shunting. **Surg Neurol** 7(1):25–29, 1977.

WILSON CB, SPETZLER RF: Factors responsible for improved results in the surgical management of intracranial aneurysms and vascular malformations. **Am J Surg** 134:33–38, 1977.

Manuscripts Published in 1976 (4)

CHATER N, SPETZLER RF, TONNEMACHER K, WILSON CB: Microvascular bypass surgery. Part 1: Anatomical studies. **J Neurosurg** 44: 712–714, 1976.

GRATZL O, SCHMIEDEK P, SPETZLER RF, STEINHOFF H, MARGUTH F: Clinical experience with extra-intracranial arterial anastomosis in 65 cases. **J Neurosurg** 44:313–324, 1976.

SCHMIEDEK P, GRATZL O, SPETZLER RF, STEINHOFF H, ENZENBACH R, BRENDEL W, MARGUTH F: Selection of patients for extra-intracranial arterial bypass surgery based on rCBF measurements. **J Neurosurg** 44:303–312, 1976.

SPETZLER RF, CHATER N: Microvascular bypass surgery. Part 2. Physiological studies. **J Neurosurg** 45(5):508–513, 1976.

Manuscripts Published in 1975 (4)

CHATER N, SPETZLER RF, MANI J: The spectrum of cerebrovascular occlusive disease suitable for microvascular bypass surgery. **Angiology** 26(3):235–251, 1975.

SPETZLER RF, WILSON CB: Enlargement of an arteriovenous malformation documented by angiography. Case report. **J Neurosurg** 43:767–769, 1975.

SPETZLER RF, WILSON CB, GROLLMUS JM: Percutaneous lumboperitoneal shunt. Technical note. **J Neurosurg** 43:770–773, 1975.

WINESTOCK DP, SPETZLER RF, HOFF JT: Acute, post-traumatic subdural hygroma. Natural course with angiographic documentation. **Radiology** 115:373–375, 1975.

Manuscripts Published in 1974 (2)

SPETZLER RF, CHATER N: Occipital artery—middle cerebral artery anastomosis for cerebral artery occlusive disease. **Surg Neurol** 2: 235–238, 1974.

SPETZLER RF, WINESTOCK D, NEWTON HT, BOLDREY EB: Disappearance and reappearance of cerebral aneurysm in serial arteriograms. Case report. **J Neurosurg** 41:508–510, 1974.

CHAPTERS

Chapters in Press 1994 (27)

ANSON JA, SPETZLER RF: Spinal arteriovenous malformations: Surgical treatment, in Carter LP, Spetzler RF (eds): *Neurovascular Surgery*. New York, McGraw-Hill, 1995, pp 1197–1212.

ANSON JA, SPETZLER RF: Giant arteriovenous malformations, in Carter LP, Spetzler RF (eds): *Neurovascular Surgery*. New York, McGraw-Hill, 1995, pp 1017–1028.

ANSON JA, SPETZLER RF: Spinal dural arteriovenous malformations, in Awad IA, Barrow DL (eds): *Dural Arteriovenous Malformations*. Park Ridge, IL, American Association of Neurological Surgeons, 1995.

ANSON JA, SPETZLER RF: Surgery for vertebral basilar insufficiency: Extracranial, in Carter LP, Spetzler RF (eds): *Neurovascular Surgery*. New York, McGraw-Hill, 1995, pp 383–403.

BALDWIN HZ, ZABRAMSKI JM, SPETZLER RF: Infectious intracranial aneurysms, in Carter LP, Spetzler RF (eds): *Neurovascular Surgery,* New York: McGraw-Hill, pp 777–788, 1995.

FRANCIS PM, KHAYATA MH, ZABRAMSKI JM, SPETZLER RF: Carotid cavernous fistulas. Part I: Presentation and features, in Carter LP, Spetzler RF (eds): *Neurovascular Surgery.* New York, McGraw-Hill, 1995, pp 1049–1059.

FRANCIS PM, KHAYATA MH, ZABRAMSKI JM, SPETZLER RF: Carotid cavernous fistulas. Part II: Treatment, in Carter LP, Spetzler RF (eds): *Neurovascular Surgery.* New York, McGraw-Hill, 1995, 1061–1071.

GOLFINOS JG, SPETZLER RF: Use of the ISG system for 3-D craniotomy, in Gildenberg PL, Tasker RR (eds): *Textbook of Stereotactic and Functional Neurosurgery.* New York, McGraw-Hill, in press, 1995.

HAMILTON MG, ANSON JA, SPETZLER RF: Arteriovenous and other vascular malformations of the spine, in Menezes AH, Sonntag VKH (eds): *The Principles of Spinal Surgery.* New York, McGraw-Hill, in press, 1995.

HAMILTON MG, KRAUS GE, DASPIT C, SPETZLER RF: Giant aneurysms of the vertebrobasilar trunk, in Awad IA, Barrow DL (eds): *Giant Cerebral Aneurysms.* Park Ridge, IL, American Association of Neurological Surgeons, in press, 1995.

HAMILTON MG, ANSON JA, SPETZLER RF: Spinal vascular malformations, in Tindall G, Cooper P, Barrow D (eds): *The Practice of Neurosurgery.* Baltimore, Williams & Wilkins, in press, 1995.

HAMILTON MG, WASCHER TM, SPETZLER RF: Cavernous malformations of the brain stem. *International Conference: New Trends in Management of Cerebrovascular Malformations.* Verona, Italy, Springer-Verlag, 1995.

HAMILTON MG, KRAUS GE, DASPIT CP, ZABRAMSKI JM, SPETZLER RF: Giant aneurysms: Infratentorial, in Carter LP, Spetzler RF (eds): *Neurovascular Surgery,* New York, McGraw-Hill, 1995, pp 829–850.

HERMAN JM, REKATE HL, SPETZLER RF: Pediatric cerebrovascular disease, in Carter LP, Spetzler RF (eds): *Neurovascular Surgery.* New York, McGraw-Hill, 1995, pp 211–229.

HERMAN JM, HAMILTON MG, SPETZLER RF: Vein of Galen malformations: Surgical indications and techniques, in Carter LP, Spetzler RF (eds): *Neurovascular Surgery,* New York, McGraw-Hill, 1995, pp 1041–1047.

KHAYATA MH, GOLFINOS JG, WAKHLOO AK, GOVIN YP, SPETZLER RF: Balloon angioplasty for symptomatic vasospasm, in Reichman HR, Al-Mefty O (eds): *Controversies in Neurosurgery.* New York, Thieme Medical, in press, 1994.

LEVY DI, KHAYATA M, SPETZLER RF: Staged occlusion of arteriovenous malformations. *International Conference: New Trends in Management of Cerebrovascular Malformations.* Verona, Italy, Springer-Verlag, 1995.

ROSKI RA, SPETZLER RF: Carotid ligation, in Wilkins R, Rengachary SS (eds): *Neurosurgery.* New York, McGraw-Hill, in press, 1995, ed 2.

SMITH KA, SPETZLER RF: Classification of arteriovenous malformations. *International Conference: New Trends in Management of Cerebrovascular Malformations.* Verona, Italy, Springer-Verlag, 1995.

THOMPSON BG, KRAUS GE, HAMILTON MG, SPETZLER RF: Giant intracranial aneurysms, in Tindall GT, Barrow DL, Cooper PR (eds): *The Practice of Neurosurgery.* Baltimore, Williams & Wilkins, in press, 1995.

WAKHLOO AK, JOHNSON BA, KRAUS GE, SPETZLER RF: Cerebral sinus and venous thrombosis, in Carter LP, Spetzler RF (eds): *Neurovascular Surgery.* New York, McGraw-Hill, 1995, pp 1337–1363.

WASCHER TM, SPETZLER RF: Saccular aneurysms of the basilar bifurcation, in Carter LP, Spetzler RF (eds): *Neurovascular Surgery,* New York: MacGraw-Hill, pp 729–752, 1995.

WASCHER TM, SPETZLER RF: Cavernous malformations of the brain stem, in Carter LP, Spetzler RF (eds): *Neurovascular Surgery.* New York, McGraw-Hill, 1995, pp 541–555.

WASCHER TM, SPETZLER RF: Cavernous malformations affecting the region of the fourth ventricle, in Cohen AR (ed): *Surgical Disorders of the Fourth Ventricle.* Cambridge, MA, Blackwell Scientific, in press, 1995.

WASCHER TM, SPETZLER RF: Cavernous malformations of the brain stem, in Yamada S (ed): *AVMs in the Functional Areas.* New York, Futura, in press, 1995.

ZABRAMSKI JM, SPETZLER RF, PAPADOPOULOS SM, BOVILL T: Intracisternal therapy with tissue plasminogen activator for the prevention of vasospasm in patients with aneurysmal subarachnoid hemorrhage. *International Conference: New Trends in Management of Cerebrovascular Malformations.* Verona, Italy, Springer-Verlag, 1995.

ZABRAMSKI JM, SPETZLER RF: Acute medical and surgical management of severely ill aneurysm patients. *International Conference, New Trends in Management of Cerebrovascular Malformations.* Verona, Italy, Springer-Verlag, 1995.

ZABRAMSKI JM, SPETZLER RF, RIGAMONTI D: Diagnosis and management of venous angiomas. *International Conference: New Trends in Management of Cerebrovascular Malformations.* Verona, Italy, Springer-Verlag, 1995.

ZABRAMSKI JM, GREENE KA, MARCIANO FF, SPETZLER RF: Carotid endarterectomy, in Carter LP, Spetzler RF (eds): *Neurovascular Surgery*. New York: McGraw-Hill, 1995, pp 325–357.

DASPIT CP, SPETZLER RF: The petrosal approach, in Brackmann D, Shelton C, Arriaga MA (ed): *Otologic Surgery*. Philadelphia, W. B. Saunders, 1994, pp 677–689.

Chapters Published in 1993 (3)

JOHNSON PC, WASCHER TM, GOLFINOS J, SPETZLER RF: Definition and pathologic features, in Awad IA, Barrow DL (eds): *Cavernous Malformations*. Park Ridge, IL, American Association of Neurological Surgeons, 1993, pp 1–11.

WASCHER TM, SPETZLER RF: Microsurgical treatment of infratentorial cavernous malformations, in Awad IA, Barrow D (eds): *Cavernous Malformations*. Park Ridge, IL, American Association of Neurological Surgeons, 1993, pp 117–132.

ZABRAMSKI JM, SPETZLER RF: Surgery of intracranial aneurysms, in Barnett HJM, Mohr JP, Stein BP, Yatsu FM (eds): *Stroke: Pathophysiology, Diagnosis, and Management*. New York, Churchill Livingstone, 1993, ed 2, pp 1055–1092.

Chapters Published in 1992 (3)

DASPIT CP, SPETZLER RF, PAPPAS CTE: Combined subtemporal-suboccipital approach, in Smith MFW, McElveen J (eds): *Neurological Surgery of the Ear*. St. Louis, MO, C. V. Mosby, 1992, pp 90–94.

GRAHM TW, SPETZLER RF, PAPPAS CTE: Benign and skull base tumors, in Little JR, Awad IA (eds): *Reoperative Neurosurgery*. Baltimore, Williams & Wilkins, 1992, pp 77–93.

SPETZLER RF: Excision of cerebral arteriovenous malformations, in Wilson CB (ed): *Neurosurgical Procedures: Personal Approaches to Classic Operations*. Baltimore, Williams & Wilkins, 1992, pp 120–137.

Chapters Published in 1991 (1)

SPETZLER RF, HADLEY MN: Extracranial-intracranial bypass grafting: An update, in Wilkins RA (ed): *Neurosurgery Update*. New York, McGraw-Hill, 1991.

Chapters Published in 1990 (7)

PUCA A, BENES V, SPETZLER RF, ZABRAMSKI JM: Experimental cerebral arterial embolism in a new rabbit model, in Montorsi M, Zennaro F (eds): *Second World Week of Professional Updating in Sur-*

gery and in Surgical and Oncological Disciplines of the University of Milan. Bologna, Italy, Monduzzi Editore, 1990, pp 3–6.

PUCA A, SPETZLER RF, ZABRAMSKI JM, CULICCHIA F: A new primate model of focal cerebral ischemia, in Montorsi M, Zennaro F (eds): *Second World Week of Professional Updating in Surgery and in Surgical and Oncological Disciplines of the University of Milan.* Bologna, Italy, Monduzzi Editore, 1990, pp 7–11.

SONNTAG VKH, HADLEY MN, SPETZLER RF: The transoral-transclival approach to the upper cervical spine, in Sundaresan F, Schmidek HH, Schiller AL, Rosenthal DI (eds): *Tumors of the Spine: Diagnosis and Clinical Management.* Philadelphia, W. B. Saunders, 1990, pp 319–328.

SPETZLER RF, ZABRAMSKI JM: Staged embolization and resection of giant intracranial arteriovenous malformations, in Barrow DL (ed): *Intracranial Vascular Malformations.* Park Ridge, IL, American Association of Neurological Surgeons, 1990, pp 141–156.

SPETZLER RF: Normal perfusion pressure breakthrough theory in large AVMs, in Abe H (ed): *Proceedings of the 7th Annual Meeting of the Japanese Congress of Neurological Surgeons.* Sapporo, Japan, 1990.

SPETZLER RF, HADLEY MN, RAUDZENS PA: Barbiturate therapy for brain protection during temporary vascular occlusion, in Weinstein PR, Faden AI (eds): *Protection of the Brain from Ischemia.* Baltimore, Williams & Wilkins, 1990, pp 253–258.

SPETZLER RF, HADLEY MN, SONNTAG VKH: The transoral surgical approach to the upper cervical spine, in Evarts CM (ed): *Surgery of the Musculoskeletal System.* New York, Churchill Livingstone, 1990, pp 1817–1855.

Chapters Published in 1989 (3)

ROSENBAUM DM, GROTTA JC, YATSU FM, PICONE CM, PETTIGREW LC, BRATINA P, ZABRAMSKI J, SPETZLER R, LOPEZ L, MARLAR J, ELLIS D: A pilot study of nicardipine for acute ischemic stroke. The Nicardipine Study Group, in Hartmann A, Kuschinsky W (eds): *Cerebral Ischemia and Calcium.* Berlin, Springer-Verlag, 1989, pp 367–372.

SPETZLER RF, ZABRAMSKI JM: Cerebrospinal fluid fistulae: Their management and repair, in Youmans JR (ed): *Neurological Surgery: A Comprehensive Reference Guide to the Diagnosis and Management of Neurosurgical Problems.* Philadelphia, W.B. Saunders, 1989, ed 3, pp 2269–2289.

SPETZLER RF, BLOOMFIELD SM: New horizons in the management of cerebral ischemia and stroke, in Edwards MSB, Hoffman HJ (eds): *Current Neurosurgical Practice. Cerebral Vascular Disease in Chil-*

dren and Adolescents. Baltimore, Williams & Wilkins, 1989, pp 451–461.

Chapters Published in 1988 (8)

AWAD IA, SPETZLER RF, LIU SS: Pathophysiology of ischemic symptoms in patients with lesions amenable to EC-IC bypass surgery, in Gagliardi R, Benvenuti L (eds): *Controversies in EIAB for Cerebral Ischemia.* Florence, Italy, Monduzzi, Editore, 1988, pp 73–78.

AWAD IA, SPETZLER RF: Neurosurgical perspective in North America: A critical analysis of the methodology and findings of the International Cooperative EC-IC Bypass Study, in Gagliardi R, Benvenuti L (eds): *Controversies in EIAB for Cerebral Ischemia.* Florence, Italy, Monduzzi, Editore, 1988, pp 47–57.

AWAD IA, SPETZLER RF, HODAK JA: Proton magnetic resonance imaging in the evaluation of patients for EC-IC bypass surgery: Advantages and limitations, in Gagliardi R, Benvenuti L (eds): *Controversies in EIAB for Cerebral Ischemia.* Florence, Italy, Monduzzi, Editore, 1988, pp 167–172.

SPETZLER RF, NEHLS DG, AWAD IA: Vascular surgery of cerebral ischemia and infarction, in Vinken PJ, Bruyn GW, Klawans HL (ed): *Handbook of Clinical Neurology, Vascular Diseases. Revised Series.* New York, Elsevier Medical, 1988, pp 441–458.

SPETZLER RF, ZABRAMSKI JM: Operative selection of patients with arteriovenous malformations, in Suzuki J (ed): *Advances in Surgery for Cerebral Stroke.* Proceedings of the International Symposium on Surgery for Cerebral Stroke, Sendai, 1987. Tokyo, Springer-Verlag, 1988, pp 481–486.

SPETZLER RF, HADLEY MN: Extracranial-intracranial bypass for cerebral revascularization, in Suzuki J (ed): *Advances in Surgery for Cerebral Stroke.* Proceedings of the International Symposium on Surgery for Cerebral Stroke, Sendai, 1987. Tokyo, Springer-Verlag, 1988, pp 165–169.

SPETZLER RF, WILLIAMS F: Cerebral revascularization, in Suzuki J (ed): *Advances in Surgery for Cerebral Stroke.* Proceedings of the International Symposium on Surgery for Cerebral Stroke, Sendai, 1987. Tokyo, Springer-Verlag, 1988, pp 549–554.

SPETZLER RF, GRAHM TW, NEHLS DG: Overview of cerebral ischemia: Rationale for cerebral protection, in Suzuki J (ed): *Advances in Surgery for Cerebral Stroke.* Proceedings of the International Symposium on Surgery for Cerebral Stroke, Sendai, 1987. Tokyo, Springer-Verlag, 1988, pp 231–235.

Chapters Published in 1987 (1)

SPETZLER RF, NEHLS D: Cerebral protection against ischemia, in Wood JH (ed): *Cerebral Blood Flow: Physiologic and Clinical Aspects.* New York, McGraw-Hill, 1987, pp 651–676.

Chapters Published in 1986 (7)

HADLEY MN, SPETZLER RF: The transoral surgical approach to the craniocervical junction, in Samii M (ed): *Surgery in and around the Brainstem and the Third Ventricle.* New York, Springer-Verlag, 1986, pp 467–475.

MANWARING KH, MANWARING ML, HARRINGTON T, CARTER LP, SPETZLER RF: Combined intracranial pressure and multilevel continuous local cerebral blood flow monitoring: Local perfusion fluctuations, in Miller JD, Teasdale GM, Rowan JO, Galbraith SL, Mendelow AD (eds): *Intracranial Pressure VI.* Berlin, Springer-Verlag, 1986, pp 230-234.

MANWARING KH, SPETZLER RF: Head and central nervous system injury in the child, in Marcus RE (ed): *Trauma in Children.* Rockville, MD, Aspen, 1986, pp 39–56.

MOHR JP, KISTLER JP, ZABRAMSKI JM, SPETZLER RF, BARNETT HJM: Intracranial aneurysms, in Barnett HJM, Mohr JP, Stein BM, Yatsu FM (eds): *Stroke: Pathophysiology, Diagnosis, and Management.* New York, Churchill Livingstone, 1986, pp 643–677.

SPETZLER RF, ZABRAMSKI JM: Surgery of intracranial aneurysms, in Barnett HJM, Mohr JP, Stein BM, Yatsu FM (eds): *Stroke: Pathophysiology, Diagnosis and Management.* New York, Churchill Livingstone, 1986, pp 1111–1128.

SPETZLER RF, HADLEY MN, RIGAMONTI D, RAUDZENS PA, SHEDD SA: Giant basilar artery aneurysms managed under circulatory arrest, in Kikuchi H, Fukishima T, Watanabe K (eds): *Intracranial Aneurysms—Surgical Timing and Techniques.* Proceedings of the First International Workshop in Intracranial Aneurysms (IWIA), Tokyo, April 2–4, 1986. Kyoto, Japan, Nishimura, 1986, pp 292–306.

SPETZLER RF, HADLEY MN: Revascularization of the brain stem and posterior fossa, in Samii M (ed): *Surgery in and around the Brainstem and the Third Ventricle.* New York, Springer-Verlag, 1986, pp 262–269.

Chapters Published in 1985 (12)

CARTER LP, HADLEY MN, SPETZLER RF: Regional cortical blood flow during extracranial-intracranial bypass, in Spetzler RF, Carter LP,

Selman WR, Martin MN (eds): *Cerebral Revascularization for Stroke.* New York, Thieme-Stratton, 1985, pp 136–142.

HADLEY MN, MASFERRER R, ZABRAMSKI JM, SPETZLER RF: Management of vertebrobasilar insufficiency, in Spetzler RF, Carter LP, Selman WR, Martin NM (eds): *Cerebral Revascularization for Stroke.* New York, Thieme-Stratton, 1985, pp 475–482.

MARANO SR, SPETZLER RF: Vein interposition grafts for anterior circulation ischemia, in Spetzler RF, Carter LP, Selman WR, Martin NM (eds): *Cerebral Revascularization for Stroke.* New York, Thieme-Stratton, 1985, pp 591–597.

RAUDZENS PA, SPETZLER RF, CARTER LP, WILKINSON E: Cerebral electrical activity during low flow states, in Spetzler RF, Carter LP, Selman WR, Martin NM (eds): *Cerebral Revascularization for Stroke.* New York, Thieme-Stratton, 1985, pp 189–196.

ROSKI RA, SPETZLER RF: Carotid ligation, in Wilkins R, Rengachary SS (eds): *Neurosurgery.* New York, McGraw-Hill, 1985, ed 1, pp 1414–1421.

SELMAN W, SPETZLER RF, ZABRAMSKI JM: Induced barbiturate coma, in Wilkins R, Rengachary SS (eds): *Neurosurgery.* New York, McGraw-Hill, 1985, pp 343–349.

SELMAN WR, SPETZLER RF, RATCHESON R: Subarachnoid hemorrhage, in Henning RJ, Jackson DL (eds): *Handbook of Critical Care Neurology and Neurosurgery.* New York, Praeger, 1985, pp 141–168.

SELMAN WR, ZABRAMSKI JM, SPETZLER RF: The therapeutic window of barbiturate protection in focal cerebral ischemia. Ineffectiveness of enhancement of protection with DMSO or naloxone, in Spetzler RF, Carter LP, Selman WR, Martin NM (eds): *Cerebral Revascularization for Stroke.* New York, Thieme-Stratton, 1985, pp 275–281.

SPETZLER RF, ZABRAMSKI JM, ROSKI RA, SELMAN WR: Cerebral venous vascular reconstructive surgery, in Handa H, Kikuchi H, Yonekawa Y (eds): *Microsurgical Anastomoses for Cerebral Ischemia.* New York/Tokyo, Igaku-Shoin, 1985, pp 90–96.

WILKINSON E, SPETZLER RF, CARTER LP, RAUDZENS PA: Intraoperative barbiturate therapy during temporary vessel occlusion in man, in Spetzler RF, Carter LP, Selman WR, Martin NM (eds): *Cerebral Revascularization for Stroke.* New York, Thieme-Stratton, 1985, pp 397–402.

ZABRAMSKI JM, SPETZLER RF: NMR imaging in the evaluation of acute focal cerebral ischemia. Comparative analysis of RF pulse techniques, in Spetzler RF, Carter LP, Selman WR, Martin NM (eds): *Cerebral Revascularization for Stroke.* New York, Thieme-Stratton, 1985, pp 113–119.

ZABRAMSKI JM, SPETZLER RF, KAUFMAN B, YEUNG HN: Acute changes in nuclear magnetic resonance in primates during occlusion of a middle cerebral artery, in Handa H, Kikuchi H, Yonekawa Y (eds): *Microsurgical Anastomoses for Cerebral Ischemia.* New York, Igaku-Shoin, 1985, pp 291–296.

Chapters Published in 1984 (3)

SPETZLER RF, ZABRAMSKI JM: Posterior circulation bypass procedures, in Smith RR (ed): *Stroke and the Extracranial Vessels.* New York, Raven Press, 1984, pp 275–283.

SPETZLER RF, SELMAN WR: Pathophysiology of cerebral ischemia accompanying arteriovenous malformations, in Wilson CB, Stein BM (eds): *Intracranial Arteriovenous Malformations.* Baltimore, Williams & Wilkins, 1984, pp 24–31.

ZABRAMSKI JM, SPETZLER RF: NMR evaluation of acute focal cerebral ischemia, in Lassen NA, Hossmann KA, Reivich M, Agnoli A, Cahn J (eds): *Maladies et Medicaments—Drugs and Diseases.* John Libbey Eurotext Limited, 1984, vol 1, pp 155–161.

Chapters Published in 1983 (2)

SPETZLER RF: Transoral Approach to the Upper Cervical Spine, in Evarts CM (ed): *Surgery of the Musculoskeletal System.* New York, Churchill Livingstone, 1983, vol 2, pp 4:19–4:24.

SPETZLER RF, SELMAN WR, KAUFMAN B: Cerebral spinal fluid fistulae: Biomechanical, etiological, and therapeutic considerations, in Wood JH (ed): *Neurobiology of Cerebrospinal Fluid 2.* New York, Plenum Press, 1983, pp 913–926.

Chapters Published in 1982 (6)

HOPKINS LN, FEIN JM, FLAMM ES, SPETZLER RF: The role of cerebral bypass in the treatment of aneurysms, in Hopkins LN, Long DM (eds): *Clinical Management of Intracranial Aneurysms.* New York, Raven Press, 1982, pp 287–293.

ROSKI RA, SPETZLER RF: Carotid ligation in the treatment of cerebral aneurysms, in Hopkins LN, Long DM (eds): *Clinical Management of Intracranial Aneurysms.* New York, Raven Press, 1982, pp 11–20.

SELMAN WR, SPETZLER RF: Intracranial pressure monitoring after subarachnoid hemorrhage: Physiological and therapeutic considerations, in Hopkins LN, Long DM (eds): *Clinical Management of Intracranial Aneurysms.* New York, Raven Press, 1982, pp 149–154.

SPETZLER RF, WILSON CB: Dural fistulae and their repair, in Youmans J (ed): *Neurological Surgery*. Philadelphia, W.B. Saunders, 1982, ed 2, pp 2209–2227.

SPETZLER RF, SELMAN WR: Barbiturate-induced coma for the treatment of subarachnoid hemorrhage, in Hopkins LN, Long DM (eds): *Clinical Management of Intracranial Aneurysms*. New York, Raven Press, 1982, pp 155–160.

SPETZLER RF: Normal perfusion pressure breakthrough theory in clinical practice, in Hopkins LN, Long DM (eds): *Clinical Management of Intracranial Aneurysms*. New York, Raven Press, 1982, pp 161–162.

Chapters Published in 1981 (1)

SCHUSTER H, SPETZLER RF, SELMAN W: Barbiturate therapie bei fokaler zerebralir Ischamie—eine experimentelle Studie, in *Internationaler Fortbildengskurs fur klinische Anaesthesiologie*. H. Egermann, 1981, pp 29–35.

Chapters Published in 1980 (4)

SPETZLER RF, SELMAN W, WEINSTEIN P, TOWNSEND J, MEHDORN HM, TELLES D: A new model for chronic reversible cerebral ischemia, in Peerless SJ, McCormick CW (eds): *Microsurgery for Cerebral Ischemia*. Berlin, Springer-Verlag, 1980, pp 23–27.

SPETZLER RF: Cerebrospinal fluid fistulae, in Wilson CB, Hoff JT (eds): *Current Surgical Management of Neurological Disease*. New York, Churchill Livingstone, 1980, pp 243–248.

WEINSTEIN PR, MEHDORN HM, SPETZLER RF, TELLES DA: Arterial dilatation and augmentation of blood flow in experimental arteriovenous fistulas, in Peerless SJ, McCormick CW (eds): *Microsurgery for Cerebral Ischemia*. New York, Springer-Verlag, 1980, pp 215–226.

WILSON CB, PITTS L, SPETZLER RF: Cerebral aneurysms, in Wilson CB, Hoff JT (eds): *Current Surgical Management of Neurological Disease*. New York, Churchill Livingstone, 1980, 123–143.

Chapters Published in 1979 (1)

WEINSTEIN PR, MEHDORN HM, SPETZLER RF: Arterial dilatation and augmentation of blood flow in experimental arteriovenous fistulae, in *Proceedings of the Fourth International Symposium on Microsurgical Anastomoses for Cerebral Ischemia*. Berlin, Springer-Verlag, 1979.

Chapters Published in 1978 (2)

GRATZL O, SCHMIEDEK P, SPETZLER RF: Extracranial-intracranial arterial bypass for cerebral ischemia, in Krayenbuhl H, Mapses PE, Sweet WH (eds): *Progress in Neurological Surgery.* New York, S. Karger, 1978, vol 9, pp 1–29.

WILSON CB, SPETZLER RF: Intracranial aneurysms, in Hoff J (ed): *Practice of Surgery.* Hagerstown, MD, Harper & Row, 1978, pp 1–36.

Chapters Published in 1977 (2)

CHATER N, WEINSTEIN P, SPETZLER RF: Microvascular bypass for cerebral ischemia—An overview, 1966—1976, in Schmiedek P, Gratzl O, Spetzler RF (eds): *Microsurgery for Stroke.* New York, Springer-Verlag, 1977, pp 79–88.

SPETZLER RF, WING SD, NORMAN D: Evaluation of patients with cerebral ischemia using computerized tomography, in Schmiedek P, Gratzl O, Spetzler RF (eds): *Microsurgery for Stroke.* New York, Springer-Verlag, 1977, pp 195–201.

Chapters Published in 1976 (3)

CHATER N, SPETZLER RF, TONNEMACHER K: Anatomical localization of optimal middle cerebral branch for anastomosis, in Austin GM (ed): *Microneurosurgical Anastomoses for Cerebral Ischemia.* Springfield, IL, Charles C Thomas, 1976, pp 39–51.

KOOS WTH, SPETZLER RF, BÖCK FW, SALAH S: Microsurgery of cerebellopontine angle tumors, in Koos WT, Böck FW, Spetzler RF (eds): *Clinical Microneurosurgery.* Stuttgart, Georg Thieme, 1976, pp 91–112.

SPETZLER RF, CHATER NL: Microvascular arterial bypass in cerebrovascular occlusive disease, in Koos WT, Böck FW, Spetzler RF (eds): *Clinical Microneurosurgery.* Stuttgart, Georg Thieme, 1976, pp 242–246.

NONREFEREED JOURNALS

Manuscripts in Press, 1994 (1)

CHEN JW, SPETZLER RF: Current concepts in the treatment of ruptured and unruptured intracranial aneurysms. **Crit Rev Neurosurg,** in press, 1994.

Manuscripts Submitted, 1994 (6)

BEALS SP, JOGANIC EF, HAMILTON MG, SPETZLER RF: Posterior skull base transfacial approaches. **Clin Plast Surg,** submitted for publication, 1994.

LAWTON MT, SPETZLER RF: Surgical management of giant intracranial aneurysms: Experience with 171 patients. **Clin Neurosurg,** submitted for publication, 1994.

LAWTON MT, HAMILTON MG, BEALS SP, JOGANIC EF, SPETZLER RF: Radical resection of anterior skull base tumors. **Clin Neurosurg,** submitted for publication, 1994.

LAWTON M, SHETTER AG, SHAPIRO W, SPETZLER RF: Angiogenesis: A neurosurgical perspective, *Advances in Clinical Neurosciences* 4:27–43, 1994.

SONNTAG VKH, HERMAN JM, SPETZLER RF: Intramedullary tumors in adults: Recent surgical experience with 54 patients. **Spinal Surgery,** submitted for publication, 1994.

WASCHER TM, SPETZLER RF: Current concepts in aneurysmal subarachnoid hemorrhage. Critical review—Vascular neurosurgery, March 1991–August 1991. **Crit Rev Neurosurg,** submitted for publication, 1994.

Manuscripts Published in 1994 (6)

KHAYATA MH, DEAN BL, SPETZLER RF: Materials and embolic agents for endovascular treatment. **Neurosurg Clin N Am** 5(3):475–484, 1994.

LAWTON MT, SPETZLER RF: Management strategies for giant intracranial aneurysms. **Clin Neurosurg** 16(17):1–6, 1994.

MARCIANO FF, GREENE KA, JOHNSON BA, COONS SW, SPETZLER RF, REKATE HL: Management of carniopharyngioma. **BNI Quarterly** 10(2):2–12, 1994.

SPETZLER RF: Editorial. **BNI Quarterly** 10(2): Inside cover, 1994.

SPETZLER RF: Editorial. **BNI Quarterly** 10(1): Inside cover. 1994.

SPETZLER RF, HAMILTON MG, DASPIT CP: Petroclival lesions. **Clin Neurosurg** 41:62–82, 1994.

ZABRAMSKI JM, KAWAGUCHI S, SPETZLER RF: Management of brain stem cavernous malformations. **Contemp Neurosurg** 16(11):1–6, 1994.

Manuscripts Published in 1993 (12)

BEALS SP, HAMILTON MG, JOGANIC EF, SPETZLER RF: Classification of transfacial approaches in the treatment of tumors of the anterior skull base and clivus. **Plast Surg Forum** XVI:211–213, 1993.

DASPIT CP, SPETZLER RF: Vestibular neurilemmoma: Translabyrinthine approach. **BNI Quarterly** 9(3):9–13, 1993.

DRUMM DA, GREENE KA, MARCIANO FF, PRIGATANO GP, SPETZLER RF: Neurobehavioral deficits following rupture of anterior communicating artery (ACoA) aneurysms: The ACoA aneurysm syndrome. **BNI Quarterly** 9(2):2–12, 1993.

HAMILTON MG, SPETZLER RF, DASPIT CP: The combined supra- and intratentorial approach for lesions of the petrous and clival regions. **BNI Quarterly** 9(3):2–8, 1993.

HERMAN JM, HAMILTON MG, SPETZLER RF: Cerebrovascular neurosurgery. **Crit Rev Neurosurg** 3:221–228, 1993.

LAWTON MT, SHETTER AG, SHAPIRO W, SPETZLER RF: Angiogenesis factors and their clinical applications. **BNI Quarterly** 9(2):46–54, 1993.

PAPPAS CTE, RIGAMONTI D, SPETZLER RF, PITTMAN HW: Surgical treatment of extra-axial and spinal cavernous malformations. **BNI Quarterly** 9(2):61–67, 1993.

SPETZLER RF: Surgical approaches to cavernous malformations. **Neurosci Forum** 3(2):6–7, 1993.

SPETZLER RF: Editorial. **BNI Quarterly** 9(1): Inside cover, 1993.

SPETZLER RF: Editorial. **BNI Quarterly** 9(2): Inside cover, 1993.

SPETZLER RF: Editorial. **BNI Quarterly** 9(3): Inside cover, 1993.

SPETZLER RF: Editorial. **BNI Quarterly** 9(4): Inside cover, 1993.

Manuscripts Published in 1992 (13)

ANSON JA, SPETZLER RF: Clinical and radiological findings of spinal dural arteriovenous fistulas (expert commentary). **Perspect Neurol Surg** 3(1):13, 1992.

ANSON JA, SPETZLER RF: Classification of spinal arteriovenous malformations and implications for treatment. **BNI Quarterly** 8(2):2–8, 1992.

GOLFINOS JG, WASCHER TM, ZABRAMSKI JM, SPETZLER RF: The management of unruptured intracranial vascular malformations. **BNI Quarterly** 8(3):2–11, 1992.

GREENE KA, MARCIANO FF, GOLFINOS JG, SHETTER AG, LIEBERMAN AN, SPETZLER RF: Pallidotomy in the levodopa era. **Adv Clin Neurosci** (India) 2:257–281, 1992.

HERMAN JM, HAMILTON M, SPETZLER RF: Skull base neurosurgery. **Crit Rev Neurosurg** 2:257–265, 1992.

SPETZLER RF, HAMILTON MG: ACS Bulletin: What's new in surgery for 1992 (Neurosurgery). **Bull Am Coll Surgeons** 77:25–29, 1992.

SPETZLER RF: Editorial. **BNI Quarterly** 8(1): Inside cover, 1992.

SPETZLER RF: Editorial. **BNI Quarterly** 8(2): Inside cover, 1992.

SPETZLER RF: Editorial. **BNI Quarterly** 8(3): Inside cover, 1992.

SPETZLER RF: Editorial. **BNI Quarterly** 8(4): Inside cover, 1992.

SPETZLER RF: Spinal arteriovenous malformations. **Neurosurg Consult** 3(13):1–8, 1992.

WASCHER TM, SPETZLER RF: Surgical approaches to lesions involving the brain stem. **BNI Quarterly** 8(4):19–28, 1992.

WASCHER TM, GOLFINOS J, ZABRAMSKI JM, SPETZLER RF: Management of unruptured intracranial aneurysms. **BNI Quarterly** 8(1):2–7, 1992.

Manuscripts Published in 1991 (20)

ANSON JA, SPETZLER RF: Interventional neuroradiology for spinal pathology. **Clin Neurosurg** 39:388–418, 1992.

ANSON JA, SPETZLER RF: Surgical management of supratentorial arteriovenous malformations. **Neurosurg Q** 1(3):160–173, 1991.

ANSON, JA, SPETZLER RF: Vascular neurosurgery. **Crit Rev Neurosurg** 1(3):147–161, 1991.

ANSON JA, SPETZLER RF: The surgical management of brainstem hematomas (expert commentary). **Perspect Neurol Surg** 2(1):46–48, 1991.

CARTER LP, GRAHM T, ZABRAMSKI JM, DICKMAN CA, LOPEZ LJ, TALLMAN DH, SPETZLER RF: Postoperative monitoring of cerebral blood flow in patients harboring intracranial aneurysm. **Neurosurg Res** 12:214–218, 1991.

DASPIT CP, SPETZLER RF, PAPPAS CTE: Combined approach for lesions involving the cerebellopontine angle and skull base: Experience with 20 cases—Preliminary report. **Otolaryngol Head Neck Surg** 105:788–796, 1991.

FRANCIS PM, FLOM RA, ZABRAMSKI JM, SPETZLER RF: Treatment of carotid-cavernous fistulas. Part 1: Interventional neuroradiology. **BNI Quarterly** 7(3):2–8, 1991.

FRANCIS PM, ZABRAMSKI JM, SPETZLER RF, SHEDD SA, FLOMM RA: Treatment of carotid-cavernous fistulas. Part II: Surgical interventions. **BNI Quarterly** 7(4):7–15, 1991.

HARGRAVES RW, SPETZLER RF: Takayasu's arteritis: Case report. **BNI Quarterly** 7(2):20–23, 1991.

HERMAN JM, DICKMAN CA, FRAM EK, SPETZLER RF: The role of magnetic resonance and conventional angiography in the detection of internal carotid artery stenosis: Case report. **BNI Quarterly** 7(4):2–6, 1991.

McCORMICK PW, McCORMICK J, ZIMMERMAN R, SPETZLER RF: The pathophysiology of acute subarachnoid hemorrhage. **BNI Quarterly** 7(3):18–26, 1991.

McCORMICK PW, SPETZLER RF: Arteriovenous malformations of the brain. **Curr Opin Neurol Neurosurg** 4:71–75, 1991.

PUCA A, SPETZLER RF, ZABRAMSKI JM, CULICCHIA F: Cardiocirculatory arrest with hypothermia. Experimental study. **Ital J Neurol Sci** 12:49–55, 1991.

SPETZLER RF, DASPIT CP, PAPPAS CTE: Combined approach for lesions involving the cerebellopontine angle and skull base: Experience with 30 cases. **Skull Base Surg** 1(4):226–234, 1991.

SPETZLER RF, PAPPAS CTE: Management of anterior skull base tumors. **Clin Neurosurg** 37:490–501, 1991.

SPETZLER RF: Editorial. **BNI Quarterly** 7(1): Inside cover, 1991.

SPETZLER RF: Editorial. **BNI Quarterly** 7(2): Inside cover, 1991.

SPETZLER RF, DICKMAN CA, SONNTAG VKH: The transoral approach to the anterior cervical spine. **Contemp Neurosurg** 13(9):1–6, 1991.

SPETZLER RF: Editorial. **BNI Quarterly** 7(3): Inside cover, 1991.

SPETZLER RF: Editorial. **BNI Quarterly** 7(4): Inside cover, 1991.

Manuscripts Published in 1990 (11)

DOUGLAS RA, BALDWIN HZ, JOHNSON PC, SONNTAG VKH, SPETZLER RF: Recurrent spinal angioblastic meningioma of the hemangiopericytic type: A case report. **BNI Quarterly** 6(4):13–20, 1990.

GRAHM TW, SPETZLER RF, HODAK JA, FREY JL: The use of computed tomography/cortical blood flow studies to determine patient eligibility for extracranial-intracranial bypass. **BNI Quarterly** 6(3):17–21, 1990.

MASFERRER R, ZABRAMSKI JM, JOHNSON PC, SPETZLER RF: The POEMS syndrome: A case report. **BNI Quarterly** 6(2):31–34, 1990.

PAPPAS CTE, SONNTAG VKH, SPETZLER RF: Surgical anatomy of the anterior aspect of the third ventricle. **BNI Quarterly** 6(1):2–10, 1990.

SPETZLER RF: Editorial. **BNI Quarterly** 6(1): Inside cover, 1990.

SPETZLER RF: Editorial. **BNI Quarterly** 6(2): Inside cover, 1990.

SPETZLER RF: Editorial. **BNI Quarterly** 6(3): Inside cover, 1990.

SPETZLER RF, ZABRAMSKI JM: Grading and staged resection of cerebral arteriovenous malformations. **Clin Neurosurg** 36:318–337, 1990.

SPETZLER RF: Editorial. **BNI Quarterly** 6(4):Inside cover, 1990.

SPETZLER RF, GRAHM TW: The far-lateral approach to the anterior clivus and the upper cervical region. **BNI Quarterly** 6(4):35–38, 1990.

ZIMMERMAN RS, SPETZLER RF, ZABRAMSKI JM: Cerebral arterial vasospasm: An update. **BNI Quarterly** 6(3):2–9, 1990.

Manuscripts Published in 1989 (8)

LEE KS, ZABRAMSKI JM, SPETZLER RF: Superficial temporal artery aneurysms. **BNI Quarterly** 5(4):13–16, 1989.

LIU SS, HADLEY MN, COONS S, SPETZLER RF: Symptomatic granular cell tumor: Case report and review of the literature. **BNI Quarterly** 5(3):2–9, 1989.

RIGAMONTI D, UEDE T, JOHNSON PC, BOJANOWSKI WM, AWAD IA, MICHAEL KT, CARTER LP, SPETZLER RF: A new model of cerebral embolic ischemia using autologous arterial thrombus. **BNI Quarterly** 5(4):2–7, 1989.

SPETZLER RF: Editorial. **BNI Quarterly** 5(1):Inside cover, 1989.

SPETZLER RF: Editorial. **BNI Quarterly** 5(2):Inside cover, 1989.

SPETZLER RF: Editorial. **BNI Quarterly** 5(3):Inside cover, 1989.

SPETZLER RF: Editorial. **BNI Quarterly** 5(4):Inside cover, 1989.

SPETZLER RF: An overview of the international clinical literature on the use of nimodipine in subarachnoid hemorrhage. **Hosp Formul** 24D:2–7, 1989.

Manuscripts Published in 1988 (8)

HADLEY MN, SPETZLER RF: Indications for cerebral revascularization (epitome). **West J Med** 149(3):323–324, 1988.

HADLEY MN, SPETZLER RF: Contemporary application of the extracranial-intracranial bypass for cerebral revascularization. **Contemp Neurosurg** 9(25):1–6, 1988.

SPETZLER RF: Editorial. **BNI Quarterly** 4(1):Inside cover, 1988.

SPETZLER RF: Two technical notes for microsurgery. **BNI Quarterly** 4(2):38–39, 1988.

SPETZLER RF: Editorial. **BNI Quarterly** 4(2):Inside cover, 1988.

SPETZLER RF: Editorial. **BNI Quarterly** 4(3):Inside cover, 1988.

SPETZLER RF: Editorial. **BNI Quarterly** 4(4):Inside cover, 1988.

WILLIAMS FC JR, SPETZLER RF: Hemodynamic management in the neurosurgical intensive care unit. **Clin Neurosurg** 35:101–163, 1988.

Manuscripts Published in 1987 (7)

HADLEY MN, SPETZLER RF, BARROW DL, MARTIN NA, CARTER LP: Management of extracranial carotid artery disease. Part I: Asymptomatic carotid atherosclerosis. **BNI Quarterly** 3(2):17–26, 1987.

RIGAMONTI D, SPETZLER RF, JOHNSON PC, DRAYER BP, CARTER LP: Cerebral vascular malformations. **BNI Quarterly** 3(3):18–28, 1987.

SPETZLER RF: Editorial. **BNI Quarterly** 3(1):Inside cover, 1987.

SPETZLER RF: Editorial. **BNI Quarterly** 3(2):Inside cover, 1987.

SPETZLER RF, HADLEY MN, MARTIN NA, THOMPSON RA, WILKINSON E, RAUDZENS PA: Management of extracranial carotid artery disease. Part II. Microsurgical endarterectomy under barbiturate cerebral protection. **BNI Quarterly** 3(3):2–17, 1987.

SPETZLER RF: Editorial. **BNI Quarterly** 3(3):Inside cover, 1987.
SPETZLER RF: Editorial. **BNI Quarterly** 3(4):Inside cover, 1987.

Manuscripts Published in 1986 (12)

AWAD IA, SPETZLER RF, CARTER LP: Neurovascular strategies in surgery at the base of the skull. **BNI Quarterly** 2(1):53–62, 1986.

CARTER LP, SPETZLER RF: Review of current management of berry aneurysms (berry clipping). **BNI Quarterly** 2(4):18–23, 1986.

NEHLS DG, SPETZLER RF: A review of cerebral protection against ischemia: Part 1. **BNI Quarterly** 2(2):18–23, 1986.

NEHLS DG, SPETZLER RF: A review of cerebral protection against ischemia: Part III. **BNI Quarterly** 2(4):2–8, 1986.

NEHLS DG, SPETZLER RF: A review of cerebral protection against ischemia. Part II: Pharmacologic agents and techniques of possible benefit. **BNI Quarterly** 2(3):2–8, 1986.

RIGAMONTI D, SPETZLER RF: Early *versus* delayed operation in subarachnoid hemorrhage (epitome). **West J Med** 145:83, 1986.

SPETZLER RF, ZABRAMSKI JM: Cerebrospinal fluid fistula. **Contemp Neurosurg** 8(1):1–5, 1986.

SPETZLER RF: Editorial. **BNI Quarterly** 2(1):Inside cover, 1986.

SPETZLER RF: Editorial. **BNI Quarterly** 2(2):Inside cover, 1986.

SPETZLER RF: Editorial. **BNI Quarterly** 2(3):Inside cover, 1986.

SPETZLER RF: Editorial. **BNI Quarterly** 2(4):Inside cover, 1986.

WILKINSON E, SPETZLER RF, ARCHIBALD J: Barbiturate protection and EEG monitoring in neurovascular surgery. **BNI Quarterly** 2(2):5–10, 1986.

Manuscripts Published in 1985 (10)

BLOOMFIELD SM, SONNTAG VKH, SPETZLER RF: Pineal region lesions. **BNI Quarterly** 1(3):10–23, 1985.

MARANO SR, SPETZLER RF, CARTER LP: Autogenous saphenous vein interposition grafts for high flow augmentation of cerebral blood flow. **BNI Quarterly** 1(4):29–33, 1985.

MARTIN NA, CARTER LP, SPETZLER RF: Measurement of regional cerebral blood flow in aneurysm surgery. **Clin Neurosurg** 32(6): 79–104, 1985.

MASFERRER R, ZABRAMSKI JM, HUNT S, FLOM R, HARRINGTON T, JOHNSON P, SPETZLER RF: Cerebral amyloid angiopathy and recurrent spontaneous intracerebral hematomas. **BNI Quarterly** 1(1): 29–33, 1985.

MASFERRER R, HADLEY MN, BLOOMFIELD S, SPETZLER RF, SONNTAG VKH: Transoral microsurgical resection of the odontoid process. **BNI Quarterly** 1(3):34–40, 1985.

NEHLS DG, SPETZLER RF, SHETTER AG, SONNTAG VKH: Application of new technology in the treatment of cerebellopontine angle tumors. **Clin Neurosurg** 32(12):223–241, 1985.

SPETZLER RF: Editorial. **BNI Quarterly** 1(1):Inside cover, 1985.

SPETZLER RF: Editorial. **BNI Quarterly** 1(2):Inside cover, 1985.

SPETZLER RF: Editorial. **BNI Quarterly** 1(3):Inside cover, 1985.

SPETZLER RF: Editorial. **BNI Quarterly** 1(4):Inside cover, 1985.

Manuscripts Published in 1984 (2)

SELMAN W, SPETZLER RF: Cerebral spinal fluid fistulae. **Contemp Neurosurg** 6(14):1–6, 1984.

ZABRAMSKI JM, SPETZLER RF, SELMAN WR, HERSHEY L, ROESSMANN U: Cerebral protection during focal cerebral ischemia: Evaluation of barbiturates and naloxone in a primate model. **Clin Res Rev** 4(1):74–76, 1984.

Manuscripts Published in 1983 (1)

LITTLE JR, SPETZLER RF, ROSKI RA, SELMAN WR, ZABRAMSKI J, LESSER RP: Ineffectiveness of DMSO in treating experimental brain ischemia. **Ann NY Acad Sci** 411:269–277, 1983.

Manuscripts Published in 1982 (1)

SPETZLER RF, ZABRAMSKI JM: Revascularization of anterior and posterior circulation ischemia. **Clin Neurosurg** 29:575–593, 1982.

Manuscripts Published in 1979 (2)

SPETZLER RF: Cerebrospinal fluid fistula. **Contemp Neurosurg** 1:1–5, 1979.

WILSON CB, SPETZLER RF: Operative approaches to aneurysms. **Clin Neurosurg** 26:232–247, 1979.

Manuscripts Published in 1978 (1)

SPETZLER RF, WILSON CB, WEINSTEIN P, MEHDORN M, TOWNSEND J, TELLES D: Normal perfusion pressure breakthrough theory. **Clin Neurosurg** 25:651–672, 1978.

BOOK REVIEWS

1993 (1)

HAMILTON MG, SPETZLER RF: **J Neurosurg** 78:847–848, 1993. Review of Laligam NS, Janecka IP (eds): *Surgery of Cranial Base Tumors.* New York, Raven Press, 1993.

1987 (2)

SPETZLER RF: **J Neurosurg** 68:155, 1987. Review of Aaslid R (ed): *Transcranial Doppler Sonography*. New York, Springer-Verlag, 1986.

SPETZLER RF: **Neurosurgery** 22(4):795, 1988. Review of Sundt TM (ed): *Occlusive Cerebrovascular Disease Diagnosis and Surgical Management*. Philadelphia, W.B. Saunders, 1987.

1986 (1)

SPETZLER RF: **J Neurosurg** 65:422, 1986. Review of Fein JM, Flamm ES (eds): *Cerebrovascular Surgery*. New York, Springer-Verlag, 1985, vol 3.

1984 (3)

SPETZLER RF: **J Neurosurg** 60:1323–1324, 1984. Review of Greenhalgh RM, Rose FC (eds): *Progress in Stroke Research 2*. London, Pitman Books Limited, 1983.

SPETZLER RF: **Surg Neurol** 21:96–98, 1984. Review of Ojemann RG, Crowell RM (eds): *Surgical Management of Cerebrovascular Disease*. Baltimore, Williams & Wilkins, 1983.

SPETZLER RF: **Neurosurgery** 14(1):118–119, 1984. Review of Barnett HJM (ed): *Neurologic Clinics: Cerebrovascular Disease*. Philadelphia: W.B. Saunders, 1983, vol 1.

1982 (2)

SPETZLER RF: **Surg Neurol** 17:236, 1982. Review of Carney AL, Anderson EM (eds): *Advances in Neurology: Diagnosis and Treatment of Brain Ischemia, CT Brain Blood Flow, Brain Hemodynamics, Carotid and Vertebral Artery Surgery*. New York, Raven Press, 1981, vol 30.

SPETZLER RF: **Neurosurgery** 10(4):540, 1982. Review of Samii M, Jannetta PJ (eds): *The Cranial Nerves: Anatomy, Pathology, Pathophysiology, Diagnosis, Treatment*. New York, Springer-Verlag, 1981.

1981 (1)

SPETZLER RF: **Surg Neurol** 16:471, 1981. Review of Perry MO (ed): *The Management of Acute Vascular Injuries*. Baltimore, Williams & Wilkins, 1981.

1979 (1)

SPETZLER RF: **Surg Neurol** 11(1):16, 1979. Review of Fein JM, Reichman OH (eds): *Microvascular Anastomosis for Cerebral Ischemia*. New York, Springer-Verlag, 1978.

COMMENTS

1994 (1)

HAMILTON MG, SPETZLER RF: **Neurosurgery** 35(3):362–363, 1994. Comments on Origitano TC, Al-Mefty O, Leonetti JP, DeMonte F, Reichman OH: Vascular considerations and complications in cranial base surgery.

1993 (3)

HAMILTON MG, SPETZLER RF: **Neurosurgery** 32(5):798, 1993. Comments on Findlay JM, Lougheed WM: Carotid microendarterectomy.

HAMILTON MG, SPETZLER RF: **Neurosurgery** 32(5):735–736, 1993. Comments on Robinson JR Jr, Awad IA, Magdinec M, Paranadi L: Factors predisposing to clinical disability in patients with cavernous malformations of the brain.

HAMILTON MG, WASCHER TM, SPETZLER RF: **Neurosurgery** 32(6): 931, 1993. Comments on Gerber CJ, Neil-Dwyer G, Evans BT: Posterior cerebral artery aneurysms.

1992 (1)

ANSON JA, SPETZLER RF: **Neurosurgery** 31:868, 1992. Comments on Chin LS, Raffel C, Gonzalez-Gomez I, Giannotta SL, McComb JG: Diffuse arteriovenous malformations: A clinical, radiological, and pathological description.

1990 (1)

SPETZLER RF: **Neurosurgery** 27:266, 1990. Comments on Young WL, Prohovnik I, Ornstein E, Ostapkovich N, Sisti MB, Solomon RA, Stein BM: The effect of arteriovenous malformation resection on cerebrovascular reactivity to carbon dioxide.

1989 (3)

SPETZLER RF: **Neurosurgery** 24(3):327, 1989. Comments on Burchiel KJ, Clarke H, Ojemann GA, Dacey RG, Winn HR: Use of stimulation mapping and corticography in the excision of arteriovenous malformations in sensorimotor and language-related neocortex.

ZABRAMSKI JM, SPETZLER RF: **Neurosurgery** 24(1):75–79, 1989. Comments on Batjer HH, Devous MD, Seibert GB, Purdy PD, Bonte FJ: Intracranial arteriovenous malformation: Relationship between clinical factors and surgical complications.

ZABRAMSKI JM, SPETZLER RF: **Neurosurgery** 25:429–436, 1989. Comments on Morgan MK and Sundt TM Jr: The case against staged operative resection of cerebral arteriovenous malformations.

1988 (9)

HADLEY MN, SPETZLER RF: **Neurosurgery** 22(2):296, 1988. Comments on Batjer HH, Purdy PD, Neiman M, Samson DS. Subtemporal transdural use of detachable balloons for traumatic carotid-cavernous fistulas.

SPETZLER RF, ZABRAMSKI JM: **Neurosurgery** 22(4):769, 1988. Comments on Young WL, Solomon RA, Prohovnik I, Ornstein E, Weinstein J, Stein BM. ^{133}Xe blood flow monitoring during arteriovenous malformation resection: A case of intraoperative hyperperfusion with subsequent brain swelling.

SPETZLER RF: **Neurosurgery** 23:103, 1988. Comments on Morioka T, Nishio S, Hikita T, Chung LH, Soejima T: Marked growth of an angiographically occult arteriovenous malformation: Case report.

SPETZLER RF: **Neurosurgery** 23(4):449, 1988. Comments on Zuccarello M, Yeh H-S, Tew JM: Morbidity and mortality of carotid endarterectomy under local anesthesia: A retrospective study.

SPETZLER RF: **Neurosurgery** 22(3):612, 1988. Comments on Miller BV, Loftus CM, Hiratzka LF, Laughlin DE: Technical note: *In vitro* evaluation of an in-line doppler flow-metering system for carotid artery shunts.

SPETZLER RF: **Neurosurgery** 23(6):785, 1988. Comments on Nazed M, Mandybur TI, Kashiwagi S: Oligodendroglial proliferative abnormality associated with arteriovenous malformation: Report of three cases with review of the literature.

ZABRAMSKI JM, SPETZLER RF: **Neurosurgery** 22(3):509, 1988. Comments on Batjer HH, Devous MD Sr, Meyer YJ, Purdy PD, Samson DS: Cerebrovascular hemodynamics in arteriovenous malformation complicated by normal perfusion pressure breakthrough.

ZABRAMSKI JM, SPETZLER RF: **Neurosurgery** 23(3):328, 1988. Comments on Batjer HH, Devous MD, Seibert GB, Purdy PD, Ajamani AK, Delareson M, Bonte FJ: Intracranial arteriovenous malformation: Relationships between clinical and radiographic factors and ipsilateral steal severity.

ZABRAMSKI JM, SPETZLER RF: **Neurosurgery** 23(4):489, 1988. Comments on Barrow DL: Unruptured cerebral arteriovenous malformations presenting with intracranial hypertension.

1987 (2)

SPETZLER RF, CARTER LP: **Neurosurgery** 21(5):698, 1987. Comments on Koshu K, Hirota S, Sonobe M, Takahashi S, Takaku A, Saito T,

Ushijima T: Continuous recording of cerebral blood flow by means of a thermal diffusion method using a Peltier stack.

ZABRAMSKI JM, SPETZLER RF: **Neurosurgery** 20(4):524, 1987. Comments on Weinstein PR, Anderson GG, Telles DA: Results of hyperbaric oxygen therapy during temporary middle cerebral artery occlusion in unanesthetized cats.

1985 (8)

SPETZLER RF: **Neurosurgery** 16(1):47, 1985. Comments on Bret P, Hor F, Huppert J, Lapras C, Fischer G: Treatment of cerebrospinal fluid rhinorrhea by percutaneous lumboperitoneal shunting: Review of 15 cases.

SPETZLER RF: **Neurosurgery** 16(1):60, 1985. Comments on Ahmadi J, Weiss MH, Segall HD, Schultz DH, Zee CS, Giannotta SL: Evaluation of cerebrospinal fluid rhinorrhea by metrizamide computed tomographic cisternography.

SPETZLER RF: **Neurosurgery** 16(3):320, 1985. Comments on Hubbard JL, McDonald TJ, Pearson BW, Laws ER Jr: Spontaneous cerebrospinal fluid rhinorrhea: Evolving concepts in diagnosis and surgical management based on the Mayo Clinic experience from 1970 through 1981.

SPETZLER RF: **Neurosurgery** 16(4):528, 1985. Comments on Standefer M, Little JR, Tomsak R, Furlan AJ, Zegarra H, Williams G: Improvement in the retinal circulation after superficial temporal to middle cerebral artery bypass.

SPETZLER RF: **Neurosurgery** 17(2):276, 1985. Comments on Diaz FG, Pearce J, Ausman JI: Complications of cerebral revascularization with autogenous vein grafts.

SPETZLER RF: **Neurosurgery** 17(2):323, 1985. Comments on Tranmer BI, Kindt GW: High altitude: An unusual cause of neurological deterioration in a patient with an arteriovenous malformation.

SPETZLER RF: **Neurosurgery** 17(4):563, 1985. Comments on Shirakuni T, Nagashima T, Tamaki N, Matsumoto S: Magnetic resonance imaging of experimental brain edema in cats.

SPETZLER RF: **Neurosurgery** 17(6):941, 1985. Comments on Quest DO, Correll JW: Basal arterial occlusive disease.

1984 (2)

SPETZLER RF: **Neurosurgery** 15(5):539, 1984. Comments on Wood JH Konstantinos S, Polyzoidis KS, Kee DB Jr, Prats AR, Gibby GL, Tindall GT: Augmentation of cerebral blood flow induced by hemodilution in stroke patients after superficial temporal-middle cerebral arterial bypass operation.

SPETZLER RF: **Neurosurgery** 14(1):82, 1984. Comments on Solomon RA, Michelsen WJ: Defective cerebrovascular autoregulation in regions proximal to arteriovenous malformations of the brain: A case report and topic review.

1983 (2)

SPETZLER RF: **Neurosurgery** 12(2):168, 1983. Comments on Toung T, Donham R, Lehner A, Alano J, Campbell J: Postoperative tension pneumocephalus.
SPETZLER RF: **Neurosurgery** 13(2):194, 1983. Comments on Hopkins LN, Budny JL, Castellani D: On extracranial-intracranial arterial bypass and basilar artery ligation in the treatment of giant artery aneurysms.

1982 (2)

SPETZLER RF: **Neurosurgery** 10:569, 1982. Comments on Diaz FG, Ausman JI, Pearce JE: Ischemia after ICA occlusion and EC-IC anastomosis.
SPETZLER RF: **Neurosurgery** 11(3):362, 1982. Comments on Park TS, Hoffman HJ, Humphreys RP, Chuang SH: Spontaneous cerebrospinal fluid otorrhea in association with a congenital defect of the cochlear aqueduct and Mondini dysplasia.

1981 (2)

SPETZLER RF: **Neurosurgery** 8(1):42, 1981. Comments on James HE, Tibbs PA: Percutaneous lumboperitoneal shunts.
SPETZLER RF: **Neurosurgery** 9(3):274, 1981. Comments on Weinstein PR, Reinert RL, Brittain F: Delayed thrombosis of synthetic microvascular bypass grafts.

LETTERS

Submitted for Publication (2)

KRAUS GE, ZABRAMSKI JM, SPETZLER RF: An experimental study of cerebrovascular resistance, pressure transmission, and craniospinal compliance (Letter). **Neurosurgery** submitted for publication, 1995.
SPETZLER RF: Relationship of pressure and size to risk of hemorrhage from arteriovenous malformations (letter). **J Neurosurg,** in press, 1995.

1994 (2)

GOLFINOS JG, THOMPSON BG, ZABRAMSKI JM, SPETZLER RF: Calcium antagonists (letter). **Neurosurgery** 35(3):541–542, 1994.

SPETZLER RF, HAMILTON MG: Radiosurgery for venous angiomas (letter). **J Neurosurg** 80:173–174, 1994.

1993 (2)

SPETZLER RF, HAMILTON MG: Pressure autoregulation is intact after arteriovenous malformation (letter). **Neurosurgery** 33(4):772–774, 1993.

SPETZLER RF: Carotid endarterectomy complicated by vein patch rupture (letter). **Neurosurgery** 32(1):151–152, 1993.

1992 (1)

WASCHER TM, SPETZLER RF: Radiosurgery of arteriovenous malformations (letter). **J Neurosurg** 76(6):1045–1047, 1992.

1991 (1)

LIU SS, ZABRAMSKI JM, SPETZLER RF: Fusiform aneurysm after surgery for craniopharyngioma (letter). **J Neurosurg** 75:670–672, 1991.

1990 (2)

DICKMAN CA, MAMOURIAN A, DRAYER BP, SONNTAG VKH, SPETZLER RF: MR imaging of lateral disc herniation (letter). **J Neurosurg** 73(4):642–642, 1990.

HERMAN JM, SPETZLER RF: MR imaging in carotid artery dissection (letter). **J Neurosurg** 72:987–988, 1990.

1989 (3)

LEE KS, SPETZLER RF: Cerebral cavernous malformations (letter). **Arch Neurol** 46(12):1273, 1989.

SPETZLER RF: Venous angiomas: An underestimated cause of intracranial hemorrhage (letter). **Surg Neurol** 30:412, 1989.

SPETZLER RF: Cavernous angiomas and AVM's (letter). **J Neurosurg** 70(3):500–501, 1989.

1988 (4)

RIGAMONTI D, JOHNSON PC, SPETZLER RF, DRAYER BP: Vascular malformations and MRI (letter). **Ann Neurol** 23(2):208–209, 1988.

SPETZLER RF: AVM surgery (letter). **Neurology** 38:167–168, 1988.

SPETZLER RF: Angiographically occult intracranial vascular malformations (letter). **J Neurosurg** 69:642–644, 1988.

ZABRAMSKI JM, SPETZLER RF, SONNTAG VKH: Treatment of spinal cavernous angiomas (letter). **J Neurosurg** 69(3):476, 1988.

1987 (2)

SPETZLER RF: Ventriculoatrial shunts (letter). **Neurosurgery** 20(3): 506, 1987.

SPETZLER RF: Extracranial-intracranial bypass trial (letter). **Surg Neurol** 27:503, 1987.

1986 (1)

NEHLS DG, CARTWRIGHT M, SPETZLER RF: Experimental primate stroke model (letter). **Neurosurgery** 18(3):388–389, 1986.

1985 (2)

SPETZLER RF: Treatment of chronic cerebral ischemia (letter). **Surg Neurol** 23:201–204, 1985.

SPETZLER RF: Retinal circulation after STA-MCA bypass (letter). **Neurosurgery** 16(4):583, 1985.

1983 (3)

SPETZLER RF: Cervical-peritoneal shunt (letter). **J Neurosurg** 58:628, 1983.

SPETZLER RF, SELMAN W, ZABRAMSKI J: High dose barbiturates in nontraumatic brain swelling (letter). **Stroke** 14(5):830–831, 1983.

SPETZLER RF: Can a patent extracranial-intracranial bypass provoke the conversion of an intracranial arterial stenosis to a symptomatic occlusion (letter)? **Neurosurgery** 13(5):621, 1983.

1981 (1)

ANTON AH, SELMAN WR, SPETZLER RF: Safe pentobarbital regimen used to treat artificially induced cerebral ischemia (letter). **Surv Anesthesiol** 25:331, 1981.

1980 (1)

SPETZLER RF, SELMAN WR: Risks of barbiturate therapy (letter). **J Neurosurg** 53:581, 1980.

RESPONSES

1993 (1)

SPETZLER RF: Response to Letter to the Editor by Chaloupka JC, Viñuela F, Duckwiler GR: Perfusion pressure and risk of AVM hemorrhage. **J Neurosurg** 78:851–853, 1993.

1992 (1)

SPETZLER RF: Response to Letter to the Editor by Castillo R, Zarate A, Chavez R: Reconstruction of the temporalis muscle. **J Neurosurg** 76:336, 1992.

1991 (1)

SPETZLER RF: Response to Letter to the Editor by Parkinson D: Intracranial Carotid-Carotid Bypass. **J Neurosurg** 74:856, 1991.

1990 (1)

SPETZLER RF: Response to Letter to the Editor by Hammerschlag PE: Petrous carotid-to-intradural carotid saphenous vein graft for intracavernous giant aneurysm, tumor, and occlusive cerebrovascular disease. **J Neurosurg** 73:496–501, 1990.

1988 (1)

SPETZLER RF: Response to Letter to the Editor by Parkinson D: Staged treatment of AVM's. **J Neurosurg** 68:659–660, 1988.

1987 (4)

HADLEY MN, SPETZLER RF: Response to Letter to the Editor by Vascik JM: Management of severely impaired SAH patients. **J Neurosurg** 67:626–627, 1987.

SPETZLER RF: Response to Letter to the Editor by Leussenhop AJ: AVM grading in assessing surgical risk. **J Neurosurg** 66:638, 1987.

SPETZLER RF: Response to Letter to the Editor by Duff TA: AVM grading in assessment of surgical risk. **J Neurosurg** 66:787–788, 1987.

SPETZLER RF, MARTIN NA: Response to Letter to the Editor by Malik GM, Ausman JI, Mann R: Grading system for AVM's. **J Neurosurg** 67:473–474, 1987.

ABSTRACTS

1993

SPETZLER RF, DASPIT CP, PAPPAS CTE: The combined supra- and infratentorial approach for lesions of the petrous and clival regions: Experience with 46 cases, in Bradley WG, Crowell RM (eds): *The Year Book of Neurology and Neurosurgery,* Chicago, Mosby Year Book, 1993, pp 297–298 (abstr).

ZIMMERMAN RS, SPETZLER RF, LEE KS, ZABRAMSKI JM, HARGRAVES RW: Cavernous malformations of the brain stem, in Bradley WG,

Crowell RM (eds): *The Year Book of Neurology and Neurosurgery,* Chicago, Mosby Year Book, 1993, pp 350–351 (abstr).

CARTER LP, GRAHM T, BAILES JE, BICHARD W, SPETZLER RF: Continuous postoperative monitoring of cortical blood flow and intracranial pressure, in Bradley WG, Crowell RM (eds): *The Year Book of Neurology and Neurosurgery,* Chicago, Mosby Year Book, 1 993, pp 208–209 (abstr).

1992

SPETZLER RF, FUKUSHIMA T, MARTIN N, ZABRAMSKI JM: Petrous carotid-to-intradural carotid saphenous vein graft for intracavernous giant aneurysm, tumor, and occlusive cerebrovascular disease, in Currier RD, Crowell RM (eds): *The Year Book of Neurology and Neurosurgery,* Chicago, Mosby Year Book, 1992, pp 217–218 (abstr).

CULICCHIA F, SPETZLER RF, FLOM RA: Failure of transluminal angioplasty in the treatment of myointimal hyperplasia of the internal carotid artery: Case report, in Currier RD, Crowell RM (eds): *The Year Book of Neurology and Neurosurgery,* Chicago, Mosby Year Book, 1992, pp 232–234 (abstr).

RIGAMONTI D, JOHNSON PC, SPETZLER RF, HADLEY MN, DRAYER BP: Cavernous malformations and capillary telangiectasia: A spectrum within a single pathological entity, in Currier RD, Crowell RM (eds): *The Year Book of Neurology and Neurosurgery,* Chicago, Mosby Year Book, 1992, pp 301–302 (abstr).

RIGAMONTI D, SPETZLER RF, MEDINA M, RIGAMONTI K, GECKLEY DS, PAPPAS C: Cerebral venous malformations, in Currier RD, Crowell RM (eds): *The Year Book of Neurology and Neurosurgery,* Chicago, Mosby Year Book, 1992, pp 306–307 (abstr).

GRAHM T, WILLIAMS FC JR, HARRINGTON T, SPETZLER RF: Civilian gunshot wounds to the head: A prospective study, in Carrier RD, Crowell RM (eds): *The Year Book of Neurology and Neurosurgery,* Chicago, Mosby Year Book, 1992, pp 351–352 (abstr).

1991 (1)

RATCLIFF BJ, MASFERRER R, SPETZLER RF: Cognitive impairment and physical findings in patients with familial cavernous malformations of the brain. **Yale J Biol Med,** 1991 (abstr).

BAILES JE, SPETZLER RF, HADLEY MN, BALDWIN HZ: Management morbidity and mortality of poor-grade aneurysm patients, in Crowell RM (ed): *The Year Book of Neurology and Neurosurgery.* Chicago, Year Book Medical, 1991, pp 281–283 (abstr).

1990 (1)

SPETZLER RF, HADLEY MN, RIGAMONTI D, CARTER LP, RAUDZENS PA, SHEDD SA, WILKINSON E: Aneurysms of the basilar artery treated with circulatory arrest, hypothermia, and barbiturate cerebral protection, in DeJong RN, Currier RD, Crowell RM (eds): *The Year Book of Neurology and Neurosurgery*. Chicago, Year Book Medical, 1990, pp 285–287 (abstr).

1989 (5)

AWAD IA, CARTER LP, SPETZLER RF, MEDINA M, WILLIAMS FW: Clinical vasospasm after subarachnoid hemorrhage: Response to hypervolemic hemodilution and arterial hypertension, in DeJong RN, Currier RD, Crowell RM (eds): *The Year Book of Neurology and Neurosurgery*. Chicago, Year Book Medical, 1989, pp 294–295 (abstr).

HADLEY MN, MARTIN NA, SPETZLER RF, SONNTAG VKH, JOHNSON PC: Comparative transoral dural closure techniques: A canine model, in DeJong RN, Currier RD, Crowell RM (eds): *The Year Book of Neurology and Neurosurgery*. Chicago, Year Book Medical, 1989, pp 210–211 (abstr).

RIGAMONTI D, DRAYER BP, JOHNSON PC, HADLEY MN, ZABRAMSKI JM, SPETZLER RF: The MRI appearance of cavernous malformations (angiomas), in DeJong RN, Currier RD, Crowell RM (eds): *The Year Book of Neurology and Neurosurgery*. Chicago, Year Book Medical, pp 315–317 (abstr).

SPETZLER RF, HADLEY MN, MARTIN NA, HOPKINS LN, CARTER LP, BUDNY J: Vertebrobasilar insufficiency. I: Microsurgical treatment of extracranial vertebrobasilar disease, in DeJong RN, Currier RD, Crowell RM (eds): *The Year Book of Neurology and Neurosurgery*. Chicago, Year Book Medical, 1989, pp 279–281 (abstr).

SPETZLER RF, MARTIN NA, CARTER LP, FLOM RA, RAUDZENS PA, WILKINSON E: Surgical management of large AVM's by staged embolization and operative excision, in DeJong RN, Currier RD, Crowell RM (eds): *The Year Book of Neurology and Neurosurgery*. Chicago, Year Book Medical, 1989, pp 314–315 (abstr).

1988 (2)

AWAD IA, SPETZLER RF, HODAK JA, AWAD CA, CAREY R: Incidental subcortical lesions identified on magnetic resonance imaging in the elderly. I: Correlation with age and cerebrovascular risk factors, in DeJong RN, Currier RD, Crowell RM (eds): *The Year Book of Neurology and Neurosurgery*. Chicago, Year Book Medical, 1988, pp 209–210 (abstr).

SPETZLER RF, MARTIN NA: A proposed grading system for arteriovenous malformations, in DeJong RN, Currier RD, Crowell RM (eds): *The Year Book of Neurology and Neurosurgery*. Chicago, Year Book Medical, 1988, pp 335–336 (abstr).

1987 (5)

AWAD IA, SPETZLER RF, Johnson PC: Unidentified bright objects on magnetic resonance imaging of the brain. **Stroke** 18(1):294, 1987 (abstr).

GROTTA J, ROSENBAUM D, ZABRAMSKI J, SPETZLER R, MARLER J, PETTIGREW LC, ELLIS D, YATSU F: Blood pressure changes after cerebral infarction: Implications for therapeutic trials. **Ann Neurol** 22(1):160, 1987 (abstr).

NEHLS DG, TODD MM, SPETZLER RF: Isoflurane does not protect against focal cerebral ischaemia in primates. **Br J Surg** 74(6):531, 1987 (abstr).

RIGAMONTI D, JOHNSEN SD, SIDELL AD, TARBY TJ, DRAYER BP, JOHNSON PC, SPETZLER RF: The clinical spectrum of cavernous malformations (angiomas) in childhood. **Ann Neurol** 22:431, 1987 (abstr).

RIGAMONTI D, JOHNSON PC, DRAYER BP, SPETZLER RF: Cavernous malformation and capillary telangiectases: Two facets of the same pathological entity. **J Neuropathol Exp Neurol** 46:401, 1987 (abstr).

1986 (2)

CARTER LP, MEDINA M, WILLIAMS F, SPETZLER RF: Hypervolemic hemodilution therapy in the management of intracranial aneurysms. **Stroke** 17(1):143, 1986 (abstr).

NEHLS DG, FLOM RA, CARTER LP, SPETZLER RF: Multiple intracranial aneurysms: Determining the site of rupture. **Stroke** 17:334, 1986 (abstr).

1985 (1)

TODD MM, NEHLS DG, DRUMMOND JC, SPETZLER RF, THOMPSON R, JOHNSON P: A comparison of the protective effects of isoflurane and thiopental in a primate model of temporary cerebral ischemia. **Anesthesiology** 63(3A):A412, 1985 (abstr).

1983 (1)

ZABRAMSKI JM, SPETZLER RF, SELMAN WR, HERSHEY LA, ROESSMANN U: Naloxone improves neurologic function during, and outcome after, temporary focal cerebral ischemia. **Stroke** 14(2):123, 1983 (abstr).

1981 (1)

SELMAN WR, SPETZLER RF, ROSKI RA: Barbiturate coma: Relation of protection to timing of therapy & duration of occlusion. **Stroke** 12(1):128, 1981 (abstr).

1975 (1)

CHATER NL, SPETZLER RF: Anatomical studies of the middle cerebral artery of microvascular significance, in Handa H (ed): *Microneurosurgery,* Baltimore, University Park Press, 1975, p 82 (abstr).

PRESENTATIONS

Presentations for 1994 (18)

SPETZLER RF: Cardiac standstill for complex aneurysms. 20th Annual Richard Lende Winter Neurosurgery Conference. Snowbird, UT, January 29–February 4, 1994.

SPETZLER RF: Vessel reconstruction and bypass in skull base surgery. North American Skull Base Society. Orlando, FL, February 18–23, 1994.

SPETZLER RF: Practical Course—Combined suprainfratentorial presigmoid petrosectomy approach. North American Skull Base Society. Orlando, FL, February 18–23, 1994.

SPETZLER RF: Aneurysms of the basilar artery. Mayfield Winter Neuroscience Symposium. Aspen, CO, February 28–March 5, 1994.

SPETZLER RF: Complex AVMs of the posterior fossa. Mayfield Winter Neuroscience Symposium. Aspen, CO, February 28–March 5, 1994.

SPETZLER RF (panel discussion): Multistrategy approaches to the treatment of aneurysms and AVMs. Mayfield Winter Neuroscience Symposium. Aspen, CO, February 28–March 5, 1994.

SPETZLER RF: The combined supra- and infratentorial approach for lesions of the petrous and clival region. Mayfield Winter Neuroscience Symposium. Aspen, CO, February 28–March 5, 1994.

SPETZLER RF (panel discussion): Controversies in skull base surgery. Mayfield Winter Neuroscience Symposium. Aspen, CO, February 28–March 5, 1994.

SPETZLER RF (panel discussion): Controversies in cervical spine surgery. Mayfield Winter Neuroscience Symposium. Aspen, CO, February 28–March 5, 1994.

SPETZLER RF: The combined supra- and infratentorial approach for lesions of the petrous and clival region. Neurosurgery at Jackson Hole. Jackson Hole, WY, March 12–17, 1994.

SPETZLER RF: Vascular malformations—Nomenclature and treatment. BNI Symposium. Phoenix, AZ, March 17–19, 1994.

SPETZLER RF: 3D Microsurgical workshop—Skull base approaches. BNI Symposium. Phoenix, AZ, March 17–19, 1994.

SPETZLER RF: Management strategies of giant aneurysms. BNI Symposium. Phoenix, AZ, March 17–19, 1994.

SPETZLER RF: The combined supra- and infratentorial approach for lesions of the petrous and clival region. Annual Arnold Barnett Lecture, Wichita Society of Neuroscience. Wichita, KS, April 4–6, 1994.

SPETZLER RF (faculty member): Surgical techniques in intracranial aneurysms. Practical clinic. American Association of Neurological Surgeons. San Diego, CA, April 10–14, 1994.

SPETZLER RF (demonstrating surgeon): Surgical dissection—3D video demonstration. American Association of Neurological Surgeons. San Diego, CA, April 10–14, 1994.

SPETZLER RF (panel member): Management of petroclival meningiomas. American Association of Neurological Surgeons. San Diego, CA, April 10–14, 1994.

SPETZLER RF: The combined supra- and infratentorial approach for lesions of the petrous and clival region. Kemink Lecture, University of Michigan. Ann Arbor, MI, April 28–29, 1994.

SPETZLER RF: Posterior circulation aneurysms. Southern California Neurosurgical Society. Long Beach, CA, May 18, 1994.

SPETZLER RF: Microsurgical AVM resection: Indications, techniques, and results. The 14th Annul Meeting of the Japanese Congress of Neurological Surgeons. Sendai, Japan, May 27–29, 1994.

SPETZLER RF: Learning, advice, and enthusiasm. Commencement Address—Knox College. Galesburg, IL, June 4, 1994.

SPETZLER RF, ZABRAMSKI JM: Use of bypass for complex aneurysms. 19th Annual Meeting, Rocky Mountain Neurosurgical Society. Aspen, CO, June 12–16, 1994.

SPETZLER RF: Spinal AVMs. Second International Neurosurgical Summer Conference. Mombasa/Kenya, Africa, August 12–27, 1994.

Presentations for 1993 (52)

SPETZLER RF: Surgical management of large incisural lesions. UCLA Neurosurgery Skull Base Program. Cranial Base Workshop. Los Angeles, January 18–19 and January 23–24, 1993.

SPETZLER RF: Preservation of olfaction and prevention of CSF leakage in anterior craniofacial approaches. 19th Annual Richard Lende

Winter Neurosurgery Conference. Snowbird, UT, January 30–February 6, 1993.

SPETZLER RF: Spinal cord AVMs: Diagnosis, pathophysiology, and treatment. 20th Annual Symposium. Recent Advances in Neurology and Neurosurgery. Phoenix, AZ, March 18–20, 1993.

SPETZLER RF: 3-D Video microsurgical workshop. 20th Annual Symposium. Recent Advances in Neurology and Neurosurgery. Phoenix, AZ, March 18–20, 1993.

SPETZLER RF: Management of complex aneurysms. Winter Neurosurgical Conference. Calgary, Alberta, Canada, March 6–13, 1993.

SPETZLER RF: Diagnosis and treatment of spinal AVMs. Winter Neurosurgical Conference. Calgary, Alberta, Canada, March 6–13, 1993.

SPETZLER RF: Vertebral-basilar circuit aneurysms. 61st Annual Meeting, American Association of Neurological Surgeons. Boston, April 24–29, 1993.

KHAYATA M, DEAN B, FLOM RA, ZABRAMSKI J, SPETZLER RF: Efficacy of endovascular treatment of meningiomas: A controlled study. 61st Annual Meeting, American Association of Neurological Surgeons. Boston, April 24–29, 1993.

SPETZLER RF (moderator): Approaches and problems in the management of intracranial AVMs. 61st Annual Meeting, American Association of Neurological Surgeons. Boston, April 24–29, 1993.

SPETZLER RF (discussant): The efficacy of particulate embolization and stereotactic radiosurgery for large AVMs of the brain. 61st Annual Meeting, American Association of Neurological Surgeons. Boston, April 24–29, 1993.

SPETZLER RF (panelist): Lateral and posterior approaches to the skull base. 61st Annual Meeting, American Association of Neurological Surgeons. Boston, April 24–29, 1993.

SPETZLER RF: Neurosurgery and the carotid artery. Operative techniques to improve outcome. 61st Annual Meeting, American Association of Neurological Surgeons. Boston, April 24–29, 1993.

SPETZLER RF: Operative strategy of midline and ventricle-related supratentorial AVMs. 44th Annual Meeting of the German Society of Neurosurgery. Frankfurt, Germany, May 1–3, 1993.

SPETZLER RF (visiting professor): Skull base approaches to the clivus. University of Maryland, School of Medicine. Baltimore, May 4–5, 1993.

SPETZLER RF (visiting professor): Pathophysiology and treatment of spinal AVMs. Tri-State Neurosurgery Conference, University of Pittsburgh. Pittsburgh, May 27, 1993.

JOHNSON BA, DRAYER BP, WASCHER TM, ZABRAMSKI JM, SPETZLER

RF: The natural history of familial cavernous malformations: A prospective clinical and MR imaging trial. American Society of Neuroradiology. Vancouver, BC, May 1993.

SPETZLER RF (Charles A. Elsberg Lecturer): Spinal AVMs. Columbia University. New York, June 1, 1993.

HAMILTON MG, SPIESER BL, KHAYATA MH, SHELTER AG, SPETZLER RF: The role for radiosurgery in the management of cerebral arteriovenous malformations. Rocky Mountain Neurosurgical Society Scientific Program, 28th Annual Meeting. Bigfork, MT, June 13–17, 1993.

ZIMMERMAN CG, ZERICK WR, SPETZLER RF, SONNTAG VKH: Transoral odontoidectomy. Update: Report of 105 cases. Rocky Mountain Neurosurgical Society Scientific Program, 28th Annual Meeting. Bigfork, MT, June 13–17, 1993.

SPETZLER RF: Midfacial approaches for tumors. Kasdan Neurosurgical Research Forum. Bermuda, June 26–30, 1993.

SPETZLER RF (visiting professor): Combined approaches to tumors of the petrous ridge. University of Miami. Miami, June 1, 1993.

SPETZLER RF (Arthur A. Ward lecturer and visiting professor): Management and pathophysiology of spinal AVMs. University of Washington. Seattle, August 10–12, 1993.

SPETZLER RF: Revascularization in skull base and vascular surgery. The decade of the brain. An International Conference. Washington, DC, September 10–14, 1993.

SPETZLER RF: Transfacial approaches to the skull base, role and perspectives. European Skull Base Society, 1st Congress. Riva del Garda, Italy, September 25–30, 1993.

SPETZLER RF: Internal carotid artery problems in lesions in the skull base: Surgical management. European Skull Base Society, 1st Congress. Riva del Garda, Italy, September 25–30, 1993.

SPETZLER RF: Systematic approach to the entire clivus. European Skull Base Society, 1st Congress. Riva del Garda, Italy, September 25–30, 1993.

SPETZLER RF: Management of large tumors of the clival region. European Skull Base Society, 1st Congress. Riva del Garda, Italy, September 25–30, 1993.

SPETZLER RF: Surgical management of meningiomas. Congress of Neurological Surgeons, 43rd Annual Meeting. Vancouver, BC, October 2–7, 1993.

SPETZLER RF: Techniques in aneurysm surgery. Congress of Neurological Surgeons, 43rd Annual Meeting. Vancouver, BC, October 2–7, 1993.

SPETZLER RF (moderator): Controversies in clinical management (panel discussion). Congress of Neurological Surgeons, 43rd Annual Meeting. Vancouver, BC, October 2–7, 1993.

SPETZLER RF: Anterior circulation aneurysms (video luncheon). Congress of Neurological Surgeons, 43rd Annual Meeting. Vancouver, BC, October 2–7, 1993.

APOSTOLIDES PJ, ZIMMERMAN CG, ZERICK WR, SPETZLER RF, SONNTAG VKH: Transoral odontoidectomy update: Report of 105 cases. Congress of Neurological Surgeons, 43rd Annual Meeting. Vancouver, BC, October 2–7, 1993.

SPETZLER RF: Normal perfusion breakthrough—A 15-year retrospective. Joint Section on Cerebrovascular Surgery Workshop, Congress of Neurological Surgeons, 43rd Annual Meeting. Vancouver, BC, October 2–7, 1993.

HAMILTON MG, SPETZLER RF: Giant cerebral aneurysms treated with circulatory arrest, hypothermia, and barbiturate cerebral protection. Congress of Neurological Surgeons, 43rd Annual Meeting. Vancouver, BC, October 2–7, 1993.

FRANCIS PM, ZABRAMSKI JM, SPETZLER RF: The use of 3% sodium chloride (NaCL) in the management of vasospasm from aneurysmal subarachnoid hemorrhage. Congress of Neurological Surgeons, 43rd Annual Meeting. Vancouver, BC, October 2–7, 1993.

SMITH KA, SPETZLER RF: Supratentorial-occipital interhemispheric approach for medial temporal lobe lesions. Congress of Neurological Surgeons, 43rd Annual Meeting. Vancouver, BC, October 2–7, 1993.

LAWTON MT, HAMILTON MG, SPETZLER RF: Management of deep AVMs: Thalamus, basal ganglia, and brain stem. Congress of Neurological Surgeons, 43rd Annual Meeting. Vancouver, BC, October 2–7, 1993.

KHAYATA MH, WALLACE RC, FLOM RA, ZABRAMSKI JM, SPETZLER RF: Comparison of arteriovenous malformation embolization with glue versus particles. Congress of Neurological Surgeons, 43rd Annual Meeting. Vancouver, BC, October 2–7, 1993.

GREENE KA, MARCIANO FF, DICKMAN CA, COONS SW, JOHNSON PC, BAILES JE, SPETZLER RF: Anterior communicating artery aneurysm paraparesis syndrome: Clinical manifestations and pathologic correlates. Congress of Neurological Surgeons, 43rd Annual Meeting. Vancouver, BC, October 2–7, 1993.

HAMILTON MG, SPETZLER RF: The prospective application of a grading system for arteriovenous malformations. Congress of Neurological Surgeons, 43rd Annual Meeting. Vancouver, BC, October 2–7, 1993.

SPETZLER RF: The role of microsurgery in the treatment of cerebral arteriovenous malformations. Arizona Neurological Society. Tucson, AZ, October 9, 1993.

SPETZLER RF (coordinator): Cerebral arteriovenous malformations. World Federation of Neurosurgical Societies. Acapulco, Mexico, October 17–22, 1993.

SPETZLER RF: Spinal AVMs (video seminar). World Federation of Neurological Societies. Acapulco, Mexico, October 17–22, 1993.

Spetzler RF (coordinator): Management of giant cerebral arteriovenous vascular malformations. World Federation of Neurological Societies. Acapulco, Mexico, October 17–22, 1993.

SPETZLER RF: Thalamic and brain stem arteriovenous malformations (video seminar). World Federation of Neurological Societies. Acapulco, Mexico, October 17–22, 1993.

SPETZLER RF: Vascular surgery: Brain stem cavernous malformations. World Federation of Neurological Societies. Acapulco, Mexico, October 17–22, 1993.

SPETZLER RF: Multimodality management of cerebral arteriovenous malformations. International Society for Pediatric Neurosurgery, 21st Annual Scientific Meeting. Phoenix, AZ, October 24–28,1993.

SPETZLER RF: Transfacial approach to the skull base with emphasis on preservation of olfaction. American Academy of Neurological Surgery. Phoenix, AZ October, 27–31, 1993.

SPETZLER RF (visiting professor): Skull base approaches for petro-clival lesions. Montreal Neurological Sciences Symposium. Montreal, Quebec, November 4–5, 1993.

SPETZLER RF (visiting professor): The management of vascular malformations. Montreal Neurological Sciences Symposium. Montreal, Quebec, November 4–5, 1993.

SPETZLER RF: Surgical management of AVMs. CNS tumors and cerebrovascular lesions: Modern management. The 18th Annual Neurosurgery Postgraduate Course. San Francisco, December 3, 1993.

SPETZLER RF: Vascular problems in skull base surgery. Modern management. The 18th Annual Neurosurgery Postgraduate Course. San Francisco, December 3, 1993.

Presentations for 1992 (59)

SPETZLER RF: Combined approach (tumors of the skull base round table). French Society of Neurosurgery. Chamonix, France, January 21, 1992.

SPETZLER RF: Surgery of giant aneurysms (Problems on Vascular Neurosurgery Round Table). French Society of Neurosurgery. Chamonix, France, January 23, 1992.

Spetzler RF: American experience in the treatment of intracranial aneurysms. French Society of Neurosurgery. Chamonix, France, January 24, 1992.

Spetzler RF: Combined approach to CP angle and clivus. UCLA Cranial Base Surgery Workshop. Los Angeles, January 30, 1992.

Spetzler RF (panelist): Cerebellopontine Angle Surgery Round Table. UCLA Cranial Base Surgery Workshop. Los Angeles, January 30, 1992.

Spetzler RF: Far lateral approach to anterior foramen magnum tumors. UCLA Cranial Base Surgery Workshop. Los Angeles, January 31, 1992.

Spetzler RF: Natural history and management of cavernous malformations. XVIIth International Joint Conference on Stroke and Cerebral Circulation. Phoenix, AZ, February 1, 1992.

Spetzler RF: Vascular malformation of brain. Cleveland Clinic Foundation. Cleveland, OH, February 7–8, 1992.

Spetzler RF: Management of brain tumor: Clinical and surgical techniques. Cook County Graduate Course. Chicago, February 9, 1992.

Spetzler RF (panel moderator): Results of invasive evaluations and surgery on internal carotid arteries. North American Skull Base Society Meeting. Acapulco, Mexico, February 16–18, 1992.

Spetzler RF (panel moderator): Far lateral approach to the anterior clivus and the upper cervical region. North American Skull Base Society Meeting. Acapulco, Mexico, February 16–18, 1992.

Spetzler RF (panel moderator): Combined approach for lesions involving the cerebellopontine angle and skull base: Experience with 30 cases. North American Skull Base Society Meeting. Acapulco, Mexico, February 16–18, 1992.

Spetzler RF (panel moderator): Reconstruction of ICA. North American Skull Base Society Meeting. Acapulco, Mexico, February 16–18, 1992.

Spetzler RF: Complex basilar artery aneurysm treated under cardiac standstill. Japanese Conference on Surgery for Cerebral Stroke. Nagoya, Japan, March 3–4, 1992.

Spetzler RF: Dilemma of intraoperative ruptured basilar artery aneurysm. Japanese Conference on Surgery for Cerebral Stroke. Nagoya, Japan, March 3–4, 1992.

Spetzler RF: Symptomatic dolichoectatic vertebral artery. Japanese Conference on Surgery for Cerebral Stroke. Nagoya, Japan, March 3–4, 1992.

Spetzler RF: Classification of vascular malformations. Japanese Conference on Surgery for Cerebral Stroke. Nagoya, Japan, March 3–4, 1992.

SPETZLER RF: Management of symptomatic carotid artery occlusion. Japanese Conference on Surgery for Cerebral Stroke. Nagoya, Japan, March 3–4, 1992.

SPETZLER RF: Management of anterior cervical intra-medullary arteriovenous malformations. Japanese Conference on Surgery for Cerebral Stroke. Nagoya, Japan, March 3–4, 1992.

SPETZLER RF: Cavernous malformations of the brain stem. Japanese Conference on Surgery for Cerebral Stroke. Nagoya, Japan, March 3–4, 1992.

SPETZLER RF: Combined approach for clivus tumors. Korean Society for Cerebrovascular Disease. Seoul, Korea, March 6–7, 1992.

SPETZLER RF: Cardiac standstill for complex aneurysms. Korean Society for Cerebrovascular Disease. Seoul, Korea, March 6–7,1992.

SPETZLER RF: Management of giant aneurysms. Korean Society for Cerebrovascular Disease. Seoul, Korea, March 6–7, 1992.

SPETZLER RF: Sixth Annual Magnetic Resonance Imaging Conference, Barrow Neurological Institute, Phoenix, AZ, March 7–11, 1992.

SPETZLER RF: Spinal AVM. Recent advances in neurology and neurosurgery. 19th Annual Symposium, Barrow Neurological Institute. Phoenix, AZ, March 12–14, 1992.

SPETZLER RF (panelist): Incidental vascular lesions, judgments, techniques, and special aspects of management. 60th Annual Meeting, American Association of Neurological Surgeons. San Francisco. April 11–16, 1992.

SPETZLER RF (panelist): Technical refinements in the surgery of vascular lesions of the posterior circulation. 60th Annual Meeting, American Association of Neurological Surgeons. San Francisco, CA, April 11–16, 1992.

SPETZLER RF (panelist): Vertebrobasilar aneurysms. 60th Annual Meeting, American Association of Neurological Surgeons. San Francisco, CA, April 11–16, 1992.

SPETZLER RF (panelist): Problems and management of occipital/parietal AVMs. 60th Annual Meeting, American Association of Neurological Surgeons. San Francisco, CA, April 11–16, 1992.

SPETZLER RF: Practical course on techniques in aneurysm surgery. 60th Annual Meeting, American Association of Neurological Surgeons, San Francisco, CA, April 11–16, 1992.

SPETZLER RF (visiting professor): Combined approach for clival tumors. University of Virginia Health Sciences Center. Charlottesville, VA, May 14–16, 1992.

SPETZLER RF: Development of departmental organization and leadership. The Society of Neurological Surgeons, 83rd Meeting in the 72nd Year. Louisville, KY, May 17–20, 1992.

SPETZLER RF: Extirpation of arteriovenous malformations: A preventable cause of stroke. 11th Mayfield Lecturer at Neuroscience Symposium. Cincinnati, OH, May 28–29, 1992.

SPETZLER RF: 3-D videotape review and discussion—Advanced neurosurgical techniques in cerebrovascular disease. 11th Mayfield Lecturer at Neuroscience Symposium. Cincinnati, OH, May 28–29, 1992.

SPETZLER RF: Intracisternal therapy with tissue plasminogen activator for the prevention of vasospasm in patients with aneurysmal subarachnoid hemorrhage. New Trends in Management of Cerebro-Vascular Malformations. Verona, Italy, June 8–12, 1992.

SPETZLER RF: Acute medical and surgical management of severely ill patients. New Trends in Management of Cerebro-Vascular Malformations. Verona, Italy, June 8–12, 1992.

SPETZLER RF: EC-IC bypass: Current role in giant aneurysms. New Trends in Management of Cerebro-Vascular Malformations. Verona, Italy, June 8–12, 1992.

SPETZLER RF: Classification of cerebral AVMs. New Trends in Management of Cerebro-Vascular Malformations. Verona, Italy, June 8–12, 1992.

SPETZLER RF: Management of high flow AVMs. New Trends in Management of Cerebro-Vascular Malformations. Verona, Italy, June 8–12, 1992.

SPETZLER RF: Staged occlusions of giant AVMs. New Trends in Management of Cerebro-Vascular Malformations. Verona, Italy, June 8–12, 1992.

SPETZLER RF: Management of brain stem cavernous malformations. New Trends in Management of Cerebro-Vascular Malformations. Verona, Italy, June 8–12, 1992.

SPETZLER RF: Management of venous angiomas. New Trends in Management of Cerebro-Vascular Malformations. Verona, Italy, June 8–12, 1992.

SPETZLER RF: Far lateral approach. First International Skull Base Congress. Hanover, West Germany, June 14–20, 1992.

SPETZLER RF: Vessel reconstruction in skull base surgery. First International Skull Base Congress. Hanover, West Germany, June 14–20, 1992.

SPETZLER RF: Combined supra and infratentorial approach for lesions of the petrous and clival regions. Kasdon Neurosurgical Research Forum. Camp Denali, Alaska, July 20–24, 1992.

SPETZLER RF: Vascular malformations: Classifications and treatment. Kasdon Neurosurgical Research Forum. Camp Denali, Alaska, July 20–24, 1992.

SPETZLER RF (visiting professor): Surgery and classification of high flow cerebral lesions. Indiana University. Indianapolis, IN, September 18–19, 1992.

SPETZLER RF: Surgery and classification of high flow cerebral lesions. Western Neurosurgical Society Meeting. Whistler, BC, Canada, September 20–23, 1992.

SPETZLER RF: Neurovascular surgical advances in the treatment of stroke. 13th Annual Current Concepts in Critical Care Medicine. Scottsdale, AZ, September 26, 1992.

JOHNSON BA, DRAYER BP, WASCHER TM, ZABRAMSKI JM, SPETZLER RF: The variable and dynamic MRI appearance of cavernous malformations. Western Neuroradiological Society. San Francisco, October 1992.

SPETZLER RF: Giant AVMs. XXV Congress Latino Americano de Neurocirurgia. La Paz, Bolivia, October 4–9, 1992.

SPETZLER RF: Techniques in aneurysm surgery. Congress of Neurological Surgeons. Washington, DC, October 31–November 5, 1992.

SPETZLER RF: Management of arteriovenous malformations. Microsurgery *versus* radiosurgery. Congress of Neurological Surgeons. Washington, DC, October 31–November 5, 1992.

SPETZLER RF: Use of frameless stereotactic navigational device during resection of skull base lesions. Congress of Neurological Surgeons. Washington, DC, October 31–November 5, 1992.

SPETZLER RF: Cerebral vascularization before, during, or after surgery. Congress of Neurological Surgeons. Washington, DC, October 31–November 5, 1992.

SPETZLER RF: Intracranial vertebral endarterectomy via the far lateral approach. Congress of Neurological Surgeons. Washington, DC, October 31–November 5, 1992.

SPETZLER RF: Transoral approach to the upper cervical spine. 5th Annual Spine Workshop, Barrow Neurological Institute. Scottsdale, AZ, November 15–17, 1992.

SPETZLER RF: Transoral approach. 5th Annual Spine Workshop, Barrow Neurological Institute. Scottsdale, AZ, November 15–17, 1992.

SPETZLER RF (visiting professor): Spinal arteriovenous malformations. Their diagnosis and treatment. The University of Chicago. Chicago, November 18–20, 1992.

Presentations for 1991 (16)

SPETZLER RF: Classification of vascular malformations. Parts I & II: Richard Lende Winter Neurosurgery Conference. Snowbird, UT, February 3, 1991.

SPETZLER RF: The far lateral approach to the anterior clivus and the upper cervical region. North American Skull Base Society. Lake Buena Vista, FL, March 1, 1991.

SPETZLER RF: Combined approach for lesions involving the cerebellopontine angle and skull base: Experience with 30 cases. North American Skull Base Society. Lake Buena Vista, FL, March 2, 1991.

SPETZLER RF (panelist): Reconstruction after cranial base surgery. Reconstruction of ICA. North American Skull Base Society. Lake Buena Vista, FL, March 3, 1991.

SPETZLER RF: Clinical aspects of intracranial aneurysms. 5th Annual Barrow Neurological Institute Magnetic Resonance Imaging Conference. Phoenix, AZ, March 19, 1991.

SPETZLER RF: Classification of vascular malformations. 18th Annual Barrow Neurological Institute Symposium. Recent Advances in Neurology and Neurosurgery. Phoenix, AZ, May 21, 1991.

SPETZLER RF: 3D video microsurgical workshop. 18th Annual Barrow Neurological Institute Symposium. Recent Advances in Neurology and Neurosurgery. Phoenix, AZ, May 21, 1991.

SPETZLER RF (chairman): Dynamics of cerebral circulation in AVM. 9th European Congress on Neurosurgery. Moscow, USSR, June 24, 1991.

SPETZLER RF, ZIMMERMAN RS, LEE KS, ZABRAMSKI JM, HARGRAVES RW: Cavernous malformations of the brain stem. 9th European Congress on Neurosurgery. Moscow, USSR, June 24, 1991.

ZABRAMSKI JM, SPETZLER RF, LEE KS, PAPADOPOULOS SM: Phase I trial of tissue plasminogen activator for the prevention of vasospasm in patients with aneurysmal subarachnoid hemorrhage. 9th European Congress on Neurosurgery. Moscow, USSR, June 24, 1991.

SPETZLER RF (visiting professor): SUNY, Buffalo, NY, July 18, 1991.

SPETZLER RF: Relationship of AVM size to risk of rupture. Neurosurgical Research Forum 7th Annual Meeting. Newport, RI, July 23, 1991.

SPETZLER RF: Three-dimensional video imaging of microsurgical carotid endarterectomy and spinal cord AVM surgery. Congress of Neurological Surgeons. Orlando, FL, October 1991.

SPETZLER RF: Oral board exams. Houston, TX, November 1991.

SPETZLER RF: 4th Annual Spine Workshop, Barrow Neurological Institute. Phoenix, AZ, November 14–16, 1991.

SPETZLER RF: Mt. Fuji Workshop on Cerebrovascular Disease. Maui, HI, November 23–26, 1991.

Presentations for 1990 (36)

SPETZLER RF: Petrosectomy for clivus meningioma. Cranial Base Surgery Workshop. The UCLA Neurosurgery Skull Base Program. Los Angeles, January 18, 1990.

SPETZLER RF: Skull base procedure. Cranial Base Surgery Workshop, The UCLA Neurosurgery Skull Base Program. Los Angeles, January 18, 1990.

GRAHM TW, SPETZLER RF: Transcranial doppler and aneurysmal subarachnoid hemorrhage. Richard Lende Winter Neurosurgery Conference. Snowbird, UT, February 4, 1990.

ZABRAMSKI JM, ZIMMERMAN RS, HARGRAVES R, SPETZLER RF, CULICCHIA F: Cardiac standstill and hypothermia—An evaluation of time and temperature. Richard Lende Winter Neurosurgery Conference. Snowbird, UT, February 4, 1990.

SPETZLER RF, ZABRAMSKI JM: Cardiac standstill in primates and homo sapiens. Richard Lende Winter Neurosurgery Conference. Snowbird, UT, February 4, 1990.

ZIMMERMAN RS, SPETZLER RF: Surgery for cavernous malformations of the brain stem. Richard Lende Winter Neurosurgery Conference. Snowbird, UT, February 7, 1990.

SPETZLER RF: Combined approach for lesions involving the clivus and CPA—Experience with 23 cases. North American Skull Base Society. Los Angeles, February 20, 1990.

SPETZLER RF: Transoral approach to the odontoid. 7th Saudi Annual Neurosciences Symposium. Riyadh, Saudi Arabia, February 11, 1990.

SPETZLER RF: Spinal cord arteriovenous malformations. 7th Saudi Annual Neurosciences Symposium. Riyadh, Saudi Arabia, February 12, 1990.

SPETZLER RF: Transcallosal approach to tumor excision. 17th Annual Barrow Neurological Institute Symposium. Recent Advances in Neurology and Neurosurgery. Phoenix, AZ, March 9, 1990.

SPETZLER RF, HEROS RC, SAMSON DS (faculty): Surgical approaches for intracranial aneurysms. The 58th Annual Meeting of the American Association of Neurological Surgeons. Nashville, TN, April 29, 1990.

BARROW DL, FOX AJ, SPETZLER RF (panelist): Dural AVMs. The 58th Annual Meeting of the American Association of Neurological Surgeons. Nashville, TN, April 30, 1990.

SPETZLER RF, DASPIT CP, PAPPAS CTE: Combined approach for lesions involving the clivus and cerebellopontine angle: Experience with 23 cases. The 58th Annual Meeting of the American Association of Neurological Surgeons. Nashville, TN, April 30, 1990.

RIGAMONTI D, MARTIN N, SPETZLER RF (panelist): Occult vascular malformations. The 58th Annual Meeting of the American Association of Neurological Surgeons. Nashville, TN, May 2, 1990.

LEE KS, SPETZLER RF: Surgical management of cavernous malformations of the brain stem (poster presentation). The 58th Annual Meeting of the American Association of Neurological Surgeons. Nashville, TN, May 3, 1990.

ZIMMERMAN RS, HARGRAVES RW, ZABRAMSKI JM, SPETZLER RF: Cardiac standstill and hypothermia: An evaluation of time and temperature (poster presentation). The 58th Annual Meeting of the American Association of Neurological Surgeons. Nashville, TN, May 3, 1990.

HARGRAVES RW, ZIMMERMAN RS, ZABRAMSKI JM, GRAHM TW, SPETZLER RF: SAH in patients over 60 years of age (poster presentation). The 58th Annual Meeting of the American Association of Neurological Surgeons. Nashville, TN, May 3, 1990.

SPETZLER RF: Complex giant basilar artery aneurysms treated under cardiac standstill. International Symposium on Processes of the Cranial Midline. Vienna, Austria, May 21, 1990.

SPETZLER RF: Management of brain stem cavernomas and their association with venous malformations. International Symposium on Processes of the Cranial Midline. Vienna, Austria, May 22, 1990.

PUCA A, SPETZLER RF, ZABRAMSKI JM, CULICCHIA F: Hypothermic circulatory arrest: A useful adjunct in the treatment of basilar artery aneurysm. Experimental study. International Symposium on Processes of the Cranial Midline. Vienna, Austria, May 23, 1990.

SPETZLER RF, DASPIT CP, PAPPAS CTE: Combined approach for lesions involving the clivus and cerebellopontine angle: Experience with 23 Cases. International Symposium of Processes of the Cranial Midline. Vienna, Austria, May 25, 1990.

SPETZLER RF, GRAHM TW: Far-lateral approach to the inferior clivus and the upper cervical region. International Symposium of Processes of the Cranial Midline. Vienna, Austria, May 25, 1990.

SPETZLER RF, SONNTAG VKH: The transoral approach to the odontoid region. International Symposium of Processes of the Cranial Midline. Vienna, Austria, May 25, 1990.

ZIMMERMAN RS, SPETZLER RF: Microsurgery of cavernous malformations of the brain stem. 10th International Symposium on Microsurgery for Cerebral Ischemia. San Francisco, CA, July 14, 1990.

SPETZLER RF: Special Conference. Society of Neurological Surgery of Western AC, 60th Congress. Puerto Vallarta, Mexico, August 4, 1990.

SPETZLER RF: Cerebral bypass: Complicated and unique problems of management. 1990 Annual Kasdon Neurosurgical Research Forum. Westwater Canyon and Telluride, CO, August 11, 1990.

SPETZLER RF: Subtemporal approach to the region of the basilar artery: Anatomical and surgical aspects. 18th Brazilian Congress of Neurosurgery, 5th Brazilian Congress of Functional Neurosurgery. Porto Alegre, Brazil, September 9, 1990.

SPETZLER RF: Supra- and infratentorial approach to the petroclival region. 18th Brazilian Congress of Neurosurgery, 5th Brazilian Congress of Functional Neurosurgery. Porto Alegre, Brazil, September 9, 1990.

SPETZLER RF: Transoral approach to the odontoid. 18th Brazilian Congress of Neurosurgery, 5th Brazilian Congress of Functional Neurosurgery. Porto Alegre, Brazil, September 10, 1990.

SPETZLER RF, ALVES A: Cerebral protection. 18th Brazilian Congress of Neurosurgery, 5th Brazilian Congress of Functional Neurosurgery. Porto Alegre, Brazil, September 11, 1990.

SPETZLER RF: Giant aneurysms of the posterior circulation: Technical and surgical aspects. 18th Brazilian Congress of Neurosurgery, 5th Brazilian Congress of Functional Neurosurgery. Porto Alegre, Brazil. September 12, 1990.

SPETZLER RF: Intraoperative monitoring with transcranial Doppler *versus* EEG monitoring. 63rd Annual Clinical Assembly of Osteopathic Subspecialists. Los Angeles, October 30, 1990.

SPETZLER RF: Transcranial bypass at the Barrow Neurological Institute, 63rd Annual Clinical Assembly of Osteopathic Subspecialists. Los Angeles, October 30, 1990

SPETZLER RF (lecturer): Combined approach for skull base lesions. 1990 J. Garber Galbraith Neurosurgical Society. Birmingham, AL, November 16, 1990.

SPETZLER RF (faculty): Spinal arteriovenous malformations. J. Garber Galbraith Neurosurgical Society. Birmingham, AL, November 16, 1990.

SPETZLER RF: Classification of vascular malformations. Surgical Grand Rounds Lecture. Birmingham, AL, November 17, 1990.

Presentations for 1989 (31)

RAUDZENS P, MATTHEWS M, SPETZLER R: Transcranial Doppler monitoring of MCA velocity during carotid endarterectomy compared with EEG and SSEP. Richard Lende Winter Neurosurgery Conference. Snowbird, UT, February 5, 1989.

SPETZLER RF: Tumors of the clivus. Richard Lende Winter Neurosurgery Conference. Snowbird, UT, February 1, 1989.

CARTER LP, DICKMAN C, SPETZLER RF: ICP-CBF monitoring in head trauma. Richard Lende Winter Neurosurgery Conference. Snowbird, UT, February 8, 1989.

CULICCHIA F, ZABRAMSKI JM, SPETZLER RF: Electrocortical somatosensory responses predict outcome from focal cerebral ischemia: Results in a reliable new primate model of stroke. Richard Lende Winter Neurosurgery Conference. Snowbird, UT, February 10, 1989.

ZABRAMSKI JM, CULICCHIA F, SPETZLER RF: Hypervolemic hemodilution improves outcome in a primate model of focal cerebral ischemia. Richard Lende Winter Neurosurgery Conference. Snowbird, UT, February 10, 1989.

SPETZLER RF: Vertebral artery aneurysms. International Symposium on Intracranial Aneurysms. Omaha, NE, March 31, 1989.

SPETZLER RF (moderator): Spinal AVM's. The Annual Meeting of the American Association of Neurological Surgeons. Washington, DC, April 3, 1989.

BAILES JE, SPETZLER RF, HADLEY MN, BALDWIN HZ, ZABRAMSKI JM (panelists): Management morbidity and mortality of Hunt and Hess grades IV and V aneurysm patients. The Annual Meeting of the American Association of Neurological Surgeons. Washington, DC, April 4, 1989.

FITZPATRICK BC, JOHNSON PC, DRAYER BP, SPETZLER RF (panelists): Correlation of postmortem magnetic resonance images and neuropathological findings in 23 patients with gliomas. The Annual Meeting of the American Association of Neurological Surgeons. Washington, DC, April 4, 1989.

CARTER LP, GRAHM TM, ZABRAMSKI JM, LOPEZ LJ, TALLMAN DH, SPETZLER RF: Postoperative monitoring of cerebral blood flow in patients with intracranial aneurysms (poster session). The Annual Meeting of the American Association of Neurological Surgeons. Washington, DC, April 6, 1989.

GUTHKELCH AN, CARTER LP, IACONO RP, SHETTER A, SPETZLER RF, CASSADY JR, CETAS TC, ROSSMANN K, LULU B, LUTZ W, SHIMM D,

STEA B, OBBENS E, HODAK J: A phase I trial of ferromagnetic induction hyperthermia combined with brachytherapy for high-grade cerebral astrocytomas (poster session). The Annual Meeting of the American Association of Neurological Surgeons. Washington, DC, April 6, 1989.

SPETZLER RF: Surgical treatment of masses at the base of the skull. 41st Annual Meeting of the American Academy of Neurology. Chicago, IL, April 13–19, 1989.

SPETZLER RF: Classification of vascular lesions. Kasdon Neurological Research Forum. Sedona, AZ, April 22–24, 1989.

SPETZLER RF, ZABRAMSKI JM: Hypothermic arrest with barbiturate coma in a primate model. Neurosurgical Satellite: Surgical Research Society (British Isles). Windsor, England, June 15, 1989.

ZABRAMSKI JM, SPETZLER RF: New model of temporary focal ischemia in the primate: Experience with hemodilution and NMDA/receptor antagonist. Neurosurgical Satellite: Surgical Research Society (British Isles). Windsor, England, June 15, 1989.

SPETZLER RF: Surgical approach to the third ventricle and its surrounding lesions. 48th Annual Meeting of the Japan Neurosurgical Society. Morioka City, Japan, September 21, 1989.

SPETZLER RF: Approaches to the third ventricle—anterior and posterior. 48th Annual Meeting of the Japan Neurosurgical Society. Morioka City, Japan, September 27, 1989.

SPETZLER RF: Intravascular neurosurgery. 48th Annual Meeting of the Japan Neurosurgical Society. Morioka City, Japan, September 27, 1989.

SPETZLER RF: Treatment of deep seated arteriovenous malformations. 48th Annual Meeting of the Japan Neurosurgical Society. Morioka City, Japan, September 27, 1989.

SPETZLER RF: Treatment of hardly manageable AVM. 48th Annual Meeting of the Japan Neurosurgical Society. Morioka City, Japan, September 29, 1989.

SPETZLER RF: Spinal cord AVMs. Ramathibodi Hospital, Bangkok, Thailand, October 4, 1989.

SPETZLER RF: Cerebral AVMs. Siriraj Hospital, Bangkok, Thailand, October 6, 1989.

SPETZLER RF: Transcranial Doppler sonography in cerebral vasospasm. 9th International Congress of Neurological Surgery. New Dehli, India, October 9, 1989.

SPETZLER RF: Management of giant AVMs. 9th International Congress of Neurological Surgery. New Dehli, India, October 9, 1989.

SPETZLER RF: EEG monitored brain protection and intraoperative angiography. 9th International Congress of Neurological Surgery. New Dehli, India, October 10, 1989.

SPETZLER RF: Incidental deep seated arteriovenous malformations. 9th International Congress of Neurological Surgery. New Dehli, India, October 10, 1989.

SPETZLER RF (chairperson): Trends in management of AVMs. 9th International Congress of Neurological Surgery. New Dehli, India, October 11, 1989.

SPETZLER RF: The surgical challenge. 9th International Congress of Neurological Surgery. New Dehli, India, October 11, 1989.

SPETZLER RF (panel discussion): Cardiac standstill for complex basilar artery aneurysm. International Symposium on Vascular Lesions of the Brain (a Satellite Conference of the 9th ICNS). Trivandrum, India, October 15, 1989.

SPETZLER RF, ZABRAMSKI JM: Vascular malformations of the brain: An overview (keynote address). International Symposium on Vascular Lesions of the Brain (a Satellite Conference of the 9th ICNS). Trivandrum, India, October 16, 1989.

SPETZLER RF: Normal perfusion pressure breakthrough syndrome: Recent concepts. International Symposium on Vascular Lesions on the Brain (a Satellite Conference of the 9th ICNS). Trivandrum, India, October 16, 1989.

Presentations for 1988 (36)

SPETZLER RF: Tumors of the tentorial incisura. 14th Annual Richard Lende Winter Neurosurgery Conference, Cliff Conference Center. Snowbird, UT, January 30–February 6, 1988.

SPETZLER RF: Surgical management of spinal AVMs. Joint Section on Disorders of the Spine and Peripheral Nerves of the American Association of Neurological Surgeons and Congress of Neurological Surgeons. Phoenix, AZ, February 16–20, 1988.

RIGAMONTI D, UEDE T, JOHNSON PC, BOJANOWSKI WM, MICHAELS KT, CARTER LP, SPETZLER RF: Cerebral embolic infarction: BNI model (poster presentation). 13th International Joint Conference on Stroke and Cerebral Circulation. San Diego, CA, February 18–20, 1988.

HADLEY MN, SPETZLER RF, ZABRAMSKI JM: Efficacy of IV nimodipine in the treatment of focal cerebral ischemia in a primate model. Workshop: Preclinical studies with nimodipine. Rye Brook, NY, March 1–9, 1988.

SPETZLER RF: Classification of AVM's and management of giant AVM's. 10th South African International Neurosurgical Congress. Johannesburg, South Africa, March 21–23, 1988.

SPETZLER RF: Cardiac standstill for complex basilar artery aneurysms. 10th South African International Neurosurgical Congress. Johannesburg, South Africa, March 21–23, 1988.

SPETZLER RF: Spinal AVM's. 10th South African International Neurosurgical Congress. Johannesburg, South Africa, March 21–23, 1988.

SPETZLER RF: Extra and intracranial management of basilar artery ischemia. 10th South African International Neurosurgical Congress. Johannesburg, South Africa, March 21–23, 1988.

ZABRAMSKI JM, SPETZLER RF: Why classify arteriovenous malformations? III International Symposium and Workshop on Microsurgery. Caracas, Venezuela, March 22, 1988.

SPETZLER RF (guest professor): Spinal cord AVM's. A new perspective. The Dana Foundation Visiting Professor, College of Physicians & Surgeons of Columbia University. New York, NY, May 19, 1988.

RIGAMONTI D, SPETZLER RF, DRAYER BP, JOHNSON PC, HOENIG-RIGAMONTI K: Cerebral cavernous malformations (angiomas) and stroke. AAN Scientific Program, 40th Annual Meeting of the Academy of Neurology. Cincinnati, OH, April 13–17, 1988.

RIGAMONTI D, SPETZLER RF, DRAYER BP, RIGAMONTI KH, MEDINA M: Cerebral venous malformations (angiomas). AAN Scientific Program, 40th Annual Meeting of the Academy of Neurology. Cincinnati, OH, April 13–17, 1988.

RIGAMONTI D, SPETZLER RF, HOENIG-RIGAMONTI D, MEDINA M, ELSNER HJ: Venous malformations: Their association with cavernous malformations. 1988 Annual Meeting, American Association of Neurological Surgeons. Toronto, Ontario, Canada, April 24–28, 1988.

GRAHM TW, WILLIAMS FC, HARRINGTON T, SPETZLER RF: Civilian gunshot wounds to the head: A prospective study. 23rd Annual Meeting, Rocky Mountain Neurosurgical Society. Lake Tahoe, NV, June 12–16, 1988.

BAILES JE, SPETZLER RF: Management of occluded internal carotid arteries. 23rd Annual Meeting, Rocky Mountain Neurosurgical Society. Lake Tahoe, NV, June 12–16, 1988.

BALDWIN HZ, HADLEY MN, ZABRAMSKI JM, SPETZLER RF, CARTER LP: Posterior circulation aneurysms: Management and outcome. 23rd Annual Meeting, Rocky Mountain Neurosurgical Society. Lake Tahoe, NV, June 12–16, 1988.

SPETZLER RF: Management of spinal cord arteriovenous malformations. 23rd Annual Meeting, Rocky Mountain Neurosurgical Society. Lake Tahoe, NV, June 12–16, 1988.

ZABRAMSKI JM, SPETZLER RF: Hypervolemic hemodilution in the treatment of acute stroke: Results of the pentastarch study. 23rd Annual

Meeting, Rocky Mountain Neurosurgical Society. Lake Tahoe, NV, June 12–16, 1988.

HADLEY MN, ZABRAMSKI JM, SPETZLER RF, RIGAMONTI D, FIFIELD MS, JOHNSON PC: Intravenous nimodipine in the treatment of focal cerebral ischemia. 23rd Annual Meeting, Rocky Mountain Neurosurgical Society. Lake Tahoe, NV, June 12–16, 1988.

SPETZLER RF (moderator): Acute cerebral ischemia. Microsurgery for cerebral ischemia. 9th International Symposium. Detroit, MI, July 7, 1988.

SPETZLER R, YASHIMOTO L, AUER L, *et al.:* Session one (round table). Microsurgery for cerebral ischemia, 9th International Symposium. Detroit, MI, July 7, 1988.

CAPLAN L, AUSMAN J, ROBERTSON J, SPETZLER R, GEORGE B: Session two (round table). Microsurgery for cerebral ischemia, 9th International Symposium. Detroit, MI, July 7, 1988.

AUSMAN J, SCHMIEDEK P, CAPLAN L, SPETZLER R, WALKER M, TILLEY B: Session two (round table). Discussion and plans for future studies. Microsurgery for cerebral ischemia. 9th International Symposium. Detroit, MI, July 8, 1988.

SPETZLER RF: Management of giant arteriovenous malformations. 34th Annual Meeting of the Western Neurosurgical Society. Laguna Niguel, CA, September 12, 1988.

AWAD IA, SPETZLER RF, HODAK JA: Magnetic resonance imaging in minor brain ischemia. 4th Toronto stroke Workshop. Toronto, Ontario, Canada, September 14–16, 1988.

SPETZLER RF: Will the carotid endarterectomy trials settle the main issues? 1st International Guillain-Barre Syndrome Symposium, American Neurological Association. Philadelphia, October 5, 1988.

SPETZLER RF: EEG monitored brain protection and intraoperative angiography. 9th International Congress of Neurological Surgery. Dehli, India, October 8–13. 1988.

SPETZLER RF, SONNTAG VKH: Transoral approach. 1st Annual Spine Workshop. Phoenix, AZ, November 10–12, 1988.

AWAD IA, SPETZLER RF, JOHNSON PC: Chronic cerebrovascular disease: The impact of age and vascular risk factors on brain parenchyma. Washington, DC, November 14–17, 1988.

SPETZLER RF: Surgery for vertebrobasilar ischemia. Postgraduate Course Neurosurgery Update, Harvard Medical School. Boston, November 15, 1988.

SPETZLER RF: Neurovascular perioperative care. Postgraduate Course Neurosurgery Update, Harvard Medical School. Boston, November 15, 1988.

SPETZLER RF: Vertebrobasilar aneurysms. Postgraduate Course Neurosurgery Update, Harvard Medical School. Boston, November 15, 1988.

SPETZLER RF: Large convexity AVM's. Postgraduate Course Neurosurgery Update, Harvard Medical School. Boston, November 15, 1988.

SPETZLER RF: Spinal AVM's. Postgraduate Course Neurosurgery Update, Harvard Medical School. Boston, MA, November 15, 1988.

SPETZLER RF (panelist): Aneurysms and AVM's. Postgraduate Course Neurosurgery Update, Harvard Medical School. Boston, MA, November 15, 1988.

ONOFRIO B, LONG D, ACKERMAN R, SPETZLER RF (panelists): Benign tumors and cerebrovascular surgery. Postgraduate Course Neurosurgery Update, Harvard Medical School. Boston, MA, November 15, 1988.

Presentations for 1987 (47)

SPETZLER RF: Treatment of spinal arteriovenous malformations. Joint Section on Spinal Disorders AANS/CNS. Boca Baton, FL, January 17, 1987.

HADLEY MN, SPETZLER RF, FIFIELD MS, BICHARD WD, HODAK JA: The effect of nimodipine on intracranial pressure and cerebral perfusion pressure. Richard Lende Winter Neurosurgery Conference. Snowbird, UT, January 31–February 7, 1987.

HADLEY MN, SPETZLER RF, MARTIN NA, FIFIELD MS, BICHARD WD, MCCORMICK JM, SONNTAG VKH, JOHNSON PC: Transoral dural closure techniques. Richard Lende Winter Neurosurgery Conference. Snowbird, UT, January 31–February 7, 1987.

SPETZLER RF: Base of the skull tumors—Surgical approaches. Richard Lende Winter Neurosurgery Conference. Snowbird, UT, January 31–February 7, 1987.

SPETZLER RF: Introduction. 1st Annual Barrow Neurological Institute Magnetic Resonance Imaging Conference. Phoenix, AZ, February 22, 1987.

SPETZLER RF: Vascular malformations: Clinical. 1st Annual Barrow Neurological Institute Magnetic Resonance Imaging Conference. Phoenix, AZ, February 22, 1987.

SPETZLER RF: Aneurysm and AVM. 14th Annual Symposium, Barrow Neurological Institute Neurology & Neurosurgery of the Aging. Phoenix, AZ, February 26, 1987.

AWAD IA, SPETZLER RF, JOHNSON PC: "Unidentified bright objects" on magnetic resonance imaging of the brain. 12th International Joint

Conference on Stroke and Cerebral Circulation. Tampa, FL, February 26–28, 1987.

SPETZLER RF (moderator): 14th Annual Symposium, Barrow Neurological Institute, Neurology & Neurosurgery of the Aging. Phoenix, AZ, February 27, 1987.

SPETZLER RF: Cardiac arrest for giant basilar artery aneurysms. Winter Conference in the Bugaboos. Banff, Alberta, Canada, March 7, 1987.

HADLEY MN, SPETZLER RF, MARTIN NA, FIFIELD MS, BICHARD WD, McCORMICK JM, SONNTAG VKH, JOHNSON PC: Comparative transoral dural closure techniques: A canine model. Federation of Western Societies of Neurological Sciences. San Diego, CA, March 29–April 1, 1987.

HADLEY MN, SPETZLER RF, FIFIELD MS, BICHARD WD, HODAK JA: The effect of nimodipine on intracranial pressure: Volume-pressure studies in a primate model. Federation of Western Societies of Neurological Science. San Diego, CA, March 29–April 1, 1987.

SPETZLER RF: Pathophysiology and treatment of spinal arteriovenous malformations. Grand Rounds, University of Nebraska Medical Center. Omaha, NE, April 15, 1987.

SPETZLER RF: Transoral approach to the cervicomedullary junction. Keegan Lecture, University of Nebraska Medical Center. Omaha, NE, April 15, 1987.

SPETZLER RF: Normal Perfusion pressure breakthrough. 7th Annual Meeting of the Japanese Congress of Neurological Surgeons. Sapporo, Japan, May 14, 1987.

SPETZLER RF: Indications of bypass surgery. 7th Annual Meeting of the Japanese Congress of Neurological Surgeons. Sapporo, Japan, May 15, 1987.

SPETZLER RF: Transoral approach to the skull base lesions. 7th Annual Meeting of the Japanese Congress of Neurological Surgeons. Sapporo, Japan, May 16, 1987.

SPETZLER RF: Removal of intramedullary AVM in cervicomedullary junction. Video presentation. International Symposium on Surgery for Cerebral Stroke. Sendai, Japan, May 25, 1987.

SPETZLER RF: Extracranial/intracranial bypass for cerebral revascularization. Round table discussion—Bypass surgery. International Symposium on Surgery for Cerebral Stroke. Sendai, Japan, May 25, 1987.

SPETZLER RF: Overview of cerebral ischemia: Rationale for cerebral protection. Round table discussion—Scientific basis for cerebral infarction. International Symposium on Surgery for Cerebral Stroke. Sendai, Japan, May 25, 1987.

SPETZLER RF: Operative selection of patients with arteriovenous malformations. Round table discussion—Surgical treatment of deep seated or large AVM. International Symposium on Surgery for Cerebral Stroke. Sendai, Japan, May 27, 1987.

SPETZLER RF: Cerebral revascularization. Round table discussion—Revascularization in the acute stage of cerebral infarction. International Symposium on Surgery for Cerebral Stroke. Sendai, Japan, May 27, 1987.

SPETZLER RF (discussant): Surgical neuroangiography: Past, present, and future, by Flom RA. 1987 Annual Meeting, The Arizona Medical Association, Inc. Phoenix, AZ, June 4, 1987.

RIGAMONTI D, JOHNSON PC, DRAYER BP, SPETZLER RF: Cavernous malformation and capillary telangiectases: Two facets of the same pathological entity. Annual Meeting of the American Association of Neuropathologists. Seattle, WA, June 13, 1987.

RIGAMONTI D, PAPPAS C, BOJANOWSKI M, MEDINA M, LIU SS, JOHNSON PC, SONNTAG VKH, SPETZLER RF: Hemangioblastomas. 22nd Annual Meeting, Rocky Mountain Neurosurgical Society. Deer Valley, UT, June 21–25, 1987.

HADLEY MN, SPETZLER RF, FIFIELD MS, BICHARD WD, HODAK JA: The effect of nimodipine on intracranial pressure: Volume pressure studies in a primate model. 22nd Annual Meeting, Rocky Mountain Neurosurgical Society. Deer Valley, UT, June 21–25, 1987.

LIU SS, SPETZLER RF, MEDINA M, JOHNSON PC, HADLEY MN: Primary lymphomas. 22nd Annual Meeting, Rocky Mountain Neurosurgical Society. Deer Valley, UT, June 21–25, 1987.

WILLIAMS FC, AWAD IA, SPETZLER RF, CARTER LP: Early surgery for midline aneurysms. 22nd Annual Meeting, Rocky Mountain Neurosurgical Society. Deer Valley, UT, June 21–25, 1987.

RIGAMONTI D, DRAYER BP, JOHNSON PC, SPETZLER RF: Cavernous malformations. 22nd Annual Meeting, Rocky Mountain Neurosurgical Society. Deer Valley, UT, June 21–25, 1987.

HADLEY MN, SPETZLER RF, MARTIN NA, FIFIELD MS, BICHARD WD, MCCORMICK JM, SONNTAG VKH, JOHNSON PC: Comparative transoral dural closure techniques: A canine model. 22nd Annul Meeting, Rocky Mountain Neurosurgical Society. Deer Valley, UT, June 21–25, 1987.

RIGAMONTI D, REKATE H, PITTMAN H, SPETZLER RF: Cavernous malformations (angiomas) in children. 1987 Annual Meeting of the International Society for Paediatric Neurosurgery. New York, July 12–16, 1987.

SPETZLER RF, HADLEY MN, SONNTAG VKH: The transoral approach to the anterior superior cervical spine: A review of 26 cases. 8th European Congress of Neurosurgery. Barcelona, Spain, September 6–11, 1987.

SPETZLER RF, HADLEY MN, RIGAMONTI D: Complex aneurysms of the basilar artery treated with circulatory arrest, hypothermia, and barbiturate cerebral protection. 8th European Congress of Neurosurgery. Barcelona, Spain, September 6–11, 1987.

SPETZLER RF, MARTIN NA, CARTER LP, FLOM RA, RAUDZENS PA, WILKINSON E: Surgical management of large AVMs by staged embolization and operative excision. 8th European Congress of Neurosurgery. Barcelona, Spain, September 6–11, 1987.

SPETZLER RF: Intradural pathology. Transoral approach to the skull base. Seminar, 8th European Congress of Neurosurgery. Barcelona, Spain, September 6–11, 1987.

SPETZLER RF (guest speaker): Cerebral angiomas—classification and surgery. Neurochirurgische Klinik, Der Universitat Erlangen-Nurnberg. Erlangen, West Germany, September 17, 1987.

SPETZLER RF (speaker): Symposium: Therapeutic options in intracranial arteriovenous malformations. 1987 Annual Meeting of the Western Neuroradiological Society. Scottsdale, AZ, October 10, 1987.

SPETZLER RF: Transoral approach to ventral extradural cervicomedullary junction pathology. Congress of Neurological Surgeons. Baltimore, October 25, 1987.

SPETZLER RF: The future of carotid endarterectomy for symptomatic occlusive disease. Congress of Neurological Surgeons. Baltimore, October 25, 1987.

SPETZLER RF: Role of hemodynamic monitoring in the neurosurgical ICU. Congress of Neurological Surgeons. Baltimore, October 26, 1987.

SPETZLER RF: Neurosurgical subspecialization: To fellowship or not to fellowship. Congress of Neurological Surgeons. Baltimore, October 27, 1987.

SPETZLER RF: Approaches to the anterior third ventricle. Congress of Neurological Surgeons. Baltimore, October 28, 1987.

SPETZLER RF (guest lecturer): The transoral approach for the craniocervical junction. The E. Harry Botterell Visiting Lecturer in Neurosurgery. November 17, 1987.

SPETZLER RF (round table discussant): Timing of aneurysm surgery—Does it really make a difference? The E. Harry Botterell Visiting Lecturer in Neurosurgery. November 17, 1987.

SPETZLER RF: Management and classification of AVM's. Royal College Lecture, Toronto Neurological Society. The E. Harry Botterell Visiting Lecturer in Neurosurgery. November 17, 1987.

RIGAMONTI D, SPETZLER RF: Cerebral venous malformations in children. 16th Winter Meeting of the Pediatric Section of the American Association of Neurological Surgeons. Chicago, IL, December 8–11, 1987.

RIGAMONTI D, REKATE HA, SPETZLER RF, HOENIG-RIGAMONTI K, MEDINA MK, EPSTEIN MA: Cerebral venous malformations in children. 16th Winter Meeting of the Pediatric Section of the American Association of Neurological Surgeons. Chicago, IL, December 8–11, 1987.

Presentations for 1986 (47)

SPETZLER RF: A new classification for AVMs. 12th Annual Richard Lende Winter Neurosurgery Conference. Snowbird, UT, February 2, 1986.

SPETZLER RF: Giant arteriovenous malformations. 12th Annual Richard Lende Winter Neurosurgery Conference. Snowbird, UT, February 2, 1986.

SPETZLER RF: Hemodilution in vasospasm. 11th International Joint Conference on Stroke and Cerebral Circulation. San Francisco, CA, February 6, 1986.

CARTER LP, MEDINA M, WILLIAMS F, SPETZLER RF: Hypervolemic hemodilution therapy in the management of intracranial aneurysms. 11th International Joint Conference on Stroke and Cerebral Circulation. San Francisco, CA, February 8, 1986.

SPETZLER RF: Approaches to the base of the skull. Midas Rex Neurosurgical Symposium. Scottsdale, AZ, February 25, 1986.

SPETZLER RF (moderator): Current issues in neurology and neurosurgery. 13th Annual Barrow Neurological Institute Symposium. Scottsdale, AZ, February 27, 1986.

CARTER LP, SPETZLER RF: Research in cerebrovascular disease. 13th Annual Barrow Neurological Institute Symposium. Scottsdale, AZ, February 28, 1986.

SPETZLER RF, CARTER LP: Surgical intervention in cerebrovascular disease. 13th Annual Barrow Neurological Institute Symposium. Scottsdale, AZ, February 28, 1986.

AWAD IA, SPETZLER RF, JOHNSON PC, HODAK JA, CAREY R: Incidental lesions noted on magnetic resonance imaging of the brain—An index of chronic cerebrovascular disease. The Research Society of Neurological Surgeons. Phoenix, AZ, March 6, 1986.

HADLEY MN, MARTIN NA, SPETZLER RF: The transoral approach to the brain stem: Clinical and experimental considerations. The Research Society of Neurological Surgeons. Phoenix, AZ, March 5, 1986.

SPETZLER RF: Transoral approach to the upper cervical spine and clivus. The 3rd Biennial American-European Neurosurgical Winter Conference. Davos, Switzerland, March 11, 1986.

SPETZLER RF: AVM classification. The 3rd Biennial American-European Neurosurgical Winter Conference. Davos, Switzerland, March 13, 1986.

SPETZLER RF: Management of giant AVMs. The 3rd Biennial American-European Neurosurgical Winter Conference. Obergurgl, Austria, March 17, 1986.

SPETZLER RF: Management of CSF leaks. The 3rd Biennial American-European Neurosurgical Winter Conference. Obergurgl, Austria, March 18, 1986.

SPETZLER RF (visiting professor): Grading of arteriovenous malformations. Sapporo Medical College. Sapporo, Japan, April 1, 1986.

SPETZLER RF (visiting professor): Management of giant arteriovenous malformations. Sapporo Medical College. Sapporo, Japan, April 1, 1986.

SPETZLER RF: Extra-intracranial arterial bypass in the management of giant internal carotid aneurysms. 1st International Workshop on Intracranial Aneurysms. Tokyo, April 4, 1986.

SPETZLER RF: Giant basilar aneurysms managed under circulatory arrest. 1st International Workshop on Intracranial Aneurysms. Tokyo, April 4, 1986.

SPETZLER RF (visiting professor): Grading of arteriovenous malformations. Tokai University Medical Center. Bohseidai, Japan, April 5, 1986.

SPETZLER RF (visiting professor): Management of giant arteriovenous malformations. Tokai University Medical Center. Bohseidai, Japan, April 5, 1986.

SPETZLER RF: EC-IC bypass. New Mexico Neurological/Neurosurgical Society Meeting. Albuquerque, NM, April 11, 1986.

WILLIAMS F, AWAD IA, SPETZLER RF, CARTER LP: Neurological complications after nonpenetrating trauma to the cervical carotid artery. American Association of Neurological Surgeons. Denver, CO, April 13–17, 1986.

SPETZLER RF: Carotid endarterectomies. American Association of Neurological Surgeons Annual Meeting. Denver, CO, April 15, 1986.

SPETZLER RF: Anterior circulating aneurysms. American Association of Neurological Surgeons Annual Meeting. Denver, CO, April 16, 1986.

SPETZLER RF: CSF fistulae. American Association of Neurological Surgeons Annual Meeting. Denver, CO, April 17, 1986.

SPETZLER RF, AWAD IA: The future of EC-IC bypass surgery. 38th Annual Meeting, American Academy of Neurology. New Orleans, LA, April 21–May 3, 1986.

SPETZLER RF: The use of the EC-IC bypass. 38th Annual Meeting, American Academy of Neurology. New Orleans, LA, May 2, 1986.

SPETZLER RF: Cardiac standstill for complex giant aneurysms. Trends in Neurosurgery Meeting. Vienna, Austria, May 16, 1986.

SPETZLER RF: A new classification for arteriovenous malformations. Trends in Neurosurgery Meeting. Vienna, Austria, May 16, 1986.

SPETZLER RF: Management of normal perfusion pressure breakthrough in giant AVMs. Trends in Neurosurgery Meeting. Vienna, Austria, May 16, 1986.

SPETZLER RF (moderator): Revascularization after the bypass study. Trends in Neurosurgery Meeting. Vienna, Austria, May 17, 1976.

SPETZLER RF: Reflections on the EC-IC bypass. Neurosurgical Research Forum. Cape Cod, MA, May 22–26, 1986.

SPETZLER RF (visiting professor): Management of giant AVMs. Tucson Medical Center. Tucson, AZ, June 4, 1986.

SPETZLER RF: Magnetic resonance imaging impact on tumor diagnosis. Arizona Medical Association 1986 Annual Meeting. Tucson, AZ, June 5, 1986.

SPETZLER RF (visiting professor): New AVM classification. University of Alberta. Edmonton, Alberta, Canada, June 21, 1986.

SPETZLER RF: Grading of arteriovenous malformations. 21st Annual Meeting, The Rocky Mountain Neurosurgical Society, Inc. Keystone, CO, June 23, 1986.

SPETZLER RF (moderator): 21st Annual Meeting, The Rocky Mountain Neurosurgical Society, Inc. Keystone, CO, June 24, 1986.

SPETZLER RF: Giant AVMs. 21st Annual Meeting, The Rocky Mountain Neurosurgical Society, Inc. Keystone, CO, June 25, 1986.

SPETZLER RF: Present indications for bypass. 3rd Toronto Stroke Workshop. Toronto, Ontario, September 5, 1986.

SPETZLER RF (chairman): Session III: Carotid plaques and neck bruits. 3rd Toronto Stroke Workshop. Toronto, Ontario, September 5, 1986.

SPETZLER RF: Present indications for carotid edarterectomy. 3rd Toronto Stroke Workshop. Toronto, Ontario, September 5, 1986.

SPETZLER RF: Approaches to the base of the skull. Midas Rex Neurosurgical Symposium. New Orleans, LA, September 13, 1986.

HADLEY MN, MARTIN NA, SPETZLER RF, FIFIELD MS, BICHARD WD, MCCORMICK JM, SONNTAG VKH, JOHNSON PC: Comparative transoral closure techniques: A canine model. Congress of Neurological Surgeons. New Orleans, September 14–19, 1986.

AWAD IA, SPETZLER RF, LIU SS, HADLEY MN: Pathophysiology of ischemic symptoms in patients with lesions amenable to EC-IC bypass surgery. 8th International Symposium on Microsurgical Anastomosis for Cerebral Ischemia. Florence, Italy, September 14–17, 1986.

AWAD IA, SPETZLER RF, HODAK JA: Proton magnetic resonance imaging in the evaluation of patients for EC-IC bypass surgery—Advantages and limitations. 8th International Symposium on Microsurgical Anastomosis for Cerebral Ischemia. Florence, Italy, September 14–17, 1986.

SPETZLER RF (moderator): Surgical therapy of skull base tumors. 36th Annual Meeting, Congress of Neurological Surgeons, New Orleans, September 16, 1986.

SPETZLER RF, HADLEY MN: Complex aneurysms of the basilar artery treated with circulatory arrest, hypothermia, and barbiturate cerebral protection. Annual Meeting of the American Academy of Neurological Surgery. Sea Island, GA, November 6, 1986.

Presentations for 1985 (35)

SPETZLER RF: Historical aspects of cerebrovascular disorders. 8th Annual Winter Symposium on Cerebrovascular Diseases. Grand Junction, CO, January 23–25, 1985.

SPETZLER RF: Posterior cerebral circulation: What is vertebral basilar insufficiency and what can be surgically treated? 8th Annual Winter Symposium on Cerebrovascular Diseases. Grand Junction, CO, January 23–25, 1985.

SPETZLER RF: Overview of carotid artery surgery. 8th Annual Winter Symposium on Cerebrovascular Diseases. Grand Junction, CO, January 23–25, 1985.

SPETZLER RF: Surgery for subarachnoid hemorrhage. 8th Annual Winter Symposium on Cerebrovascular Diseases. Grand Junction, CO, January 23–25, 1985.

SPETZLER RF: The future of neurosurgery for stroke: Brain protection and resuscitation. 8th Annual Winter Symposium on Cerebrovascular Diseases. Grand Junction, CO, January 23–25, 1985.

SPETZLER RF: Barbiturates and microendarterectomy. 11th Annual Richard Lende Winter Neurosurgery Conference. Snowbird, UT, January 26–February 2, 1985.

SPETZLER RF: Transcallosal approach for midline lesions. 11th Annual Richard Lende Winter Neurosurgery Conference. Snowbird, UT, January 26–February 2, 1985.

SPETZLER RF: Posterior fossa craniotomy with one burr hole. Midas Rex Conference. Scottsdale, AZ, February 8–10, 1985.

SPETZLER RF: Transcallosal tumor surgery. 12th Annual Barrow Neurological Institute Symposium. Scottsdale, AZ, February 11, 1985.

SPETZLER RF (moderator): Tumors of the central nervous system. 12th Annual Barrow Neurological Institute Symposium. Scottsdale, AZ, February 12, 1985.

SPETZLER RF: Revascularization of the brain stem. International Symposium on Surgery In and Around the Brain Stem and the Third Ventricle. Hanover, West Germany, February 18–23, 1985.

SPETZLER RF: Surgery of processes affecting midbrain and basal ganglia. International Symposium on Surgery In and Around the Brain Stem and the Third Ventricle. Hanover, West Germany, February 18–23, 1985.

SPETZLER RF: Transoral approach to foramen magnum and clivus. International Symposium on Surgery In and Around the Brain Stem and the Third Ventricle. Hanover, West Germany, February 18–23, 1985.

SPETZLER RF: Neurosurgical management of posterior fossa ischemia. 37th Annual Meeting, Southern Neurosurgical Society. Scottsdale, AZ, February 27–March 3, 1985.

SPETZLER RF: Brain revascularization surgery. 6th Annual Vail Clinical Brain Conference. Vail, CO, March 11–15, 1985.

SPETZLER RF: Management of arteriovenous malformations. 6th Annual Vail Clinical Brain Conference. Vail, CO, March 11–15, 1985.

SPETZLER RF: Aneurysm management. 6th Annual Vail Clinical Brain Conference. Vail, CO, March 11–15, 1985.

SPETZLER RF: Intraventricular lesions. 6th Annual Vail Clinical Brain Conference. Vail, CO, March 11–15, 1985.

SPETZLER RF: Extxacranial-intracranial bypass. American Association of Neurological Surgeons Annual Meeting. Atlanta, GA, April 21–25, 1985.

SPETZLER RF: Staged management of giant AVMs. 76th Meeting, The Society of Neurological Surgeons. Phoenix, AZ, May 5–8, 1985.

SPETZLER RF: Perioperative therapy of patients with ruptured aneurysms. Neurosciences Society Meeting. Tulsa, OK, May 15, 1985.

SPETZLER RF: Posterior fossa revascularization. 1st International Neurosurgical Summer Conference. Mombasa, Kenya, June 16, 1985.

SPETZLER RF: Giant basilar aneurysms: Hypothermia and extracorporal circulation. 1st International Neurosurgical Summer Conference. Mombasa, Kenya, June 17, 1985.

SPETZLER RF: Transoral approach to the odontoid. 1st International Neurosurgical Summer Conference. Mombasa, Kenya, June 18, 1985.

SPETZLER RF: Giant AVMs and their management. 1st International Neurosurgical Summer Conference. Mombasa, Kenya, June 18, 1985.

SPETZLER RF: Management of spinal fluid leak. 1st International Neurosurgical Summer Conference. Mombasa, Kenya, June 20, 1985.

SPETZLER RF: Staged embolization and excision of giant AVMs. 8th International Congress of Neurological Surgery. Toronto, Ontario, Canada, July 12, 1985.

SPETZLER RF: Staging of AVMs. Management of perfusion-pressure breakthrough. Giant aneurysms and the bypass. The 3rd Annual Stonwin Medical Conference on Subarachnoid Hemorrhage. New York, July 16, 1985.

SPETZLER RF: Tumors involving major vessels. Neurosurgical Research Forum. Santa Fe, NM, September 5, 1985.

SPETZLER RF: Intracranial hemorrhage: Pathophysiology, medical diagnosis and management related to aneurysms, vascular malformations, and other spontaneous hemorrhage. Pilot Program of the Neuroscience Nursing Graduate Program, Barrow Neurological Institute. Phoenix, AZ, October 22, 1985.

SPETZLER RF: Surgical treatment of hemorrhagic stroke. Stroke Update '85, St. Joseph's Hospital and Medical Center. Phoenix, AZ, October 26, 1985.

SPETZLER RF: Microsurgical endarterectomy under barbiturate protection: A prospective study. American Academy of Neurological Surgery Annual Meeting. Houston, TX, October 28, 1985.

Presentations for 1984 (33)

SPETZLER RF: Management of head trauma. Yavapai Community Hospital. Prescott, AZ, January 5, 1984.

SPETZLER RF: Barbiturate protection in cerebral ischemia. Barrow Neurological Institute. Phoenix, AZ, January 26, 1984.

SPETZLER RF: Clinical value of NMR. 10th Annual Richard Lende Winter Neurosurgery Conference. Snowbird, UT, January 28–February 4, 1984.

SPETZLER RF: Surgery on AVMs. 11th Annual Barrow Neurological Institute Symposium. Scottsdale, AZ, February 13–15, 1984.

SPETZLER RF, ZABRAMSKI JM: NMR imaging: Pulse technique and early detection of focal ischemic injury. 9th International Joint Conference on Stroke and Cerebral Circulation. Tampa, FL, February 16–18, 1984.

SPETZLER RF: Therapy of cerebrovascular disease. Federation of Western Societies of Neurological Science. Napa, CA, February 23–26, 1984.

SPETZLER RF: Cerebral revascularization. Desert Samaritan Hospital. Mesa, AZ, February 29, 1984.

SPETZLER RF: Transoral/transclival approaches for brain stem compressing lesions. 2nd Biennial American-European Neurosurgical Winter Conference. St. Moritz, Switzerland, March 12, 1984.

SPETZLER RF: Clinical usefulness of NMR. 2nd Biennial American-European Neurosurgical Winter Conference. St. Moritz, Switzerland, March 12, 1984.

SPETZLER RF: Giant cerebral AVMs. 2nd Biennial American-European Neurosurgical Winter Conference. St. Moritz, Switzerland, March 12, 1984.

SPETZLER RF: Transcallosal approach. Microsurgical Research Institute. San Francisco, April 6, 1984.

SPETZLER RF: Techniques for giant aneurysms. American Association of Neurological Surgeons. San Francisco, April 11, 1984.

SPETZLER RF: Clinical role of NMR technology in the neurosurgical patient. American Association of Neurological Surgeons. San Francisco, April 8–12, 1984.

SPETZLER RF: Neurosurgical management of stroke. Internal Medicine Grand Rounds, St. Joseph's Hospital and Medical Center. Phoenix, AZ, April 18, 1984.

SPETZLER RF: Management of focal ischemia in primates. UCSD Medical Center. San Diego, CA, May 3, 1984.

SPETZLER RF: Current status and indication of EC-IC bypass surgery. Neurosciences Grand Rounds of UCSD Medical Center. San Diego, CA, May 4, 1984.

SPETZLER RF: Evolution of edema following cerebral ischemia as monitored by NMR scanning. Research Society of Neurological Surgeons. Chicago, May 23–26, 1984.

SPETZLER RF: Management of posterior fossa ischemia. Rocky Mountain Neurosurgical Society. Colorado Springs, CO, June 6–10, 1984.

SPETZLER RF (visiting professor): Cerebrovascular disease. Lecture, Dent Institute. Buffalo, NY, July 1–9, 1984.

SPETZLER RF: Physiology and therapy of focal ischemia. 4th Annual Clinical Neuroanesthesia Conference. San Diego, CA, August 17–21, 1984.

SPETZLER RF: Case: Occlusive vascular disease (and EEG monitoring). 4th Annual Clinical Neuroanesthesia Conference. San Diego, CA, August 17–21, 1984.

SPETZLER RF: Case: Cerebral aneurysm and subarachnoid hemorrhage. 4th Annual Clinical Neuroanesthesia Conference. San Diego, CA, August 17–21, 1984.

SPETZLER RF, HADLEY MN: Management of posterior fossa cerebral ischemia. 30th Annual Meeting, Western Neurosurgical Society. Colorado Springs, CO, September 9–12, 1984.

SPETZLER RF: The use of regional cerebral blood flow in aneurysm surgery. 34th Annual Meeting, Congress of Neurological Surgeons. New York, September 30–October 5, 1984.

SPETZLER RF: Application of new technology in the treatment of cerebellopontine angle tumors. 34th Annual Meeting, Congress of Neurological Surgeons. New York, September 30–October 5, 1984.

SPETZLER RF: Management of posterior fossa cerebral aneurysms. Congress of Neurological Surgeons—Post Congress Scientific Meeting. Berlin, Germany, October 6–13, 1984.

SPETZLER RF: Transoral odontoid resection. Congress of Neurological Surgeons—Post Congress Scientific Meeting. Berlin, Germany, October 6–13, 1984.

SPETZLER RF, HADLEY MN, MASFERRER R, CARTER LP, *et al.*: Management of vertebrobasilar insufficiency. 7th International Symposium on Microsurgical Anastomoses for Cerebral Ischemia. Phoenix, AZ, October 14–17, 1984.

SPETZLER RF, CARTER LP: Management of unclippable giant aneurysms (poster presentation). 7th International Symposium on Microsurgical Anastomoses for Cerebral Ischemia. Phoenix, AZ, October 14–17, 1984.

SPETZLER RF: Medullary cervical junction—NMR evaluation and comprehensive diagnosis with tomography and metrizamide CT supplementation. 70th Scientific Assembly of the Radiological Society of North America. Washington, DC, November 1984.

SPETZLER RF: Microendarterectomy under barbiturate anesthesia. Symposium on Contemporary Neurosurgery. Amelia Island, FL, November 14–17, 1984.

SPETZLER RF: Surgical management of posterior fossa ischemia. Symposium on Contemporary Neurosurgery. Amelia Island, FL, November 14–17, 1984.

SPETZLER RF: Indications and methods of carotid artery ligation. Symposium on Contemporary Neurosurgery. Amelia Island, FL, November 14–17, 1984.

Presentations for 1983 (19)

SPETZLER RF (visiting professor): Cerebral protection from ischemia, Thomas Jefferson University. Philadelphia, January 6–7, 1983.

SPETZLER RF: Endarterectomy using barbiturate anesthesia, antiplatelet protection and the microscope—A prospective study. 9th Annual Richard Lende Winter Neurosurgery Conference. Salt Lake City, UT, February 1, 1983.

ZABRAMSKI JM, SPETZLER RF, SELMAN WR, HERSHEY LA, ROESSMANN U: Naloxone improved neurologic function during, and outcome after, temporary focal cerebral ischemia. 8th International Joint Conference on Stroke and Cerebral Circulation. San Diego, CA, February 11, 1983.

SPETZLER RF: Surgical management of cerebrovascular disease. Conference on Stroke, St. Joseph's Hospital. Loraine, OH, February 19, 1983.

SPETZLER RF: Reconstructive intracranial surgery. Vascular Conference, Cleveland Clinic Foundation. Cleveland, OH, March 4, 1983.

SPETZLER RF (visiting professor): Barbiturate, protection in the primate. University of Wisconsin at Madison. Madison, WI, March 23–24, 1983.

SPETZLER RF (visiting professor): Cerebrovascular disease. Medical College of Wisconsin. Milwaukee, WI, March 25, 1983.

SPETZLER RF: Current thoughts on cerebral revascularization in strokes. State Medical Society Meeting of Wisconsin. Milwaukee, WI, March 25, 1983.

SPETZLER RF: New ideas in the treatment of subarachnoid hemorrhage. Practical Approaches to Critical Care Neurology and Neurosurgery Symposium. Cleveland, OH, April 15, 1983.

ZABRAMSKI JM, SPETZLER RF, SELMAN WR, HERSHEY LA, ROESSMANN U: Cerebral protection during focal cerebral ischemia: Evaluation of naloxone and barbiturates in a primate model. 1983 Annual Meeting of The American Association of Neurological Surgeons. Washington, DC, April 15, 1983.

SPETZLER RF, ZABRAMSKI JM, SELMAN WR, VANDERVEER C: Evaluation of antiplatelet therapy and barbiturate protection during carotid endarterectomy: A prospective study. 1983 Annual Meeting of The American Association of Neurological Surgeons. Washington, DC, April 15, 1983.

SPETZLER RF: Recent advances in the surgical approach to the stroke prone patient. Medicine, 1983. Cleveland, OH, May 4, 1983.

SPETZLER RF: Surgical management of vascular disease. Booth Memorial Medical Center Seminar in Current Trends in the Management of Cerebrovascular Disease, May 10, 1983.

SPETZLER RF: Influence of naloxone on recovery from cerebral ischemia. Workshop on Reperfusion of Ischaemic Tissues. University of Newcastle upon Tyne, England, May 19, 1983.

BONSTELLE CT, ZABRAMSKI JM, SPETZLER RF: Evaluation of effect of nifedipine upon basilar artery spasms in a canine model. 69th Scientific Assembly of The Radiological Society of North America, 1983.

SPETZLER RF: TAPE: Indication and techniques for revascularizing anterior circulation. **Neurosurg Rev** 1282(1):1983.

SPETZLER RF: TAPE: The stroke prone patient—Recent surgical advances. **Audio-Digest Surg** 30(14):July 27, 1983.

SPETZLER RF (visiting professor): What's new in microvascular neurosurgery. University of Vienna. Vienna, Austria, December 3–12, 1983.

SPETZLER RF: Extracranial-intracranial arterial bypass. Current Perspectives in Cerebrovascular Disease, The Arizona Medical Association. Phoenix, AZ, December 14, 1983.

Presentations for 1982 (27)

SPETZLER RF: Management of giant AVM. 8th Annual Richard Lende Winter Neurosurgery Conference. Snowbird, UT, January 31, 1982.

SPETZLER RF (chairman): Microsurgery of the sellar region study section. Conference on Cerebrovascular Disease and Posterior Fossa Pathology. Vienna, Austria, March 21, 1982.

SPETZLER RF: Intracranial aneurysms: Variations on a theme. Conference on Cerebrovascular Disease and Posterior Fossa Pathology. Vienna, Austria, March 22, 1982.

SPETZLER RF: Giant AVMs with normal perfusion pressure breakthrough. Conference on Cerebrovascular Disease and Posterior Fossa Pathology. Vienna, Austria, March 23, 1982.

SPETZLER RF: Pineal tumors—Supracerebellar approach. Conference on Cerebrovascular Disease and Posterior Fossa Pathology. Vienna, Austria, March 26, 1982.

SPETZLER RF (visiting professor): A third ventricular mass. St. Luke's Hospital, Cleveland, Ohio, April 17, 1982.

SPETZLER RF: Neurosurgery update: Aneurysms. American Academy of Neurology, Washington, DC, April 25, 1982.

ROSKI RA, SPETZLER RF: Middle cerebral artery perfusion pressure in occlusive cerebrovascular disease. Annual Meeting of the American Association of Neurological Surgeons. Honolulu, HI, April 26, 1982.

SPETZLER RF (panelist): Management of carotid aneurysms. Annual Meeting of the American Association of Neurological Surgeons. Honolulu, HI, April 19, 1982.

SPETZLER RF (panelist): Management of giant and complex aneurysms. Annual Meeting of the American Association of Neurological Surgeons, Honolulu, HI, April 29, 1982.

SPETZLER RF: The protection from cerebral ischemia by pharmacologic agents. Ohio State Neurosurgical Society Meeting, May 4, 1982.

SPETZLER RF: Indications and techniques for revascularizing anterior circulation. 12th Annual Neurosurgery Postgraduate Course, University of California. San Francisco, June 4, 1982.

SPETZLER RF: Cerebral protection. 12th Annual Neurosurgery Postgraduate Course, University of California. San Francisco, June 4, 1982.

SPETZLER RF: Management of normal perfusion pressure breakthrough in giant AVMs. 12th Annual Neurosurgery Postgraduate Course, University of California. San Francisco, June 4, 1982.

SPETZLER RF, HYDE-ROWAN D, ROSKI RA, *et al.*: Cerebral venous vascular reconstruction surgery. 6th International Symposium on Microsurgical Anastomoses for Cerebral Ischemia. Kyoto, Japan, September 13, 1982.

SPETZLER RF, ZABRAMSKI JM, KAUFMAN B, *et al.*: Acute NMR changes in primates following MCA occlusion. 6th International Symposium on Microsurgical Anastomoses for Cerebral Ischemia. Kyoto, Japan, September 15, 1982.

SPETZLER RF: Cerebrospinal fluid rhinorrhea/otorrhea. 32nd Annual Meeting, Congress of Neurological Surgeons. Toronto, Ontario, Canada, October 5, 1982.

SPETZLER RF, ZABRAMSKI JM, KAUFMAN B, YEUNG HN: NMR changes in primate cerebral focal ischemia. 32nd Annual Meeting, Congress of Neurological Surgeons. Toronto. Ontario, Canada, October 7, 1982.

SPETZLER RF, SELMAN WR, ZABRAMSKI JM: Management of the "normal perfusion pressure breakthrough phenomenon" in giant AVMs. 32nd Annual Meeting, Congress of Neurological Surgeons. Toronto, Ontario, Canada, October 7, 1982.

KAUFMAN B, HOPKINS A, SPETZLER RF, YEUNG HN, KRAMER D, HINSHAW W, BRATTON C, BONSTELLE C: NMR imaging of mesencephalic hind brain in cerebellar anatomy: Normal and abnormal. 12th Symposium Neuroradiologicum. Washington, DC, October 10–16, 1982.

SPETZLER RF, KAUFMAN B, ZABRAMSKI JM, YEUNG HN, KRAMER D, CRUMRINE RC, HINSHAW W, ALFIDI R: NMR demonstration of acute brain infarcts in primates following middle cerebral artery occlusion. 12th Symposium Neuroradiologicum. Washington, DC, October 10–16, 1982.

KAUFMAN B, MIRALDI F, SPETZLER RF, YEUNG HN, KRAMER H, HIN-

SHAW W, BONSTELLE C, ALFIDI R: Movement of paramagnetic field. 12th Symposium Neuroradiologicum. Washington, DC, October 10–16, 1982.

KAUFMAN B, HOPKINS A, SPETZLER RF, YEUNG HN, HINSHAW W, BONSTELLE C, BRATTON C, RATCHESON RA: 3-D NMR imaging of posterior fossa in medullary-cervical junction abnormalities. RSNA. Chicago, November 1982.

SPETZLER RF: Giant aneurysms. Symposium on Contemporary Neurosurgery. Boca Baton, FL, November 18, 1982.

SPETZLER RF: Transoral odontoid resection. Symposium on Contemporary Neurosurgery. Boca Baton, FL, November 19, 1982.

SPETZLER RF: Large AVM with perfusion pressure breakthrough. Symposium on Contemporary Neurosurgery. Boca Baton, FL, November 19, 1982.

SPETZLER RF: Large graft bypass. Symposium on Contemporary Neurosurgery. Boca Baton, FL, November 20, 1982.

Presentations for 1981 (27)

SPETZLER RF: Barbiturate protection in primates and man. 7th Annual Richard Lende Winter Neurosurgery Conference. Snowbird, UT, February 4, 1981.

RHODES RS, SPETZLER RF, ROSKI RA: Improved neurologic function post CVA with extracranial-intracranial arterial bypass. 42nd Annual Meeting of the Society of University Surgeons. Hershey, PA, February 12–14, 1981.

SPETZLER RF, ROSKI RA: A combination of STA-MCA bypass and staged internal carotid artery occlusion for the treatment of giant internal carotid artery aneurysms. 6th International Joint Conference on Stroke and Cerebral Circulation. Los Angeles, February 13, 1981.

ROSKI RA, SPETZLER RF, NULSEN FE: Comparison of late complications for internal carotid *versus* common carotid artery ligation. 6th International Joint Conference on Stroke and Cerebral Circulation. Los Angeles, February 13, 1981.

SELMAN WR, ROSKI RA: Barbiturate coma: Relation of protection to timing of therapy and duration of occlusion. 6th International Joint Conference on Stroke and Cerebral Circulation. Los Angeles, February 14, 1981.

SPETZLER RF: Management of cerebral ischemia. Neurosurgery Grand Rounds, Cleveland Clinic. Cleveland, OH, March 11, 1981.

SPETZLER RF: Variations of the EC-IC (anterior and posterior circulations). Central Neurosurgical Society Meeting. Chicago, March 21, 1981.

SPETZLER RF: Extra-intracranial bypass. "Cardiology 1981," Western Pennsylvania Hospital. Pittsburgh, March 22, 1981.

SPETZLER RF: Thoughts on cerebral ischemia. Columbia University College of Physicians and Surgeons. New York, April 2, 1981.

MATJASKO J, WURM H, SPETZLER RF, FERGUSON G (panelists): Intraoperative monitoring. American Association of Neurological Surgeons Meeting. Boston, April 7, 1981.

SPETZLER RF (discussant): Holographic reconstruction of neuroradiogram. American Association of Neurological Surgeons Meeting. Boston, April 9, 1981.

SPETZLER RF: Barbiturate, induced coma for focal cerebral ischemia in primates. 17th Annual Meeting, Society of University Neurosurgeons. London, Ontario, Canada, May 8, 1981.

SPETZLER RF: Indications and technique for transoral approach to C1-2. American Academy of Orthopaedic Surgeons, Treatment of Adult Spinal Disorders. Cleveland, OH, May 12, 1981.

SPETZLER RF: Indications for posterior *vs.* anterior approach to the cervical disc. American Academy of Orthopaedic Surgeons, Treatment of Adult Spinal Disorders. Cleveland, OH, May 12, 1981.

SPETZLER RF: Regional cerebral blood flow following middle cerebral artery occlusion and barbiturate therapy in baboons. 10th International Symposium on Cerebral Blood Flow and Metabolism. St. Louis, MO, June 22, 1981.

SPETZLER RF, SELMAN WR, REDFORD J, ROSKI RA, DABB B, ANTON A, CASCORBI H: Intraoperative barbiturate protection during temporary vessel occlusion in man. International Symposium on Cerebrovascular Diseases: New Trends in Surgical and Medical Aspects. Garda Lake, Italy, July 3, 1981.

SPETZLER RF: Treatment of communicating hydrocephalus. Symposium of Hydrocephalus. Munich, Germany, July 12, 1981.

SPETZLER RF, RHODES RS, ROSKI RA: High flow extracranial to intracranial bypass. 7th International Congress of Neurological Surgery. Munich, Germany, July 16, 1981.

SELMAN WR, SPETZLER RF, ROSKI RA: Therapeutic barbiturate-induced coma for focal cerebral ischemia: Relation of response to timing of therapy and duration of occlusion. 7th International Congress of Neurological Surgery. Munich, Germany, July 17, 1981.

SPETZLER RF (visiting professor): Pharmacologic protection for cerebral ischemia. Dent Neurologic Institute of Millard Fillmore Hospital. Buffalo, NY, August 7, 1981.

SPETZLER RF: Cerebral protection during ischemia. University of New York. Buffalo, NY, August 14, 1981.

SPETZLER RF: Subarachnoid hemorrhage. Lakewood Hospital. Lakewood, OH, September 30, 1981.

SPETZLER RF: Variations on a theme. American College of Surgeons. San Francisco, October 16, 1981.

SPETZLER RF, ZABRAMSKI JM: Revascularization of anterior and posterior circulation ischemia. Congress of Neurological Surgeons. Los Angeles, October 21, 1981.

SELMAN WR, ROSKI RA, SPETZLER RF, CRUMRINE RC, JACKSON D: Cerebral blood flow during MCA occlusion and barbiturate coma in primates: Analysis of radiolabeled microspheres. Congress of Neurological Surgeons. Los Angeles, October 22, 1981.

KAUFMAN B, ROESSMANN U, SPETZLER RF: Transforaminal cerebellar ectopia. Radiological Society of North America. Chicago, November 16, 1981.

KAUFMAN B, ROESSMANN U, SPETZLER RF: Classification of craniovertebral junction abnormalities. Radiological Society of North America. Chicago, November 16, 1981.

Presentations for 1980 (43)

SPETZLER RF: Techniques of lumboperitoneal shunting. Heyer-Schulte meeting, LaCosta Hotel & Spa, Rancho LaCosta. Carlsbad, CA, January, 1980.

SPETZLER RF: Extracranial-intracranial arterial anastomosis in the treatment of giant aneurysms. 6th Annual Richard Lende Winter Neurosurgery Conference. Snowbird, UT, February 2–7,1980.

SPETZLER RF: What's new in the treatment of stroke. Lutheran Medical Center Seminar. Cleveland, OH, March 12, 1980.

SPETZLER RF: Posterior fossa vascular compression syndromes. American Association of Neurosurgical Nurses of Northeast Ohio. Cleveland, OH, March 13, 1980.

ROSKI RA, SPETZLER RF, NULSEN FE: Late ischemic complications of carotid ligation in the treatment of intracranial aneurysms. American Association of Neurological Surgeons Annual Meeting. New York, April 21, 1980.

SPETZLER RF, SCHUSTER H, ROSKI RA: EIAB in the treatment of giant ICA aneurysms. American Association of Neurological Surgeons Annual Meeting. New York, April 21, 1980.

SELMAN WR, SPETZLER RF: Therapeutic management of prolonged barbiturate coma. American Association of Neurological Surgeons Annual Meeting. New York, April 23, 1980.

YAMADA S, ZINKE DE (SPETZLER RF: discussant): Surgical treatment of arteriovenous malformations (AVMs) in the functional areas: Correlation with CBF. American Association of Neurological Surgeons Annual Meeting. New York, April 23, 1980.

KRICHEFF I, SPETZLER RF, CLARK WK, SUGAR O (panelists): CT scan diagnosis in neurosurgery. American Association of Neurological Surgeons Annual Meeting. New York, April 24, 1980.

SELMAN WR, SPETZLER RF: Barbiturate control of ischemic edema: Comparison of effect on permanent and temporary middle cerebral artery occlusion in baboons. Ohio State Medical Association Annual Meeting. Cincinnati, OH, May 13, 1980

SELMAN WR, SPETZLER RF: Therapeutic barbiturate induced coma for control of ICP after middle cerebral artery occlusion: Relation to duration of occlusion (First Prize). 5th Annual Neuroscience Residents' Day, Rainbow Babies and Children's Amphitheater. Cleveland, OH, May 15, 1980.

SELMAN WR, SPETZLER RF: Therapeutic barbiturate induced coma for focal cerebral ischemia: Relationship of protection to timing of therapy. 5th Annual Neuroscience Residents' Day, Rainbow Babies and Children's Amphitheater. Cleveland, OH, May 15, 1980.

SPETZLER RF: Long-term effects of carotid artery ligation. Aneurysm Patient Seminar. Niagara Falls, NY, June 12, 1980.

SPETZLER RF: Intracranial pressure and subarachnoid hemorrhage: Implications, monitoring, and control. Aneurysm Patient Seminar. Niagara Falls, NY, June 13, 1980.

SPETZLER RF: Barbiturate coma. Aneurysm Patient Seminar. Niagara Falls, NY, June 13, 1980.

SPETZLER RF: Normal perfusion pressure breakthrough theory in clinical practice. Aneurysm Patient Seminar. Niagara Falls, NY, June 13, 1980.

SPETZLER RF: EC-IC and ligation-cerebral perfusion. Aneurysm Patient Seminar. Niagara Falls, NY, June 14, 1980.

SPETZLER RF: Bypass surgery and carotid ligation for aneurysms. Panel discussion: The role of cerebral bypass in the treatment of aneurysms. Aneurysm Patient Seminar. Niagara Falls, NY, June 14, 1980.

SPETZLER RF: Transoral odontoid removal. Philippine General Hospital, Sino-American Neurosurgery Study Tour, June 23, 1980.

SPETZLER RF: Extracranial-intracranial aneurysm. Philippine General Hospital, Sino-American Neurosurgery Study Tour, June 23, 1980.

SPETZLER RF: Cerebrovascular disease. Peking, Sino-American Neurosurgery Study Tour, June 26, 1980.

SPETZLER RF: Normal perfusion pressure theory. Peking, Sino-American Neurosurgery Study Tour, June 26, 1980.

SPETZLER RF: Barbiturates for clinical use. Beidahai, Sino-American Neurosurgery Study Tour, June 28, 1980.

SPETZLER RF: Microsurgery for aneurysms. Tiaryin, Sino-American Neurosurgery Study Tour, June 30, 1980.

SPETZLER RF: Extracranial-intracranial bypass. Tiaryin, Sino-American Neurosurgery Study Tour, June 30, 1980.

SPETZLER RF: Variation on a theme. Shanghai, People's Republic of China, Sino-American Neurosurgery Study Tour, July 2, 1980.

SPETZLER RF: Variation of Extracranial-intracranial bypass. Shanghai, People's Republic of China, Sino-American Neurosurgery Study Tour, July 2, 1980.

SPETZLER RF: Embolization and surgery for large AVMs. Shanghai, People's Republic of China, Sino-American Neurosurgery Study Tour, July 3, 1980.

SPETZLER RF: CSF leaks. Hong Kong, Sino-American Neurosurgery Study Tour, July 7, 1980.

SPETZLER RF: Revascularization for aneurysms. Hong Kong, Sino-American Neurosurgery Study Tour, July 8, 1980.

SPETZLER RF: Surgical approaches to improving cerebral perfusion. Current Concepts of Medical-Surgical Management of Cerebral Vascular Disease Conference, Lakewood Hospital. Lakewood, OH, September 10, 1980.

SPETZLER RF, ROSKI RA: Middle cerebral artery perfusion pressure in cerebral ischemia. 5th International Symposium on Microvascular Anastomoses for Cerebral Ischemia. Vienna, Austria, September 15, 1980.

SPETZLER RF, SELMAN WR: Barbiturate control of ischemic intracranial pressure. 5th International Symposium on Microvascular Anastomoses for Cerebral Ischemia. Vienna, Austria, September 15, 1980.

SPETZLER RF, ROSKI RA, SELMAN WR: Variations on a theme. 5th International Symposium on Microvascular Anastomoses for Cerebral Ischemia. Vienna, Austria, September 15, 1980.

SPETZLER RF, SCHUSTER H, ROSKI RA: EIAB in the treatment of giant ICA aneurysms. 5th International Symposium on Microvascular Anastomoses for Cerebral Ischemia. Vienna, Austria, September 16, 1980.

ROSKI RA, SPETZLER RF: Late complications of carotid ligation in the treatment of intracranial aneurysms. 5th International Symposium on Microvascular Anastomoses for Cerebral Ischemia. Vienna, Austria, September 16, 1980.

SPETZLER RF, KOPANIKY D, CUANTE S, MODIC M, ROSKI RA, BONS-TELLE C: By-pass surgery—Variations on a theme. Exhibit, 30th Annual Meeting, Congress of Neurological Surgeons. Houston, TX, October 5–10, 1980.

SPETZLER RF: Identification and management of CSF fistulae. 30th Annual Meeting, Congress of Neurological Surgeons. Houston, TX, October 9, 1980.

SELMAN WR, SPETZLER RF: Therapeutic barbiturate induced coma for focal cerebral ischemia: Relation of response to timing of therapy and duration of occlusion. 30th Annual Meeting, Congress of Neurological Surgeons. Houston, TX, October 9, 1980.

SPETZLER RF: The microscope in cervical disc excision. American Academy of Orthopaedic Surgeons, The Spine—Surgery and Rehabilitation Meeting. Kissimmee, FL, December 1, 1980.

SPETZLER RF: Surgical technique of excision of the odontoid. American Academy of Orthopaedic Surgeons, The Spine—Surgery and Rehabilitation Meeting. Kissimmee, FL, December 4, 1980.

KAUFMAN B, BOHLMAN HH, SPETZLER RF: Craniovertebral junction evaluation with metrizamide, metrizamide plus tomography, and computerized tomography with sagittal reconstruction. 8th Annual Meeting Cervical Spine Research Society. Palm Beach, FL, December 11, 1980.

SPETZLER RF, ROSKI RA, KAUFMAN B: Microsurgical approach to the anterior cervical spine. 8th Annual Meeting Cervical Spine Research Society. Palm Beach, FL, December 11, 1980.

Presentations for 1979 (25)

SPETZLER RF: Normal perfusion pressure breakthrough theory in large AVMs. 5th Annual Richard Lende Winter Neurosurgery Conference, sponsored by the University of Utah. Salt Lake City, February, 10–15, 1979.

SELMAN WR, SPETZLER RF: Transoral microsurgical odontoid resection and spinal cord monitoring. 5th Annual Richard Lende Winter Neurosurgery Conference, sponsored by the University of Utah. Salt Lake City, February 10–15, 1979.

SPETZLER RF: Neurosurgical management of stroke. Cleveland Clinic (co-sponsored with the American Association of Neurosurgical Nurses of Northeast Ohio), Changing Concepts in Neurosurgical Nursing. Cleveland, Ohio, March 9, 1979.

SPETZLER RF: Neurosurgical management of stroke. Cleveland Clinic (co-sponsored with the American Association of Neurosurgical

Nurses of Northeast Ohio), Changing Concepts in Neurosurgical Nursing. Cleveland, OH, March 9–10, 1979.

SPETZLER RF: Microsurgical treatment of arteriovenous malformation. Cleveland Clinic (co-sponsored with the American Association of Neurosurgical Nurses of Northeast Ohio), Changing Concepts in Neurosurgical Nursing. Cleveland, Ohio, March 9–10, 1979.

SELMAN WR, SPETZLER RF: Simplified shunting therapy for communicating hydrocephalus. **First Place,** Annual Resident Essay Contest. Northeast Ohio Neurosurgical Society Meeting. Cleveland, OH, March 15, 1979.

SPETZLER RF: Microsurgical technique for removal of osteophytes from the cervical spinal canal. Surgery of the Spine Indications and Techniques (course designed by Department of Orthopaedics and Rehabilitation of the University of Miami School of Medicine), Americana Hotel. Miami Beach, FL, April 5, 1979.

SPETZLER RF: CSF leaks. American Association of Neurological Surgeons Scientific Program Committee Breakfast Seminar, Annual Meeting, Century Plaza Hotel. Los Angeles, April 24, 1979.

SPETZLER RF, SPETZLER H, NULSEN FE: Holography in neurosurgery. American Association of Neurological Surgeons Annual Meeting General Scientific Session, Century Plaza Hotel. Los Angeles, April 24, 1979.

SELMAN WR, SPETZLER RF, WILSON CB, GROLLMUS JS: Percutaneous lumboperitoneal shunt: Review of 130 cases. American Association of Neurological Surgeons Annual Meeting General Scientific Session, Century Plaza Hotel. Los Angeles, April 26, 1979.

SELMAN WR, SPETZLER RF, CASCORBI HF, NULSEN FE, BRODKEY JS, CRUMRINE RC: Rational management of barbiturate induced coma. Annual Meeting of the Ohio State Neurological Surgeons Meeting. Columbus, OH, May 15, 1979.

SPETZLER RF: Microsurgical application of cerebrovascular disease. Fairview General Hospital. Cleveland, OH, May 19, 1979.

KAUFMAN B, ROESSMANN U, SPETZLER RF, NULSEN FE, BONSTELLE C: Trans-foraminal cerebellar ectopia. 17th Annual Meeting, American Society of Neuroradiology. Toronto, Ontario, Canada, May 20–24, 1979.

SPETZLER RF, RHODES RS, LIKAVEC M, ROSKI R: Subclavian artery-Middle cerebral artery-Saphenous bypass and variations on this theme. 4th Annual Meeting of the Cleveland Vascular Society, May 9, 1979.

SPETZLER RF: Recent advances in occlusive cerebral ischemia. NEONS, May 18, 1979.

SELMAN WR (speaker), SPETZLER RF: Neurophysiological monitoring of barbiturate coma. 9th International Symposium on Cerebral Blood Flow and Metabolism. Tokyo, June 5, 1979.

SPETZLER RF (moderator): Management of shunt complications. 29th Annual Meeting for Congress of Neurological Surgeons Meeting. Las Vegas, October 7–12, 1979.

SPETZLER RF, RHODES RS, LIKAVEC M, ROSKI R: Subclavian artery-middle cerebral artery saphenous vein bypass. 29th Annual Meeting of Congress of Neurological Surgeons. Los Vegas, October 7–12, 1979.

SPETZLER RF, SELMAN WR, BRODKEY JS, NULSEN FE, LORIG RJ, GOOD W: Visual evoked potentials during deep barbiturate therapy. 29th Annual Meeting of Congress of Neurological Surgeons. Las Vegas, October 7–12, 1979.

SELMAN WR, SPETZLER RF (presenter): Correlation between CO_2 and ICP with response to therapeutics. Society of Neurosurgical Anesthesia and Neurologic Supportive Care. San Francisco, October 19, 1979.

SPETZLER RF: Microsurgical application to cerebrovascular disease. Lutheran Medical Center. Cleveland, OH, Surgical Grand Rounds, October 25, 1979.

SPETZLER RF: Role of extracranial-intracranial anastomosis. Northeast Ohio Neurosurgery Society. Cleveland, OH, November 2, 1979.

SPETZLER RF, SELMAN WR, BONSTELLE C: Neuroradiologic assessment in a new model for chronic reversible ischemia in baboons. Scientific Sessions of the Society for Computerized Tomography and Neuro-Imaging (SCTNI), Ponte Vedra Club. Ponte Vedra Beach, FL, November 5, 1979.

SPETZLER RF, SCHUSTER H, NULSEN FE: Elective extracranial-intracranial arterial bypass in the treatment of giant aneurysms. Annual Meeting of American Academy of Neurological Surgery. Memphis, TN, November 7–10, 1979.

KAUFMAN B, ROESSMANN U, SPETZLER RF, NULSEN FE, BONSTELLE C: Trans-foraminal cerebellar ectopia. Cervical Spine Research Society. Cambridge, MA, December 8, 1979.

Presentations for 1978 (21)

SPETZLER RF: IC/EC bypass. Northeast Ohio Vascular Society-Rainbow Babies and Children's Amphitheater. Cleveland, OH, January 24, 1978.

OWEN M, SPETZLER RF: Blue nevus syndrome. 6th Annual Interim

Meeting, Pediatric Section of American Association of Neurological Surgeons. Cleveland, OH, February 2–4, 1978.

SPETZLER RF: Cauda equina electrical monitoring. 6th Annual Interim Meeting, Pediatric Section of American Association of Neurological Surgeons. Cleveland, OH, February 2–4, 1978.

SPETZLER RF (program coordinator): Lesions of sella and parasellar area and cerebral vascular disease, Winter Seminar. Davos, Switzerland/St. Anton, Austria, February 10–25, 1978.

SPETZLER RF: Surgical anatomy of the sellar region. Winter Seminar. Davos, Switzerland, February 12, 1978.

SPETZLER RF: Review of the surgical merit of the frontal approach of sella and parasellar area. Winter seminar. Davos, Switzerland, February 14, 1978.

DEROME P, SPETZLER RF: Hypersecreting pituitary adenomas. Winter Seminar. Davos, Switzerland, February 15, 1978.

SPETZLER RF: Pathophysiology of cerebral infarction. Winter Seminar. St. Anton, Austria, February 19, 1978.

SPETZLER RF: Anatomical-physiological consideration of extracranial to intracranial arterial bypass. Winter seminar. St. Anton, Austria, February 20, 1978.

KOOS W, SPETZLER RF: Technique of cerebral revascularization surgery. Winter Seminar. Davos/St. Anton, Austria, February 20, 1978.

SPETZLER RF: Special problems associated with subarachnoid hemorrhage. Winter seminar. Davos/St. Anton, Austria, February 22, 1978.

SPETZLER RF: Spinal cord injury—acute care-medical/surgical management. American Association of Neurosurgical Nurses of Northeast Ohio. Cleveland, OH, March 21, 1978.

SPETZLER RF: Spinal cord injury—acute care-medical/surgical management. Physicians' Radio Station. Cleveland, OH, March 21, 1978.

SPETZLER RF, WEINSTEIN P, MEHDORN M: New model for chronic reversible cerebral ischemia. Annual Meeting American Association of Neurological Surgeons. New Orleans, April 24, 1978.

SPETZLER RF: Experimental cerebral blood flow studies. Clinical Neurosciences Didactic Lecture Series, Cleveland Clinic. Cleveland, OH, May 6, 1978.

SPETZLER RF, WEINSTEIN PR, SELMAN WR: Reversible cerebral ischemia. 4th International Symposium on Microsurgical Anastomoses for Cerebral Ischemia, The University of Western Ontario. London, Ontario, Canada, September 6, 1978.

WEINSTEIN PR, MEHDORN HM, SPETZLER RF: Arterial dilatation and augmentation of blood flow in experimental arteriovenous fistulae. 4th International Symposium on Microsurgical Anastomoses for Cerebral Ischemia, The University of Western Ontario. London, Ontario, Canada, September 7, 1978.

SPETZLER RF (moderator), APFELBAUM RI (speaker): Television, movie, and still photography through the operating microscope. 28th Annual Meeting, Congress of Neurological Surgeons. Washington, DC, September 28, 1978.

WILSON CB, SPETZLER RF: Operative approaches to aneurysms. 28th Annual Meeting, Congress of Neurological Surgeons. Washington, DC, September 28–29, 1978.

SPETZLER RF: Cerebral revascularization. Lakewood Hospital. Lakewood, OH, October 11, 1978.

SPETZLER RF, SELMAN W, BROWN RH: Transoral cervical odontoid decompression and spinal cord monitoring. 6th Annual Meeting Cervical Spine Research Society. Baltimore, November 30–December 2, 1978.

Presentations for 1977 (8)

SPETZLER RF: Percutaneous shunting techniques. San Francisco Neurological Society. Oak Knoll, CA, January 19, 1977.

SPETZLER RF: Ondine's curse. Sierra Neurosurgical Society. February 18–21, 1977.

SPETZLER RF: Lumbo-peritoneal shunting in the diagnosis and treatment of normal pressure hydrocephalus. Federation of Western Societies of Neurological Science. Mazatlan, Mexico, February 24–27, 1977.

WILSON CB, U HOI SANG, SPETZLER RF (presenter): Microsurgical treatment of intracranial vascular malformation. American Association of Neurological Surgeons, Sheraton Centre. Toronto, Ontario, Canada, April 24–28, 1977.

SPETZLER RF (discussant): (a) Genetic control of brain tumor growth. C. Albright and T. Gill (b) Evaluation of glucose metabolism in experimental cerebral neoplasm with 2-deoxy-D-glucose, radioautography. Alteman L, Kindt G, McGauley J. American Association of Neurological Surgeons, Sheraton Centre. Toronto, Ontario, Canada, April 24–28, 1977.

WILSON CB, SPETZLER RF: Results of 250 transsphenoidal operations for pituitary tumors. San Francisco Neurological Society, Silverado Lodge. Napa, CA, May 21–22, 1977.

HOFF JT, PITTS LH, SPETZLER RF, WILSON CB: Barbiturates for protection from cerebral ischemia in aneurysm surgery. 8th International Symposium on Cerebral Function, Metabolism, and Circulation, Lasses N (ed). Copenhagen, June, 1977.

SPETZLER RF, WEINSTEIN PR: Alterations in blood flow through an experimental cerebral arteriovenous fistula. 27th Annual Meeting, Congress of Neurological Surgeons, Inc., San Francisco Hilton. San Francisco, October 9–14, 1977 (Annual Resident Award, October 13, 1977).

Presentations for 1976 (5)

SPETZLER RF: Regional cerebral blood flow before and after cerebral revascularization. Microneurosurgery Course, VA Hospital. San Francisco, March 1–5, 1976.

SPETZLER RF: Percutaneous lumbo-peritoneal shunting. 6th Annual Neurosurgery Postgraduate Course. San Francisco, May 20–27, 1976.

SPETZLER RF, WILSON CB: Management of recurrent CSF rhinorrhea. 6th Annual Neurosurgery Postgraduate Course. San Francisco, May 20–27, 1976.

SPETZLER RF, WING SD, NORMAN D: Evaluation of patients with cerebral ischemia using computerized tomography. 3rd International Symposium on Microneurosurgical Anastomoses for Cerebral Ischemia. Rottach-Egern, West Germany, June 28–30, 1976.

SPETZLER RF: Closing comments. 3rd International Symposium on Microneurosurgical Anastomoses for Cerebral Ischemia. Rottach-Egern, West Germany, June 28–30, 1976.

Presentations for 1975 (2)

SPETZLER RF: A shunt for the diagnosis of normal pressure hydrocephalus. Televised Neurology Grand Rounds, University of California. San Francisco, June, 1975.

SPETZLER RF, WILSON CB: A new approach to the diagnosis of normal pressure hydrocephalus. Congress of Neurological Surgeons. Atlanta, October, 1975.

Presentations for 1974 (1)

SPETZLER RF, CHATER NL: Blood flow measurements of superficial temporal artery-middle cerebral artery bypass procedure. Cushing Meeting, April, 1974.

Presentations for 1973 (3)

SPETZLER RF, CHATER NL: Middle cerebral artery anatomical studies. International Symposium on Neurosurgery through the Microscope,

Mt. Sinai School of Medicine, City University of New York. New York, June 12, 1973.

CHATER NL, SPETZLER RF: Alternative blood supply for cerebral microvascular bypass. International Symposium on Neurosurgery through the Microscope, Mt. Sinai School of Medicine, City University of New York. New York, June 12, 1973.

CHATER NL, SPETZLER RF: Anatomical studies of cerebral cortical vasculature of microvascular surgical significance. International Congress of Neurosurgery Symposium on Microneurosurgery. Kyoto, Japan, October 1973.

Contents

Preface v
Honored Guests ix
Officers of the Congress of Neurological Surgeons xi
Contributors xiii
Biography of Robert F. Spetzler, M.D. xvii
Bibliography of Robert F. Spetzler, M.D. xix

CHAPTER 1

The Winds of Change

Richard A. Roski, M.D., F.A.C.S. 1

———————————— I ————————————

GENERAL SCIENTIFIC SESSION I
EMERGING HEALTH CARE REFORM

CHAPTER 2

The Politics of Health Care Reform

Henry Desmarais, M.D., M.P.A. 15

CHAPTER 3

Medicine in Transition: Strategies for Change

David E. Vogel, M.S. 23

CHAPTER 4

Health Reform: Past, Present, and Future

Helen L. Smits 30

CHAPTER 5

Uniting Surgeons in Response to Healthcare Reform

Paul A. Ebert, M.D., F.A.C.S. 37

———————————— II ————————————

GENERAL SCIENTIFIC SESSION II
CONTROVERSIES IN SKULL BASE SURGERY

CHAPTER 6

Radical Resection of Anterior Skull Base Tumors *(Honored Guest Lecture)*

Michael T. Lawton, M.D., Mark G. Hamilton, M.D.C.M.,
  Stephen P. Beals, M.D., Edward F. Joganic, M.D., and
  Robert F. Spetzler, M.D. 43

CHAPTER 7

Management of Anterior Cranial Base and Cavernous Sinus
  Neoplasms with Conservative Surgery Alone or in Combination
  with Fractionated Photon or Stereotactic Proton Radiotherapy

Robert G. Ojemann, M.D., Allan F. Thornton, M.D., and
  Griffith R. Harsh IV, M.D. 71

CHAPTER 8
Stereotactic Radiosurgery of Anterior Skull Base Tumors
L. Dade Lunsford, M.D., Thomas C. Witt, M.D.,
    Douglas Kondziolka, M.D., M.Sc., FRCS(C), and
    John C. Flickinger, M.D. 99
CHAPTER 9
Techniques of Carotid Reconstruction
Takanori Fukushima, M.D., D.M.Sc. 119
CHAPTER 10
Is Carotid Artery Reconstruction Mandatory?
Chandranath Sen, M.D., and David Segal, M.D. 135
CHAPTER 11
The Cavernous Carotid Artery: Preservation is the Best
    Means of Reconstruction
Alfred P. Bowles, Jr., M.D., and Ossama Al-Mefty, M.D. 154
CHAPTER 12
Intra-operative Neurophysiologic Monitoring in Neurosurgery:
    Benefits, Efficacy, and Cost-Effectiveness
Aage R. Møller, Ph.D. 171
CHAPTER 13
Neurophysiologic Monitoring during Cranial Base Surgery:
    Is it Necessary?
Laligam N. Sekhar, M.D., F.A.C.S., Ghassan Bejjani, M.D.,
    Peter Nora, M.D., and Pedro L. Vera, Ph.D. 180
CHAPTER 14
Intra-operative Monitoring is Not Essential
Leonard I. Malis, M.D., F.A.C.S. 203

———————————————III———————————————

GENERAL SCIENTIFIC SESSION III
CONTROVERSIES IN THE MANAGEMENT OF
CEREBROVASCULAR MALFORMATIONS

CHAPTER 15
Natural History of Giant Intracranial Aneurysms
    and Indications for Intervention
Daniel L. Barrow, M.D., and Cargill Alleyne, M.D. 214
CHAPTER 16
Surgical Management of Giant Intracranial Aneurysms:
    Experience with 171 Patients *(Honored Guest Lecture)*
Michael T. Lawton, M.D., and Robert F. Spetzler, M.D. 245
CHAPTER 17
Endovascular Management of Giant Intracranial Aneurysms
Scott C. Standard, M.D., Lee R. Guterman, Ph.D., M.D.,
    Tamerla D. Chavis, M.D., Mary Duffy Fronckowiak, Ph.D.,
    Kevin J. Gibbons, M.D., and L. Nelson Hopkins, M.D. 267

CHAPTER 18
Therapy of AVM's: A Decision Analysis
Wink S. Fisher III, M.D. 294
CHAPTER 19
Role of Embolization in the Management of
    Arteriovenous Malformations
Takashi Yoshimoto, M.D., Akira Takahashi, M.D.,
    Hiroyuki Kinouchi, M.D., Ph.D., Kazuo Mizoi, M.D., and
    Hidefumi Jokura,M.D. 313
CHAPTER 20
Radiosurgery for Arteriovenous Malformations
William A. Friedman, M.D. 328
CHAPTER 21
Surgical Treatment of Intracranial Arteriovenous Malformations
    with an Analysis of Cost-Effectiveness
Eric S. Nussbaum, M.D., Roberto C. Heros, M.D., and
    Paul J. Camarata, M.D. 348

IV

GENERAL SCIENTIFIC SESSION IV
MANAGEMENT OF LOW GRADE GLIOMAS

CHAPTER 22
Brain Tumor Gene Therapy in Mice with a Novel "Suicide" Gene:
    The Cyclophosphamide-activating CYP2B1 Gene
E. Antonio Chiocca, M.D., Ph.D. 370
CHAPTER 23
Surgery for Low-Grade Glioma: Rationale for Early Intervention
Charles B. Wilson, M.D., and Michael D. Prados, M.D. 383
CHAPTER 24
Low-Grade Glioma: The Case for Delayed Surgery
J. Gregory Cairncross, M.D. 391
CHAPTER 25
Surgical Issues in the Management of Supratentorial
    Low-Grade Gliomas
Patrick J. Kelly, M.D., F.A.C.S. 399
CHAPTER 26
Functional Mapping-guided Resection of Low-Grade Gliomas
Mitchel S. Berger, M.D., F.A.C.S. 437
CHAPTER 27
Management of Low-Grade Gliomas: Results of Resections
without Electrocorticography
Itzhak Fried, M.D., Ph.D. 453

CHAPTER 28
Brain Astrocytomas: Biopsy, Then Irradiation
L. Dade Lunsford, M.D., F.A.C.S., Salvador Somaza, M.D.,
   Douglas Kondziolka, M.D., M.Sc., F.R.C.S.(C), and
   John C. Flickinger, M.D. 464

CHAPTER 29
Radical Resection for the Treatment of Glioma
Edward R. Laws, Jr., M.D., F.A.C.S. 480

CHAPTER 30
The Low-Grade Glioma Debate: Evidence Defending
   the Position of Early Radiation Therapy
Edward G. Shaw, M.D. 488

CHAPTER 31
Management of Low-Grade Gliomas: Radiation Therapy
   at Time of Recurrence
Joseph M. Piepmeier, M.D., F.A.C.S., and Murat Gunel, M.D. . . 495

———————————————— V ————————————————

SESSION V

CHAPTER 32
Interactive Audience Participation
Mark N. Hadley, M.D. 508

1

The Winds of Change

RICHARD A. ROSKI, M.D., F.A.C.S.

When Hunt Batjer and I first sat down with the Annual Meeting Committee more than a year ago, he suggested that the theme for this year's meeting should be "the winds of change." With Chicago known as the "Windy City," and with neurosurgery facing a turbulent and rapidly changing health care environment, "the winds of change" seem to appropriately describe both the situation and location in which neurosurgery finds itself today. It is this turbulent and changing health care environment that I would like to address today. To do so, I will first review how American medicine arrived at these unsettled times, and then I will evaluate two major issues that confront us today—managed care and health care reform. Finally, I will explain what neurosurgery has done and what it must do to survive in these difficult times.

FINANCIAL EVOLUTION OF AMERICAN HEALTH CARE

Let us start by reviewing the financial evolution of our health care system. It has gone through tremendous changes in the last 100 years. As practitioners, we naturally look with pride on the technical and scientific advances that have taken place within our own specialty. These developments, however, only partially explain the unprecedented changes that have profoundly influenced American health care. Notwithstanding technology, the financial restructuring of American medicine has provided the framework for the innovative advances in our health care system, but at the same time this reimbursement system has brought us to the brink of crisis.

In 1971, John G. Veneman, while serving the Nixon administration as Undersecretary of the Department of Health, Education and Welfare, stated that "in the past, decisions on health care delivery were largely professional ones. Now those decisions will be largely political" (7). I submit that in the 1990s those health care delivery decisions will now be largely financial. Just prior to the turn of the century, there were no financial intermediaries between the physician and patient. Direct payment by the patient forced physicians to price their services competitively. Hospitals were financed by the community to provide indigent or charity care while most other care was provided in the home. Obviously, the way physicians and hospitals are paid has changed dramatically over the years. This is one of several key issues that we will review as we see how money has flowed into and through the health care system.

Health Insurance Industry

The genesis of the health insurance industry in this country was one of the major financial turning points in American medicine. Early in this century, indemnity plans that reimbursed patients for their hospital services were introduced. These plans continued to grow during World War II. They preserved free choice of physician and hospital while maintaining the traditional concept of payment for services directly by the patient. Two important health insurance alternatives—prepaid health plans and service benefit plans—soon developed. The first physician-directed prepaid health plan was introduced in Los Angeles in 1929 by Donald Ross and H. Clifford Loos. The most widely known prepaid health plan, however, was developed in 1933 by a young innovative surgeon named Sidney Garfield. He provided medical care on a prepaid basis for workers building an aqueduct across the dessert to Los Angeles. Subsequently, he provided similar services to men working on the Grand Coulee Dam for Henry Kaiser. During World War II, when tens of thousands of workers moved to California in defense industry-related jobs, Kaiser transplanted the prepaid plan to shipyards in the San Francisco area and to other West Coast plants. Other companies saw the Kaiser system as an attractive worker benefit, and in 1945 the Permanente Health Plan began enrolling employees from non-Kaiser groups. The Kaiser Permanente Health Plan was the first to guarantee total medical services on a prepaid basis and would provide the framework for many subsequent managed care plans. At about the same time, a second alternative, the service benefit plan, provided reimbursement directly to the hospital. The most notable service benefit plan was the nonprofit Blue Cross plan that started in 1929 by insuring the faculty at Baylor University in Dallas, Texas. The Blue Cross plans also maintained free choice of physician and hospital, but the payment for hospital services was removed from the hands of the patient.

Despite the initial objection from physicians, indemnity insurers expanded the health insurance market by providing reimbursement for both physician and hospital services. The Blue Shield plans were developed to allow the "Blues" to compete in both the physician and the hospital reimbursement markets. Meanwhile, as these plans developed, the patients were gaining access to more and more insurance money to cover medical costs. This naturally equated with improved reimbursement for both hospitals and physicians. As the general flow of money into health care increased, less and less of these funds passed through the hands of patients.

Government Involvement

In the first half of this century, the government had little direct impact on the delivery of health care in this country. Meanwhile, other industrialized nations developed national systems of compulsory sickness insurance. For example, Germany had a plan in place as early as 1883. President Truman, and virtually every president thereafter, proposed some form of national health insurance for the United States, although none has yet materialized. Inevitably, the Federal government's financial support for medicine began to expand during the post-World War II era. The actual commitment of general revenue funds was most noticeable in the area of medical research. The newly created National Institutes of Health had a research budget of $180,000 in 1945, which would mushroom to $400 million by 1960 and over $11 billion in 1994. In 1946 the Hospital Survey and Construction Act was signed into law. Commonly known as the Hill-Burton Act, it provided massive construction funds for community hospitals throughout the country.

MEDICARE

A dramatic turning point in the Federal government's financial involvement in health care occurred on July 30, 1965. The law signed by President Johnson included (a) a Democratic plan for compulsory hospital insurance under Social Security, known as Part A of Medicare, (b) a revised Republican program for voluntary insurance to cover physicians' charges, known as Part B of Medicare, and (c) an additional layer, known as Medicaid, which expanded the subsidies to the states to provide medical care for the poor. This was arguably the most significant single event in the financial evolution of American health care. The increased funding provided through the Medicare and Medicaid systems produced restructuring of health care financing.

INTERMEDIARIES

Intermediaries were needed both to administer the Medicare plan and to provide an interface between the Federal government and all health care providers. The Blue Cross and Blue Shield Plans functioned in many locations as the intermediaries for Medicare. They reimbursed hospitals on a cost-plus basis, rather than at a negotiated rate. Hospitals were allowed to include accelerated depreciation and the cost of residency training in their charges. They could even depreciate assets paid for by the Federal government through the Hill-Burton Act.

With the hospital's cost the major determinant of Medicare reimbursement, it was an ideal time for hospitals both to build and to invest in new high-technology equipment. Consequently, dramatic growth in the hospital infrastructure ensued. These changes made the Federal government a principal source of funding for the entire health care system. Few could have foreseen the financial impact that the government would eventually have on health care.

GOVERNMENT COST CONTAINMENT

It soon became apparent that the Federal government had to control the spiraling costs associated with the Medicare and Medicaid programs. At its inception, the projected costs for Medicare Part A would be $5.7 billion by the year 1980; instead, those costs increased to $25.6 billion. The differences between projections and actual costs demonstrated how difficult it was to predict future costs in a system as uncertain and changing as health care. Many today are once again concerned about the government's ability to project future costs realistically relating to any of the currently proposed health care reform plans.

In 1983, the government implemented The Medicare Prospective Payment System in an attempt to constrain rising hospital costs. Reimbursement to the hospitals was based on a DRG or Diagnosis-related Group. This program provided the hospital with set reimbursement, depending on the patient's admitting diagnosis. Under this system, larger hospitals were able to average out their expenses or to shift their costs to other insurers. However, some of the smaller hospitals were unable to shift their costs and, consequently, went out of business.

To control physician costs, in 1992 Congress enacted the Resource-based Relative Value System, or RBRVS. This relative value scale was developed by Professor Hsiao at Harvard University with extensive help from organized medicine. The RBRVS fee schedule incorporates three components in the calculation of the total relative value unit, or RVU, for each Current Procedural Terminology (CPT) code. They are the work RVU, the practice expense RVU, and the professional liability or malpractice RVU. The work RVU is the only component for which actual resource-based studies were performed; the other two were derived from historical data. Each of the three components is multiplied by a geographic conversion factor and then summed. A dollar amount or fee is then determined by multiplying the total RVU by a dollar conversion factor.

The present debate regarding the RBRVS fee schedule centers around whether or not Congress will authorize funding for a resource-based study of the practice expense RVU and around what will happen in the upcoming Federally mandated 5-year review of the RBRVS system. Neurosurgery as a discipline has continuously complained about certain aspects of the RBRVS system. One such complaint relates to the compression of values that occurred when the final RBRVS schedule was presented. Of greater concern have been the periodic modifications that the Health Care Financing Administration (HCFA) has made to the RBRVS scale. The manner in which the fee schedule has been modified has produced significant aberration from the initial RBRVS concept, and those modifications will continue to impact all of us as the RBRVS fee schedule becomes more widely accepted by private insurance carriers.

Soon, several hundred of you will be sent surveys from Dr. Robert Florin. These surveys will provide us with essential data regarding the RBRVS work values that will be necessary for the 5-year review process. This data is crucial in our effort to undo the compression of the RBRVS system and, hopefully, to change some of the modifications that have been made to the scale. I cannot emphasize enough the importance of your input in this survey process.

Employer Pressure

As the Federal government acted to provide coverage to the unemployed, the aged, and the needy, the private sector has also increased coverage for employees and dependents. With the expansion of coverage, demand for medical services outstripped supply, in both the public and private sectors. This resulted in prices increasing far faster than the cost of living, and neither the public nor private sectors could finance the increases without some method of cost containment. As the Federal government worked to contain rising Medicare and Medicaid costs, hospitals and physicians shifted charges to the private sector, producing yet another realignment of the flow of dollars into the health care system. Consequently, employers were faced with escalating medical insurance premiums and, thus, demanded improved methods of cost containment from their health care providers.

Up to this point, incentives for physicians were not focused on cost savings. Conversely, there was a variety of factors that influenced physicians to increase services and fees, to make expensive referrals, and to practice defensive medicine. With these misdirected incentives, medicine was unable to contain spiraling costs or to address the issues of cost-effective treatment or allocation of resources.

MANAGED CARE

The door was opened for nonmedical administrators to step in and "manage" how health care services are to be used. Because increased utilization meant increased costs for employers and insurers under fee-for-service reimbursement, it was believed that increasing costs would never be reversed unless utilization incentives were altered. This awoke the sleeping giant. "Managed care," the foundation of which was based purely on cost savings, was embraced by the insurance industry. Employers' demand for cost containment has produced an explosion in the managed care market. HMO- and PPO-managed care products currently comprise one-third of this country's health insurance market, and that figure is expected to grow to one-half by the year 2000. California's experience is indicative of this trend: In 1993 75% of Californians with health insurance were in a managed care plan, while its 5 million Medi-Cal participants began shifting over into managed care plans as well.

Let's look more closely at managed care. The recent annual report from the Physician Payment Review Commission defines managed care as ". . . any system of health service payment or delivery arrangements where the health plan attempts to control or coordinate use of health services by its enrolled members in order to contain health expenditures, improve quality or both. Arrangements often involve a defined delivery system of providers with some form of contractual arrangement with the plan" (4). This definition, however, is much too simplistic to describe the current managed care environment. Managed care today is not just a contractual arrangement, but rather, it incorporates layers of nonmedical managers who have become responsible for overseeing decisions regarding patient care. These managers use statistical comparisons and protocols to guide them in evaluating medical decisions. Unfortunately, there has not been a good assessment of how this process will impact quality of care or the doctor-patient relationship. In this regard, I urge you to read Dr. Theodore Cooper's 1989 Cushing Oration entitled, "Who Manages the Managers" (1). Dr. Cooper pointed out in his address that analysts felt that containment of expenditures in all parts of the health care system could be achieved by altering physician behavior. The intervention of nonmedical managers, by design, limits the physician's ability to make independent decisions regarding patient care and at the same time severely compromises the physician-patient relationship. This environment is in stark contrast to our tradition of physician-directed care. Dr. Cooper recommends that physicians be placed back in the role of overseeing the medical decisions that are made by the nonmedical managers.

IPAs, PPOs, HMOs, and fully integrated delivery systems have introduced external controls of how medicine is practiced. The concept of managed care seemed reasonable at the outset, with the elimination of unnecessary testing and tight utilization controls. Significant savings were obtained, and there was hope that our scarce supply of health dollars would be better dispersed. Recent trends, however, have shown that managed care is not the remedy for this country's health care problems. As managed care has escalated, our former ideas about peer review and credentialing processes have changed. Physicians are no longer being evaluated on just treatment. Clinical outcome has become the leading gauge by which their success will be evaluated.

The term "economic credentialing" is already used in many areas of the country to describe the shift from previous credentialing criteria to credentialing that is based solely on financial criteria. Managed care has focused on cost containment by trimming waste, but as competition has increased, plans with primary care physician gatekeepers have developed. These physicians are often reimbursed on a capitated basis, and their compensation is determined by the number of tests ordered or the amount of speciality care they utilize. Consequently, there is concern that the influence of financial gain, by denying access to specialty care, may lead to inappropriate rationing of health care. The entire system of rewards is turning upside down. Behaviors that were rewarded in a fee-for-service environment will be punished in a capitation environment. Hospital executives formerly successful at filling beds, nurturing profit centers, generating charges, building extensive inpatient campuses and recruiting specialists are no longer employed. In their place are individuals who know how to negotiate with managed care payers, keep patients out of the hospital, manage the organization as a cost center, develop integrated relationships with physician groups, build a strong primary care base, and manage risk.

As the managed market has become more competitive, there has been a dramatic shift toward consolidation. While the total number of HMO enrollees in the country has continued to grow, the number of HMOs has started to decline. The smaller or less competitive HMOs are either going out of business or are being acquired by larger HMO networks. It is clear that there is an increasing frequency of non profit HMOs converting to profit-seeking organizations. The increased number of profit-seeking HMOs has resulted in a growing share of premium dollars allocated for administrative overhead and profits. The health care premium dollars now pass into the hands of large, corporate managed care bureaucracies with a corresponding decline in money spent directly on the patient, on reimbursement to the physician, or on improvement of the health care infrastructure.

In a 1994 *Harvard Business Review* article, "Making Competition in Health Care Work," authors Teisberg, Porter, and Brown discuss many of the flaws in how we have looked at competition in our country's health care market (8). The idea of "managed competition" espoused by the current administration has all too often lead to the development of large monopolies, such as we are now seeing in the HMO market. These monopolies have tended to stifle competition and have suppressed the innovative spirit that has made American medicine the best in the world. More importantly, if medical care decisions are to be based solely on statistical norms and protocols, quality of care can only move toward mediocrity. Michael Porter, the second author of the article, is very well known in the business world because of his works on competitive advantage. He and others have stressed that the foundations for competition in business are the ongoing processes of continuous quality improvement and cost reduction. These are terms that many of you have already heard in quality assessment work within your own hospitals. The key to making these processes work, however, is innovation. Any system that undermines the importance of competition within the health care market, impedes innovation, and leads us to mediocrity in medical care can only lead to failure.

NATIONAL HEALTH CARE REFORM

Let us now turn to the debate over national health care reform. As the American health care system has grown, so has its cost to society. Total expenditures in the United States for health care were $69 billion in 1970; by 1980 they had grown to $230 billion; by 1992 they had more than tripled to $800 billion; and by the year 2000 they are expected to reach $1.7 trillion. During Truman's administration our health care expenditures comprised only 4% of the gross domestic product; by 1970 that figure was up to 7.3%; it reached 14.5% of GDP in 1992; and it is projected to reach 19% by the year 2000 (3). It is the rapidly rising health care costs that have fueled the Federal government's present push for national health care reform. The stated objectives of health care reform today are to constrain rising costs, to increase access, and to ensure quality of care.

Containing the escalating costs of health care and providing care to the estimated 37 million uninsured people in this country are not the issues of debate by organized medicine or society in general. The crucial issues in the debate focus on how to pay for those changes and how to provide competition within the health care market so as to control costs without diminishing access to medical care of choice. Congress, of course, is still entrenched in the health care debate. I do not anticipate radical reform this year. The issue, however, will not go away. Much work yet has to be done to improve our present system without destroying those qualities that have made it great.

CHALLENGES FOR NEUROSURGERY

As physicians, and as an organization of neurosurgeons, we face two large problems: the uncertain impending national health care reform that continues to be debated in Congress and the restrictive effects of the expanding managed care market. We have a responsibility to address these issues to create change in this rapidly evolving environment. Just as the innovative neurosurgical leaders of our past have lead the way in the technical advances in medicine, we must now become the leaders in the financial restructuring of our health care system.

Fundamental services that must be provided by organized neurosurgery are education of the membership on health care issues, access to an improved communication network with vital data, and critical responses to proposed governmental regulations. As in any meaningful endeavor, a solid educational foundation is of paramount importance. Both of our national organizations are working diligently to provide the educational framework needed to guide and direct neurosurgeons in the issues of health care reform and managed care.

Educational Role

The AMA series, "Medicine in Transition," provides an excellent resource for understanding the managed care market and the physicians' role in the development of integrated health care systems (2). Both the Congress of Neurological Surgeons (CNS) and the American Association of Neurological Surgeons (AANS), along with the Joint Managed Care Task Force, have provided several courses and manuals to better educate neurosurgeons about managed care. I think today's General Scientific Session further highlights the importance that the CNS places on the need to expand our knowledge in this area. The CNS and the AANS will continue to increase the number, the availability, and the quality of the educational programs that will help prepare neurosurgeons to lead the way in health care reform. You as individual neurosurgeons, however, must avail yourself of those opportunities. The days of solely concerning ourselves with improving our technical skills are gone. Our involvement in creating change in the delivery of health care is equally as important as our surgical prowess.

Communication

Communication and data are also becoming increasingly essential tools for working in the current health care environment. They are being aggressively researched. The joint CNS/AANS Computer Task Force has begun to address the communication and informational data needs of neurosurgery. The COSIN (Clinical Outcomes Studies in Neurosurgery) office has been established by the CNS to provide technical support for clinical outcome studies in neurosurgery. The AANS has an active committee working on guideline and outcomes development. All of these efforts will help to provide the coordinated information services that we will need to compete in the future.

Response to Governmental Regulations

The activities of the Washington Committee have significantly escalated this past year. The Key Person Program, which develops close ties for organized neurosurgery with our Federal legislators, has greatly increased its efforts over the last year. The Washington Committee has continued to monitor and respond to the proposed changes in the RBRVS fee schedule and to other rulings proposed by HCFA. Through the Washington office, both the AANS and the CNS have joined the Patient Access to Specialty Care Coalition, and both support the Patient Protection Act (HR4527). The Washington Committee will continue to monitor and respond to all proposed governmental regulations pertaining to health care.

Role of the Individual Neurosurgeon

What can the individual neurosurgeon do? How can each of us help to restructure the health care market in our respective local environments? There is no cookbook answer to these questions. The true potential for lasting health care reform lies in our hands. Sidney Garfield had no blueprint when he developed a prepaid health plan for Henry Kaiser back in 1933, yet the effects of his innovative ideas have been felt by all of us. It is difficult, however, to face the risks and uncertainties associated with forging into uncharted waters. Change is never easy but initiating change can be absolutely frightening. This health care transformation will be difficult and complicated, but it may help us to remember the simple but profound words of a famous childhood author. In this book *Oh, The Places You'll Go!,* Theodor Geisel, better known as Dr. Seuss, encourages us as only he can (5):

> You have brains in your head
> You have feet in your shoes
> You can steer yourself any direction you choose
> You're on your own
> and you know what you know
> and YOU are the guy who'll decide where to go

Keeping these words in mind can help us to challenge the current health care delivery system as we strive to develop a better one. We must be ready to lead our colleagues in this time of uncertainty.

Let's look at some specific areas that we individually can address. Teisberg, Porter, and Brown in their article on competition in health care listed four key elements necessary for any lasting cure for the U.S. health care system. They are: corrected incentives to spur productive competition, universal coverage to secure economic efficiency, relevant information to ensure meaningful choice, and vigorous innovation to guarantee dynamic improvement.

CORRECTED INCENTIVES

To correct the incentives for physicians, we must critically evaluate the effects of fee-for-service payment and crisis management, as well as the current movement toward capitated reimbursement and disease prevention. As long as our incentive for reimbursement continues to be based solely on sickness, rather than wellness, health care costs will continue to rise. We must get away from those misdirected incentives that have encouraged us to do more procedures, order more tests, and practice defensive medicine. It is important for us to realize that we are on common ground with our primary care colleagues in this realignment of physician incentives. One of my local primary care physicians has aptly expressed this idea by saying that "Physicians have more in common with each other than with any hospital or insurance company" (Langley W, personal communication, 1994). Primary care physicians control the flow of patients in the nonmanaged care market. That control has been dramatically enhanced in the managed care market as primary care physicians have been made the gatekeepers in some tightly controlled managed care plans. By working with primary care physicians, our leadership in the development of integrated delivery systems is still possible. By working against other physicians, we will fail to have any voice in this evolving health care system. We must, however, address these issues soon. At the AANS Annual Meeting in

San Diego, Dr. Jacque J. Sokolov told us in his address, "The Role of the Surgical Specialist in the Future of Health Care," that the development of integrated delivery systems must begin while physicians still have the capital to undertake such projects (6). He outlined for us the popular movement toward integrated delivery systems, but he made it very clear that the large amount of capital necessary to finance such endeavors may not be available to us much longer. If we wish to maintain any control or ownership of these developing health care systems, we must be ready to act now and must not wait until we are facing huge corporate monopolies against which will we be unable to compete.

UNIVERSAL COVERAGE

Universal coverage, which is currently being proposed by the present administration, is still a central issue in the ongoing health care debate. The inefficiencies within our health care system produced by uncompensated care would be eliminated by providing coverage for all Americans. Most, if not all of the national medical societies, support universal coverage. It would be beneficial not only for medicine, but also and more importantly, it would be advantageous for society as well. The focus in the debate, however, is whether society can afford universal coverage in the form in which it has presently been proposed. Financing of universal coverage, whether by employer mandate or individual mandate, is still undecided. We must continue to work at the local and state levels to ensure that health care benefits are provided to a broader segment of our society.

MEANINGFUL DATA

As patients become better-educated consumers of health care services, meaningful data, which include costs and effectiveness of treatments, will allow them to make informed choices about their care. The outcome data from individual practices will become essential marketing information for physicians as they negotiate with managed care plans and other insurers. As an example, if we wish to become the primary caregivers to patients with spine disorders we will need to prove that we can provide the most cost effective care with the best outcomes. To be useful, that data must relate to and be provided by individual practices. National norms are unlikely to give good practitioners an upper hand in competitive markets. Computerization, software upgrades, and practice consolidations can help us to generate meaningful data that we can use in managed care negotiations. With the ongoing work for the development of a national neurosurgical computer online system, you will be able to share, pool, and compare data with other neurosurgical colleagues. This data can be used to augment the guidelines that are also being developed at the national level.

INNOVATION

Managed competition, as it has been proposed, may assist in the management of health care but does not lead to competition within the health care market. Communities that already have a high penetration of managed care have witnessed the trend of HMOs combining into even larger monopolistic entities. These large, managed care corporations stifle innovation in the delivery of health care. If we do not put innovation back into the health care delivery system, we will see the entire system move toward unacceptable mediocrity. Neither managed competition as it has been proposed nor any component of the health care reform plans being debated in Congress will solve our present financial health care crisis. Managed care, capitation payments, and integrated delivery systems define the parameters within which we must presently work. Understanding and working in such a system is essential for our immediate survival. Those concepts, however, will not sustain our health care system.

CONCLUSION

Redirecting physician incentives, providing universal coverage, improving access to meaningful information, and providing innovation are the key components to solving this crisis. Those changes must focus on true competition and innovative ideas, which we must provide. In the past, the innovation in health care has come from physicians, and physicians must provide it in the future. Now is the time for action. Once again, we can use the words of Theodor Geisel to inspire us:

> So . . .
> Be your name Buxbaum or Bixby or Bray
> or Mordaci Ali Van Allen O'Shea,
> You're off to great places!
> Today is your day!
> Your mountain is waiting!
> So . . . get on your way!

No one could put it more clearly or succinctly than Dr. Seuss. Take his words to heart. The challenge lies before us, and the opportunities are endless. Just as Sidney Garfield revolutionized health care delivery more than 60 years ago, now is the time to introduce revolutionary changes of our own. Do not sit idly by while our health care system further deteriorates. Allow yourselves to be the innovative leaders that will give this country a new and better system of health care delivery. So remember, your mountain is waiting! Get on your way!

REFERENCES

1. Cooper T: Who manages the managers. **J Neurosurg** 71:311–315, 1989.
2. Medicine in Transition: A series produced by the Doctors Resource Service of the American Medical Association. Chicago, AMA, 1994.
3. Physician Payment Review Commission: *Annual Report to Congress,* 1993, p 1.
4. Physician Payment Review Commission: *Annual Report to Congress,* 1994, p 484.
5. Seuss, Dr. (Theodor Geisel): *Oh, The Places You Will Go!* New York, Random House, 1990.
6. Sokolov JJ: The role of the surgical specialist in the future of health care. The Richard C. Schneider Lecture. Presented at the Annual Meeting of the American Association of Neurological Surgeons, San Diego, 1994.
7. Starr P: *The Social Transformation of American Medicine.* New York, Basic Books, 1982, p 393.
8. Teisberg EO, Porter ME, Brown GB: Making competition in health care work. **Harvard Bus Rev** July-August:131–141, 1994.

I

General Scientific Session I—Emerging Health Care Issues in 1994

2

The Politics of Health Care Reform

HENRY DESMARAIS, M.D., M.P.A.

The health care reform debate in 1994 has been wildly unpredictable, and there has been considerable associated morbidity and mortality. As an added precaution, I placed a call to Washington to the Senate Democratic cloakroom just before I delivered this address to find out what was on the legislative agenda for that day. They have a tape recording, giving that information, and it is updated very regularly. What I heard kind of surprised me, and I scribbled it all down and would like to share it with you. The legislative program for the day in the United States Senate: heavens crumble; men turn into dogs; the sky rains blood; the dead walk among the living. Both Democratic and Republican leadership meet with the administration in a closed summit. They emerge with a patched-up health care plan that will pass a little later in the day!

As you might imagine, that was not on the tape recording, but it was a health care reform timetable that was published a little earlier this year by Natwest Securities Corporation, investment banking firm. The truth obviously is a little bit different. There is one old saying about Capitol Hill that goes as follows: "Congress does two things best, overreact and nothing." Well, in health care reform this time, we got nothing. From nothing, I had to make something; I had to make a speech. So I would like to cover three objectives with this address. I want to focus on the issues and controversies that confronted the administration and the Congress; I want to look more particularly at the political dimensions of the debate; and finally I would like to speculate about the future of health care reform. I'll be doing all of this as an outsider, because I'm not in the Congress now; I'm not in the administration; and I'm also an outsider in the sense that I consult with a wide range of clients who have a great variety of views about most health care reform issues. This will contrast with the presentations of Helen Smits, an insider, and Paul Ebert, from the College of Surgeons.

The issues and controversies I would like to focus on are money, money, money, and power; or, more eloquently, financing of health care reform, provider revenue issues, graduate medical education, and roles and responsibilities.

FINANCING HEALTH CARE REFORM

From the financing perspective, here is a menu of things the Congress was considering as means for financing the wonderful reforms. The first option was cuts in Medicare and Medicaid spending. In effect they were planning to cut current Medicare expenditures for current benefits, for example, payments to neurosurgeons, and in return to use some of that money to provide additional benefits such as prescription drugs. That was the contract they were trying to enter into with the beneficiary community.

Employer mandate was the other controversial financing option, that is, sending the bill to the employers and having them pay health insurance coverage for their workers and families. Individual mandate would have required sending it to each and every family, and we would have helped some of them along if they were unable to afford purchasing a policy.

DEFINING BENEFITS AND PROVIDERS

Next, there was the issue of the insurance benefits package. It was to be a simple standardized package facilitating comparison shopping and was to be available to as many people as possible. Unfortunately, that would have increased, in an ever-increasing way, the cost of coverage. Then, people who were providing care today to the uninsured, such as community health centers and migrant health centers, feared they might be left out and insisted on requiring every health insurance plan in the country to have a contractual relationship with them, to send them money, and to make sure that they would continue to stay in business. It was not long before academic health centers felt the same way. They wanted some kind of special accommodation from the Congress that would guarantee that they could continue to do what they are doing today and that they would not be shut out by insurance companies and managed care organizations.

Of course, cost containment is a very fundamental part of a number of the health care reform plans. This last issue also relates to the question of "any willing provider." This flows from the issue that managed care organizations tend to create closed panels or networks of providers and leave other people outside, when the other providers left outside want to get in. So, those left outside petition the Congress, as they have in many states, indicating that if they are willing to meet certain baseline criteria, and if they are willing to live by certain conditions and the rules of a particular health plan, there should be no reason for a health plan to shut them out. In fact a number of states have already passed "any willing provider" laws. Sometimes, the laws only apply to pharmacies; sometimes they only apply to some kinds of insurance policies and not necessarily to health maintenance organizations.

At any rate, let's explore this issue a little bit further. When I consider the various perspectives, putting the patient's perspective first, obviously it is nice if he or she has an unlimited choice of providers. Yet, another added concern or issue is the price of the insurance policy, and it may be that the cost of that premium may be related to the number of physicians in the network or the physicians that are part of any closed panel. From a health plan perspective, plans are told by employers and others that they will receive a certain amount of money each month, and for that sum they must provide health care benefits to employees and make sure they are given quality care. Also, the government indicates it is planning to issue report cards on each one of the health plans to show how well they are doing, summarizing their performance, etc. So from the insurer's perspective, they want to have some control over which providers, which physicians, which nurse practitioners, etc., will be allowed in their particular plan.

What about the "in-network" physicians? Well, those providers may be in favor of a closed network because they are on the inside and they are able to participate and care for the enrollees of that particular plan. They may have gotten there by offering discounts from their normal fees, so they are going to be extremely concerned about how many patients they will be able to care for because they recognize that only so many operations will be needed. What about the out-of-network physicians? Well, they are concerned, of course, because they're out of favor and it may be more difficult or almost impossible for a particular patient to get access to them, depending on which plan the patient belongs to and which gatekeeper mechanism is in place.

What about the primary payers? Well, they want "value"; they want to keep the cost of coverage low, as low as possible. They also want to keep their employees or enrollees happy, which requires quality and a certain level of choice. They are in a little bit of a bind. The government is also in a bind because the Congress is being buffeted from all sides: by those who want unlimited choice; by the whole contingent wanting to keep costs down; and by those who want to keep the administration of the program simple. There may be some interest in limiting the number of contracts, physician plan contracts, that must be entered into and negotiated, etc.

Having discussed the issues and perspectives, what about the policy options? The first option is very simple. It requires every single health plan in the country to deal with any willing provider. In general, people who favor this approach view the requirements as twofold: qualification as a licensed physician, with the possible added specification of Board certification, etc., and also willingness to accept the price or payment level the plan is willing to pay for particular procedures. I might add that those offering the plan may have a different perspective because they're not only concerned about price but also about the volume of services, because that affects total expenditures. Another option being discussed, or that has been discussed, is to require every plan to have a point-of-service option so that at any point in time a particular patient can decide to go out of network to see any physician of his or her choice. More than likely the patient will have to pay a little bit more in terms of cost sharing, but he or she will have the right at any moment, at any time, to see any provider. A third option is to allow each person or each family at any moment in time to select from a number of different options, some of which provide the point-of-service option or fee for service, some of which allow them to go to any particular provider. The fourth option is one that has been championed by the American Medical Association and others: it is to impose certain procedural safeguards. So if a health plan, for example, decides to exclude a neurosurgeon from a network, it would have to provide adequate notice, and an opportunity for review the decision, appeal the decision, etc. Sometimes, this process gets rather elaborate, depending on the particular option in question.

Obviously, we can always fall back on the status quo which would leave the whole reform process to market forces. It would be confusing and would impose continued difficulty, but it would be likely for the pendulum to swing back and forth, maybe ending up somewhere in the middle of the spectrum.

GRADUATE MEDICAL EDUCATION

We have heard discussed the need to reduce the total number of residency programs in the United States, and the goal of many, though not necessarily the Clinton administration, was to maintain the total number of residency positions at 110% of the number of medical and osteopathic graduates in the United States. (We are currently exceeding 140%, with international medical graduates filling the additional residency positions.) There has also been a call for more primary care residency positions. In fact, many plans have called for 55% of all residency positions to be devoted to primary care, including obstetrics and gynecology, and only 45% to be devoted to nonprimary care specialties. At the same time, there have been calls for a dramatic increase in the number of physician assistants and nurse practitioners.

Finally, we must consider the cost of medical education. It has been suggested that every insurer be required to pay a share of the cost, as well as to institute various reforms that in some cases, would mean paying less to certain hospitals. This would require converting to a national payment rate system. However, what would the implications of that be? When we consider the total number of current PGY1 positions (just under 25,000), the 55:45 requirement would reduce that figure to just under 19,000—a fairly dramatic decline. There would be an even more dramatic reduction effect on the residency outflow. In primary care, there would be a net increase in graduating residents, from the current level of about 9,400 to about 10,300, achieving the desired objectives of 55% of the total. The output of nonprimary care residencies would decline from the current 15,000 to approximately 8,400—roughly a 43% decline. This is the degree of change being discussed by some experts. They would not propose implementation immediately but would phase the changes in over 3 to 5 years but with similar eventual impact.

The specific situation for neurological surgery deserves separate consideration. There are currently 96 residency programs with 808 total residents enrolled, as reported in 1993. In 1983, there were about 666 residency positions. When we examine what HMOs do, or at least what some HMOs do, we begin to realize what it might mean in the future when we talk about reducing the number of residency positions for non-primary care, and we begin to understand the implications that might have for neurosurgery. Some HMOs, including the Group Health Cooperative of Puget Sound, are employing far fewer neurosurgeons per 100,000 people in the plan, than the current rates of practicing neurosurgeons in the general U.S. population. Other HMOs, such as Kaiser Portland, employ very close to the current U.S. rate of neurosurgeons per 100,000. What would be the overall implications for neurosurgical manpower requirements if we integrated the rates of all current major plans? While some of the patients in these HMOs are no doubt going out of network for some of their care, in particular for specialty care, the overall implications for the specialty are inescapable.

POWER AND CONTROLLING THE REFORM AGENDA

The final issue to be discussed relates to power and the roles of various parties in driving the process of reform. Will the government, the insurance companies, the provider community, etc., dictate the scope and pace of reform? Was the Federal government going to adopt a single global health reform plan and impose it? Or were states going to be left with greater flexibility to choose their own system? Large employers generally have not favored state flexibility, in view of the variability of policies and procedures likely to emerge. Similarly, insurance companies want to avoid lobbying and waging legislative battles in 50 different state capitals, instead of engaging in a single debate at the national level.

Another source of tension between roles and responsibilities pits individual health plans *versus* the health insurance purchasing cooperatives, or "HIPC's." The latter were originally going to be new entities created to facilitate the purchase of insurance by individuals and small businesses because, in theory, by banding them together and allowing them to join a purchasing cooperative, they would have more market clout and would be able to get a better deal. Now, health plans were very comfortable if the purchasing cooperatives collected premiums and shared information, but they did not want these purchasing cooperatives to have negotiating powers. They did not want these purchasing cooperatives to have the power to exclude any health plans. Last but not least, as for the struggle between health plans and health providers for as to who was going to have the power; were physicians going to be allowed to join together to negotiate collectively and if so we would provide some exemptions to anti-trust laws or were we going to adopt an "any willing provider" statute as discussed earlier?

All these tensions produced a menu of wide ranging options for health care reform. Everything from a single payor Canadian style system; to expanding Medicare beyond the aged and disabled under Medicare part C; to the Clinton plan which provided universal coverage and essentially used an employer mandate to do that along with cost containment features; and down more toward the bottom we have more incremental reforms just changing insurance rules a little bit, or maybe introducing modest subsidies to a few people. These latter options promised to go slow and did not claim to deliver universal coverage.

This sort of menu was closely examined by conservatives and liberals as they considered particular plans. Well, what happened to health care reform? It died. Who's responsible? Well, my favorite answer to that question was in the New York Times, September 1994, in a news analysis by Robin Toner which states, "As in murder on the Orient Express, most of the suspects had their hands in the knife at one time or another, a divided Democratic party on Capitol Hill, an over reaching Clinton administration, a fiercely partisan class of Republicans, an insatiable collection of interest groups."

Let's just set that down a little bit. Here's my catalog of key considerations that affected the political dynamics. Tempus fugit (time flies), and the administration was always late. They always were going to do something by a certain day and some of us, including me, stated they weren't going to miss that date because they would look silly and they would set themselves back. And time and again they missed their dates.

MAGNUM OPUS

Magnum Opus is loosely translated a big one. Big in two ways, the bills the Clinton administration and others produced were huge in size, they were also huge in terms of the diversity of issues they attempted to resolve in a single piece of legislation. A major problem for Congress and one that proved to be one of the reasons for the downfall. Not Monticello, we know too that President William Jefferson Clinton began his inaugural journey from Monticello, Thomas Jefferson's home in Charlottesville. Those of you who've been there know that Monticello means, somewhat loosely translated from the Italian, "a small hill" or "small mountain." Well, the President's plan was not "Monticello," because he said the only thing he would accept is universal coverage. That's what he said early on, and he threatened to veto any bill that didn't provide it. I think assertion created another major problem: it demanded too much.

There were multiple procedural hurdles. Many committees, were focusing on health reform and many issues had to be resolved. There was a lack of bipartisanship. Let me quote a Democrat on this particular issue. Congressman Jim Cooper of Tennessee said "I think the administration's key mistake was not being bipartisan. They only had one Republican in America supporting their approach. They should have reached out to moderates in both parties in order to build a broad national consensus for health reform." A lack of consensus existed. There were conflicting signals from the public. The public asked for reform but also demanded that health insurance premiums not increase very much. The public wanted reform but did not want to alter their favorite features of the current system. Then, in the end, the public said "Don't do it this year. Wait." Yet, Congress continued to work on health reform. Of course, there were multiple distractions from the work at hand: everything from Whitewater to foreign affairs and even a few alleged domestic affairs. Then there was the other rate-limiting factor: the Congressional Budget Office. The Congressional Budget Office is the place where they have to estimate the financial impact of each and every one of these bills, and Congress always seemed to be too late in getting a bill ready and had to wait for the Congressional Budget Office to do its important analysis.

What about next year? Here's my list of questions. Obviously, my crystal ball and yours will be a little bit less hazy after the November elections. Quite likely, the new congress that will convene will be more Republican and more conservative. Probably not as Republican as some Republicans would like or expect or plan on, but nevertheless it will probably be very different in orientation from the current Congress. Quite likely, the administration will decide not to send forward another omnibus bill of the kind that it worked on this year.

3

Medicine in Transition: Strategies for Change

DAVID E. VOGEL, M.S.

The prospect of change is always challenging, often generating fear, anger, and frustration among those confronting it. However, change can also be viewed as opportunity, just as it can be now by physicians interested in actively participating in the development of a real system of health care.

For in truth, the United States has never had a health care "system," in the scientific sense. A true system, after all, must have rules for meeting defined goals and expectations and must provide for audits of levels of performance against those rules, together with a means for corrective action when it is needed. Historically, the so-called U.S. health care "system" has not met those criteria.

The opportunity for change now exists. Unfortunately, that opportunity also leaves physicians vulnerable to making the wrong choices from the options available to them. However, knowledge is strength, and physicians' ability to successfully manage transition lies in their ability to understand the forces that are driving it. That knowledge should help all physicians, clinical neurosurgeons among them, identify appropriate clinical practice management and develop personal strategies to position themselves for success.

A PARADIGM SHIFT

Nothing less than a major paradigm shift in health care economics is now underway, driven primarily by the increase in the percentage of gross domestic product (GDP) spent for health care services since 1965, when it stood at just 6%. Furthermore, that percentage is expected to continue to increase—from 13.6% in 1992 to 18% in the year 2000, and to 29% by 2020. With those increases, of course, come concomitantly increasing constraints on the availability of funds to address other essential needs, such as food, housing, and education; hence, the growing rhetoric that insists that limits on increases in health care spending must be imposed.

Why health care spending has increased and continues to do so is the subject of great and often-heated debate—not to mention considerable buck-passing—among both health care providers and consumers, with the list of oft-cited culprits ranging from inefficiencies in the health care system to the threat of malpractice suits and the cost of medical technology. In fact, there are virtually dozens of contributing factors, none in themselves accounting for more than a few percentage points' increase but cumulatively resulting in a major impact on total health care spending.

The rising cost of health care is the bad news that all of us already know. However, there is good news, too, and ample cause for optimism, because there is still an opportunity for the phenomenon labeled "health care reform" to be shaped primarily by market forces rather than by legislative fiat—that is, by the purchasers and providers of services themselves. While issues such as malpractice may need to be addressed through tort reform and other legislative initiatives, physicians can take the lead in resolving many others.

Those physicians interested in realizing a positive result from the change process will recognize that assigning blame is likely to be far less productive then identifying which inflationary factors they may be contributing to and determining what can be done about them. The lack of validated clinical practices and the absence of clinical outcomes data offer examples of two such issues. Development of technology to fill those gaps would be one substantial contribution to the creation of an effective U.S. health care system that physicians are both legitimately and uniquely qualified to address.

The shift from episodic, fee-for-service patient care to managing all care required by an entire population for a fixed revenue—a process typically referred to as "global budgeting," or "capitation"—is another important trend reshaping the health care economic paradigm. Threatening on the surface, it offers another opportunity in disguise.

To replace a system that provides incentives to raise fees and produce a maximum number of services, the marketplace is seeking to convert fee-for-service health care to a reimbursement system that fixes revenues at a specific amount per person per year and per month. The change is an important one to understand, because it shifts the focus from revenue enhancement to cost center management, the major cost centers in managed care organizations being physicians, hospitals, and other providers. To be responsive, providers must become integrally involved in the process of managing resources within the fixed-revenue environment, a process that involves a mind-set far different from the one that has traditionally guided physicians in their practices. The relevant goal today is no longer to focus on identifying ways in which to generate more revenues but on determining how to participate in managing resources more effectively.

Fixing revenues to providers on a per-person per-month basis also means that providers are assuming risk. However, assuming risk without at the same time developing the capability to manage risk is a sure-fire formula for clinical and financial failure, another reason why providers would be well advised to seize the opportunity to become actively involved in developing systems that will contribute to effective risk management.

THE FUNDAMENTAL ISSUE

Although much of the discussion of the need for health care reform has focused on the cost of care, it is important to recognize that cost is only one of the issues driving change. In fact, what the health care market is seeking is not cost control, *per se,* but *value* for the health care dollars that are spent. Specifically, the market is asking for:

- Maximization of clinical quality, as measured by outcomes.
- Maximization of patient service, as measured by statistically valid patient surveys and other objective standards.
- Minimization of total health care costs per person per year, as measured by health insurance premiums.

How best to measure and manage the clinical quality objectives is one of the most challenging questions of all, for to do so requires sophisticated clinical decision-making support systems beyond the capability of most individual physicians to develop and operate. Many physicians are finding the answer in becoming affiliated with larger organizations that have sufficient resources to meet those essential systems support and other infrastructure needs.

IMPLICATIONS FOR NEUROLOGIC SURGEONS

The demand for value maximization and the resultant systemization of health care have many implications for neurosurgeons, among them, changes in their relationship with their key partners in health care.

Patients (or the employers who typically pay their health care bills) will be shopping for the best values in care, seeking out physicians who can not only provide value but also can prove that they do.

Primary care physicians will become the neurologic surgeon's primary "customers," as more patients participate in managed care organizations and as managed care mechanisms make primary care physicians the overseers of patients' care.

Hospitals will be less interested in establishing relationships with neurosurgeons as their focus shifts from revenue enhancement to resource management within a fixed-revenue environment.

Relationships among neurosurgeons themselves will also be affected as the number of neurosurgical procedures per 1,000 population declines, and competition for the shrinking patient pool intensifies.

Meanwhile, as traditional relationships undergo these alterations, neurosurgeons will be experiencing the need to define their role within the new, broadly integrated health care structures that are now taking shape. Given this trend to attempt to integrate all of the sometimes disparate and conflicting components of health care into a single seamless system that can be managed and held accountable for the care it provides, the challenge for neurosurgeons is to determine how they can respond productively.

One thing is certain: Yesterday's survival strategies no longer apply.

NEW LEADERSHIP NEEDS

If neurosurgeons must rethink practice management objectives, they also would be well advised to look with renewed objectivity at the way in which they respond to change. A new health care paradigm demands new approaches to health care leadership.

Historically, physician leadership has manifested itself primarily in efforts to protect the *status quo*. In a changing world, attempts to maintain the status quo are doomed to failure. Consider this case in point:

In 1988, 150 physicians from throughout a large state met to discuss their options in the wake of the threat they perceived from changes in the health care environment. As a result of that discussion, a decision was made to organize a statewide individual practice association (IPA).

The physicians had three objectives in establishing the IPA:

- To retain control of the health care environment.
- To maximize their influence in it.
- To preserve the practice of fee-for-service medicine.

A relatively low entry fee was established to encourage participation in the IPA by as many physicians in the state as possible, the rationale being that the more physicians that participated, the more leverage those physicians could exert in influencing health care. Ultimately, several thousand physicians joined the IPA, knowing no more about it than its objectives. In this way, more than $1.5 million was raised, and the new statewide IPA was off and running.

Or was it?

Two years and many thousands of physician-hours later, with $1.5 million spent on writing bylaws and articles of incorporation, drafting physician contracts, and developing a detailed fee schedule, the organization had yet even to begin putting in place the systems that would be essential to achieving a positive impact on clinical outcomes, patient satisfaction, and health care costs.

Even worse, with prospective customers already skeptical of the value of the organization because of the motives underlying its creation, there was little market demand for the services the IPA offered.

Small wonder, then, that by 1991, with the organization out of money and many physicians questioning its viability, the effort was abandoned.

Although some IPA, physician-hospital organizations (PHOs), hospital networks, and other provider-sponsored organizations have been successful, the fate of the IPA in this tale is becoming increasingly common. Health care providers are understandably feeling mounting pressure to respond to the forces driving change in health care today. Unfortunately, their responses all too often take a form that dooms their efforts to failure. In their diagnosis of the situation, they recognize the symptoms but too often design an inappropriate and ineffective treatment plan.

While many physicians are responding effectively to changes in the health care environment, too many others are responding ineffectively, or even counterproductively, investing their energies and other resources in the always futile effort to resist social and economic trends.

Viability in any industry requires responsiveness to the marketplace. For that reason, enlightened physicians and other providers in some markets have come to realize that their interests, and the interests of their patients, are best served by responding to what the market is demanding. The lessons for our friends in the failed IPA should be clear: resources invested in finding ways to respond to market demands are likely to realize a better return than those invested in resisting them. Change is the only constant in life, and in any industry it is those who understand the need to evolve *with* change who profit from it.

Consider, then, how the physicians who established the above-cited IPA might have achieved a different outcome.

IDENTIFYING THE REAL ISSUES

Retaining control was the overriding objective in the case of the failed IPA, but is *control* the issue to which physicians should be addressing themselves today? Rarely, except as a short-term strategy, has the attempt to control a market through the establishment of monopolies, barriers, or other artificial means worked. Thus, organizing physicians for the purpose of resisting change (whether that purpose is stated or not) is almost always doomed to failure.

Consider how different the outcome might have been if physicians who established the IPA had defined *viability* as their objective. If they had, they would have focused on devising ways to better produce the value sought by prospective purchasers of care. Recognizing that the fixed-revenue health care environment will inevitably demand better management of resources, the organizers of the IPA might have invested in developing the tools needed to accomplish that objective. Dollar for dollar, $1.5 million invested in systems to monitor patient outcomes, measure patient satisfaction, and document positive impact on the cost of care might have represented far better protection for the physicians' futures. By striving to achieve the value maximization sought by consumers, they are far more likely to have realized the rewards of a steady flow of patients, as well as the fair and reasonable compensation that could be expected to follow.

In short, instead of investing in resisting change, they could have invested in making it work for them.

DESIGNING APPROPRIATE RESPONSES

The ill-fated IPA suffered not only from a failure of vision but also of appropriate organizational design. The flaws inherent in the design would probably have doomed it to failure, whatever its objectives had been.

While the goal of the IPA was to enroll as many physician members as possible, as soon as possible, that goal in itself undermined its eventual success. In fact, when a large number of physicians joined before the organization had established founding principles, set up basic operating guidelines and standards, or arrived at any real understanding of the essential changes required to have an impact on quality, service, and cost, the organization practically guaranteed that it would never take the steps necessary to deal with those difficult matters. It is much easier, after all, to avoid these knotty issues and deal with the more immediate and more readily resolved issues related to fees and contracts.

A common misunderstanding among physicians in developing physician organizations is that bigger is better. While large democratic organizations may be important to the realization of certain objectives, they do not necessarily lend themselves well to every purpose. Although they may be suited to undertaking activities that require consensus of a large broad-based constituency such as the medical staff of a hospital, their very size makes them cumbersome when it comes to making the kind of effective, timely decisions required to survive in a competitive environment.

Even when an organization's leadership can move in a timely manner, constituents are typically not as knowledgeable about the organization's basic business as is its leadership; most members simply lack the time and other resources needed to build the information base it takes to make sound decisions. A democratic organization's leadership may, of course, sometimes muster the courage to make sound but unpopular business decisions. When it does so, however, it is likely to find itself no longer the leadership come the next election.

Thus, while a democratic, broad-based organization may be most effective when it comes to exercising political clout, an organization dedicated to helping a group of professionals navigate the treacherous and fast-moving shoals of the changing health care environment may best be served by one that is smaller and more nimble. Similarly, the more locally focused the organization, the more responsive it is likely to be to marketplace demands. Health care is, after all, a personal, local matter that is more effectively managed at the doctor-patient interface. Hence, organizations that are smaller and closer to that interface often can provide better support than those that are larger and more remote.

REASONS FOR OPTIMISM

There is a moral to every story, and the moral to the tale of the failed IPA is clear: No business can succeed when it tries to resist the market rather than respond to it, and bigger is not better when responsiveness is the goal. Openness, responsiveness, and agility are the attributes that are the best survival strategies for organizations—and for individual physicians as well. Fortunately, physicians are an extremely intelligent, highly motivated group of individuals. These attributes should equip them to make intelligent choices when they have good information and the incentive to learn—and economic realities, present and future, should provide powerful incentives to learning, indeed.

In the last analysis, viability requires determining whether to be part of the problem or part of the solution. Few would question that there are problems in the health care system today; the market would not be demanding change if there were not. The choices for physicians are to cling steadfastly to the way things have been or to direct their energies toward defining the way things might be.

Working together, physicians have awesome potential to response to the market's demand for maximum value for the health care dollar. It is urgent that neurosurgeons exert leadership by working to find ways to improve patient outcomes, patient satisfaction, and total cost per person per year. That is what the public is demanding, and it is only through their responsiveness to those demands that neurosurgeons can ensure their own viability.

4

Health Reform: Past, Present, and Future

HELEN L. SMITS

The obvious objective of this address is to review with you the status of health reform: what happened to date, what I personally expect will happen now, and what I think those of you in practice should expect both in the political sense, and equally importantly, in the sense of where health reform will go even without legislative change. Finally, I would like to talk specifically about the practice of neurosurgery and some of the issues that the graduate medical education provisions in both the President's and other bills present for you as a specialty.

A POSTMORTEM OF THE HEALTH SECURITY ACT OF 1994

As I'm sure you all know, less than 1 year ago, President Clinton presented to Congress a fully written bill for health reform. In fact, these same weekends last year, I spent most of my time in the office with many other people in the process of last-minute review of the legislation. As you know, nothing was passed in the U.S. Congress, although there were certainly times during the summer when it looked like a bill would pass, particularly if we hadn't been working so hard against the clock and if there hadn't been so many distractions within the legislative schedule.

Everyone has his or her own version of what went wrong, and I think it is worth listening to the different versions as you make up your own mind. For those of you that are interested, there is a story in this Monday morning's *New York Times* (October 3, 1994) about some of the First Lady's opinions. My views from watching the process very closely in Washington is that first of all, the plan that emerged in October 1993 was a fully developed bill which had been produced in a relatively secretive environment. Now, there were hundreds of people involved; it was not, in terms of Washington, really very secretive; The fact of the bill being given to Congress in such a manner tended to mute legislative support, because even those members of both houses who were most strongly in favor of the bill had not worked for the issues themselves and did not have a passionate commitment to every detail. They had not been in on the negotiations and the compromising themselves.

One of the interesting things about the bill is that, as one critic described it, it was not modular, that is, it was a piece of legislation that hung together very well, but when you tried to take one part out, for example, if you tried to take out the alliances where people would buy health insurance, you then had to make a lot of changes in other parts of the bill. So you had a very comprehensive bill where it wasn't easy to, as Congress puts it, "tweek it." It wasn't easy to make small changes, and that, I think, turned out to be a major barrier. Finally, the bill tried to deal in a very honest way with a wide range of perceived problems within the health care system, rather than with the core issues of cost of care and access to care that had first brought the Clintons to their focus on health reform. In speaking about it I used to describe it as really six or seven bills rolled together and, frankly, I think that over time worked against it.

It is widely known that the Clinton bill contained major provisions with respect to graduate medical education, provisions that in any ordinary year would compose a very substantive bill in and of themselves. It also contained somewhat less noticeable but equally important provisions regarding the privacy of health care information and the sharing of health care claims information from private plans with the government and among each other so that we would all understand in better detail what's happening in the health care system. There were also major provisions to increase access to care in certain underserved parts of the country. The result was a bill that in many senses was overwhelming; it took a tremendous amount of time to grasp it all and it became difficult, I think, not to be against one part of it. As the various opposition groups rolled into action that worked very much against it. In terms of what the public thought, the bill's complexity helps to explain why this bill did not pass in a period when all polls showed that most Americans believed there ought to be health care reform and there ought to be universal coverage.

In the big picture, the bill was seen, correctly or incorrectly, as too much government. Since I work for the agency that runs Medicare, I found it particularly amusing that the same people who attacked this bill as too much government also were very firm about insisting that Medicare not change substantially. Somehow, the fact that Medicare is a government-run health care program disappeared in the debate. Not that I am arguing that Medicare ought to run health insurance for the entire country, but it does present some evidence that the government can do reasonably well at managing a major insurance plan. Another issue that the negative interest groups pressed on very hard was that of cost. They maintained that the estimated costs were understated and the bill would become an enormous tax burden in the long run. Finally, I think those who were opposed to it very effectively played the theme in the American mind of "If I'm a little worse off at the moment, then it must be bad for me, or it must be bad overall." So the second wave of the famous Harry and Louise television commercials focused on the healthy young person whose insurance premiums would go up if there was universal community rating. What is ironic about this implication is that the young man would have been paying those higher premiums for something he can not buy now. He would have been paying them for guaranteed lifetime coverage and the promise that he would never lose coverage no matter what illness he developed. If the same young man goes out on the open market and tries to buy that kind of coverage, he will not be able to find it, certainly not at anywhere near the price for which it would be available to him if there were community rating and universal coverage. However, the sense that there would be short-term increase in costs for some people had a great deal of influence.

Obviously, part of the reason this bill did not pass is that a lot of money was spent on opposing it by interest groups. It is interesting that the press continued, throughout the whole fight, to talk about opposition "from doctors and hospitals." I am really very proud that the medical profession, with varying attitudes and with varying degrees of enthusiasm, came out very strongly in support of the general concepts of reform. My experience from meeting with doctors around the country and talking to doctors in all specialties is that physicians are tired of a lack of universal coverage. There are tired of the extremely uncomfortable ways in which our insurance system affects patients, and they would prefer to work in a system where you did not have to make very painful cost trade-offs because this patient's coverage is missing or is about to be taken away.

The support from the physician community was certainly there in terms of universal coverage but was not concerted or focused enough to stand up to the pressure of other interest groups. Obviously the most powerful and successful of the opposing interest groups were the small insurance companies now writing health insurance. This was coupled with the stance of small and large businesses; although you did not hear much from them specifically, they were important. These businesses saw the extra cost of providing health insurance as damaging to their cost effectiveness in various ways.

THE IMMEDIATE FUTURE OF HEALTH REFORM

What is going to happen now? That is obviously everybody's next question. What will happen in a political sense obviously depends very much on the upcoming midterm election in November 1994. One of the interesting phenomena that was reported moderately well, not extremely well, in the press, was the effort over the last few months by a group calling itself "mainstream" and called by some people the "rump group." This was a bipartisan group in the Senate who tried to write a smaller but still very significant bill that would have at least moved towards significant improvements in coverage. Watching that process certainly suggested that if those same people had had control of the situation 2 or 3 months earlier, we might have had a very different outcome.

The bill that evolved from their efforts included significant insurance reform, eliminating denial for pre-existing conditions, and guaranteeing insurance portability upon changing employment. There was also movement toward more general community rating, although not for everyone, and toward subsidies for the poorest families. There were a variety of versions proposed, some with subsidies for all children in families with low incomes, some with subsidies for full families. There were also some pieces of the original bill, particularly in the area of information sharing and privacy, that seemed to have generated bipartisan consensus. Some of the people who worked hardest on that, like Senator Durenberger, will not be back; some others may not be back, depending on how the vote goes. So whether that particular set of ideas crystallizes a new movement in the next Congress will really depend, I think, on individuals: on who comes back, that is, how much the people who come to the House and the Senate feel committed to health care, and on what their personalities are like. Both of these factors may have as much to do with whether there is a bill next session as the actual count of the number of Democrats *versus* Republicans.

There remain within the Republican party some fairly strong groups who are committed to the idea that we need to do something about the health care system, at least in the general areas that President Bush indicated, and many current senators support. Certainly, if something does pass, it would be a modest first step, and it would not include any significant increase in the Federal government's involvement in health care.

That is the politics of the matter, but what about the rest of the system? The important thing to remember is that there were two sources of pressure that brought us here in the first place. They were the rapidly rising cost of care and particularly the impact of that cost on our ability to fund government programs, coupled with the increasing distress of a very articulate part of the voting public about loss of access to care, loss of insurance, and fear of loss of insurance. Those issues are not going away. The economy is better; some of the people who were afraid that they were going to lose insurance didn't lose it or got it back again but, in aggregate, fewer Americans are insured today, even with a very robust economy, than were insured 3 years ago under a weaker economy.

You may hear some stories claiming that the inflation rate for health care has abated. That is not true. The real inflation rate, that is the inflation in the health care sector, when you subtract the inflation in the rest of the economy, is pretty much the same. The inflation rate of health care is still rising 2.5 to 3.5% faster than inflation in the rest of the economy. This increase is not devastating in any one year, but over time it will shift an increasing segment of the cost of the total economy into health care and will cause increasing problems and pressure on all of the remaining elements of the economy to try to support it. One of the principles of the President's bill was that cost control, in this case, market-based cost controls, and competition were possible only in a setting where everyone was covered. Unfortunately, in a setting in which there are many uninsured people, one of the ways to make the most money and to be the most cost effective is to avoid anyone with bad insurance or minimal insurance. What we are going to see from the field is what we are seeing right now: a continued increase in large systems of care and large organized plans and a continued increase in the number of uninsured, which is probably fairly gradual at present, but which very likely will come back very uncomfortably whenever the next recession arises.

We also will continue to see the very interesting phenomenon of state variability. You have probably noticed, and some of you may even practice in, states where waivers have been granted. These are waivers to the states of the technical rules of Medicaid, in order to urge or require Medicaid beneficiaries to go into managed care and also to take the savings that result from organized systems of care and put them into expansions of coverage. I think the fact that states as different as Florida and Tennessee and Washington and Ohio all want to receive waivers is a very clear sign that there is continued public pressure in favor of increasing coverage. This will result in continued variation in precise regulations across various states, along with differences in practice rules and differences in how things are paid for. That presents a problem for many people whose practice crosses state lines. I happen to be at this moment in the part of New Jersey that is right across the border from Pennsylvania and right across the border from New York and trying to practice and see patients in a setting like this is difficult now and will get even more difficult with state variability.

One thing that the President can do for the states is to offer them flexibility in experimenting with health care reform, and certainly one of the long-term hopes for health care reform is that a few states will do it in ways that seem to work well and that appear to offer lessons that could then be applied nationally.

HEALTH REFORM AND NEUROSURGERY

I was struck by the fact that when my staff prepared material for me for this address, they gave me a whole lot of interesting general things but nothing specific about neurosurgeons. So I asked for some additional material and received almost endless faxes over the weekend, telling me more about neurosurgery than I wanted to know. Basically, the bottom line is that in 1980, when the Graduate Medical Education National Advisory Council, looking at graduate medical education, made estimates of the need for certain specialties, neurosurgery was regarded as an oversupplied speciality, quite significantly oversupplied in terms of the number of new residents. In fact, you as neurosurgeons have gone through a fairly rapid rise, as have many other specialties, between 1980 and now, suggesting at least that the increased number of residents is probably related more to the local need for residents to help with the work than it is to the national need for fully received neurosurgeons. I have been there; I was running a teaching hospital just before I came to the government and the pressure on all sides to keep the residency group at a given size or even expand it were very considerable. I do think that you probably have some of the best available ways of measuring whether your specialty is oversupplied or not. That is: how it is for people leaving residency positions to enter either into an agreement with an existing group or to locate some place where there is a real promise of the kind of volume of activity that is necessary to keep a neurosurgeon active and skilled.

I know that there are a number of fields, like anesthesia, that very recently, 3 or 4 years ago, were scoffing at the estimates of oversupply that are now facing the situation of new graduates unable to find work. Anesthesiologists, as you know, mostly go into groups and many graduating residents have been unable to find work that pays within the range of salaries that a newly trained resident could have commanded 4 years ago. People are starting out new for a great deal less than was available quite recently. Those are worrisome trends, as it certainly is not fair to young people to fully train them for specialties in which they would not be able to practice.

High-paying specialties like neurosurgery will be increasingly squeezed by the large systems of care as the health care environment as a whole becomes more and more organized. I would urge you again to look very carefully at the reality in the numbers, the real numbers you have seen in terms of work for your new graduates, and to give some very careful consideration to whether some shrinkage in residency size over the next few years would not be appropriate for you, regardless of what happens with graduate medical education payment. I do think, frankly, that there also is a very significantly possibility that there will be some arrangement in which at least Medicare payment and, quite possibly, payment from other payers for residency would be tied to the type of residencies in a given consortium or a given medical school, rather than the current arrangement, whereby any legitimate certified residency receives the funding from Medicare, regardless of the specialty. These and other trends will surely not spare the field of neurosurgery, regardless of what form will finally characterize future health care reform.

5

Uniting Surgeons in Response to Healthcare Reform

PAUL A. EBERT, M.D., F.A.C.S.

I was asked today to address the issue of uniting surgeons' responses to questions about health system reform. I assumed by the nature of the request that it was made on a positive basis and that we do believe that there is some value in having surgeons attempt to articulate as united a response as possible to questions about most national health issues. Certainly, for good or for bad, the lay public, government, and many of our colleagues seem to consider medicine as having three general classifications of physicians. There seem to be those who provide primary care, those who provide specialty care, and surgeons. Clearly we all recognize that surgeons are specialists, but with today's general terminology that defines specialist, it seems to apply more to the category
of medial specialist. Maybe this is not all bad, because with the current dialogue emphasizing primary care and less specialty care, surgeons seem to have been somewhat immunized by the fact that we have not greatly proliferated in number over the past 20 years. Now, I think up to this point surgeons *per se,* in what has to be considered some of the more infantile efforts to characterize the socioeconomics affecting medical care, have stayed fairly close together. In general, what has been good or bad for one surgical specialty has been pretty much generally accepted as such for and has had similar impact on other surgeons.

I will attempt to identify some factors that might cause surgeons not to be united. I think much depends on how we particularly practice and, in many specialties, such as neurosurgery, cardiac surgery, etc., there is a defined medical specialty counterpart from which many referrals generate. Most cardiac surgeons, for example, receive almost all of their referrals from cardiologists. Neurosurgeons probably do not have quite that high a referral base from neurologists but, at the same time, many major medical centers have a tendency to group departments or divisions of neurosciences and put together essentially everyone dealing with illnesses related to the nervous system. Thus, it could be logically said that neurosurgeons might be better off if they aligned their responses to questions about health reform with those of their medical counterparts, such as the neurologists. Although this suggestion sounds attractive to several of the surgical specialties, there are many in surgical specialties who essentially have a large component of office practice or nonsurgical consultation or even direct access to patients on a primary care basis and, thus, are not as easily categorized into major anatomically or physiologically based, commonly oriented services.

A second difficulty that applies to all of medicine, and especially to all surgeons, is that we across the nation have what must be considered a geographic timetable. There are some of you in the audience today who are probably very satisfied with your practice setting; there are some who have been more influenced by managed care; and there are others who feel more impacted by state or Federal government. Thus, the so-called geographic timetable of health system change across the United States has a major impact as to how much or how little each of you want major organizations to suggest health policy alterations. Also, the particular practice setting in which each of you functions makes a considerable difference as to your opinion of the importance of various factors affecting the delivery of care. Some surgeons in major clinics have almost no contact with billing, CPT codes, or day-to-day finances concerning the activities of their clinic. Others, as individual practitioners, are faced with these dilemmas on a minute-to-minute basis. We constantly note, even among each individual specialty, that there is often considerable interest or disinterest about many subjects based on how subspecialized a particular surgical specialty has become.

On the other hand, there are many areas of interest common to all areas of surgery. Surgeons, without question, have much in common in terms of their training, history, and heritage. Although I recognize that residency training in surgery has changed over the years, most surgical specialities still have some basic roots in a year or two of common training. The length and intensity of training in most surgical specialties is much greater than they are among our medical specialty or primary care colleagues. We all use a hospital or ambulatory surgical center, so we have a common bond that ties us to the quality and efficiency of the operating room environment and always has made issues relating to this area of interest common to every surgeon, regardless of specialty. Thus, it has always been relatively easy to obtain agreement and unity among surgeons in terms of dealing with the hospital administration, ambulatory surgery staff, anesthesiologists, and operating room nurses because, as usual, what was good for one surgical specialty was usually good for the other.

The recognition of the efforts in the early 1980s of many of our medical colleagues to create a relative value scale that clearly was more advantageous to the office practitioner than to the surgical specialists did much to unite surgeons. Although there were differences among surgical specialities as to whether or how to actively participate in the study, there was certainly unification of opinion among surgeon that the methodology being used contained many flaws. Fortunately or unfortunately, the opinion that much of the methodology proposed by the AMA/Harvard Study would not be useable turned out to be true. Thus, a resource-based relative value scale was created that essentially related only to the time of contact between patient and physician or surgeon. The value scale, considered by most surgeons to be somewhat unfavorable, probably has greatly united us, and we have come forth with a single voice on positions related to health policy. One might logically ask why a single unified position can not be addressed to all physicians in all disciplines of medicine, so that we as a group would not be compartmentalized or partitioned in the health system debate. Unfortunately, when we look at each specialty or each major section of medicine, there seems always to be some portion of reimbursement that is inadequate. In today's world, where no new monies are forthcoming, only redistribution seems to obtain priority. It is fair to say that the surgical profession did not initiate, nor has it ever articulated, ideas or concepts to affect redistribution to the betterment or favor of surgeons. This has clearly been an issue in which we, as surgeons, have been the target.

It is clear that we as doctors have many positive attributes that may contribute to what are sometimes considered faults that keep us from exercising a unified voice or opinion. All doctors are trained to be independent and have confidence in their own decision making. Surgeons probably receive more emphasis on this than other physicians, because many of our decisions and recommendations deal with the life or death of a patient or certainly incur the possibility of a major operative procedure. To have the confidence and assurance to make these serious recommendations, surgeons *per se* have to be independent and generally not afraid to express their opinions. Thus, I believe it is fair to say that most surgeons believe they are equally correct in issues and matters outside the realm of direct surgical consultation. When opinions on health policy are sought, we get many zero and 100 responses but not too many in the 40 to 60 category. It is not difficult to understand how surgeons feel about most issues. Another fault of the surgical profession in being unable to unite on many issues is the fact that there are few issues that are central to all surgeons. Most issues seem to affect one specialist or one site of practice more than they do others. This could be the result of geography or could simply be related to the type and method by which we practice, but it is very obvious that if the issue does not bother us, it is very doubtful that we will take any strong position one way or the other, or even bother to respond to a particular question or query. Now, one could probably say that these same issues affect the entire field of medicine, and I think in most ways they do. I just happen to believe that surgeons are often more forceful in their opinion and, at the same time, less interested in an issue if it does not directly affect them.

It is of interest that today there are more than 70 physician organization represented by some form of consultant or lobbyist or which have offices in Washington, DC. Twenty-four surgical societies in DC have either offices or hired lobbyists. This situation certainly arises from the interest in recognition by members of all surgical specialities that we must have input and information in order to have an avenue by which our opinions can be expressed. The difficulty that comes from this multispecialty is not related as much to interaction of the surgical societies as it is to the lobbyist or consultant. Many of these individuals have different opinions as to how certain policy should be addressed. Some are quite experienced in health care matters, and others have few, if any, other clients in the health care arena. Thus, we often find that it is really not you and I as surgeons who are discussing an issue; it is our secondary agents, whose opinions and egos must also be recognized and often satisfied. True, the American College of Surgeons has tried to host periodic meetings with officers and staff of each specialty organization, as well as with the lobbyists of the surgical speciality societies in DC, to attempt to discuss socioeconomic issues of concern to the surgical profession.

Over the years, the College has attempted to develop programs that would benefit all surgeons. In 1993, the College instituted a reimbursement hotline that all surgical specialists can use to get information on how best to use the CPT codes. Also, managed care symposia were initiated in 1993 and have been attended by all types of surgical specialists. Probably one of the most successful, as well as educational, unifying programs has been the College's program to bring surgeons from various states to meet their representatives and senators. These meetings have usually been organized through individual chapters of surgeons, and certainly all types of surgical specialists have attended and participated. Let me ad lib for a moment and simply emphasize the amount of money that surgical societies, as well as other medical societies, have spent for consultants and lobbyists in Washington. I must ask, except for informational return, what has that dollar brought us? Clearly, there have been several victories: the definition of surgical services; the maintenance of some payment for assistants at surgery; and, of course, the Medicare Volume Performance Standard, which has been beneficial to all surgeons in the reimbursement of Medicare patients. Obviously, we probably could have simplified and united our responses if we concentrated our efforts in one consulting firm. However, we at the College have always been willing to share whatever information we have and offer the availability of our particular consulting firm to all surgeons, regardless of their specialty or whether particular societies had their own representatives. Without doubt, advice from a single consultant probably simplifies the problem of attempting to come forth with a unified response to most issues.

Future suggestions for unifying opinions and positions among the surgical specialists so that we may be more effective in the health system debate should improve. I actually believe that it is going to be easier in coming years to singularly identify positions that are clearly beneficial to the patient and positions by which surgeons would clearly unite. I say this because surgical practice *per se* has not changed as much in many settings as has medical practice. Surgeons are not being asked to deny the provision of treatments, as are some primary care physicians in a managed care setting. I recognize that patients may not be sent to us as quickly or as frequently in these situations, but at the same time when they are sent, we are asked to do what we would normally do for these patients. Thus, I believe surgeons will have an easier time providing true quality care and can articulate the importance of quality to their patients. Also, I believe the means of communication among surgical specialties are much better today than they were a decade ago. Each specialty is interested and recognizes the need to have an interest in our health system. Informal meetings between societies, the College, and the leadership of all surgical specialties will tend to form confidences and, undoubtedly, more comfort in supporting positions that oftentimes do not always particularly affect a particular specialist. At the same time, it still seems logical and, from my own personal experience in the past 8 years, that it is very rare that there is much disagreement among surgical specialists. Oftentimes, disagreement is not over the issue or the principle involved, but basically a discussion of when and how best to lend our support to particular political positions. At the same time, I do not believe that unification can be mandatory, because if a position is derogatory to a particular specialty, there is no logic that the specialty should support it. However, it is unusual that, concerning an issue that does not affect a particular specialty, for that specialty to take a distant and remote position, rather than believing that if it helps the majority of other surgical specialists, it is probably worth the support.

Thus, as we approach the reform of the health care system in the twenty-first century, surgeons need to be better informed and to express their opinions. Obviously, the more unified we can be in expressing our opinions, the stronger voice we have both within medicine as well as in the national health debate. I believe we all recognize that historically, even though surgery may have had somewhat of a common trunk, the direction of surgical specialities over the past one hundred years has been to be somewhat isolated and independent. They have focused mainly on the fact that a particular area of knowledge required specific education. Result are better and education and knowledge can progress more rapidly when absorbed in a more concentrated form. Thus, when we approach issues now such as health policy or any socioeconomic events that affect our entire surgical profession, it is without question, somewhat of a reversion of our past hundred years of experience to decide that in these arenas, we may be better as a unified group as, in my opinion, no component of surgery will have a significant voice unless it is a single voice expressed by all surgeons. As I stated earlier, whether we like it or not, the public regards surgeons as surgeons and, thus we best be able to respond to dilemmas in the public arena as surgeons and with a unified voice.

II

General Scientific
Session II—Controversies
in Skull Base Surgery

6

Radical Resection of Anterior Skull Base Tumors

MICHAEL T. LAWTON, M.D., MARK G. HAMILTON, M.D.C.M.,
STEPHEN P. BEALS, M.D., EDWARD F. JOGANIC, M.D.,
AND ROBERT F. SPETZLER, M.D.

Honored Guest Lecture

PART I: THE TRANSFACIAL APPROACHES

Introduction

Tumors of the anterior cranial fossa and clivus can be resected completely through transfacial routes of exposure (4–8, 10, 11, 13–17, 19, 22–25, 27, 28, 32, 35, 36, 39–42, 44–47, 51, 53, 56, 57, 59–62). These exposures provide safe avenues through areas of complex anatomy where critical structures were once considered insurmountable obstacles for curative resection. Paul Tessier *et al.* (58) established the principles for the correction of congenital facial anomalies. He demonstrated that intracranial and extracranial surgical exposures can be combined without undue risk of infection; that the orbits can be osteotomized; that the globes can be moved without causing blindness; and that the facial bones can be stripped of periosteum, osteotomized, repositioned, and still survive. Transfacial disassembly widely exposes the midline skull base for visualization of tumors and critical structures. Direct anterior approaches to the midline skull base and anterior cranial fossa have potentially important advantages, compared to lateral approaches, for the surgical management of certain lesions. First, access is obtained through the relatively avascular midline plane. Second, the surgical approach is directed straight at the bulk of the lesion, and the surgical working distance is reduced. Third, vital neurovascular structures, the temporomandibular joint, and the muscles of mastication are avoided. Finally, facial incisions are seldom needed because of the wide exposure that is possible with facial degloving.

Building on our preliminary clinical experience with transfacial exposures, the authors have found it helpful to organize transfacial approaches into six "levels." This classification system, which is based on selecting the most appropriate angle of approach to the anatomic site of the tumor (Table 6.1, Figs. 6.1–6.8) (5, 6, 17) can help the surgeon to plan appropriate surgical strategies for lesions of this region (Fig. 6.1).

Classification of Transfacial Approaches

The anatomic site of tumors or other lesions of the anterior cranial fossa and clivus (midline skull base) guides the selection of a surgical

TABLE 6.1
Transfacial Approaches to Anterior Skull Base and Clivus: Classification Scheme

Level	Name	Anatomic Sites of Lesions
I	Transfrontal	Anterior cranial fossa (Fig. 6.2)
II	Transfrontal nasal	Anterior cranial fossa, nasopharynx, clivus tumors with anterior growth (Fig. 6.3)
III	Transfrontal-nasal-orbital	Large anterior cranial fossa or nasopharyngeal lesions, clivus tumors with anterior growth (Figs. 6.3, 6.4, and 6.8)
IV	Transnasomaxillary	Nasopharyngeal lesions, large clivus lesions that extend anteriorly, posteriorly, or inferiorly (Fig. 6.5)
V	Transmaxillary	Clivus lesions with superior and inferior extensions, small nasopharyngeal lesions(Figs. 6.6 and 6.8)
VI	Transpalatal	Lower clivus region lesions (Fig. 6.7)

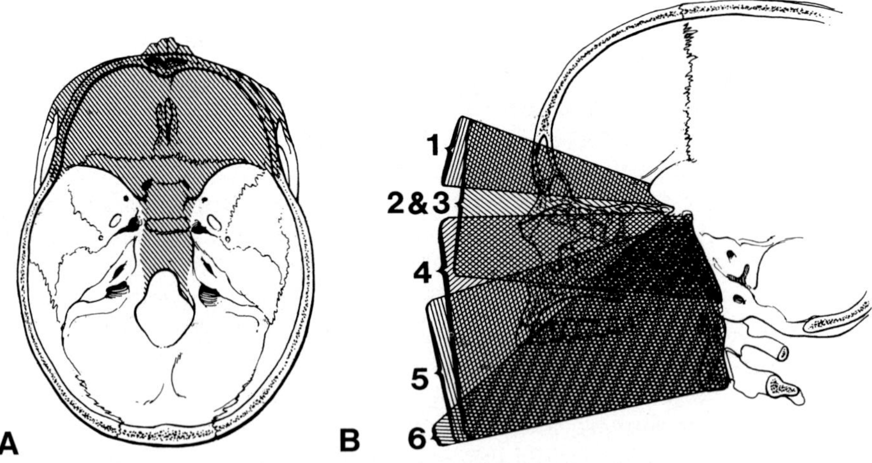

FIG. 6.1 (**A**) Scope of tumor sites in the anterior skull base and clivus that can be exposed by transfacial routes. (**B**) Summation of the six different levels of approach, demonstrating that the anatomic site of the tumor and direction of growth determine the level of transfacial exposure. The overlapping exposure shared by these exposures allows flexibility in choosing the best angle of surgical approach. [Reproduced with permission from (6).]

approach. The skull base has a kyphotic configuration that is approximately perpendicular to the vertical plane of the face. This general principle dictates that tumors with an anterior extension be approached from a superior approach through the frontal-nasal region (levels I to IV); posteriorly located tumors with more superior exten-

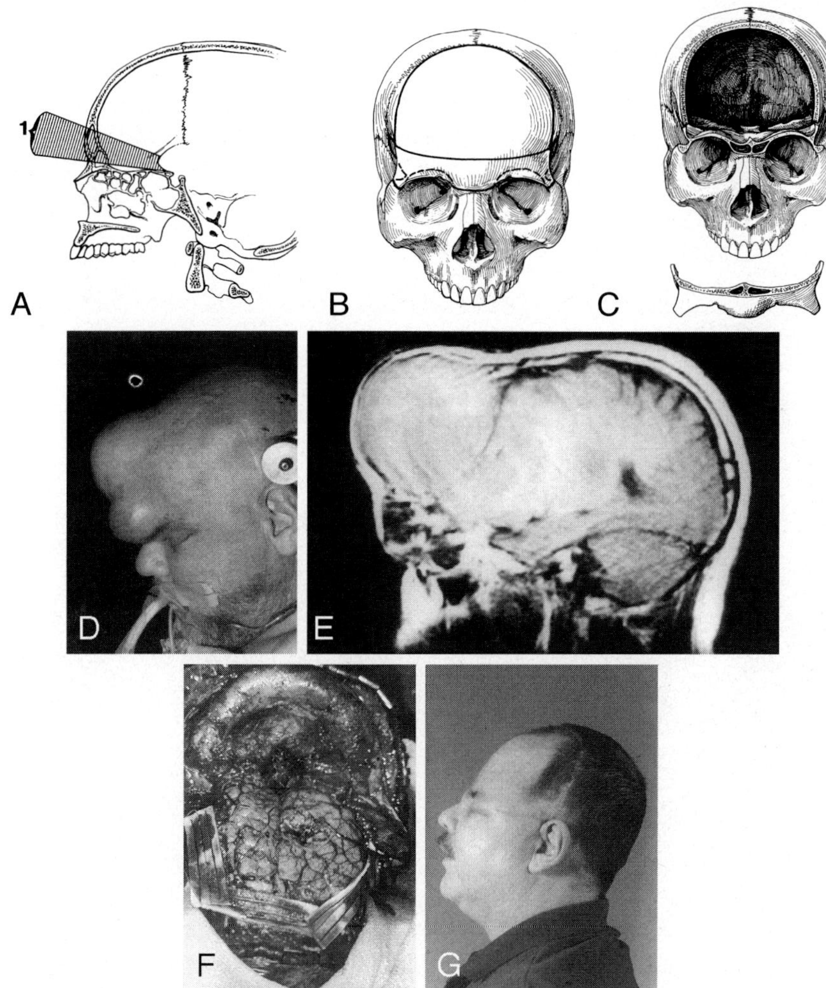

FIG. 6.2 (**A**) Level I **transfrontal** exposure from anterior cranial fossa and cribriform lesions. (**B** and **C**) level I exposure requires osteotomy of the supraorbital bar. A 35-year-old man (**D**) presented with the malignant fibrous histiocytoma shown on a sagittal T1-weighted MRI (**E**). A level I transfrontal approach was used to resect the lesion (**F**). The patient is shown 3 months after resection (**G**). [Reproduced with permission from (6).]

sion, especially behind the sella turcica, should be accessed through a more inferior or transmaxillary surgical approach (levels IV to VI).

To aid in the decision-making process, transfacial surgical exposures have been classified into six levels (Table 6.1 and Figs. 6.1–6.7) (5, 6, 17). The first three approaches (levels I to III) build on the supraorbital

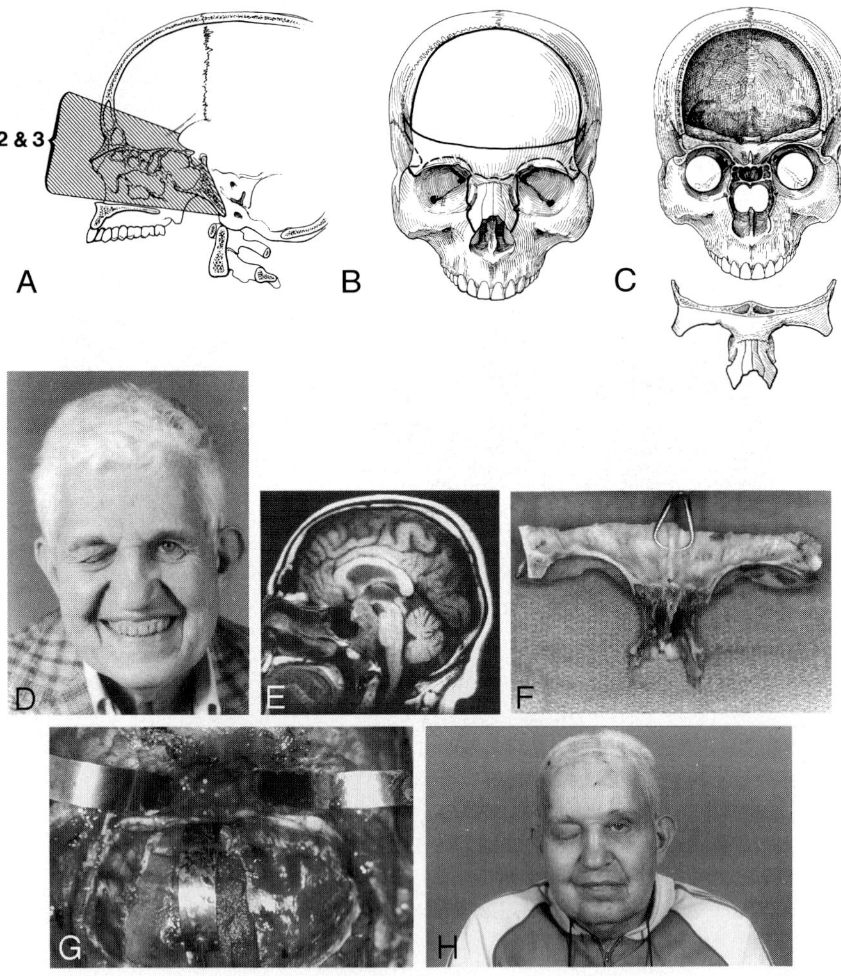

FIG. 6.3 (A) Level II **transfrontal-nasal** exposure for anterior approach to the anterior cranial fossa and clivus. This exposure is identical to that used for the level III approach. (B and C) Level II exposure requires removing the frontonasal unit. A 68-year-old man (D) presented with a recurrent clivus chordoma shown on a sagittal T1-weighted MRI (E). Level II transfrontal-nasal approach (F) was used to resect the lesion (G). The patient is shown 1 month after resection (H). [Reproduced with permission from (6).]

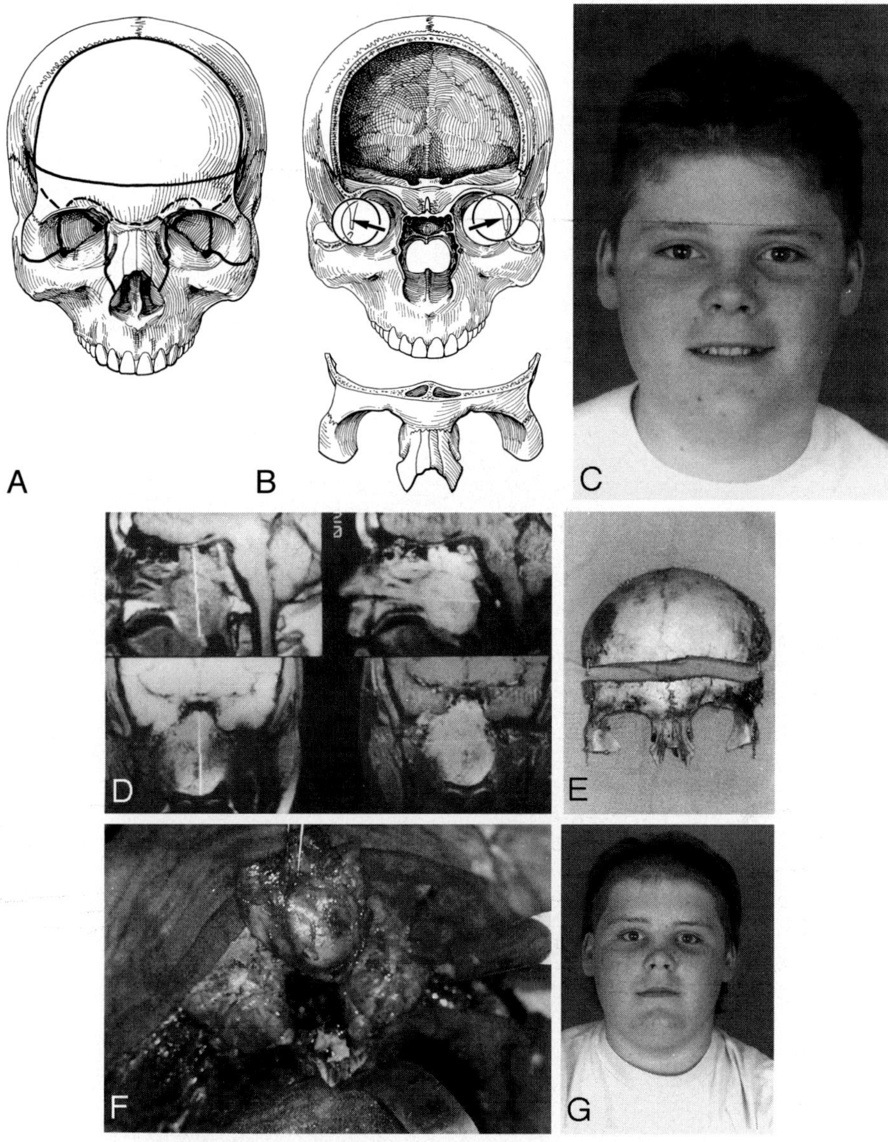

FIG. 6.4 Level III **transfrontal nasal-orbital** exposure for larger anterior cranial fossa and clivus lesions. This level of approach is similar to that of level II (see Fig. 6.3A). However, this approach provides a wider exposure by allowing lateral retraction of the globes. (**A** and **B**) Level III exposure includes the lateral orbital walls on the frontonasal fragment (frontal nasal-orbital unit). A 16-year-old boy (**C**) presented with state II angiofibroma of the nasopharynx shown on sagittal and coronal MRIs without and with gadolinium. (**D**) After preoperative embolization of the tumor, a level III transfrontal-nasal-orbital approach (**E**) was used to resect the lesion (**F**). The patient is shown 1 month after resection (**G**). [Reprinted with permission from (6).]

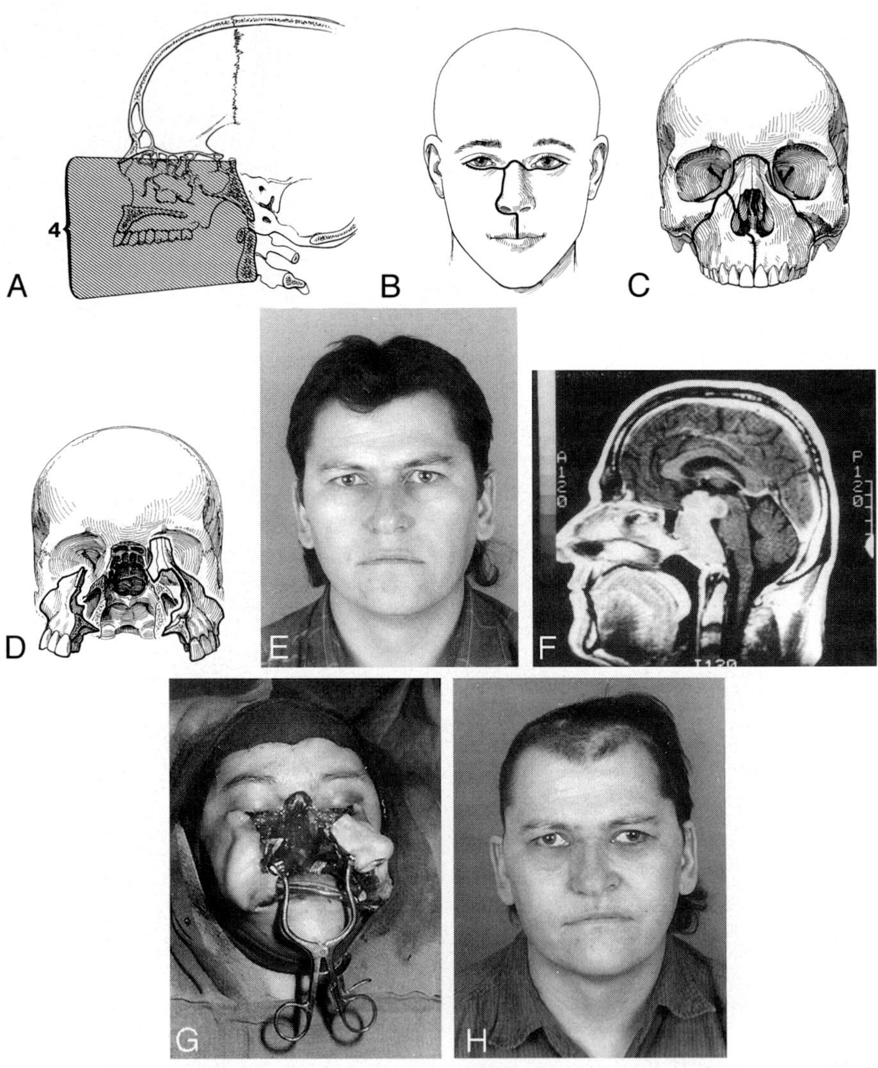

FIG. 6.5 (**A**) Level IV **nasomaxillary** osteotomy yields a wide exposure of the entire central skull base from the radix to the cervical spine. A similar degree of exposure usually can be obtained with a combination of the level III and level V exposures. (**B**) Incisions for the transmaxillary approach. (**C** and **D**) Level IV exposure requires a Le Fort II osteotomy. A 26-year-old man (**E**) presented with a large clival tumor shown on a sagittal T1-weighted MRI with gadolinium (**F**). Level IV transnasomaxillary approach was used to resect the lesion (**G**). The patient is shown 3 months after resection (**H**). [Reprinted with permission from (6).]

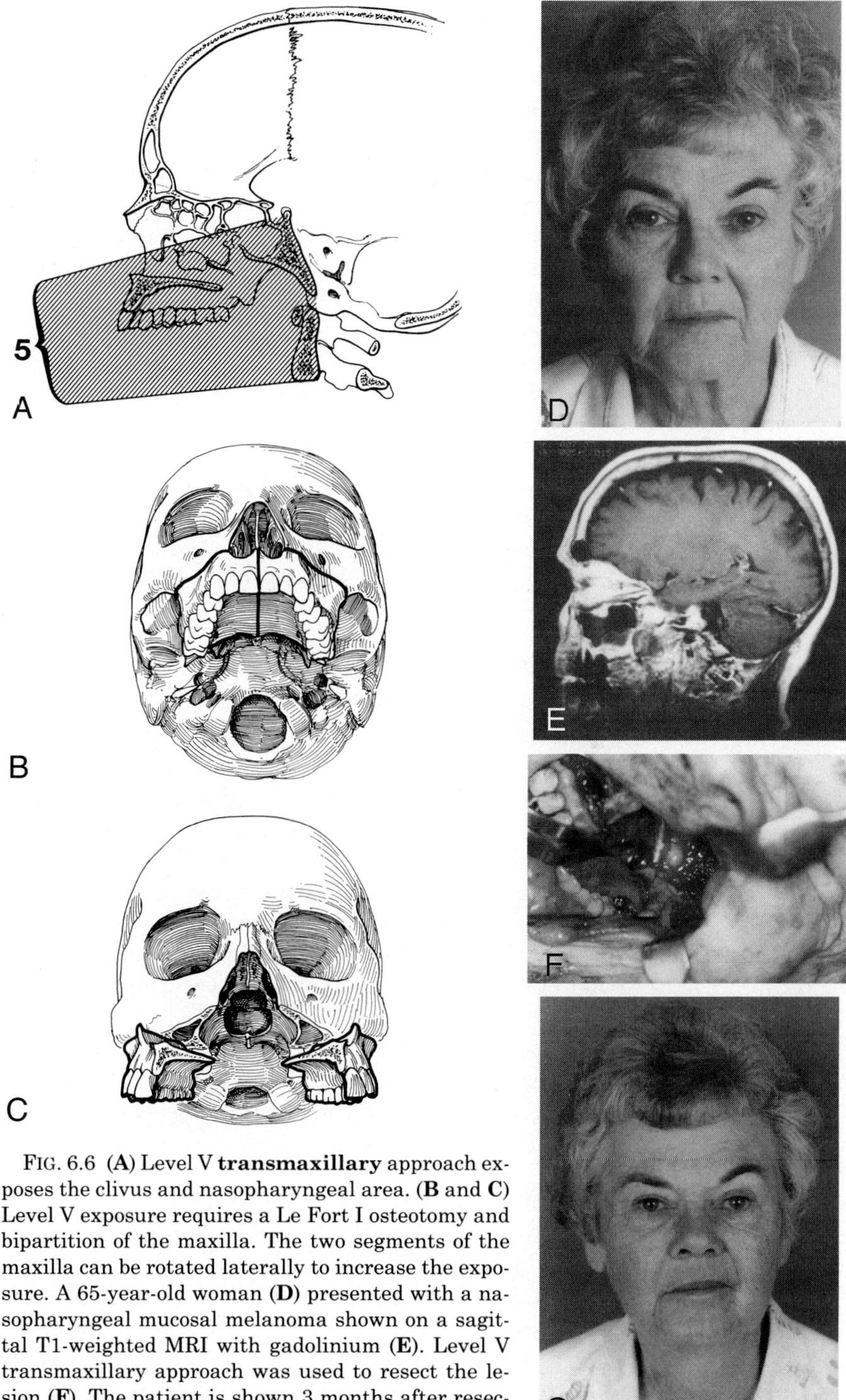

FIG. 6.6 (**A**) Level V **transmaxillary** approach exposes the clivus and nasopharyngeal area. (**B** and **C**) Level V exposure requires a Le Fort I osteotomy and bipartition of the maxilla. The two segments of the maxilla can be rotated laterally to increase the exposure. A 65-year-old woman (**D**) presented with a nasopharyngeal mucosal melanoma shown on a sagittal T1-weighted MRI with gadolinium (**E**). Level V transmaxillary approach was used to resect the lesion (**F**). The patient is shown 3 months after resection (**G**). [Reproduced with permission from (6).]

bar (Figs. 6.2–6.4 and 6.8). Subfrontal access that is achieved by removal of the supraorbital bar is extended vertically to include the entire midline skull base to the craniocervical junction by removing the nasal complex and medial orbital walls on the supraorbital bar. Greater horizontal exposure is achieved by adding the lateral orbital walls and orbital roofs to the frontal nasal fragment. Greater posterior exposure with level II and III approaches can be achieved with a circumferential cribriform plate osteotomy (Figs. 6.9 and 6.10) that allows for retraction of the cribriform plate. Its preservation also has the advantage of diminishing the risk of a cerebrospinal fluid (CSF) leak, simplifying skull base reconstruction, and saving olfaction. Preservation of the cribriform plate is an option when the region is not involved with tumor.

The final three approaches (levels IV to VI) provide various degrees of exposure to the posterior skull base through the maxilla. The level IV approach exposes the entire midline skull base; the level V approach exposes the lower half; and the level VI approach exposes the lower third of the skull base.

LEVEL I: TRANSFRONTAL APPROACH

Indications. This approach is used to access tumors of the anterior cranial fossa and those that extend into the superior orbital region (Fig. 6.2) (28).

Technique. A bicoronal scalp incision is used to achieve this exposure. Its position must be posterior enough to permit an adequate length of frontogaleal flap to be dissected for reconstruction of the skull base. After the radix and upper orbits have been exposed, the temporalis muscles are reflected, and a bifrontal craniotomy is performed. The dura is dissected from the anterior cranial fossa, and the supraorbital bar is removed to facilitate exposure of the anterior cranial fossa and cribriform plate.

After tumor resection, the skull base is reconstructed, trying to achieve a watertight separation from the nasopharynx with local flaps and cranial autografts. Fibrin glue can be used to seal the suture lines further.

LEVEL II: TRANSFRONTAL—NASAL APPROACH

Indications. This approach is used to expose the anterior cranial fossa, nasopharynx, clivus, and tumors that grow anteriorly (Fig. 6.3). A level II exposure also is useful for exposing tumors that extend into the superior, medial, and posterior aspects of the orbit. Compared to the level I approach, additional exposure is achieved by retaining the nasal and medial orbital wall complex on the supraorbital bar.

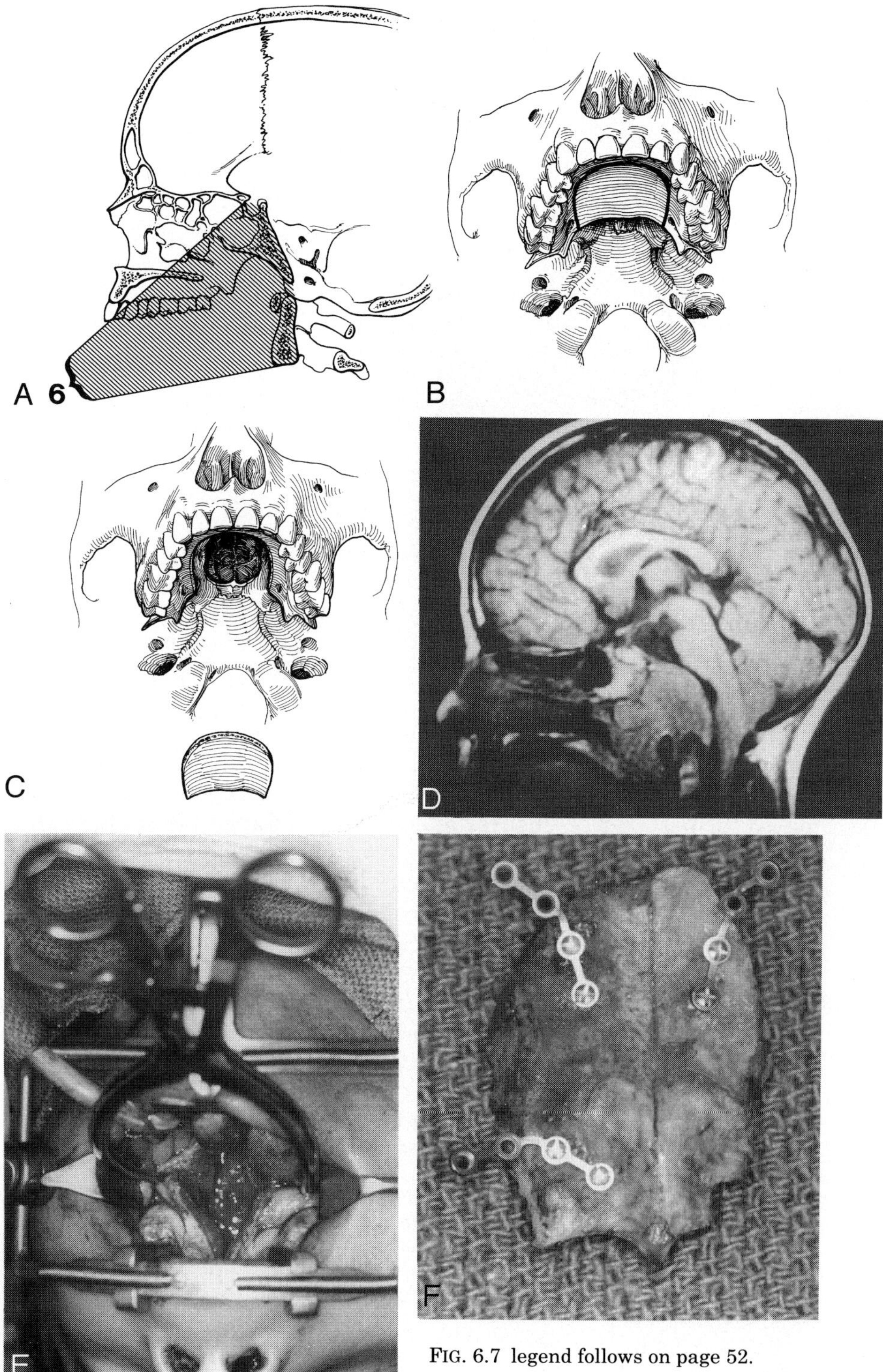

FIG. 6.7 legend follows on page 52.

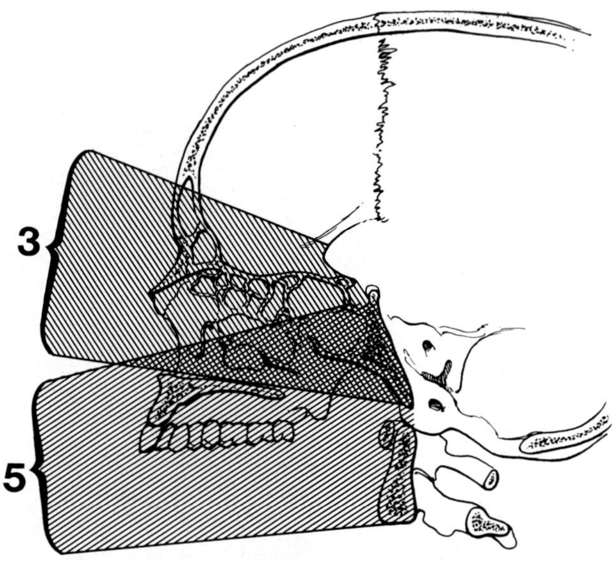

FIG. 6.8 A combination of level III and level V approaches exposes most of the anterior skull base and clivus. The combination of the two approaches is illustrated with the cribriform plate preserved. [Reproduced with permission from (6).]

Technique. While providing wide access to the nasopharynx, as well as to the ethmoid and sphenoid sinuses, the transfrontal-nasal approach is a direct anterior approach to the clivus. A bicoronal incision, placed far posteriorly, ensures adequate local flaps to reconstruct the skull base. The flap is reflected anteriorly, exposing the radix, nasal bones, and nasal process of the maxilla, as well as stripping the periorbita. The medial canthal ligaments are taken down, and the upper lateral canthal cartilages are detached from the nasal bones. The nasolacrimal duct is exposed and preserved. A fragment of bone can be retained on the medial canthal ligament to facilitate subsequent transnasal wiring. A bifrontal craniotomy and dural dissection are performed, and the supraorbital bar and nasal orbital complex are osteotomized and removed.

After the tumor has been resected, the frontal nasal fragment is re-

FIG. 6.7 (**A**) Level VI **transpalatal** approach accesses the lower clivus and upper cervical region. (**B** and **C**) Level VI exposure requires an osteotomy of the palate. A 9-year-old girl presented with a clivus chordoma shown on sagittal T1-weighted MRI (**D**). Level VI transpalatal approach was used to resect the lesion (**E**). The palatal fragment is rigidly affixed with microplates and screws after tumor resection (**F**). [Reproduced with permission from (6).]

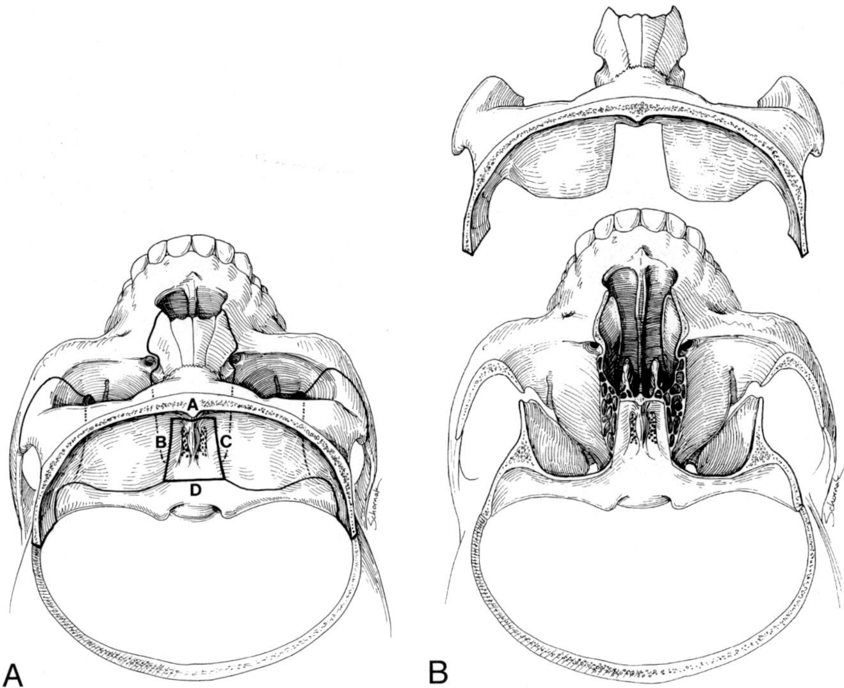

FIG. 6.9 (**A**) Illustration of the frontal skull anatomy, demonstrating the initial circumferential cribriform plate osteotomies. *A*, anterior osteotomy; *B* and *C*, parasagittal osteotomy; *D*, posterior osteotomy through the planum sphenoidale. The *additional lines* indicate osteotomy cuts for removal of the frontonasal-orbital unit. (**B**) All osteotomy cuts, except for *D*, are performed to allow removal of the frontonasal-orbital unit. [Reproduced with permission from (6).]

turned to its anatomic position. Rigid fixation with small plates and screws is preferred. The skull base is reconstructed as needed with local flaps and cranial autografts. The upper lateral cartilages must be reattached to the nasal bones, and the medial canthal ligaments are repaired by transnasal wiring.

LEVEL III: TRANSFRONTAL-NASAL-ORBITAL APPROACH

Indications. Large anterior cranial fossa or nasopharyngeal lesions and clival lesions with anterior extension can be accessed through a level III exposure (Figs. 6.4 and 6.8). Similar to the level II approach, the level III approach is augmented by including the lateral orbital wall and orbital roofs on the frontal nasal fragment. Consequently, the globes can be retracted laterally.

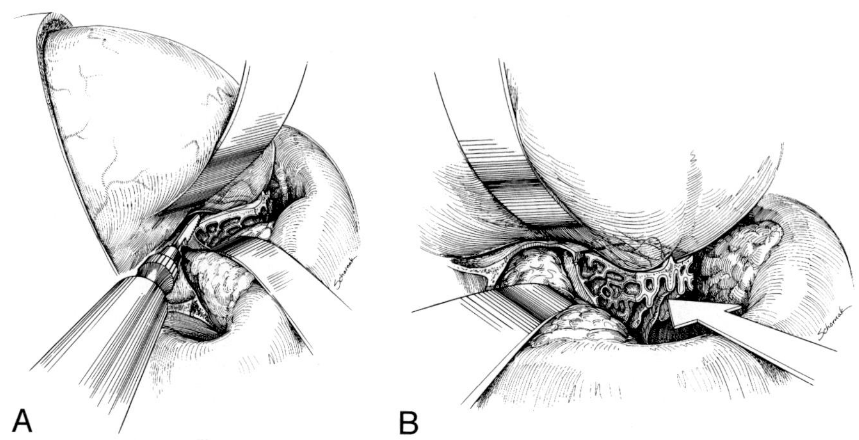

FIG. 6.10 (**A**) The final osteotomy cut (*D*, planum sphenoidale, in Figure 6.9A) is performed with appropriate retraction of the dura of the frontal lobe and paranasal soft tissues. (**B**) After the trabeculae have been divided and a generous cuff of mucosa has been left intact, the intact cribriform plate unit is released from the skull base. [Reproduced with permission from (6).]

Technique. The method of dissection is identical to that used in the level II approach. The osteotomy includes the lateral orbital walls from the level of the infraorbital fissure as part of the supraorbital fragment. Most of the superior orbital roof also can be included in the fragment to facilitate the lateral retraction of the globes (Figs. 6.4 and 6.8).

CRIBRIFORM PLATE PRESERVATION

Indications. When one is performing a level II or III approach to a tumor that does not involve the cribriform plate, the integrity of the cribriform plate and olfactory nerves can be preserved. This technique permits greater posterior exposure while simplifying reconstruction of the skull base. It thereby reduces the risk of CSF leak and preserves olfaction (Figs. 6.9 and 6.10) (52).

Technique. The craniotomy for the level II or III approach is performed in the usual fashion. Fixation plates are preregistered before the craniotomy is performed and before the frontonasal-orbital bar is removed. After CSF has been drained with a spinal drain, the dura is separated from the orbital roofs, and the frontonasal-orbital area is exposed as described. Osteotomies are performed to remove the frontonasal or frontonasal-orbital unit, leaving the cribriform plate exposed (Fig. 6.9)(52). Under direct vision, an osteotomy is performed posterior to the cribriform plate through the planum sphenoidale (Fig.

6.10). The final cut is made through the ethmoid bone and nasal mucosa. Care is taken to preserve a generous cuff of nasal mucosa attached inferiorly to the cribriform plate (Fig. 6.10). This final maneuver completes the separation of the cribriform plate from all bony connection and leaves it attached to the base of the frontal dura with the olfactory nerve rootlets left intact. The frontal lobes, with the dura intact, can be elevated generously to access the involved area. The cribriform plate is reattached to the supraorbital-nasal bar with stainless steel wires. The remainder of the craniotomy is reconstructed as described for levels I, II, or III.

LEVEL IV: TRANSNASOMAXILLARY APPROACH

Indications. Wide exposure of the entire central skull base region can be achieved through the transnasomaxillary approach, which is produced with a Le Fort II osteotomy. This approach can be used for large nasopharyngeal and clival lesions, particularly those that extend anteriorly, posteriorly, inferiorly, superiorly, or in all four directions (Fig. 6.5).

Technqiue. A modified Weber-Ferguson incision (Fig. 6.5) is extended across the radix and along the subciliary margin on the lower lid on the opposite side. After skeletal exposure, a Le Fort II osteotomy is performed. The osteotomy crosses just medial to the infraorbital foramen and nasolacrimal duct. Although the nasolacrimal duct usually can be preserved, excess retraction of the fragments can disrupt it. If extreme retraction is needed, the nasolacrimal ducts can be cannulated, transected, and then repaired over the tubes. The nasal fragment is divided at the nasal process of the maxilla on one side, and the palate is split at the midline, yielding two fragments. The nasal soft-tissue complex remains intact and is retracted with the fragment. The approach can be performed from either side, depending on which side can provide the best angle of exposure for the tumor. Fixation plates are preregistered by passive adaptation and application before the osteotomy. After tumor resection, reassembly is accomplished with the previously prepared plates and an acrylic interdental splint fabricated from dental models. The splint is left in place after surgery to add stability to the fixation. Intermaxillary fixation is not used. Incisions must be repaired meticulously to yield the best possible aesthetic results.

LEVEL V: TRANSMAXILLARY APPROACH

Indications. Small clival lesions with superior, posterior, and inferior extensions and small-to-moderate nasopharyngeal lesions can be accessed through this approach; this is accomplished through a Le Fort I osteotomy with or without a palatal split (Figs. 6.6 and 6.8).

Technique. An intraoral approach is utilized through an upper buccal sulcus incision. The anterior maxilla is prepared for a Le Fort I osteotomy. If a palatal split is required, the midline is incised through the oral mucosa and the soft palate to one side of the uvula. The Le Fort I osteotomy is then performed and split in the midline to the back of the soft palate (Fig. 6.6) (7, 45, 49). The two maxillary fragments can then be rotated laterally to expose the clivus. After tumor resection, reassembly is performed with prepared interdental splints and preregistered fixation plates.

LEVEL VI: TRANSPALATAL APPROACH

Indications. This approach exposes the lower clival and upper cervical regions for resection of small tumors by removing the hard palate and splitting the soft palate (Fig. 6.7).

Technique. The palate is approached through both the nasal floor and oral mucosa. The upper buccal sulcus is incised, allowing the nasal floor to be approached extramucosally. The incision is made through the midline of the oral mucosa and through the soft palate to one side of the uvula. Mucoperiosteal flaps are elevated from the palatal surface to the alveolar margin around the greater palatine foramen to the maxillary tuberosity. The septum is separated from the nasal groove along the nasal floor. A reciprocating saw is used around the margin of the palate against the alveolar edge, just medial to the greater palatine foramen. Cuts are made in the lateral nasal wall into the antra with an osteotome. The bony palate is lifted out, and the soft-tissue portions are retracted. The vomer and perpendicular plate of the ethmoid are removed with a rongeur for further exposure (Fig. 6.7).

After tumor resection, preregistered microplates on the bone fragment (attached to the oral surface of the palatal fragment) are used for rigid fixation. The soft tissue is closed with absorbable sutures.

General Treatment Techniques

Patients with lesions affecting the anterior skull base and clivus are assessed by a careful history and physical examination, followed by computed tomography (CT) and magnetic resonance imaging (MRI) of the cranium and neural structures (34). Angiography is performed, if needed for diagnosis, preoperative assessment of involved vessels, or a therapeutic option (*e.g.,* preoperative tumor embolization). Postoperative CT is obtained for all patients, MRI in most patients. Preoperatively, the patient is counseled by the surgical team and a dedicated craniofacial nurse. Patients undergoing level V or VI approach have an acrylic splint of their teeth fashioned preoperatively to aid in reconstruction and to eliminate the need for arch bars in referencing the mandibular arch.

When indicated, prophylactic postoperative lumbar spinal drainage is instituted for 3 days to avoid unwanted CSF leakage through the transfacial surgical operative site. All patients receive antibiotic prophylaxis (intravenous cefuroxime (1.5 g) before surgery and for three postoperative doses or every 8 hours until CSF drainage is discontinued) and prophylaxis for deep-vein thrombosis (*e.g.,* graduated leg stockings, intermittent pneumatic leg compression) (18).

Patients are positioned supinely on the operating table, and three-pin skull fixation is used to secure the head. The skull pins are positioned posterior to the ears when a bicoronal scalp incision is required. For level IV to VI approaches, the endotracheal tube is secured to the lower dentition with 26-gauge wire to ensure a secure airway. The ISG localizing wand (ISG Technologies, Mississauga, Ontario, Canada) is used for all patients undergoing tumor resection. Temporary tarsorrhaphy sutures of 5-0 cardiovascular silk are placed in the eyelids to protect the corneas. A 1-cm strip of hair is shaved when a bicoronal incision is required, followed by infiltration of the intended incision with a mixture of Marcaine and epinephrine. For appropriate patients an epinephrine mixture is infiltrated into the upper buccal sulcus and mucosa in the anterior maxillary region. The anterior scalp flap (for levels I to III) is reflected by microneedle dissection (15), which is more hemostatic and preserves the important pericranial and temporalis tissues for possible use as flaps. When tissue dissection is completed, all osteotomy lines are marked with a sterile pencil, and the intended bone fragments are preregistered with fixation plates to ensure anatomic reconstruction of the facial units after disassembly. Bifrontal craniotomy flaps are performed using the Midas Rex drill (Midas Rex Pneumatic Tools, Fort Worth, TX), while all orbital osteotomies are performed with a reciprocating saw.

After tumor resection, reassembly is performed. If needed, the skull base and orbital walls can be reconstructed with split cranial grafts, which can be harvested from the inner table of the bifrontal bone flap. Sealing the intracranial and extracranial interface is important in level I to III approaches, particularly if the dura has been entered. Depending on the location and size of the defect, the seal can be achieved with regional flaps, such as those taken from pericranial, frontogaleal, and temporalis muscle. Such flaps should be inset and sutured into place after replacement of the supraorbital bar complex. If the cribriform plate has been sacrificed, it is ideal to place a flap on the nasal and intracranial side of the bone graft. If the cribriform plate has been preserved, a single flap is used to cover the osteotomy defect, and the cribriform plate is reattached to its anatomic site with wire fixation. Fibrin glue can be used to seal the flap margins to obtain a watertight closure. The upper lateral nasal cartilage must be reattached to the caudal margins of the nasal bones to prevent saddlenose deformity, and the medial canthal ligament is repaired by transnasal wiring.

After tumor resection through transmaxillary approaches, defects in the sella turcica, sphenoid, or clivus can be filled with a dermal fat graft or bone graft before mucosal closure. A palatal fistula can occur if reapproximation of the palatal mucosa is not meticulous. No nasal pack is required after these approaches (levels IV to VI). The dental splint should be left intact between 10 and 14 days. Routine oral care for a Le Fort I osteotomy is used. The patient is kept on a liquid diet for 4 weeks, then on a soft diet for 4 weeks, and then returned to a normal diet at 8 weeks. Patients with a level VI approach can be advanced to a normal diet much faster.

Summary of Clinical Experience

Between February 1990 and June 1994, 32 patients (19 males and 13 females) underwent a transfacial surgical approach to treat lesions involving the anterior skull base and clivus. Their mean age was 37.7 years (range, 7 to 71 years).

Lesions included a wide spectrum of tumor pathologies (Table 6.2), although chordoma and angiofibroma were the most common. Altogether 41 levels were utilized; level 1, $n = 1$; level II, $n = 2$; level III, $n = 14$; level IV, $n = 2$; level V, $n = 14$; and level VI, $n = 8$. Twenty-three patients underwent a single transfacial operation, using one level; five patients underwent a single transfacial operation, using a combination of levels III and V; and four patients underwent two transfacial operations, each using one level (two for tumor recurrence (chordoma, fibrosarcoma), one for repair of CSF leak, and one for repositioning of bone fragments). Gross total resection was possible in 30 of these 32 patients.

Complications related to treatment occurred in 14 patients and included six CSF leaks (four patients treated with lumbar drains, two treated with surgical procedures), two strokes (one related to a C3-C5 bypass; one related to erosion of a central-line catheter through the vessel), two superficial wound infections (one surgically treated, one treated with antibiotics), and two small palatal fistulae (both surgically repaired). Two patients experienced transient pituitary dysfunc-

TABLE 6.2
Lesion Type for Transfacial Surgery

Lesion Type	No. of Patients
Chordoma[a]	7
Angiofibroma	4
Craniocervical anomalies/instability	4
Pituitary adenoma	2
Meningioma	2
Adenocystic carcinoma	2
Fibrosarcoma[a]	2
Melanoma	1
Ossifying fibroma	1
Inflammatory clival mass	1
Malignant fibrous histiocytoma	1
Myxochondrosarcoma	1
Neurofibroma of cranial nerve V2	1
Odontogenic myxoma	1
Papillary adenocarcinoma	1
Osteochondrosarcoma	1
Osteoma	1
CSF leak	1
Malpositioned bone fragment	1
Orbitomaxillary encephalocele	1

[a]One patient underwent repeated craniofacial surgery for tumor recurrence.

tion; two had cranial nerve deficits; and the nasolacrimal duct was injured in one patient (repaired). Permanent neurologic morbidity associated with treatment occurred in three patients (9%). No deaths were related directly to surgery.

The length of follow-up was a mean of 11.3 ± 11.6 months (range, 0.5 to 40.7 months). At the last follow-up examination, the Glasgow Outcome Scale (GOS) was used to classify patients' outcome (26): 20 patients were classified as good; 4 patients were classified as having moderate disability; 3 patients were classified as having severe disability; and 5 patients had died. The 27 surviving patients have been followed for a mean of 11.7 ± 12.2 months (range, 0.5 to 40.7 months), and the five patients who died were followed for a mean of 9.0 ± 7.9 months after surgery (range, 0.9 to 18.7 months). Three patients died after their tumors recurred (two had metastatic disease (melanoma, malignant fibrous histiocytoma), and one with local disease (chordoma). One patient died from fungal meningitis 15 months after surgery, and one patient died 3 weeks after surgery from an airway obstruction and respiratory arrest after vomiting while in a halo brace.

CASE REPORT

This patient illustrates the spectrum of transfacial exposure possible when level III and level V exposures are combined. A 16-year-old boy sought treatment after 3 years of frequent nosebleeds, sinus congestion, and anosmia. His physical examination was normal, except for the anosmia. Nasal endoscopy revealed a tumor mass, and CT revealed a large enhancing nasal-paranasal mass consistent with juvenile angiofibroma (Fig. 6.11). Preoperative angiography and tumor embolization were performed. A gross total resection of tumor was accomplished, using a combination of level III and level V approaches with preservation of the cribriform plate. Postoperative MRI confirmed complete tumor removal. The patient's postoperative course was unremarkable, and he had no postoperative deficits. Olfaction returned after 4 weeks.

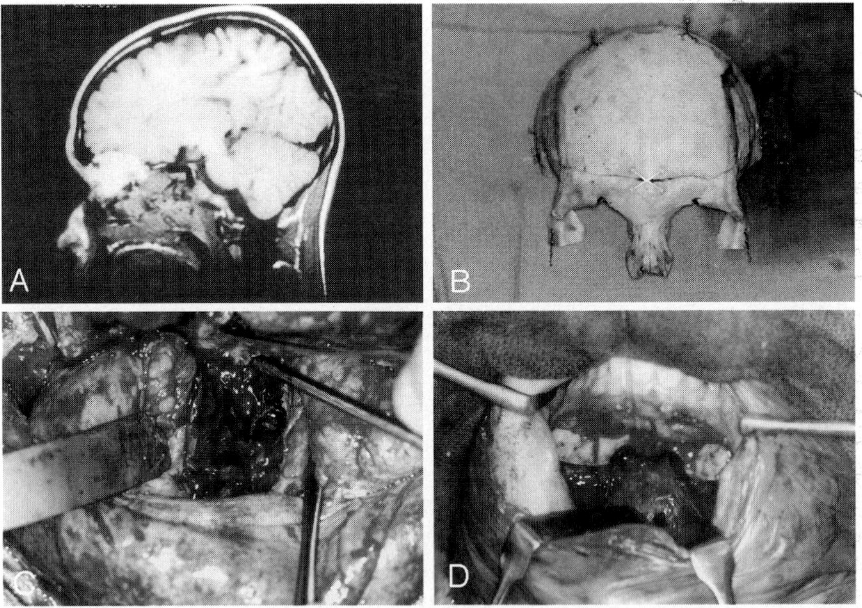

FIG. 6.11 Sixteen-year-old patient with angiofibroma who underwent combined level III and level V approaches with preservation of the cribriform plate. The tumor was resected completely. (A) Preoperative MRI, demonstrating large enhancing paranasal mass. Intraoperative photographs of (B) frontonasal-orbital unit and (C) the extended exposure of the tumor obtained with the level III approach. The retractor blade is positioned upon the medial aspect of the left globe. (D) Intraoperative photograph, demonstrating the extended exposure of the tumor obtained with the level V approach. [Reproduced with permission from (6).]

Discussion

Deep-seated lesions of the anterior skull base and clivus remain significant treatment challenges. Many benign and malignant tumors can occur in this region. The complex and critical anatomy of this region can accord increased difficulties for both surgeon and patient. When surgical resection is an important component of the treatment regimen, tumor resection must be maximized while morbidity is minimized. These two goals can be accomplished by using appropriately selected transfacial approaches (6, 15, 17, 32, 46). Transfacial approaches are best performed by a multidisciplinary team composed of a neurosurgeon, a craniofacial surgeon, an otolaryngologist, and an interventional neuroradiologist. A multidisciplinary team expands the possible surgical approaches that are available to deal with these complex lesions.

Most of the transfacial techniques reported here have been described previously. No logical organizational scheme, however, has been available to help the surgeon choose the most suitable transfacial approach for an individual lesion. Several features must be considered when selecting a transfacial approach: (*a*) the location and size of the lesion, (*b*) the tumor type and its biologic behavior, (*c*) the patient's age, and (*d*) the surgeon's preference and experience. From our experience with these transfacial exposures in 32 patients, we developed a classification system that uses the anatomic site of the lesion to direct the selection of the surgical approach with the best working angle. The anatomic location of the lesion is the most important factor determining the surgical approach. The six transfacial surgical approaches described by the authors' classification system provide extensive access to the anterior skull base and clivus. Furthermore, the exposures overlap enough to permit flexibility in dealing with other factors, such as tumor location and sizes, when selecting a surgical procedure (Fig. 6.1).

These transfacial exposures also may be combined to provide an overlapping spectrum of exposure to a suitably located lesion. The combination of level III and level V approaches provides extensive exposure of the anterior skull base and clivus. Other potential combinations include level II and level V or level II or III and level VI. Furthermore, these transfacial exposures can be combined with other intracranial approaches, simultaneous or staged, to deal with all aspects of a particular lesion (as was done in 10 of our 32 patients). This feature is particularly important to deal effectively with lesions that extend into the intradural compartment. For example, we do not advocate a transfacial approach to treat a clival meningioma. However, a transfacial exposure, combined with an intradural procedure such as a pterional craniotomy, may allow gross total resection of a tumor that is primarily extradural but has an intradural extension (e.g., chordoma). The decision to use a single- or multiple-stage procedure will also reflect the type of tumor, its size, the patient's age, and the patient's general physical condition.

With the exception of the level IV approach, all of these techniques provide surgical access without a facial incision. This advantage reduces patient morbidity. Although two of our patients underwent surgery via a level IV approach, we have learned that combining the level III and level V approaches during the same operation usually provides the same degree of surgical exposure and spares the patient a facial incision. The level IV approach, however, can be useful with extensive tumors and should not necessarily be abandoned. The level V approach (Le Fort I osteotomy) should be raised to the infraorbital foramen in children to avoid the tooth buds. An alternative is to use the level VI approach (transpalatal) to access the lower skull base and to avoid maxillary osteotomy.

The authors' preliminary experience illustrates how this classification system can guide the selection of the appropriate surgical approach based on the desired angle of surgical exposure for an approach to the anterior skull base or clivus. This classification system is simple and useful for planning treatment. The level III and level V approaches have become the "workhorses" of the authors' skull base team: either alone or in combination, these levels provide access to most parts of the anterior skull base and clivus. However, the flexibility of selecting a level I or level II approach in place of a level III approach, or a level VI approach in place of level V approach, greatly enhances the ability to individualize treatment.

Finally, the issue concerning the role of surgical treatment for aggressive tumors of the anterior skull base and clivus has not been addressed by the series presented here. These surgical approaches provide an excellent opportunity to achieve complete resection of a benign tumor such as an angiofibroma. However, the role for aggressive surgical resection has not been established for lesions like chordomas or nasopharyngeal melanomas: a gross total resection, with clear margins, was achieved in all three patients in this series who died from either local or metastatic tumor recurrence. Therefore, while the technical feasibility of comprehensive tumor resection has been demonstrated, the role for such treatment in specific tumor types (and the role for adjuvant therapy) must be defined by future prospective clinical trials.

PART II: INTERNAL CAROTID ARTERY SACRIFICE

Introduction

Anterior skull base tumors frequently encase the internal carotid artery (ICA) (2, 12, 30, 31, 33, 48–50). Because complete resection is the objective of most tumor operations, the surgeon must decide how to manage this artery. Some tumors can be dissected cleanly from the artery and resected completely with carotid preservation (2). Other tumors, however, adhere to or invade the artery and cannot be resected totally without injuring it (30, 33, 48–50). The choice between preserving the ICA and resecting a tumor subtotally or sacrificing the ICA to obtain a complete resection is difficult and controversial. Furthermore, the issue of whether to reconstruct the ICA after sacrifice is also controversial. This section reviews our experience with ICA sacrifice and presents our strategy for managing the ICA in the radical resection of anterior skull base lesions.

Clinical Material and Methods

In an experience with more than 300 anterior skull base tumors treated between 1988 and 1994, the ICA was sacrificed and revascularized in 10 patients. There were five women and five men with an average age of 48 years (range, 31 to 72 years).

Four patients presented with untreated tumors. Six patients sought treatment for recurrent tumor after being treated elsewhere. All six of these patients previously underwent surgical resection of their tumors, with multiple resections in four patients. Five patients received radiation therapy, and none received chemotherapy.

Five patients presented with symptoms of mass effect and neural compression. Two patients had progressively worsening pain; two had episodes of excessive nasopharyngeal bleeding; and one had transient ischemic attacks related to occlusion of the ICA by tumor. All 10 patients had cranial nerve deficits but normal motor function.

Eight tumors were located in and around the cavernous sinus, and two were found in the infratemporal fossa. Eight tumors were located on the right side, and two were on the left side. Angiography demonstrated encasement of the ICA with luminal narrowing in nine patients; one patient had complete ICA occlusion.

Pathologic examination of tumor specimens revealed the following diagnoses: five squamous cell carcinomas, two adenoid cystic carcinomas, one mucoepidermoid carcinoma, one malignant meningioma, and one benign meningioma.

Results

All lesions were approached through a standard frontotemporal craniotomy. Additional exposure was gained through an infratemporal fossa approach in three patients, through a radical neck dissection in two patients, and through a transfacial approach in one patient. Six patients underwent staged resections of tumor. The tumors were resected totally in five patients and subtotally in five patients.

All 10 patients had their ICA sacrificed as part of a radical tumor resection; revascularization was performed in all patients. Five patients were given a bypass before tumor resection during the same operation; five were given a bypass first, followed by tumor resection in a second-stage operation. Revascularization procedures included five cervical ICA-MCA saphenous bypasses (including one on the contralateral side for a complication), one cervical-to-supraclinoid ICA saphenous bypass, three petrous-to-supraclinoid (C3-C5) bypasses, and two bonnet bypasses (contralateral (STA)-to-ipsilateral MCA) (54).

Surgical complications occurred in five patients. One occluded bypass graft caused a cerebral infarction. During transfacial tumor resection in another patient, the contralateral ICA was injured with delayed formation and rupture of a pseudoaneurysm and cerebral infarction. Other complications included one wound infection, one necrotic muscle flap with formation of an orocutaneous fistula, and one CSF leak.

No patients died for reasons related to their surgical treatment. Four patients experienced neurologic deterioration associated with treatment. Two of these patients recovered to their neurologic baseline at a later follow-up examination (mean length of follow-up, 0.8 year).

Discussion

BENIGN SKULL BASE TUMORS

Most anterior skull base neoplasms—meningioma, nerve sheath tumors, pituitary adenoma, and juvenile angiofibroma—are benign (48). Many of these tumors can be resected completely without sacrifice of the ICA. DeMonte *et al.* (12) preserved the ICA in all 41 patients with cavernous sinus meningiomas and achieved total resection in 31 (76%) patients. In his review of clinoidal meningiomas, Al-Mefty (2) concluded that the presence of an arachnoid membrane between the ICA and the tumor determines whether dissection of the vessel from the tumor is possible; complete ICA encasement by the tumor does not prevent total resection. However, meningiomas that encase the ICA without this intervening arachnoidal layer adhere to the adventitia and cannot be resected completely without sacrificing the ICA. The 76% total resection rate in DeMonte's series demonstrates that a protective arachnoidal membrane is usually present around meningiomas; therefore, the majority of these benign tumors can be resected completely while preserving the ICA. Other benign tumors, such as pituitary adenomas, neurilemomas, and angiofibromas, are more likely than meningiomas to be dissected free of the ICA (31).

Residual benign tumor left around the ICA to preserve it could potentially invade the vessel wall and compromise the integrity of the artery. However, benign tumors tend not to invade the ICA to such an extent. Kotapka *et al.* (30) studied ICAs encased by cavernous sinus meningiomas in 19 patients, with luminal narrowing in all but 2. Eight of these patients' ICAs were infiltrated by tumors to the outer adventitia (five patients) and to the media through adventitia (three patients). Apparently, meningiomas invade the carotid wall but only to a limited extent. Residual tumor on the ICA after resection, therefore, does not threaten the integrity of the vessel. Tumor debulking is often sufficient to restore lumenal patency.

Residual benign tumor around the ICA could potentially increase the incidence of tumor recurrence. Because the risk of tumor recurrence decreases with more extensive surgical resection (1) the recurrence rate should be lower in patients whose carotid arteries are sacrificed than in patients whose carotid arteries are preserved. However, two series of patients with cavernous sinus meningiomas that were aggressively resected, either with (50) or without ICA resection (12), had recurrence rates that were strikingly similar. Sen and Sekhar (50) treated 17 patients with tumor and ICA resection, totally resecting the tumors of 76% of the patients. The symptomatic radiographic recurrence rate was 8% after total tumor resection and 25% after subtotal tumor resection. In comparison, DeMonte *et al.* (12) achieved the same gross total resection rate in 41 patients without carotid resection. In this series, the rates of recurrence were 3% and 20%, after total and subtotal resections, respectively. Therefore, ICA resection in the treatment of meningiomas of the anterior skull base does not appear to lower the rate of recurrence.

The lack of ICA invasion by residual tumor and the lack of improvement in the tumor recurrence rate with carotid resection argue for preserving the ICA when dealing with benign skull base tumors. ICA preservation is the practice at our institution. Furthermore, the risk of complication from elective ICA occlusion is around 10%, even with revascularization (Lawton MT, Spetzler RF, 1995). This risk cannot be justified in the treatment of benign lesions. Although total resection is the goal of this surgery, subtotal resection of a benign tumor is considered safe. However, patients with residual tumor are followed carefully for recurrence with serial neurologic and imaging examinations.

MALIGNANT SKULL BASE TUMORS

An ICA surrounded by a malignant tumor is managed differently than one surrounded by a benign tumor. First, because malignant tumors can invade adjacent structures, metastasize, and cause death, oncologic principles of radical resection with tumor-free margins must be adhered to more strictly. Second, the risks of ICA sacrifice are justified when compared to the dismal prognosis of patients with malignant neoplasms.

Our treatment strategy is based on the invasive behavior of malignant tumors. Malignant neoplasms tend to invade the ICA wall directly and can lead to frank ICA rupture (21, 29, 37, 55), which differs from benign neoplasms that invade the ICA superficially and do not precipitate rupture. Because ICA rupture can cause potentially life-threatening hemorrhage, an artery involved with a malignant tumor is best resected. The risk of an ICA rupture invaded by malignant intracranial tumor is unknown. However, it is likely to be similar to the risk of rupture of an ICA invaded by malignant cervical tumor—which is 17 to 18% (20, 21, 29). Furthermore, most of these ICAs rupture within 6 months (21, 29). Therefore, when dealing with malignant neopolasms, the risk of ICA preservation and subsequent rupture exceeds the risk of ICA sacrifice with revascularization.

The effect of ICA resection on tumor recurrence and the survival of patients is difficult to determine because no prospective randomized studies have examined this issue. Malignant tumors are more difficult to resect than benign tumors, with total resection rates of 55 and 86%, respectively (48). Recurrence after total resection also is increased with malignant tumors (25 *versus* 6%). ICA sacrifice permits en bloc resection of the cavernous sinus and, therefore, a better chance at disease-free margins of resection (3). However, it is unclear whether aggressive resection extends a patient's survival significantly (43). A prospective randomized clinical study may identify a subgroup of patients in whom survival is extended by radical tumor resection. At the least, radical tumor resection should attempt to relieve local symptoms and decrease the rate of intracranial recurrence.

ARTERY RECONSTRUCTION OF THE ICA

ICA resection produces a risk of ischemic complications. Morbidit for elective ICA resection without reconstruction for neck carcinomas ranges from 0 to 45%, and mortality ranges from 0 to 31% (9). Consequently, the surgeon must determine that the patient has either the collateral circulation to tolerate ICA sacrifice, or the surgeon must restore cerebral blood flow with a bypass graft. Diagnostic studies, such as the balloon occlusion test and xenon computed tomographic-cerebral blood flow (Xe CT-CBF), identify patients who are unlikely to tolerate ICA sacrifice and who will require revascularization (33, 49, 50). These provocative tests may cause temporary and permanent ischemic deficits, and their rate of false-negatives ranges from 7 to 30% (38, 50). Therefore, we tend to revascularize patients whose ICA has been sacrificed.

The revascularization procedure is performed immediately before the tumor is resected or in a preceding surgical stage. Intraoperative somatosensory evoked potentials (SSEPs) are used routinely during the anastomosis. Changes in SSEPs alert the surgeon that the patient is not tolerating the temporary ICA occlusion, and ICA perfusion should be maintained during proximal anastomosis by suturing the bypass graft to the external carotid artery.

The indications for revascularization are controversial. Although we limit ICA sacrifice and revascularization to patients with malignant tumors that encase the ICA, Sen and Sekhar do not perform bypasses for malignant neoplasms (50). In contrast, only one patient in our series (10%) had an ICA resected for a benign tumor. This patient had a meningioma that completely occluded the ICA and caused transient ischemic attacks. Complete ICA occlusion permitted resection of the artery with a benign tumor, but the ischemic symptoms indicated that cerebral blood flow was inadequate and needed augmentation with a bypass graft.

CONCLUSION

The transfacial approaches give the surgeon wide exposure for resecting skull base lesions. The classification system, using six levels, helps plan the best surgical strategy. Our experience with the transfacial approaches has been associated with acceptably low rates of morbidity and mortality. Our small experience with carotid sacrifice reflects our practice of preserving the ICA whenever possible. We recommend preserving the ICA with benign tumors because they do not invade the artery, or they invade it to a limited extent. In contrast, we recommend radical tumor resection and sacrifice of the ICA with malignant tumors, because they directly threaten the integrity of the ICA and a patient's survival. The ICA should not be considered a limitation to radical tumor resection, because the ICA can be safely reconstructed with an appropriate bypass procedure.

REFERENCES

1. Adegbite AB, Khan MI, Paine KW, *et al.:* The recurrence of intracranial meningiomas after surgical treatment. **J Neurosurg** 58:51–56, 1983.
2. Al-Mefty O: Clinoidal meningiomas. **J Neurosurg** 73:840–849, 1990.
3. Al-Mefty O: Management of the cavernous sinus and carotid siphon. **Otolaryngol Clin N Am** 24:1523–1533, 1991.
4. Anand VK, Harkey LH, Al-Mefty O: Open-door maxillotomy approach for lesions of the clivus. **Skull Base Surg** 1:217–224, 1991.
5. Beals SP, Hamilton MG, Joganic EF, *et al.:* Posterior cranial base transfacial approaches. **Clin Plast Surg,** in press, 1995.
6. Beals SP, Joganic EF: Transfacial exposure of anterior cranial fossa and clival tumors. **BNI Q** 8:2–18, 1992.
7. Belmont JR; The Le Fort I osteotomy approach for nasopharyngeal and nasal fossa tumors. **Arch Otolaryngol Head Neck Surg** 114:751–754, 1988.
8. Blacklock JB, Weber RS, Lee Y, *et al.:* Transcranial resection of tumors of the paranasal sinuses and nasal cavity. **J Neurosurg** 71:10–15, 1989.
9. Brennan JA, Jafek BW: Elective carotid artery resection for advanced squamous cell carcinoma of the neck. **Laryngoscope** 104:259–263, 1994.
10. Crockard HA: The transmaxillary approach to the clivus, in Sekhar LN, Janecka IP (eds): *Surgery of Cranial Base Tumors.* New York, Raven Press, 1993, p 235.
11. deFries HO, Deeb ZE, Hudkins CP: A transfacial approach to the nasal-paranasal cavities and anterior skull base. **Arch Otolaryngol Head Neck Surg** 114:766–769, 1988.
12. DeMonte F, Smith HK, Al-Mefty O: Outcome of aggressive removal of cavernous sinus meningiomas. **J Neurosurg** 81:245–251, 1994.
13. Derome PJ: The transbasal approach to tumors invading the base of the skull, in Schmidek HH, Sweet WH. (eds): *Operative Neurosurgical Techniques.* Orlando, FL, Grune & Stratton, 1988, p 619.
14. Derome PJ, Bisot A, Monteil JP, *et al.:* Management of cranial chordomas, in Sekhar LN, Schramm VLJ (eds): *Tumors of the Cranial Base: Diagnosis and Treatment.* Mount Kisco, NY, Futura, 1987, p 607.
15. Farnworth TK, Beals SP, Manwaring KH, *et al.:* Comparison of skin necrosis in rats by using a new microneedle electrocautery, standard-size needle electrocautery, and the Shaw hemostatic scalpel. **Ann Plast Surg** 31:164–167, 1993.
16. Fujitsu K, Saijoh M, Aoki F, *et al.:* Telecanthal approach for meningiomas in the ethmoid and sphenoid sinuses. **Neurosurgery** 28:714–719, 1991.
17. Hamilton MG, Herman JM, Beals SP, *et al.:* The role of transfacial exposure in treatment of tumors of the anterior skull base and clivus. **Skull Base Surg** 3 (Suppl): 91–93 (abstr).
18. Hamilton MG, Hull R, Pineo G: Venous thromboembolism in neurosurgery and neurology patients: A review. **Neurosurgery** 34:280-296, 1994.
19. Haughey BH, Wilson JS, Barber CS: Massive angiofibroma: A surgical approach and adjunctive therapy. **Otolaryngol Head Neck Surg** 98:618–624, 1988.
20. Hiranandani LH: The management of cervical metastasis in head and neck cancers. **J Laryngol Otol** 85:1097–1126, 1971.
21. Huvos AG, Leaming RH, Moore OS: Clinicopathologic study of the resected carotid artery. An analysis of sixty-four cases. **Am J Surg** 126:570–574, 1973.
22. Jackson IT, Marsh WR, Bite U, *et al.:* Craniofacial osteotomies to facilitate skull base tumour resection. **Br J Plast Surg** 39:153–160, 1986.

23. Jackson IT, Marsh WR, Hide TA: Treatment of tumors involving the anterior cranial fossa. **Head Neck Surg** 6:901–903, 1984.
24. James D, Crockard HA: Surgical access to the base of skull and upper cervical spine by exterior maxillotomy. **Neurosurgery** 29:411–416, 1991.
25. Janecka IP, Sen CN, Sekhar LN, *et al.:* Facial translocation: A new approach to the cranial base. Otolaryngol **Head Neck Surg** 103:413–419, 1990.
26. Jennett B, Bond M: Assessment of outcome after severe brain damage. A practical scale. **Lancet** 1:480–484, 1975.
27. Kaplan MJ, Jane JA, Park TS, *et al.:* Supraorbital rim approach to the anterior skull base. **Laryngoscope** 94:1137–1139, 1984.
28. Kawakami K, Yamanouchi Y, Kubota C, *et al.:* An extensive transbasal approach to frontal skull-base tumors. Technical note. **J Neurosurg** 74:1011–1013, 1991.
29. Kennedy JT, Krause CJ, Loevy S: The importance of tumor attachment to the carotid artery. **Arch Otolaryngol** 103:70–73, 1977.
30. Kotapka MJ, Kalia KK, Martinez AJ, *et al.:* Infiltration of the carotid artery by cavernous sinus meningioma. **J Neurosurg** 81:252–255, 1994.
31. Lanzino G, Hirsch WL, Pomonis S, *et al.;* Cavernous sinus tumors: Neuroradiologic and neurosurgical considerations on 150 operated cases. **J Neurosurg Sci** 36:183–196, 1992.
32. Lauritzen C, Vallfors B, Lilja J: Facial disassembly for tumor resection. **Scand J Plast Reconstr Surg** 20:201–206, 1986.
33. Linskey ME, Sekhar LN, Sen C: Cerebral revascularization in cranial base surgery, in Sekhar LN, Janecka IP (eds): Surgery of Cranial Base Tumors. New York, Raven Press, 1993, p 45.
34. Lund VJ, Howard DJ, Lloyd GA, *et al.:* Magnetic resonance imaging of paranasal sinus tumors for craniofacial resection. **Head Neck** 11:279–283, 1989.
35. Mann WJ, Gilsbach J, Seeger W, *et al.:* Use of a malar bone graft to augment skull-base access. **Arch Otolaryngol** 111:30–33, 1985.
36. Maran AG: Surgical approaches to the nasopharynx. **Clin Otolaryngol** 8:417–429, 1983.
37. McCready RA, Miller SK, Hamaker RC, et al.; What is the role of carotid arterial resection in the management of advanced cervical cancer? **J Vasc Surg** 10:274–280, 1989.
38. McIvor NP, Willinsky RA, TerBrugge KG, *et al.:* Validity of test occlusion studies prior to internal carotid artery sacrifice. **Head Neck** 16:11–16, 1994.
39. Miller HS, Petty PG, Wilson WF, *et al.:* A combined intracranial and facial approach for excision and repair of cancer of the ethmoid sinuses. **Aust N Z J Surg** 43:179–183, 1973.
40. Munro, IR, Bruce, DA, Fearon JA. Transfacial Approach for Tumours of the Midline Skull Base. Abstract in *Plastic Surgery 1992 Excerpta Medica from International Congress Series 937.* III:60, 1992.
41. Panje WR, Dohrmann GJ III, Pitcock JK, *et al.:* The transfacial approach for combined anterior craniofacial tumor ablation. **Arch Otolaryngol Head Neck Surg** 115:301–307, 1989.
42. Persing JA, Jane JA, Levine PA, *et al.:* The versatile frontal sinus approach to the floor of the anterior cranial fossa. Technical note. **J Neurosurg** 72:513–516, 1990.
43. Prasad S, Janecka IP: Efficacy of surgical treatments for squamous cell carcinoma of the temporal bone: A literature review. **Otolaryngol Head Neck Surg** 110:270–280, 1994.

44. Price JC: The midface degloving approach to the central skull base. **Ear Nose Throat J** 65:174–180, 1986.
45. Sandor GK, Charles DA, Lawson VG, *et al.:* Transoral approach to the nasopharynx and clivus using the Le Fort I osteotomy with midpalatal split. **Int J Maxillofac Surg** 19:352–355, 1990.
46. Sataloff RT, Bowman C, Baker SR, *et al.:* Transfacial resection of intracranial tumor. **Am J Otol** 9:222–228, 1988.
47. Schramm VL Jr, Myers EN, Maroon JC: Anterior skull base surgery for benign and malignant disease. **Laryngoscope** 89:1077–1091, 1979.
48. Sekhar LN, Ross DA, Sen C: Cavernous sinus and sphenocavernous neoplasms: Anatomy and surgery, Sekhar LN, Janecka IP (eds): **Surgery of Cranial Base Tumors.** New York, Raven Press, 1993, p 521.
49. Sekhar LN, Sen CN, Jho HD: Saphenous vein graft bypass of the cavernous internal carotid artery. **J Neurosurg** 72:35–41, 1990.
50. Sen C, Sekhar LN: Direct vein graft reconstruction of the cavernous, petrous, and upper cervical internal carotid artery: Lessons learned from 30 cases. **Neurosurgery** 30:732–743, 1992.
51. Shah JP, Galicich JH: Surgical approach to carcinoma of the nasal cavity and paranasal sinuses with extension to the base of the skull. **Clin Bull** 82:61–66, 1978.
52. Spetzler RF, Herman JM, Beals S, *et al.:* Preservation of olfaction in anterior craniofacial approaches. **J Neurosurg** 79:48–51, 1993.
53. Spetzler RF, Pappas CTE: Management of anterior skull base tumors. **Clin Neurosurg** 37:490–501, 1991.
54. Spetzler RF, Roski RA, Rhodes RS, *et al.:* The "bonnett bypass." Case report. **J Neurosurg** 53:707–709, 1980.
55. Suarez CN, Estervan Solano JM, Buron Martinez G, *et al.:* Invasion of the carotid artery in tumours of the head and neck. **Clin Otolaryngol** 6:29–37, 1981.
56. Sundaresan N: Craniofacial resection for paranasal sinus tumors. **Indian J Cancer** 16:74–79, 1994.
57. Sundaresan N, Shah JP: Craniofacial resection for anterior skull base tumors. **Head Neck Surg** 10:219–224, 1988.
58. Tessier P, Guiot G, Rougerie J, *et al.:* Cranio-naso-orbito-facial osteotomies. Hypertelorism (French). **Ann Chir Plast** 12:103–118, 1967.
59. Uttley D, Moore A, Archer DJ: Surgical management of midline skull-base tumors: A new approach. **J Neurosurg** 71:705–710, 1989.
60. Van Buren JM, Ommaya AK, Ketcham AS: Ten years' experience with radical combined craniofacial resection of malignant tumors of the paranasal sinuses. **J Neurosurg** 28:341–350, 1968.
61. Wei WI, Lam KH, Sham JS: New approach to the nasopharynx: The maxillary swing approach. **Head Neck** 13:200–207, 1991.
62. Wood GD, Stell PM: The Le Fort I osteotomy as an approach to the nasopharynx. **Clin Otolaryngol** 9:59–61, 1984.

7

Management of Anterior Cranial Base and Cavernous Sinus Neoplasms with Conservative Surgery Alone or in Combination with Fractionated Photon or Stereotactic Proton Radiotherapy

ROBERT G. OJEMANN, M.D., ALLAN F. THORNTON, M.D., AND GRIFFITH R. HARSH IV, M.D.

INTRODUCTION

The Scientific Program Committee of the Congress of Neurological Surgeons asked that we discuss conservative resection and radiotherapy for anterior cranial base and cavernous sinus neoplasms. In the 27th edition of *Dorland's Medical Dictionary,* published in 1988, the definition of "conservative" is "designed to preserve health, restore function and repair structures by non-radical methods, as conservative surgery." We believe it is the goal of every neurosurgeon to accomplish these results. We would define conservative surgery for anterior cranial base and cavernous sinus neoplasms as a procedure that is planned to restore and preserve function, attempting to combine the lowest possible risks with the maximum benefit to the patient. In many patients this will mean removal of the entire tumor. However, in some it will be better to leave a segment of tumor that might be involved with important functional structures and, then, either follow the patient with clinical examination and imaging or administer radiotherapy.

Radical surgery for tumors in these locations also is used to restore and preserve function. However, a more aggressive attempt is made to totally remove a complex tumor by methods such as a more extensive craniofacial exposure, resection and graft of the internal carotid artery, and excision and graft of nerves in the cavernous sinus. Inherent in these procedures is a risk of disability. The expectation would be that the higher risk of surgically induced morbidity would more often be offset by a lower risk of morbidity from a reduced incidence of tumor recurrence or from not having to use radiotherapy. To date, our experience indicates that conservative surgery complemented, when indicated, by radiotherapy, is the preferred treatment for most patients. As surgeons become more skilled and procedures are more highly refined, a more radical operation may be indicated.

Planning a treatment program requires a detailed evaluation of the history, findings, and radiographic studies. The treatment options are carefully considered, along with pertinent questions (43, 45–47): What is the expected natural history of the tumor? What are the chances of the recommended treatment improving or relieving the patient's symptoms and preventing future disability? What are the risks of the treatment? Do the benefits of the planned treatment outweigh those risks? What is the patient's age and functional status? What are the patient's hopes and expectations from the planned treatment? Addressing this last question, Pelligrino (52), in his Cushing Oration to the American Association of Neurological Surgeons in 1983, said, "A biomedically good decision is one that is scientifically correct, but it is not automatically a good decision from the patient's point of view. It must be placed within the context of the patient's life situation and his (her) value system. It must square with what the patient thinks worthwhile, given the circumstances and choices illness forces upon him (her)." Kassirer (31), in an editorial in *The New England Journal of Medicine* in 1994 entitled, "Incorporating Patient's Preferences into Medical Decisions," noted "that good clinical decisions require an understanding of how patients view certain outcomes."

Application of these principles to the choice of therapy must be individualized for the particular patient and his/her tumor. Although the ideal goal of surgery is complete removal of the tumor, a number of factors may dictate either nonsurgical treatment or an operation that may leave some portion of the tumor. Factors favoring a more conservative approach include (*a*) advanced age of a patient, (*b*) minimal or nonprogressive symptoms, (*c*) a quiescent or slowly growing tumor with an indolent natural history, (*d*) tumor location in which surgical manipulation causes high risk of morbidity, and (*e*) greater predictability of outcome in comparison with that of newer treatments whose long-term results have not yet been established.

This chapter focuses on tumors of the anterior cranial base with intracranial extension and on tumors of the cavernous sinus. It includes a discussion of meningiomas, with benign and atypical pathology, arising from the olfactory groove, tuberculum sellae, floor of the frontal fossa, optic sheath, medial sphenoid wing, and cavernous sinus. Excluded are meningiomas predominantly involving the clivus or petrous bone and only secondarily extending into the cavernous sinus. Other tumors discussed include chondrosarcoma, chordoma, esthesioneuroblastoma (olfactory neuroblastoma), sinus carcinoma with intracranial extension, trigeminal neuroma primarily located in the cavernous sinus, and epidermoid. Pituitary tumors growing into the cavernous sinus have not been included.

In this chapter results of patients treated by surgery are those of the senior author over a 15-year period (1978–1992). Some of these patients have been included in previous publications (39–43, 44, 48, 49). The result of radiotherapy for patients treated by the Radiation Oncology Service at the Massachusetts General Hospital (MGH) are presented separately. In the earlier years of this series, more patients received photon radiotherapy. Because of advantages that will be discussed later, fractioned stereotactic proton radiotherapy, combined with a 30% component of photon irradiation, is now used more frequently. This latter group includes some of the patients who received radiotherapy in the surgical series presented in this chapter, as well as patients whose initial surgical treatment was done by other members of the staff or by other physicians who referred the patient for the therapy. The other patients in the surgical series who had radiotherapy received photon treatment, occasionally at other institutions.

GENERAL ASPECTS OF TREATMENT

Surgery

The surgical principles for removal of anterior skull base and cavernous sinus tumor have been presented in our previous publications (39–42, 44, 48, 49) and in those of other surgeons (1, 3, 4, 11, 17, 25, 34, 36, 57, 59, 61, 64, 65). Craniofacial procedures are discussed in another chapter. Reference will be made to appropriate publications in the discussion of individual tumors, but it is not the purpose of this chapter to discuss the technical details of the operations, which were extensively presented in volume 40 of *Clinical Neurosurgery* (44).

Most patients are given steroids for at least 48 hours before the operation and for a longer period when there is significant brain edema. Postoperatively, the steroids are tapered over 5 days or longer, depending on the degree of cerebral edema and the patient's condition. For most procedures an anticonvulsant medication is started. Intravenous antibiotics are given before the operation and for 24 hours after the procedure, or longer if a lumbar drain is in place. After induction of anesthesia and insertion of a catheter in the bladder, 10 to 20 mg furosemide are given and 100 g of mannitol administered intravenously during the exposure if required for brain relaxation. If there is a strong probability of a CSF leak, a lumbar drain is placed after the induction of anesthesia.

The terms used to record the extent of tumor removal are: total (T), removal of all visible tumor; radical subtotal (RST), small fragments of tumor are left adherent to important structures; and subtotal (ST), extensive removal with a portion of the capsule remaining. The terms used to designate outcome are: good (G), free of major neurologic deficit, with ability to return to previous level of activity; fair (F), independent but unable to return to full activity because of new or preoperative neurologic deficit from which patient did not fully recover; and poor (P), dependent with major neurologic deficit.

Fractionated Stereotactic Proton Therapy

BACKGROUND

Conventional photon radiotherapy has been shown to arrest the growth of some cranial base meningiomas (8, 13, 24, 66, 72). However, this therapy may be constrained from delivering tumoricidal does to meningiomas and other anterior cranial base neoplasms by the dose-limiting tissues of the visual system, particularly the optic chiasm, as well as the frontal and temporal lobes. Proton irradiation offers the potential to deliver substantially higher does to the target tissues while respecting accepted dose constraints on critical normal tissues.

First proposed by Robert Wilson in 1946 (74), the clinical use of proton radiotherapy has concentrated on tumors with well-defined margins in close approximation to dose-limiting structures. Lawrence *et al.,* at the University of California cyclotron in Berkeley, accumulated experience with proton irradiation of pituitary adenomas (68). Extensive experience with ocular melanomas (37), clivus and cervical chordomas (7, 62), and chondrosarcomas of the cranial base (7; Liebsch NJ, Ojemann RG, Renard L, *et al.,* manuscript in preparation, 1995) suggests that protons offer decided clinical advantages over photon modalities.

The advantages of proton radiotherapy are entirely provided by the physical properties of the beam. The finite range of penetration of protons is affected by both the initial beam energy and the electron density of the absorbing material. The rapid increase in the rate of energy loss near the end of the range of a proton particle results in a well-defined volume of increased dose, known as the Bragg peak. By appropriate distribution of proton energies, the Bragg peaks may be grouped so as to provide a uniform 100% isodose across the target and a near-zero dose deep to the target. Additionally, the long distance from the last source scatterer of the cyclotron to the patient's skin results in nearly nondivergent beam edges. This lack of divergence results in a rapid falloff of dose at the edge of the field, facilitating accurate treatment of tumors near critical structures.

TREATMENT PLANNING

Accurate treatment with particle irradiation requires accurate dosimetry, reflecting the correct prediction of proton absorption within the scattering material. Such dosimetry relies on complex algorithms, largely ray-tracing in design, to provide information on the likely patterns of scattering and absorption of incident protons. Computer modeling through beam's-eye view (BEV) perspectives provides enhanced recognition of the relative positions of tumor, target, and critical structure volumes. The combination of accurate algorithms and computer-aided image reconstruction techniques offers the ability to reconstruct CT data in any plane (*e.g.*, coronal parasellar perspective) and display composite dose deposited on that plane from a combination of beam directions and energies (18, 20). Such 3-dimensional treatment planning systems are available at a growing number of facilities and provide the opportunity to maximize the therapeutic ratio of radiotherapy in the treatment of parasellar tumors (67).

Targeting is based on CT volume definition, complemented by magnetic resonance imaging (MRI) information. Customarily, both high-quality preoperative and postoperative contrast-enhanced CT scans, using 3-mm slices through the region to be studied, are performed in the immobilized treatment position for planning purposes. MRI is routinely incorporated in the target definition process and is especially useful in defining postoperative volumes at risk, particularly in the parasellar regions. MRI is also relied on to define optic chiasm and tract locations.

TREATMENT PROGRAM

In the MGH fractionated proton program, the Harvard Cyclotron is used for all proton treatments. Using the 160-MeV synchrocyclotron beam generated by this facility, field of up to 30 cm in diameter can be treated with dose rates ranging from 8 to 15 cGy/min to depths of up to 17 cm. To minimize skin entrance reactions, a 30% component of photon irradiation is used, planned with the same 3-dimensional software as used with proton therapy. Although equipment and shielding for photon therapy is conventional in design, the use of rigid immobilization and routine incorporation of fiducial markers aids in setup and restricts these photon treatments to the minimum necessary to treat intended volumes.

Patients are treated in positions offering maximal daily reproducibility. This often necessitates the supine position for photon treatments and the sitting position for proton treatments, utilizing mask immobilization devices complemented by denture-based restraint devices. However, conventional supine positions may be used where lateral or superior (vertex) beams are intended. Proper localization of appropriate tumor target volumes requires excellent reproducible immobilization and correlation of imaging studies. To achieve this, fiducials implanted within the skull and a mask immobilization system incorporating external fiducials, similar to currently accepted markers for stereotactic radiosurgical treatment, are used.

PREVENTION OF COMPLICATIONS

Optic Pathways Injury. Although extensive data exist on the effects of radiation on the eye, most experimental data pertain to large single fractions of beta applicator irradiation. There are few studies of pathologic changes associated with clinical doses of radiation to the eye. Data pertinent to the clinical situation must be extracted from a few series that include patients treated over a considerable period of technological changes in radiotherapy.

The lens is the most radiation-sensitive structure. Thickening of the posterior capsule frequently occurs following irradiation (16). Complications related to the retina and optic nerve are more significant consequences of irradiation. Shukovsky and Fletcher (60) reported that 7 of 15 patients treated for sinus carcinoma developed retinal degeneration after receiving 7000 cGy. Chan and Shukovsky (14) subsequently described two cases in a series of 22 patients irradiated with up to 6000 cGy who developed retinal blindness. Five of 18 patients with pituitary adenomas and craniopharyngiomas treated by Harris and Levine (26) with 4500 cGy in 6 weeks developed blindness, while Aristizabal and Caldwell (6) noted that 22% of pituitary tumor patients treated with 250-cGy fractions *versus* 12% treated with the same dose, using 200-cGy fractions, developed blindness. Surprisingly, Wara *et al.* (71) reported that eight patients developed radiation retinopathy, of whom four received less than 5000 cGy in 6 weeks.

Two major classes of radiation injury, differentiated primarily by times of onset, occur in the optic nerve and chiasm (53). The first, retrobulbar optic neuropathy, presents within the first 18 months following irradiation, often with sudden visual loss. The fundoscopic examination may often be normal or show pallor in only one sector. The injury is usually confined to the chiasm or adjacent optic nerve. The second ischemic optic neuropathy usually occurs years following radiation and manifests a slowly progressive course (55). Fundoscopic examination may show disc pallor and edema with or without splinter hemorrhages. This injury usually involves the intraorbital optic nerve.

Both types of radiation optic neuropathy involve hyaline occlusion of small vessels, resulting in gliosis, demyelination and, ultimately, necrosis (73).

Tolerance of the intracranial visual system to irradiation exhibits dose- and fraction-size dependence that differs from that of soft tissue. However, empirical data of chiasma and optic nerve tolerance are largely limited to anecdotal case reports involving pituitary and brain irradiation. The period of greatest risk for these chronic changes to the visual system is between 6 months and 5 years following irradiation, although shorter intervals have been reported.

Reviews involving contemporary photon radiation techniques and fractionation suggest that approximately 20% of optic nerves exposed to doses greater than 6000 cGy will develop radiation injury (51). A review of 74 patients undergoing irradiation to the visual system suggests that the sigmoid dose-response curve is steep between 5000 and 6000 cGy (76). Tolerance of the optic chiasm is conventionally considered to be between 5000 cGy and 5500 cGy. Recommendation is made to reduce the length of irradiated optic nerve to a minimum. Efforts at the MGH and Harvard Cyclotron Laboratory have tested the hypothesis that optic nerve radiation tolerance may be increased through precise stereotactic irradiation of limited lengths of optic nerve on a fractionated basis. A review of patients treated with proton stereotactic methods suggests that portions of the optic nerve may be safely irradiated to doses of 6800 cGy on 180 cGy/day fractionation (69).

In summary, the current dose constraints for optic structures are as follows: The retinal portion of the globe is constrained to receive no more than 5940 cGy; limited segments of the optic nerves may receive up to 6800 cGy if treated in 180 cGy/day fractions (70); the chiasm should receive no more than 5580 cGy in 180-cGy daily fractionation.

Brain Necrosis. Central nervous tissues demonstrate limited capacity for repopulation or repair after radiation damage. Overall treatment time is less important than the amount of radiation delivered per treatment in determining the risk of radiation damage. The volume of brain irradiated also contributes to the risk of late cerebral damage. Fractionated stereotactic proton irradiation allows an increased dose of irradiation to be delivered through: (*a*) maximizing tolerance of normal brain, using small daily fractions of irradiation and (*b*) minimizing irradiated volumes through stereotactic precision. As an example, complex parasellar tumors may be irradiated with adjacent normal temporal and frontal regions receiving doses only 30% of those with conventional photon irradiation.

Empirical evidence of the advantages of fractionated stereotactic irradiation is forthcoming from analysis of complication rates of patients treated for skull base sarcomas at the MGH. A 5-year prospective assessment of neuropsychologic late effects in patients treated for skull base sarcomas with doses exceeding 7000 cGy has recently been completed. This work demonstrates no evidence of cerebral, including temporal lobe, dysfunction when limited-field irradiation is delivered on a fractionated basis.

Endocrine Deficiencies. During radiotherapy for tumors of the parasellar region, both the pituitary and the hypothalamus are likely to be within the field of irradiation. In one series of patients with either paranasal sinus or nasopharyngeal carcinoma (54), 86% of all patients ($n = 110$) developed endocrine deficiencies. The majority (83%) of these demonstrated hypothalamic deficiency, with a significant minority showing evidence of anterior pituitary dysfunction, with prolactinemia the most common. Such complications are often subtle and require both baseline and pretreatment evaluation, as well as careful follow-up.

Osteonecrosis. Radiation damage to the skull base may occur. More commonly seen when doses of radiation greater than 6000 cGy are used, the combination of operative trauma and radiation-induced fibrosis increases the risk of bony damage (33). Any reduction in volume of irradiated tissue achieved through stereotactic irradiation methods translates into decreased rates of osteoradionecrosis (9).

MEDICAL THERAPY

Corticosteroids are frequently used to palliate neurologic symptoms caused by edema secondary to tumor compression or invasion of neural structures. They lack tumoricidal activity. Side effects and loss of efficacy preclude their long-term use.

The progesterone blocker mifepristone (RU486) has been evaluated in the treatment of meningiomas. Initial clinical trials were disappointing because of inability to show a significant sustained response and the occurrence of frequent side effects (23). Presently, a more extensive trial is in progress. Chemotherapy has not played a part in the treatment of chordomas, chondrosarcomas, or schwannomas. The use of chemotherapy in treating esthesioneuroblastoma is discussed under Esthesioneuroblastoma (Olfactory Neuroblastoma).

OBSERVATION

Not every patient with an anterior skull base tumor or cavernous sinus tumor needs an operation. In some patients, periodic clinical evaluation and MRI provide an appropriate course of action. Indications for this form of management include: (*a*) absence of symptoms, (*b*) a long history of stable symptoms, (*c*) mild symptoms or a medically controlled seizure disorder, (*d*) very slowly progressing symptoms in an elderly patient, and (*e*) patient preference. Worsening of symptoms or radiographically demonstrable tumor growth usually warrant treatment.

OLFACTORY GROOVE MENINGIOMA

Management

MRI defines the extent of the tumor, the edema in the surrounding brain, the relationship of the tumor to the optic nerves and anterior cerebral arteries, and any extension into the ethmoid sinus (41, 44). Angiography is rarely needed because MRI usually provides all of the information required. Preoperative embolization is not indicated.

The indications for surgical treatment are worsening neurologic symptoms such as altered mental function, headache, and/or disturbance in vision. Occasionally, a seizure disorder is the only symptom, and in that circumstance there is usually edema in the surrounding brain. Surgery should be considered in an asymptomatic patient with edema in the adjacent brain or MRI findings that the meningioma is near the optic nerves (48). Usually, total removal of the tumor can be achieved. Occasionally, a small fragment of tumor is left on the internal carotid or anterior cerebral artery.

For patients with large tumors, the authors have preferred to use a bifrontal craniotomy (41, 44). This approach is associated with the least amount of retraction on the frontal lobes. It provides direct access to all sides of the tumor and allows decompression of the tumor while working along the base of the skull to interrupt the blood supply. Guthrie *et al.* (25) and Long (36) also preferred bifrontal exposure. For smaller tumors, a right subfrontal lateral-to-medial approach from over the orbital roof may be used (41, 44). Hassler and Zentner (27) used a pterional approach. Logue (34), Symon (64), and Solero *et al.* (61) used either method of exposure and may resect part of the frontal lobe.

Radiation therapy has not been recommended as a primary treatment. However, it has been used after subtotal removal and in the treatment of recurrence.

Results

In this surgical series there were 20 patients with olfactory groove meningioma (Table 7.1). This group included 15 females and 5 males,

TABLE 7.1
Olfactory Groove Meningioma: Surgical Series

Treatment		T	T and RT	RST
No. of patients		18	1[a]	1
Follow-up scan		13[b]	1	1
Years		1–14[c]	6	6
Growth		0	0	0
Status at last evaluation	G	17[b]	1	1
	F	0	0	0
	P	0	0	0
	D	1	0	0

[a]See text.
[b]Four patients were lost to follow-up after 1 to 2 years.
[c]Mean = 5.6 years.

ranging from 23 to 73 years of age, with 3 over 70 years of age. Complete removal was accomplished in 18 patients. One patient had a radical subtotal removal with a small fragment left on the internal carotid artery.

Nineteen of the patients had a good result. There was one postoperative death. In more than 300 operations for all meningiomas done over the same time period as those for the patients reported on in this chapter, there were only two postoperative deaths. One occurred in the case of a patient with an olfactory groove meningioma due to pulmonary embolus (44). In other reported series the operative mortality has also been low (27, 64).

The incidence of complications was also low and did not interfere with eventual recovery. In this series, one patient had a cerebrospinal fluid leak through the ethmoid sinus that required transethmoidal repair; one patient developed a wound infection that cleared up; and one 71-year-old woman required treatment of a subdural hygroma with a subdural-peritoneal shunt. Patients exhibiting disturbance in mental function and personality changes preoperatively or transiently in the postoperative period usually recovered completely. Patients exhibiting preoperatively visual symptoms generally recovered, and headache was relieved in these patients.

Olfactory groove meningiomas have not recurred in the patients followed-up with periodic MRI or CT scans. Chan and Thompson (15) found no recurrence of resected tumors (Simpson, grade I and II) during an average 9-year follow-up.

The results of radiotherapy are presented in Table 7.2. There have been no complications.

TABLE 7.2
Olfactory Groove Meningioma: Radiotherapy Series

Type of Radiotherapy		Photon	Proton
No. of patients		1	3
Prior surgery	T	1[a]	0
	ST	0	3
Dose	cGy	5860	5040
			5940
			6480[b]
Follow-up scan		1	3
Years		6	2,4,4
Growth		0	0
Status at last evaluation	G	1	3
	F	0	0
	P	0	0
	D	0	0

[a]Gross total removal of recurrent atypical meningioma.
[b]Atypical meningioma.

TUBERCULUM SELLAE MENINGIOMA

Management

MRI depicts the tumor and its relationship to the optic nerves, the chiasm, the internal carotid artery and its branches (42, 44). Angiography is usually unnecessary, and there is no indication for embolization.

The indication for surgical treatment is, usually, worsening vision. Surgical removal of the tumor provides the best chance for relief of symptoms and the highest possibility of curing the patient. Surgery should also be considered for an asymptomatic patient because of the likelihood of developing visual loss in the future. A conservative strategy dictates leaving small fragments of tumor attached to a critical structure that might be injured by their removal. Examples include tumors that do not easily separate from the internal carotid or anterior cerebral arteries and tumors encasing optic nerves, the optic chiasm, and their delicate blood supply.

In general, the authors prefer to use a right subfrontal exposure elevating the frontal lobe anterior to the sphenoid wing (40, 42, 44, 48). A left subfrontal exposure is used when the tumor bulk is greater on that side. Very large tumors may require a bifrontal exposure. Guthrie *et al.* (25), Andrews and Wilson (5), and Grisoli *et al.* (22) used the right subfrontal approach unless visual loss was greater on the left side. Logue (34) and Symon (64) used a unilateral right subfrontal exposure but approached the tumor along the midline. Al-Mefty and Smith (4) used a unilateral supraorbital exposure. For large tumors, Al-Mefty *et al.* (2) used a bifrontal craniotomy. Symon (64) resected a portion of the frontal lobe. The optic canal may need to be opened to complete the removal of the tumor.

Radiation therapy is recommended unless total removal is achieved. It is also used for recurrent tumor not previously irradiated. Doses of 5580 cGy in 180-cGy fractions are recommended.

Results

In this series, there were 18 patients who had an operation for tuberculum sella meningioma (Table 7.3). Fifteen females and three males ranged from 20 to 77 years of age; three were over 70 years of age. The indication for surgery in all but two patients was worsening vision. These two patients had frontal lobe syndromes. Sixteen of the eighteen patients had a good outcome after surgery. A fair result occurred in a female who had previously had four operations for her tumor before the authors saw her. Mild frontal lobe symptoms did not improve, and vision was worse. The poor result was in a 73-year-old woman with a severe frontal lobe syndrome that did not improve. After operation, vision was improved in 12, unchanged in 4, and worse in only 2. Two patients had transient changes in mental function that resolved. When diabetes insipidus occurred, it was transient.

Radical subtotal removal left a small fragment of tumor adherent to the internal carotid or anterior cerebral arteries or to the optic nerves

TABLE 7.3
Tuberculum Sella Meningioma: Surgical Series

Treatment		T	RST	RST and RT	ST	ST and RT
No. of patients		8	4	3	1	2
Follow-up scan		6	2	3	0	2
Years		2–12[a]	4,7	5,5,6	0	5,6
Growth		0	0	1[b]	0	1
Status at last evaluation[d]	G	7	4	2	1	2
	F	0	0	0	0	1[c]
	P	1[c]	0	0	0	0
	D	0	0	1[b]	0	0

[a]Mean = 6.3 years.
[b]Atypical meningioma that recurred after RT. See text.
[c]These patients had preoperative frontal lobe syndrome that did not improve.
[d]Five patients were lost to follow-up: good result, one total, two radical subtotal, and one subtotal removal; fair result, one total removal.

or chiasm. Subtotal removal was necessary in two patients with recurrent tumors in which the optic and arterial structures were encased in the tumor. It was also considered prudent to use subtotal removal in one elderly patient (21).

The results are recorded in Tables 7.3 and 7.4. There has been no recurrence after total removal. One patient had an atypical meningioma growing under his optic nerve into the optic canal. He did well for 5 years after radical subtotal removal and photon radiotherapy. The tumor then recurred with rapid growth. He did not improve with further surgery and died from tumor recurrence. One patient with subtotal removal had the optic nerves and chiasm encased in tumor. Following photon radiotherapy there was a reduction in the size of the tumor and a dramatic improvement in vision in one eye. A second patient showed deterioration in vision 5 years after subtotal removal and was given photon therapy at another institution. The authors now would usually recommend radiotherapy after any subtotal removal.

Patients in the series of Symon and Rosenstein (65), Andrews and Wilson (5), and Al-Mefty and Smith (4) also showed good results from surgery. A long history of visual impairment does not preclude good recovery, but improvement is more likely when the history is of relatively short duration (21).

The results of the authors' radiotherapy series are recorded in Table 7.4. Four of the patients are from the surgical series. There have been no complications.

TABLE 7.4
Tuberculum Sellae Meningioma (Radiotherapy Series)

Type of Radiotherapy		Photon	Proton
No. of patients		3	3
Prior surgery	RST	2	1
	ST	1	2
Dose	cGy	4500	5000
		4500	5400
		5000	5600
Follow-up scan		3	3
Years		5,5,6	2,3,6
Growth		1[a]	0
Status at last evaluation	G	2	3
	F	0	0
	P	0	0
	D	1[a]	0

[a]See text.

FLOOR OF FRONTAL FOSSA

Management

These meningiomas arise from the dura over the orbital roof and compress and/or cause edema in the adjacent frontal lobe. The diagnosis is established by MRI; angiography is not needed. The indications for operation are headache or frontal lobe symptoms. A lateral subfrontal approach is used to achieve total removal of the tumor. Radiation therapy has not been indicated.

Results

In this series, there were two patients. The indication for treatment in both was persistent headache. Both were females, ages 51 and 63 years, respectively. Total tumor removal was achieved, and both patients resumed their preoperative level of activity. There has been no recurrence.

OPTIC SHEATH MENINGIOMAS

Management

MRI clearly outlines the extent of this tumor (44); angiography is not needed. Decisions regarding treatment are difficult when the patient still has useful vision. In general, we have deferred surgery in patients with useful vision and in those with poor vision and tumor confined to the orbit. We reserve surgery for patients with poor vision and either intracranial extension or increasing orbital symptoms. Wright *et al.* (75) have emphasized the more aggressive nature of these tumors in younger patients and have recommended surgery for these patients. It is usually possible to remove the tumor completely but, if necessary, a small fragment of tumor is left if it is growing into the back of the globe, or if it is densely adherent to the internal carotid artery. The surgical approach is through a frontal-temporal craniotomy and orbital exploration (35).

Since the prognosis for vision is so poor with either observation or surgery, radiation therapy has been used in patients with worsening but still useful vision (32, 38). Long-term results remain to be evaluated.

Results

Fifteen patients had 16 operations for removal of an optic sheath meningioma, usually because of intracranial extension (Table 7.5). There were 13 females and 2 males, ranging from 16 to 65 years of age. All had poor or absent vision preoperatively, and all made a good recovery, except for their visual deficits. All intracranial tumor was re-

TABLE 7.5
Optic Sheath Meningioma (Surgical Series)

Treatment		T	RST	ST and RT
No. of patients		10	5	1[a]
Follow-up scan		9	4	1
Years		1–10[b]	2–10[c]	2
Growth		0	0	0
Status at last evaluation	G	9	5	1
	F	0	0	0
	P	0	0	0
	D	1[a]	0	0

[a]This patient had bilateral tumors and is also included in the total removal group. See text.
[b]Mean = 4.2 years.
[c]Mean = 5.1 years.

moved in 14 of these patients. One patient had a radical subtotal removal with a small piece of tumor left adherent to the internal carotid artery. Four patients had a small amount of tumor left at the back of the globe, but there has been no growth from these residual pieces.

Postoperatively, every patient had ptosis and some extraocular muscle paresis, but these symptoms usually recovered within a few months. There was one complication, a cerebrospinal fluid leak from an ethmoid air cell, which was repaired with a transethmoid approach.

The results are recorded in Table 7.5. There has been no recurrence. One patient, a 30-year-old man, had complete removal of an optic sheath meningioma. In less than a year, a tumor in the other optic sheath developed and began to cause visual loss. Exploration disclosed an optic sheath meningioma; a biopsy was performed and the optic canal decompressed. This tumor has been treated with 4500-cGy photon radiotherapy, and there has been no change over 2 years.

Good results following operation have been reported by others (10, 38, 56). In one report of 32 patients in whom it was thought total removal had been accomplished, three tumors recurred, and all of them were described as showing an infiltrative pattern of growth (19). Kennerdell *et al.* (32) reported that of six patients treated with radiation therapy (5400 to 5500 cGY), five had improvement in visual acuity, with follow-up ranging from 3 to 7 years.

MEDICAL SPHENOID WING (CLINOIDAL)

Management

These meningiomas involve the region of the anterior clinoid, adjacent medial sphenoid wing, superior orbital fissure, and cavernous sinus. They may grow into the orbit. The tumor often encases the internal carotid, proximal middle, and anterior cerebral arteries, as well as the optic nerve, and may compress or provoke edema in the temporal or frontal lobes.

MRI outlines the extent of the tumor and shows the relationship to the arterial structures and the extent of constriction of the internal carotid artery (44). MRI often shows the location of the optic nerves and chiasm. Angiography is usually needed to determine the external carotid artery blood supply and to decide if embolization of external carotid artery branches is needed.

Decisions on how to treat are often difficult to make. Prior to the development of CT and MRI and microsurgical techniques, it was difficult to remove these tumors completely. In addition, there was significant morbidity with the operation. With the development of microsurgical techniques, some of these tumors now can be radically removed. However, the relative indications for radical resection, partial removal followed by radiation therapy, or radiation therapy alone have not been defined.

Some general guidelines for the treatment of these tumors can be outlined. With mild or nonprogressive symptoms it may be appropriate to follow the patient with periodic scans and clinical examination to determine whether the lesion is growing or symptoms are progressing and to see whether the symptoms are significantly interfering with the patient's life. The indications for surgery in younger patients are worsening symptoms and/or growth seen on follow-up scans, and in older patients, a large tumor with worsening symptoms. The operation is planned to remove as much of the tumor as possible but to leave tumor that is densely adherent or encases the internal carotid artery, its branches, and/or the optic nerve, or is growing into the cavernous sinus or superior orbital fissures. Radiotherapy is used in older patients with small- and medium-sized tumors with worsening symptoms and for all ages with regrowth after subtotal removal.

The operative approach is similar to that used for tuberculum sella meningioma but with more temporal exposure. It may be necessary to open the medial aspect of the sylvian fissure to define the middle cerebral artery. The authors prefer a frontal temporal craniotomy, as do others (11, 25, 44).

Al-Mefty (1) has described a group of tumors that originate from the superior and/or lateral aspect of the anterior clinoid process. As the tumor grows, the arachnoid membrane remains intact, making microsurgical dissection from the internal carotid artery and optic nerve possible. Brotchi and Bonnal (11) also emphasize the importance of the arachnoid membrane in aiding dissection when there is arterial encasement.

Results

There were 16 patients in this surgical series, which included 12 females and 4 males, ranging from 28 to 79 years of age with two over 70 (Table 7.6). No patient had total removal because of involvement of the internal carotid artery and its branches and/or optic nerve and chiasm, or because of extension of the tumor into the cavernous sinus and/or orbit. Two patients had radical subtotal removal and 14 subtotal removal. In 15 patients there was an immediate good result. One patient had a postoperative intracerebral hemorrhage 2 weeks after surgery, apparently from a middle cerebral branch, and has permanent moderate dysphasia and hemiparesis.

The results are summarized in Table 7.6. Four of the patients who had subtotal removal have had regrowth of their tumor. Repeat surgery in three and radiotherapy in all four has been followed by arrest of growth. From the time of initial evaluation to last follow-up, only two patients had worsening vision, which was related in both patients to tumor regrowth. Vision was improved following the radical subtotal removal in two patients.

Brotchi and Bonnal (11) reported total removal in 9 of 28 patients, and 21 had no or minimal sequelae. Excellent results have been reported by Al-Mefty (1) with total removal in 20 of 27 patients.

The results of the radiotherapy series are recorded in Table 7.7; They include the six patients from the surgical series. There has been no growth in 9 of the 11 patients. One patient was lost to follow-up. One required a reoperation after 11 years. One had a small extension into

TABLE 7.6

Medial Sphenoid Wing Meningioma (Surgical Series)

Treatment		RST	ST	ST and RT
No. of patients		2	12	2 and 4[a]
Follow-up scan[b]		2	11	5
Years		7,11	2–14[c]	2–13[d]
Growth		0	4[a]	1[e]
Status at last evaluation	G	2	7[b]	6[b]
	F	0	0	0
	P	0	1	0
	D	0	0	0

[a]Four recurrences in the ST group were treated, with repeat operation in three patients and RT at 2,4,6, and 7 years.
[b]Two patients were lost to follow-up.
[c]Mean = 7.2 years.
[d]Mean = 5.6 years.
[e]Small growth in sinus (see text).

TABLE 7.7
Medial Sphenoid Wing Meningioma (Radiotherapy Series)

Type of Radiotherapy		Photon	Proton
No. of Patients		2	11
Prior surgery	ST	2	11
Dose	cGy	5000	5500–7200
		5200	M 6000
Follow-up scan[a]		2	10
Years		3,6	2–13[b]
Growth		0	2
Status at last evaluation	G	3	10
	F	0	0
	P	0	0
	D	0	1[c]

[a]One patient was lost to follow-up.
[b]Mean = 6.6 years.
[c]Unrelated cause at 6 years.

the ethmoid sinus that was removed while the intracranial tumor remains unchanged over 13 years. One patient died 6 years after treatment from an unrelated cause with no evidence of regrowth. One patient has had intermittent trigeminal pain and one worsening of a cranial nerve deficit.

CAVERNOUS SINUS MENINGIOMA

Management

Meningiomas may be localized to the region of the cavernous sinus and the immediate surrounding area, or the involvement may be part of a large tumor of the medial sphenoid wing, middle fossa, clivus, and/or petrous bone. The patients reviewed in this section are those with tumor localized to the cavernous sinus and adjacent area. Medial sphenoid wing meningomas with and without cavernous sinus involvement are discussed under Medical Sphenoid Wing (Clinoidal).

The extent of the tumor and involvement of the internal carotid artery are defined by MRI (44). When a surgical procedure is planned, angiography is needed to define the blood supply to the tumor.

The decision regarding treatment is often difficult because the symptoms may be mild or nonprogressive; the natural history may be one of minimal or no growth for long periods of time; there is risk of significant cranial nerve morbidity with surgical treatment; and the long-term results of new surgical treatments and radiation therapy modalities are unknown.

Because of these factors, guidelines for management continue to evolve. For patients less than 60 years old with worsening symptoms, the tumor is often explored. Removal is attempted when it appears feasible with a low probability of sacrificing cranial nerves and without the need to bypass the internal carotid artery. If injury to the cranial nerves or internal carotid artery appears likely, a subtotal removal is performed and radiation therapy administered. Radiotherapy is also used in older patients with worsening symptoms. Patients at any age with mild or nonprogressive symptoms are often followed-up.

The application of microsurgical techniques to the treatment of lesions in the cavernous sinus has been reviewed (3, 17, 57–59, 70). The anatomy of the cavernous sinus must be understood in order to treat these tumors. The approach used is a frontal-temporal craniotomy. As described by van Loveren *et al.* (70), the subsequent steps in the dissection depend on the direction and extent of the tumor's growth. We have resected the internal carotid artery only in the case of a malignant meningioma. Origitano *et al.* (50) have noted that the management of the internal carotid artery still places a significant limitation on cranial base surgery.

Results

The results are recorded in Table 7.8. In our surgical series, there were six patients. In only one did we think the entire tumor had been removed. The postoperative complications included two cases of third nerve palsy with one complete and one partial recovery, a wound infection, and a pulmonary embolus. Three have been given photon radiotherapy, all in the immediate postoperative period.

TABLE 7.8
Cavernous Sinus Meningioma

Treatment	Surgery			No Surgery		
	Alone	+ Photon	+ Proton	Photon	Proton	Observe
No. of patients	3	3	4	3	1	6
Dose (cGy)		4500 5200	5600–6400	4500 5000 5400	6300	
Follow-up scan	3	1[a]	4		1	6
Years	2,3,6	2	2,3,7,11		3	2–7[b]
Growth	0	0	0	0	0	1
Status at last evaluation G	3	3[a]	4	3	1	6
F	0	0	0	0	0	0
P	0	0	0	0	0	0
D	0	0	0	0	0	0

[a]One treatment at another institution, and one lost to follow-up after 1 year.
[b]Mean = 4.3 years.

Sekhar *et al.* (59) have reported total removal of 60 of 68 benign meningiomas of the cavernous sinus. Four of these have recurred. As this report was part of an overall summary of cavernous sinus tumors, the complications related to resection of meningiomas were not separately identified. However, in an earlier report of 45 patients with cavernous sinus meningiomas, 37 had a total removal of the tumor (57). The risk of permanent neurologic deficit exclusive of diplopia appeared to be low. In more than one-third of the patients the diplopia was worse, as compared to their preoperative status.

Six patients in our series have a presumed diagnosis of cavernous sinus meningioma based on MRI findings and are being followed-up without treatment. The clinical situations in which this decision was made include age and/or mild diplopia in five, intermittent trigeminal neuralgia in one, and asymptomatic tumors in two. In five of these patients the tumor and symptoms have remained stable. One patient shows minimal change on MRI but has a progressive third nerve palsy. He has declined treatment.

The results of radiotherapy are also recorded in Table 7.8. There have been no evidence of further growth and no new cranial nerve palsies.

CHONDROSARCOMA

Management

The majority of chondrosarcomas of the cranial base involve the posterior fossa, but they can occur in the ethmoid region and the cavernous sinus area by extension from the clivus (Liebsch NJ, Ojemann RG, Renard L, *et al.*, manuscript in preparation, 1995). MRI may suggest the diagnosis, but the nature of this tumor may not be established until operation. The indications for operation have been the development of an ethmoid sinus mass with extension through the cribriform plate and/or the recent onset of cranial nerve deficit.

Management includes surgery and stereotactic fractionated proton radiotherapy (Liebsch NJ, Ojemann RG, Renard L, *et al.*, manuscript in preparation, 1995). For chondrosarcomas involving the ethmoid sinus and growing intracranially, we combine a bifrontal craniotomy and lateral rhinotomy with or without a pedicle nasal flap (63). An en block resection of the area of pathology, including the dura, is done. The dura is repaired with a free pericranial graft. A separate vascularized pericranial graft is then brought over the bone defect and sutured to the dura posterior to the dural repair. The otolaryngologist places a skin graft in the roof of the nasal cavity. Nasal packs are left in place for 10 to 14 days, and a lumbar drain is used for 5 days. When the tumor is in the cavernous sinus, the approach is similar to that described for meningiomas. In some patients a gross total removal of the tumor can be done. Tumor projecting near the optic nerves or chiasm is removed, but no attempt is made to dissect the nerves in the cavernous sinus or to resect the internal carotid artery.

Results

In a series of 130 patients with low-grade chondrosarcoma of the cranial base treated with fractionated proton radiotherapy from 1974 to 1994, the authors found a local tumor control rate of 98% at 5 years (Liebsch NJ, Ojemann RG, Renard L, *et al.,* manuscript in preparation, 1995). Six of these patients had tumors involving the anterior skull base and/or cavernous sinus. The results are presented in Table 7.9. Three of these patients were in our surgical series. In one patient an en block resection of a chondrosarcoma involving the anterior cranial base with ethmoid sinus and intracranial extension was performed. The area of resection was treated with proton radiotherapy. Two patients had subtotal removal of tumor in the region of the cavernous sinus. Three other patients also had proton radiotherapy after a surgical procedure. There have been no complications in the surgical or radiotherapy series.

CHORDOMA

Management

Chordomas usually grow from the clivus into the posterior fossa. However, there can be growth into the cavernous sinus. Most patients present with a worsening cranial nerve deficit.

The management plan is to remove as much of the tumor as possible and then use fractionated stereotactic proton radiotherapy (7, 62). It is rarely possible to remove these tumors totally.

TABLE 7.9
Chondrosarcoma: Anterior Cranial Base and Cavernous Sinus

No. of patients		6
Prior surgery	RST	2
	ST	4
Proton radiotherapy	cGy	6800
Follow-up scan		6
Years		2–10[a]
Growth		0
Status at last evaluation	G	6

[a]Mean = 3.5 years.

TABLE 7.10

Chordoma: Anterior Cranial Base and Cavernous Sinus

No. of patients		7
Prior surgery	T	2
	ST	5
Proton radiotherapy	cGy	6900
Follow-up scan		7
Years		3–15[a]
Growth		2
Status at last evaluation	G	5
	D	1
	Unknown	1

[a]Mean = 8.5 years.

Results

The results of this combined therapy in our overall series have shown a local tumor control rate of 54% at 5 years. There were seven patients with anterior cranial base and cavernous sinus chordoma (Table 7.10). In this surgical series there was one patient with a chordoma involving the cavernous sinus. Subtotal removal was followed by proton radiation. There has been no growth in 10 years. Six other patients were treated after a surgical procedure. One patient died from recurrence, and one had a recurrence and has been lost to follow-up. There have been no complications from the treatment.

Sekhar *et al.* (58) reported recurrence in two of seven patients after apparent total removal and in three of five after partial removal of cavernous sinus chordomas.

ESTHESIONEUROBLASTOMA (OLFACTORY NEUROBLASTOMA)

Management

These patients present with nasal obstruction, epistaxis, or proptosis. When the nasal cavity is examined, there is a fleshy polypoid mass. CT scan defines the extent of the bony defect, and the MRI shows the soft tissue extension into the anterior fossa and/or cavernous sinus. The diagnosis is established by means of nasal biopsy. The tumor is then staged according to the system proposed by Kadish *et al.* (30).

Our management plan for patients with intracranial extension starts with two cycles of *cis*-platinum and VP16 (etoposide). If there is a good response, fractionated stereotactic proton radiotherapy (6800 cGy) is administered. This is followed by two additional cycles of chemotherapy. If there is an incomplete response to the chemotherapy, surgical resection is performed. This procedure is followed by radiotherapy and additional chemotherapy. For the surgical resection the authors use the same combination of procedures described for chondrosarcoma of the anterior cranial base. A different program of treatment has been reported (12).

Results

There were six patients in this series. All but one patient has had a complete response to the initial chemotherapy. For this patient a bifrontal craniotomy combined with a lateral rhinotomy was performed and a gross total removal of the tumor accomplished. All patients were treated with fractionated stereotactic proton radiotherapy, then with more chemotherapy. All six patients are alive and well without evidence of intracranial recurrence, but follow-up has been short, with the longest follow-up only 2 years.

SINUS CARCINOMA GROWING INTO ANTERIOR FOSSA

Management

For the surgical management of those tumors with intradural extension, the authors used a bifrontal craniotomy combined with a lateral rhinotomy as described under Chondrosarcoma (63). Careful planning of the surgical approach is needed to include prevention of CSF leak and adequate functional and aesthetic preservation (28). Tumors without intradural extension are treated with surgical removal through an ethmoid or maxillary approach, followed by fractionated stereotactic proton radiotherapy.

Results

There were three patients in this series treated with the combined surgical procedure for intradural extension, followed by radiotherapy. There were no postoperative complications.

Thirteen patients with sinus carcinoma and intracranial extension were treated with fractionated stereotactic proton radiotherapy, usually up to a dose of 7600 cGy. Eight patients had squamous cell carcinoma; five are alive with no evidence of regrowth up to 14 months after treatment. Three patients have died of metastatic disease, but two of these had no evidence of local recurrence.

Five patients had adenocystic carcinoma; four are alive with no evidence of local recurrence up to 16 months, but one has a lung metastasis. With the one death, there was good local control of the tumor.

TRIGEMINAL NEUROMA

Management

These tumors usually present with increasing facial numbness and/or trigeminal pain. The diagnosis is suggested by MRI scan, particularly if there is a small "hourglass" extension into the posterior fossa (9).

Jefferson (29) classified these tumors into three categories. Class A tumors are located primarily within the posterior fossa; Class B tumors are located primarily within the middle fossa; and Class C tumors have significant masses in both posterior and middle fossa with a thin "hourglass" bridge around the petrous apex. Class B tumors, which comprise about 50% of the total, are located in Meckel's cave and wall of the cavernous sinus with, at times, a small extension below the tentorium. These tumors are removed through a low subtemporal intradural approach, which may involve division of the zygomatic arch. A lumbar drain, in addition to the use of furosemide and mannitol, aids the exposure and minimizes complications from temporal lobe retraction. The tentorium may need to be opened to aid the dissection along the fifth nerve.

Radiotherapy has not been used in this group of patients.

Results

In this series, three patients had complete removal of a trigeminal neuroma from Meckel's cave and the wall of the cavernous sinus. All made a good recovery, with varying degrees of residual numbness.

EPIDERMOID

Management

Epidermoid tumors can involve the cavernous sinus and adjacent bone, causing abnormalities in ocular motility. The diagnosis is suggested by the typical MRI findings.

A patient with stable symptoms may be followed. The indication for surgery is worsening diplopia or headache.

Intraoperatively, the most difficult decision is usually how much of the capsule should be dissected from functional structures. Often, it may be good judgment to leave a small piece of capsule that is densely adherent (46, 47).

Results

There were two patients in this series. One presented with a partial third nerve palsy, which has worsened over a period of 10 years with no change on CT scan; he has declined surgery. The other patient had increasing unilateral frontal and orbital discomfort, which was relieved by removal of the tumor. There has been no recurrence in 4 years.

ACKNOWLEDGMENTS

The authors thank Drs. John Munzenrider, Norbert Liebsch, and Rita Linggood of the Radiation Oncology Service at the Massachusetts General Hospital, who treated many of these patients, and Jean Ojemann, who provided editorial assistance and manuscript preparation.

REFERENCES

1. Al-Mefty O: Clinoidal meningiomas, in Al-Mefty O (ed): **Meningiomas.** New York, Raven Press, 1991, pp 427–443.
2. Al-Mefty O, Holoubi A, Rifai A, *et al.:* Microsurgical removal of suprasellar meningiomas. **Neurosurgery** 16:364–372, 1985.
3. Al-Mefty O, Smith RR: Surgery of tumors invading the cavernous sinus. **Surg Neurol** 30:370–381, 1988.
4. Al-Mefty O, Smith RR: Tuberculum sella meningiomas, in Al-Mefty O (ed): *Meningiomas.* New York, Raven Press, 1991, pp 395–411.
5. Andrews BT, Wilson CB: Suprasellar mengingiomas: The effect of tumor location on postoperative visual outcome. **J Neurosurg** 69:523–528, 1988.
6. Aristizabal S, Caldwell WL: The relationship of time-dose factors to complications in the treatment of pituitary tumors by irradiation. **Int J Radiation Oncol Biol Phys** 1:24–28, 1990.
7. Austin-Seymour M, Munzenrider J, Goitein M, *et al.:* Fractionated proton radiation therapy of chordoma and low grade chondrosarcoma of the base of the skull. **J Neurosurg** 70:13–17, 1989.
8. Barbaro NM, Gutin PH, Wilson CB, *et al.:* Radiation therapy in the treatment of partially resected meningiomas. **Neurosurgery** 20:525–528, 1987.
9. Barker FG II, Ojemann RG: Surgical approach to tumors of the posterior fossa cranial nerves (excluding acoustic neuroma), in Barrow DL (ed): *Surgery of the Cranial Nerves of the Posterior Fossa.* Park Ridge, IL, AANS Publications, 1993, pp 253–274.
10. Basso AJ, Carrizo A, Kreutel A, *et al.:* Primary intraorbital meningioma, In Schmidek HH (ed): *Meningiomas and Their Surgical Management.* Philadelphia, W.B. Saunders, 1991.
11. Brotchi J, Bonnal JP: Lateral and middle sphenoid wing meningiomas, in Al-Mefty O (ed): *Meningiomas.* New York, Raven Press, 1991, pp 413–425.
12. Cantrell RW: Esthesioneuroblastoma, in Sekhar LN (ed): *Surgery of Cranial Base Tumors.* New York, Raven Press, 1993, pp 471–476.
13. Carella RJ, Ransohoff J, Newall J: Role of radiation therapy in the management of meningiomas. **Neurosurgery** 10:332–339, 1982.
14. Chan RC, Schukovksy LJ: Effects of irradiation on the eye. **Radiology** 120:673–675, 1976.
15. Chan RC, Thompson GB: Morbidity, mortality and quality of life following surgery for intracranial meningiomas. A retrospective study in 257 cases. **J Neurosurg** 60:52–60, 1984.

16. Cogan DG, Donaldson DD, Reese AB: Clinical and pathological characteristics of radiation cataract. **Arch Ophthalmol** 47:55–70, 1952.
17. Dolenc V: *The Cavernous Sinus.* New York, Springer-Verlag, 1987.
18. Fraass BA, McShan DL: 3-D treatment planning. 1. Overview of a clinical planning system, in Bruinvis IAD (ed): *The Use of Computers in Radiation Therapy.* Amsterdam, Elsevier Science Publishers BV, 1987, pp 273–276.
19. Gabibov GA, Blinkov SM, Tchorkayev VA: The management of optic nerve meningiomas and gliomas. **J Neurosurg** 68:889–893, 1988.
20. Goitein M, Abrams M, Rowell D, *et al.:* Multi-dimensional treatment planning. II. Beam's-eye view, back-projection, and projection through CT sections. **Int J Radiat Oncol Biol Phys** 9:789–797, 1983.
21. Gregorius FK, Hepler RS, Stern WE: Loss and recovery of vision with suprasellar meningiomas. **J Neurosurg** 42:69–75, 1975.
22. Grisoli F, Diaz-Vasquez P, Riss M, *et al.:* Microsurgical management of tuberculum sellae meningiomas. Results in 28 cases. **Surg Neurol** 26:37–44, 1986.
23. Grunberg SM, Weiss MH, Spitz IM, *et al.:* Treatment of unresectable meningiomas with the antiprogesterone agent mifepristone. **J Neurosurg** 74:861–866, 1991.
24. Guthrie BL, Carabell SC, Law ER Jr: Radiation therapy for intracranial meningiomas, in Al-Mefty O (ed): *Meningiomas.* New York, Raven Press, 1991, pp 253–262.
25. Guthrie BL, Ebersohl MJ, Scheithauer BW: Neoplasms of the intracranial meninges, in Youmans JR (ed): *Neurological Surgery.* Philadelphia, W.B. Saunders, 1990, pp 3250–3315.
26. Harris, JR, Levine MB: Visual complications following irradiation for pituitary adenomas and craniopharyngiomas. **Radiology** 120:167–171, 1976.
27. Hassler W, Zentner J: Pterional approach for surgical treatment of olfactory groove meningioma. **Neurosurgery** 25:942–947, 1989.
28. Janecka ID, Sekhar LN, Myers EN: Nasal/paranasal sinus carcinoma, in Sekhar LN (ed): *Surgery of Cranial Base Tumors.* New York, Raven Press, 1993, pp 497–506.
29. Jefferson G: The trigeminal neurinomas with some remarks on malignant invasion of the gasserian ganglion. **Clin Neurosurg** 1:11–54, 1955.
30. Kadish S, Goodman M, Wang CC: Olfactory neuroblastoma. **Cancer** 35:1571–1576, 1976.
31. Kassirer JP: Incorporating patient's perferences into medical decisions. **N Engl J Med** 330:1895–1896, 1994.
32. Kennerdell JS, Maroon JC, Maltor M, *et al.:* The management of optic nerve sheath meningiomas. **Am J Ophtalmol** 106:450–457, 1988.
33. Komisar A, Silver C, Kalnicki S: Osteoradionecrosis of the maxilla and skull base. **Laryngoscope** 95 (1):24–28, 1985.
34. Logue V: Sugery of meningiomas, in Symon L (ed): *Operative Sugery: Neurosurgery.* London, Butterworth, 1979, pp 128–173.
35. Long DM: Neurosurgical involvement in tumors of the orbit. **Clin Neurosurg** 32:514–523, 1984.
36. Long DM: Surgery for supratentorial meningiomas, in Long DM (ed): *Atlas of Operative Neurosurgical Technique, Vol 1: Cranial Operations.* Baltimore, Williams & Wilkins, 1989, pp 218–248.
37. Munzenrider JE, Verhey LJ, Gragoudas ES, *et al.:* Conservative treatment of uveal melanoma: Local recurrence after proton beam therapy. **Int J Radiat Oncol Biol Phys** 17:493–498. 1989.
38. Newman SA, Jane JA: Meningiomas of the optic nerve, orbit and anterior visual pathways, in Al-Mefty O (ed): **Meningiomas.** New York, Raven Press, 1991, pp 461–494.

39. Ojemann RG: Meningiomas of the basal parapituitary region. Technical considerations. **Clin Neurosurg** 27:233–262, 1980.
40. Ojemann RG: Meningiomas: Clinical features and surgical mangement, in Wilkins RH, Rengachary SS (ed): *Neurosurgery.* New York, McGraw-Hill, 1985, pp 635–654.
41. Ojemann RG: Olfactory groove meningiomas, in Al-Mefty O (ed): *Meningiomas.* New York, Raven Press, 1991, pp 383–394.
42. Ojemann RG: Surgical management of olfactory groove, suprasellar and medial sphenoid wing meningioma, in Schmidek HH (ed): *Meningiomas and Their Surgical Management.* Philadelphia, W.B. Saunders, 1991, pp 242–259.
43. Ojemann RG: Skull-base surgery: A perspective. *J Neurosurg* 76:569–570, 1992.
44. Ojemann RG: Management of cranial and spinal meningiomas. **Clin Neurosurg** 40:321–383, 1993.
45. Ojemann RG: Modern neurosurgical philosophy, in Awad IA (ed): *Philosopy of Neurological Surgery.* Park Ridge, IL, AANS Publications, 1995, pp 27–31.
46. Ojemann RG: Clinical decision making in skull base surgery, in Tindal GT, Cooper PR, Barrow DL (eds): *The Practice of Neurosurgery.* Baltimore, Williams & Wilkins, in press, 1995.
47. Ojemann RG: Black PM: Difficult decisions in managing patients with benign brain tumors. *Clin Neurosurg* 35:259–285, 1988.
48. Ojemann RG, Swann KW: Meningiomas of the anterior cranial base, in Sekhar LN, Schramm VS Jr (ed): *Tumors of the Cranial Base: Diagnosis and Treatment.* Mount Kisco, NY, Futura, 1987, pp 279–294.
49. Ojemann RG, Swann KW: Surgical management of olfactory groove, suprasellar and medial sphenoid wing meningiomas, in Schmidek HH, Sweet WH (ed): *Operative Neurosurgical Techniques.* Orlando, FL, Grune & Stratton, 1988, pp 531–544.
50. Origitano TC, Al-Mefty O, Leonnetii JP, DeMonte F, Reichman OH: Vascular considerations and complications in cranial base surgery. **Neurosurgery** 35:351–363, 1994.
51. Parsons JT, Fitzgerald CR, Hood CI, *et al.:* The effects of irradiation on the eye and optic nerve. **Int J Radiat Oncol Biol Phys** 9:609–622, 1983.
52. Pellegrino ED: "The Common Devotion": Cushing's legacy and medical ethics today. The 1983 Harvey Cushing Oration. **J Neurosurg** 59:567–573, 1983.
53. Roden D, Bosley TM, Fowbie B, *et al.:* Schatz NJ: Delayed radiation injury to the retrobulbar optic nerves and chiasm. Clinical syndrome and treatment with hyperbaric oxygen and corticosteroids. **Ophthalmology** 97 (3):346–351, 1990.
54. Samaan NA, Vieto R, Schultz PN, *et al.:* Hypothalamic pituitary and thyroid dysfunction after radiotherapy to the head and neck. **Int J Radiat Oncol Biol Phys** 8 (11):1857–1867, 1982.
55. Schatz N, Lichtenstein S, Corbet J: Delayed radiation necrosis of optic nerve and chiasm, in Glaser JS, Lawton-Smith J (eds): *Neuro-Ophthalmology.* St. Louis, CV Mosby, vol 8, chap 19, p 131.
56. Schurmann K: Meningiomas of the orbit: A personal series, in Schmidek HH (ed): *Meningiomas and Their Surgical Management.* Philadelphia, W.B. Saunders, 1991, pp 324–336.
57. Sekhar LN, Altschulen EM: Meningiomas of the cavernous sinus, in Al-Mefty O (ed): *Meningiomas.* New York, Raven Press, 1991, pp 445–460.
58. Sekhar LN, Pemeranz S, Sen C: Management of tumors involving the cavernous sinus. **Acta Neurochir Suppl** 53:101–112, 1991.
59. Sekhar LN: Ross DA, Sen C: Cavernous sinus and sphenocavernous neoplasms: Anatomy and surgery, in Sekhar LN, Janaka IP (eds): *Surgery of Cranial Base Tumors.* New York, Raven Press, 1993, pp 521–604.

60. Shukovsky LJ, Fletcher GH: Retinal and optic nerve complications in a high dose irradiation technique of ethmoid sinus and nasal cavity. **Radiology** 104 (3):629–634, 1972.
61. Solero CL, Giombini S, Morello G: Supersellar and olfactory meningioma: Report of a series of 153 personal cases. **Acta Neurochir** 67:181–194, 1983.
62. Suit HD, Goitein M, Munzenrider J, *et al.:* Definitive radiation therapy for chordoma and chondrosarcoma of base of skull and cervical spine. **J Neurosurg** 56:377–385, 1982.
63. Swearingen B, Joseph M, Cheny M, *et al.:* A modified transfacial approach to the clivus. Neurosurgery 36:101–105, 1995.
64. Symon L: Olfactory groove and suprasellar meningiomas, in Krayenbuhl H (ed): *Advances and Technical Standards in Neurosurgery, Vol 4.* Vienna, Springer-Verlag, 1977, pp 67–91.
65. Symon L, Rosenstein J: Surgical management of suprasellar meningioma. Part 1: The influence of tumor size, duration of symptoms and microsurgery on surgical outcome in 101 consecutive cases. **J Neurosurg** 61:633–641, 1984.
66. Taylor BW Jr, Marcus RB Jr, Friedman WA, *et al.:* The meningioma controversy: Postoperative radiation therapy. **Int J Radiat Oncol Biol Phys** 154:299–304, 1988.
67. Thornton AF, Gell K, Rosenthal SJ: Technical advances in the irradiation of head and neck neoplasia. *Proceedings of the Third International Conference on Head and Neck Cancer.* Amsterdam, Elsevier Science Publishers BV, 1992.
68. Tobias CA, Roberts JE, Lawrence JH, *et al.:* Irradiation hypophysectomy and related studies using 340-MeV protons and 190-MeV deutrons. Peaceful uses of atomic energy 10:95–106, 1956.
69. Urie MM, Fullerton B, Tatsuzaki H, *et al.:* A dose response analysis of injury to cranial nerves and/or nuclei following proton beam radiation therapy. **Int J Radiat Oncol Biol Phys** 23:27–39, 1992.
70. van Loveren HR, Keller JT, El-Kalliny M, *et al.:* The Dolenc technique for cavernous sinus exploration (cadaveric prosection). Technical note. **J Neurosurg** 74:837–844, 1991.
71. Wara WM, Irvine AR, Neger RE, *et al.:* Radiation retinopathy. **Int J Radiat Oncol Biol Phys** 5:81–83, 1979.
72. Wara WM, Sheline GE, Newman H, *et al.:* Radiation therapy of meningiomas. **Am J Roentgenol** 123:453–458, 1975.
73. Wigg DR, Koschel K, Hodgson GS: Tolerance of the mature human central nervous system to photon irradiation. **Br J Radiol** 54 (645):787–798, 1981.
74. Wilson RR: Radiological use of fast protons. **Radiology** 47:487–491, 1946.
75. Wright JE, McNab AM, McDonald WI: Primary optic nerve sheath meningioma. **Br J Ophthalmol** 73:960–966, 1989.
76. Young, W, Thornton A, Gebarski S, *et al.:* Radiation-induced optic neuropathy: Correlation of MRI and radiation dosimetry. **Radiology** 185:904–907, 1992.

8

Stereotactic Radiosurgery
of Anterior Skull Base Tumors

L. DADE LUNSFORD, M.D., THOMAS C. WITT, M.D.,
DOUGLAS KONDZIOLKA, M.D., M.Sc., FRCS(C),
AND JOHN C. FLICKINGER, M.D.

INTRODUCTION

Two important goals of modern skull base surgery are to improve the natural history of the tumor and to reduce the likelihood of new postoperative neurologic deficits. These goals are particularly difficult to achieve in patients with tumors of the anterior skull base. Even with advanced microsurgical techniques, the possibility of early surgical morbidity and mortality and delayed tumor regrowth remains. The three most common sources of morbidity and mortality in conventional skull base neurosurgery are injury to cranial nerves exiting the skull base, cerebrospinal fluid leakage, and injury to the carotid artery.

Secondary goals of current management of skull base tumor patients include reduction in the cost of treatment and optimization of the patient's ability to return to preoperative functional status and gainful employment. Because extensive skull base operations require the expertise of multiple surgical specialists, extended recovery periods, lengthy stays in intensive care units, and prolonged rehabilitation, the current total cost of microsurgical treatment is high. The total percentage of patients who undergo skull base microsurgery and return to work is not known.

An alternative neurosurgical approach for many patients with skull base tumors is stereotactic radiosurgery. Stereotactic radiosurgery attempts to achieve tumor control (prevention of further growth) by delivering a large, highly concentrated dose of radiation to the tumor while at the same time subjecting adjacent normal structures to a tolerable radiation dose. The high dose of radiation delivered to the tumor may arrest tumor growth, either by a direct cytotoxic effect or by inducing endothelial thickening and vessel occlusion within the tumor microvasculature.

Since 1987, the authors have used stereotactic radiosurgery for 143 patients with a variety of anterior skull base tumors. The majority of these tumors were located adjacent to the pituitary gland or the cavernous sinuses. The spectrum of tumors included meningiomas, pituitary adenomas, chordomas, chondrosarcomas, craniopharyngiomas, and metastases (Table 8.1). The authors have used stereotactic radiosurgery as a primary treatment in patients with the following associated features: the elderly; those medically unfit for a major operation secondary to concomitant systemic medical problems; those who fail balloon test occlusion of the carotid artery; those with multiple skull base tumors; those who are unable to accept the potential risk of cranial nerve dysfunction associated with microsurgery; and those who refuse microsurgical excision. The authors have also used stereotactic radiosurgery as a secondary management strategy or even in a prospective staged approach in patients with residual or recurrent tumor after microsurgical excision.

Technique

Stereotactic radiosurgery at the University of Pittsburgh is performed with high-energy photon beams using the 60-cobalt 201 source Gamma Knife (Elekta Instruments, Atlanta, GA). The authors' techniques have been thoroughly reported on elsewhere (18, 19) but will be briefly described here.

The Leksell Model G (Elekta Instruments, Atlanta, GA) stereotactic frame is applied under local anesthesia, supplemented in certain patients with a small amount of intravenous sedation as needed. General anesthesia is used for patients under the age of 14. Patients are then transported to the magnetic resonance imaging (MRI) or computed tomography (CT) unit for high-resolution multiplanar stereotactic imaging. The authors rely almost exclusively on MRI images due to their superior multiplanar resolution of the relationship of tumor to adjacent cranial nerve, vascular, and brain stem structures. The authors have not detected any significant differences between MRI-derived

TABLE 8.1
Stereotactic Radiosurgery for Tumors of the Anterior Skull Base[a]

Tumor Type	Total No. of Tumors (%)
Meningiomas	64 (45)
Pituitary tumors	55 (38)
Craniopharyngiomas	7 (5)
Metastatic tumors	7 (5)
Chordomas	7 (5)
Chondrosarcomas	3 (2)
Total	143 (100)

[a]Data from the University of Pittsburgh was compiled from August 1987 to August 1994.

stereotactic coordinates and CT-derived coordinates (14). The stereotactic images are transferred via Ethernet to a computer work station for dose planning. Measurements of the patient's skull radii are used to calculate the attenuation of the photon beams prior to reaching the target. The angle that the central beam will make with respect to the frame base is also determined and used in dose planning (29). Sources that generate photon beams penetrating the lenses of the patient's eyes during treatment are blocked to reduce the theoretical risk of delayed cataract development.

Once these measurements and the stereotactic images are entered into the computer, conformal isodose plans are generated with various combinations, 4-, 8-, 14-, and 18-mm collimator beams. The use of multiple isocenters in dose plans is essential to shape precisely the desired isodose to the tumor margin (10). The 50% isodose line most commonly conforms to the tumor margin. This line represents the point at which the slope of radiation falloff is sharpest when the Gamma Knife is used (29). Higher marginal isodoses are prescribed in those patients whose tumor margins conform to such isodoses (*e.g.,* 60%). Selective beam blocking can be used to reduce the radiation dose curves near the optic nerves, chiasm, and tracts (11) (Fig. 8.1).

Selection of maximum and marginal tumor doses is performed in conjunction with colleagues from radiation oncology and medical physics. The dose is selected by examining the relationship of the tumor volume to the dose that would be predicted by the integrated logistic formula to have a 3% chance of causing a permanent neurologic deficit (8). Dose may also be reduced if the patient has had prior fractionated radiotherapy (9), or if the tumor margin is close to the optic apparatus. The authors generally keep the dose to the optic system at no more than 8 or 9 Gy in a single fraction (7).

After the coordinates for the first isocenter have been set on the stereotactic frame, the patient is positioned in the Gamma Knife helmet for delivery of a specific dose of radiation for each isocenter. The frame is removed on completion of treatment. The patient receives an intravenous dose of methylprednisolone and is transported to an observation unit. The majority of patients are released on the same day, and the remainder are discharged the next morning.

Results

MENINGIOMAS

Stereotactic radiosurgery was performed on 64 patients with meningiomas of the anterior skull base. The anatomic distribution of these

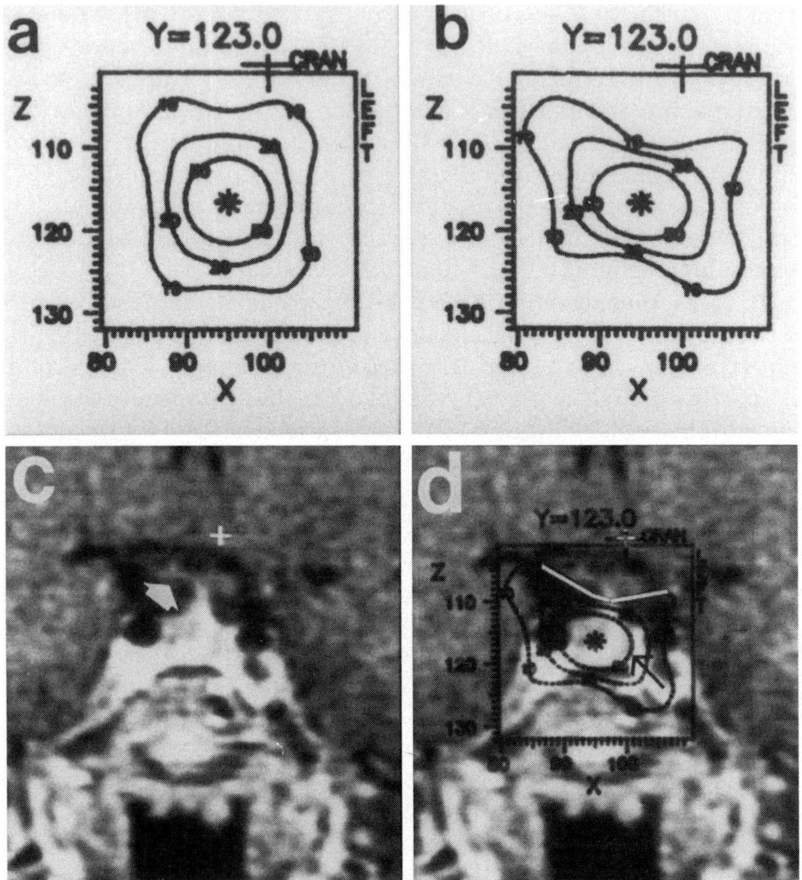

FIG. 8.1 Through selective beam blocking, peripheral isodose curves are shifted away from critical structures. (a) 10, 20, and 50% isodose curves for a single isocenter of radiation, using the 8-mm collimator beams and no selective blocking. (b) The same set of isodose curves after selectively blocking beams located at the left and rear of the helmet. (c) The optic chiasm (*arrow*) is in close proximity to the tumor. (d) Using selective beam blocking, the optic chiasm lies outside of the 10% isodose curve, while the intrasellar pituitary adenoma is enclosed within the 50% isodose line.

tumors is shown in Table 8.2. Tumors were located primarily within the cavernous sinus in 49 (76%) patients, along the floor of the anterior cranial fossa in 10 (16%) patients, extending from the cavernous sinus along the petrous apex in 3 (5%) patients, and originating from the dorsum sella in 2 (3%) patients. A neurologic deficit was present in 52 (81%) patients at the time of radiosurgery. Forty-four patients (69%)

had undergone one or more microsurgical resections of their tumor prior to radiosurgery. Eight patients underwent a gross total resection of their tumor but suffered a recurrence. Four patients (6%) received fractionated radiotherapy prior to radiosurgery. Patients varied from 12 to 86 years of age (mean, 54 years). Forty-eight (75%) of the patients were female, and 16 (25%) were male.

The dose of radiation delivered to the tumor margin varied from 10 to 20 Gy (mean, 15,38 Gy), and the maximum dose received by the tumor was 20 to 54 Gy (mean, 37 Gy). A mean number of 5 isocenters was used to create a conformal radiation dose plan for each tumor. The volume of tumor within the prescribed isodose margin ranged from 2.9 to 23.0 ml. The isodose prescribed to the tumor margin was most commonly the 50% isodose (55 of 64 cases).

Follow-up was available in 55 of 64 patients from 3 to 60 months (mean, 27 months) after radiosurgery. Patients with less than 3 months follow-up and those in whom no follow-up was available were excluded from analysis of outcome. The tumor volume response was obtained by examining serial MRI studies (Table 8.3). The tumor volume decreased in 28 patients (51%) (Fig. 8.2) and remained stable in 25 patients (45%) (Fig. 8.3), resulting in an overall tumor control rate of 96%. Tumor growth occurred in two patients at 46 and 48 months after radiosurgery; one of these patients (who had a malignant meningioma) also developed metastasis to the lung.

Follow-up clinical information and neurologic status was assessed in 28 patients who had a neurologic deficit prior to radiosurgery (Table

TABLE 8.2

Anatomic Location of Anterior Skull Base Meningiomas Undergoing Radiosurgery[a]

Location	No. of Meningiomas (%)
Cavernous sinus	49 (76)
Olfactory groove/tuberculum sella	10 (16)
Cavernous sinus/petroclival	3 (5)
Dorsum sella	2 (3)

[a]n = 64.

TABLE 8.3

Tumor Imaging Changes after Radiosurgery for Anterior Skull Base Meningiomas[a]

Tumor Volume	No. of Tumors (%)
Decreased	28 (51)
Unchanged	25 (45)
Increased	2 (4)

[a]n = 55. Mean follow-up, 27 months (range, 3 to 60 months).

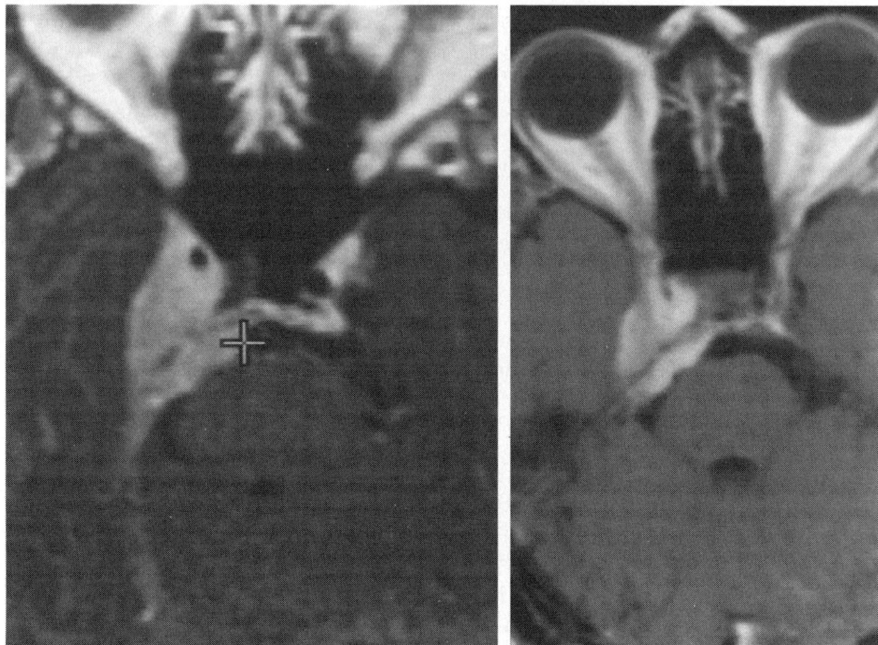

FIG. 8.2 Reduction in volume of a cavernous sinus meningioma in a patient who did not tolerate balloon test occlusion of her carotid artery. (**Left**) Tumor at the time of radiosurgery. (**Right**) 30 months after radiosurgery.

8.4). Eight patients (28%) showed improvement in neurologic function, and 19 patients (68%) remained stable after radiosurgery. One patient (4%), who had a tuberculum sella meningioma that was directly adjacent to the optic chiasm, had bilateral inferior temporal quadrantanopsia, 20/30 vision in the left eye, and 20/40 vision in the right eye at the time of radiosurgery. His tumor was treated at the 50% isodose line with a maximum dose of 33.3 Gy. Using CT images for stereotactic dose planning, the estimated dose to the optic chiasm was less than 10 Gy. Eight months after radiosurgery, he had a complete right homonymous hemianopsia, a decrease in a vision in the left eye to 20/40, and decreased acuity in the right eye to 20/200. An MRI showed no change in the size of the tumor and a new area of contrast enhancement in the inferior hypothalamus. In this patient the optic nerve most likely received a higher than tolerance dose.

Three patients who had no deficits prior to radiosurgery developed neurologic deficits afterward. One patient with a cavernous sinus meningioma extending into the middle fossa developed a left inferior

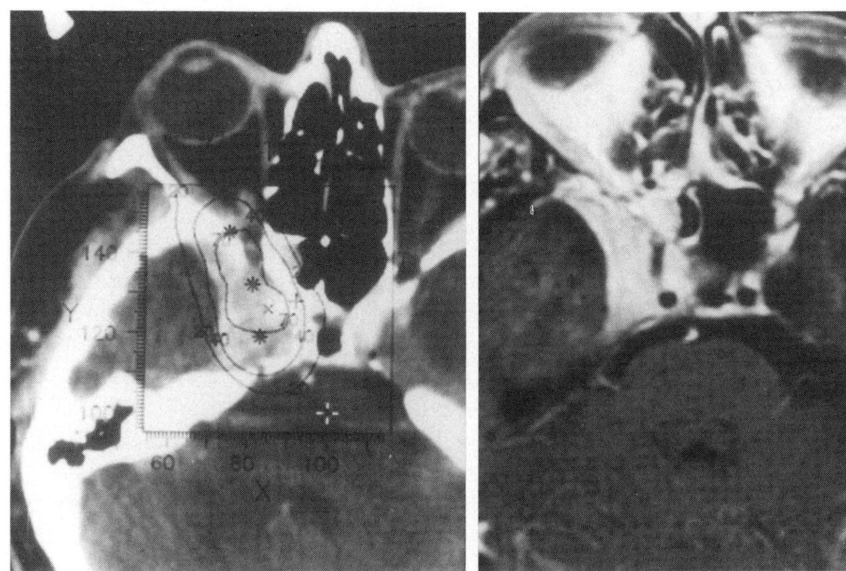

FIG. 8.3 Arrest of tumor growth in a patient with a medial sphenoid wing meningioma that recurred 2 years after "gross total removal." (**Left**) Tumor at the time of radiosurgery. (**Right**) Dormant tumor 5 years after radiosurgery.

TABLE 8.4
Clinical Status after Radiosurgery for Anterior Skull Base Meningiomas[a]

Pre-existing Neurologic Deficit[b]	No. of Patients (%)
Improved	8 (28)
Unchanged	19 (68)
Worse	1 (4)

[a]Mean follow-up, 27 months (range, 3 to 60 months).
[b]$n = 28$.

nasal quadrantanopsia and decreased acuity (20/70) in her left eye 6 months after radiosurgery. There was enhancement of her left optic nerve on MRI scan but no change in the size of the tumor. By 10 months, acuity in her left eye had improved to 20/30. The estimated dose for her optic nerve was 12.5 Gy. A second patient developed a left hemianopic defect 32 months after radiosurgery for a cavernous sinus meningioma, extending along the tentorium and into the pituitary fossa. The T2-weighted MRI scan showed high signal in the left side of the optic chiasm but no change in the size of the tumor. Her visual field deficit has remained stable at 59 months. A third patient developed a partial sixth nerve paresis 46 months after radiosurgery for a recurrent cavernous sinus/petrous apex meningioma. MRI also showed an increase in tumor volume in the cavernous sinus, tentorial notch, and middle fossa.

Three patients died during the follow-up interval. One patient (who had four previous craniotomies for a cavernous sinus meningioma) died from a seizure and respiratory failure 19 months after radiosurgery for a residual clivus meningioma. A second patient died of a myocardial infarction 8 months after radiosurgery. A third patient died 49 months after radiosurgery from a recurrent cavernous sinus malignant meningioma. Her tumor remained stable for 4 years after radiosurgery, but she subsequently developed extracranial metastases to the parapharyngeal area and to the lung. Local tumor recurrence produced multiple new cranial nerve palsies before she died.

Tumor volume decreased or was stable in 96% of patients with meningiomas. The rate of preservation or improvement in preradiosurgical neurologic status was 96%. Three of 55 patients had complications most likely related to adverse effects of radiation. One patient developed a new neurologic deficit as a consequence of tumor growth. One patient developed new deficits and died as a result of further malignant tumor growth.

These results (Table 8.5) compare favorably with the results reported in a recent series of microsurgical resection of anterior skull base meningiomas. Even with advanced microsurgical techniques and postoperative intensive care, mortality rates may be as high as 6% (6). The incidence of new postoperative cranial nerve deficits in recent surgical series ranged from 18 to 86% (5, 6, 13, 24). In an earlier report of patients with cavernous sinus meningiomas who has stereotactic radiosurgery at our institution, we found that 62% had deficits as a direct consequence of prior microsurgical resection of tumor (7). The incidence of other postoperative morbidity from CSF leak, infection, cerebral ischemia, and pulmonary emboli is also significant. Origitano *et*

TABLE 8.5
Tumor Control and Neurologic Status after Radiosurgery
Anterior Skull Base Meningiomas[a]

Tumor control	96 (53/55)
Tumor growth	4 (2/55)
Preservation of neurologic function	91 (50/55)
Decreased neurologic function	9 (5/55)
Related to radiation	5 (3/55)
Related to tumor growth	4 (2/55)

[a]n = 55. Mean follow-up 27 months (range, 3 to 60 months).

al. recently reported a 22% incidence of delayed ischemic complications in patients undergoing sacrifice of one carotid artery, even though they had passed preoperative carotid occlusion assessments (21). In such patients radiosurgery appears to be a valuable alternative. We have never observed delayed cerebral ischemia or imaging-defined vessel narrowing after radiosurgery in a patient with a cavernous sinus tumor surrounding the carotid artery.

PITUITARY TUMORS

Stereotactic radiosurgery was performed on 55 patients with pituitary adenomas. Forty-one patients (74%) had endocrine-active tumors. At the time of radiosurgery, 14 patients (26%) had a neurologic deficit related to vision and/or to the cranial nerves coursing through the cavernous sinus. The ages of the patients varied from 9 to 81 years; the mean age was 46 years. Thirty-six of the patients were female, and 19 were male. Microsurgical resection had been performed by craniotomy or via a transsphenoidal approach in 45 of the patients (82%), and fractionated radiotherapy had been delivered to 11 (20%) prior to radiosurgery.

The radiation dose to the tumor margin varied from 10 to 30 Gy (mean, 19.64), and the maximum dose received by the tumor was 20 to 60 Gy (mean, 38.16 Gy). The mean number of isocenters used to shape the final radiation dose was 3.2. The volume of tumor irradiated within the prescribed isodose margin ranged from 0.1 to 20.5 ml.

Follow-up was available in 44 of 55 patients over a period of 3 to 72 months (mean, 24 months) after radiosurgery (Table 8.6). By examining serial MRI scans, tumor volume was found to decrease in 15 patients (34%), remain stable in 27 (61%), and increase in 2 (4%) (Fig. 8.4). Detailed follow-up information regarding endocrine function was available in 32 of the 41 patients with endocrine active tumors (Table 8.7). There was a significant decrease or normalization in growth hormone levels in 9 of 14 patients (64%) with acromegaly. ACTH levels normalized or diminished in 10 of 16 patients (62%) with Cushing's disease (Fig. 8.5). The prolactin level decreased after radiosurgery in one

TABLE 8.6
Tumor Imaging Changes after Radiosurgery for Pituitary Tumors[a]

Tumor Volume	No. of Tumors (%)
Decreased	15 (34)
Unchanged	27 (61)
Increased	2 (5)

[a]*n* = 44. Mean follow-up 24 months (range, 3 to 72 months).

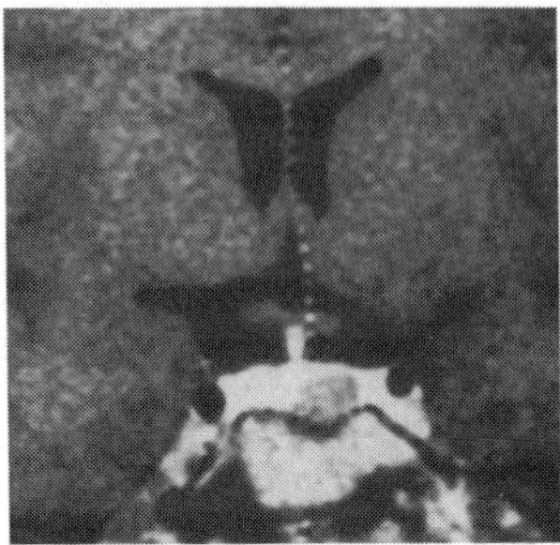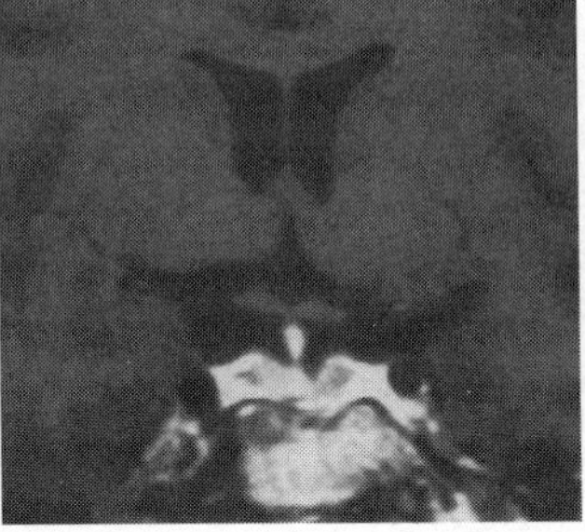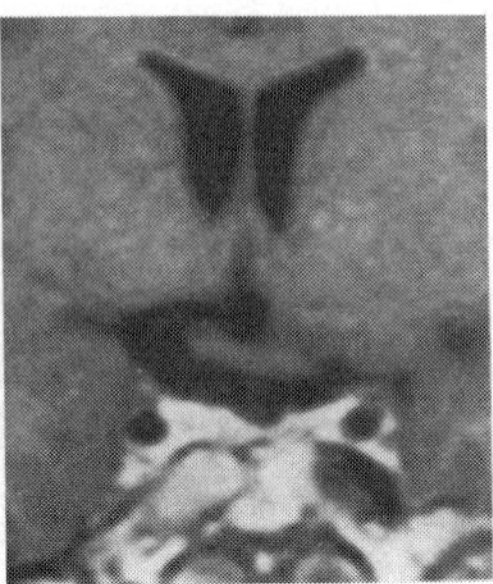

FIG. 8.4 **(Left)** Growth hormone-secreting tumor 1 month prior to radiosurgery. **(Center)** Tumor involution at 46 months after radiosurgery. **(Right)** Progressive tumor involution at 70 months after radiosurgery.

TABLE 8.7
Endocrine Function after Radiosurgery for Pituitary Tumors[a]

Serum Level	GH (%)	ACTH (%)	PRL(%)	PRL + GH (%)
Normalized or improved	9 (64)	10 (62)	1 (100)	1 (100)
Unchanged	5 (36)	6 (38)	0	0

[a] $n = 32$. Mean follow-up, 24 months (range, 3 to 72 months).

patient with a prolactinoma. Another patient with a tumor secreting both prolactin and growth hormone had a decrease in serum prolactin levels and normalization of somatomedin C levels after radiosurgery.

Nine of the 14 patients with neurologic deficits at the time of radiosurgery had clinical follow-up (Table 8.8). One patient improved; six remained stable; and two had a further decline in their neurologic function. One of the latter two patients had a previous transsphenoidal resection, a frontal craniotomy for tumor resection, and fractionated radiotherapy for an invasive endocrine-inactive tumor. He was blind in both eyes prior to radiosurgery. Five months after radiosurgery, he regained 20/25 vision in his left eye and was able to read a newspaper. His tumor had decreased in size on imaging studies. By 12 months after radiosurgery, however, his vision had deteriorated, and he developed new cognitive deficits. MRI-defined contrast enhancement developed in the hypothalamus, and he died 16 months after radiosurgery. A second patient had an invasive ACTH-secreting tumor and had undergone transsphenoidal resection twice, craniotomy twice and, eventually, fractionated radiotherapy. At the time of radiosurgery, she could count fingers in her left eye and had left sixth and third nerve palsies. Over the next 5 months, the tumor continued to grow, and she had further loss of vision in both eyes. Bilateral adrenalectomy was

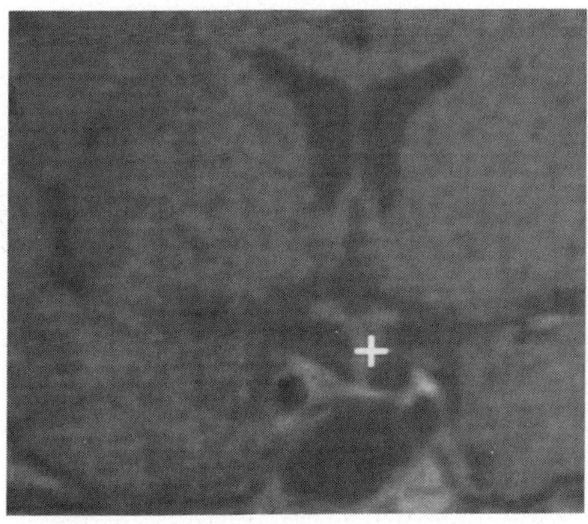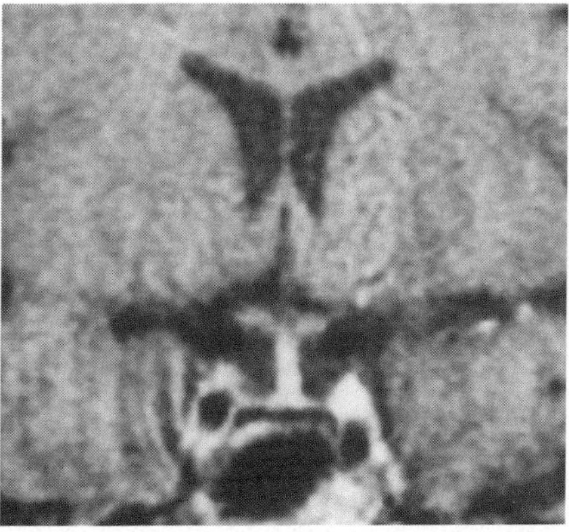

FIG. 8.5 (**Left**) ACTH-secreting adenoma in the right side of the sella at the time of radiosurgery. (**Right**) No evidence of tumor 15 months after radiosurgery. Patient had normalization of ACTH levels 6 months after radiosurgery.

TABLE 8.8
Neurologic Status after Radiosurgery for Pituitary Tumors[a]

Deficit prior to Radiosurgery[b]	No. (%)
Improved	1 (11)
Unchanged	6 (67)
Worse	2 (22)
No deficit prior to Radiosurgery[c]	**No. of Patients (%)**
Preservation of normal function	42 (95.5)
New deficit	2 (4.5)

[a]Mean follow-up, 24 months (range, 3 to 72 months).
[b]$n = 9$.
[c]$n = 44$.

performed, and she died shortly thereafter from systemic medical problems.

Two of 44 patients without deficits at the time of radiosurgery developed neurologic deficits. One patient had an endocrine-inactive macroadenoma and had undergone two prior operations and fractionated radiotherapy. This patient developed decreased visual acuity in the left eye and a right temporal visual field defect 7 months after radiosurgery; the tumor volume decreased. A second patient with an invasive ACTH-producing adenoma developed new cranial nerve deficits 7 months after radiosurgery. MRI demonstrated extensive tumor growth into the cavernous sinuses bilaterally, the sphenoid sinus, nasopharynx, and middle cranial fossa.

Control of tumor growth was achieved in 95% of patients undergoing stereotactic radiosurgery for pituitary adenomas. A significant decrease in or normalization of excessive ACTH and GH secretion was seen in 62% of patients with Cushing's disease and 64% of patients with acromegaly. Two (22%) of nine evaluable patients with pre-existing neurologic deficits deteriorated neurologically after radiosurgery. In one patient, the tumor continued to grow. In the other patient, it was difficult to determine whether tumor growth or radiation effect was responsible for the eventual deterioration in neurologic function. Both of these patients had had multiple microsurgical procedures, as well as fractionated radiotherapy, prior to radiosurgery. Two of 44 patients (4.5%) developed either new visual deficits or extraocular muscle palsies after radiosurgery. One of these complications was either radiation-related or caused by traction on the chiasm from tumor shrinkage; the other one was related to treatment failure and progressive tumor growth.

The primary goals in the surgical resection of pituitary adenomas are decompression of neural structures, resolution of endocrinopathy without producing additional endocrine insults, and prevention of regrowth of the tumor. We believe that tumors that produce visual deficits require microsurgical resection. If the tumor is at least 3 mm from the optic apparatus, then radiosurgery is another treatment option. Radiosurgery provides excellent (95%) tumor control that seems to prevent future compromise of the optic chiasm in most patients. Radiosurgery also results in improvement of endocrine dysfunction that is equivalent to the outcomes reported in recent microsurgic series. A 52 to 82% success rate for resolution of endocrinopathy has been reported for microsurgical excision of GH-secreting tumors (4, 26). The success rate for treatment of the endocrinopathy of Cushing's disease has been reported by leading centers to be 76 to 85% (20, 25) for primary tumors and 71% (23) for recurrent tumors. However, there is extensive variability in success rates among all centers nationwide; success rates of less than 60% (3) are noted. The fact that 82% of our patients already had failed attempted microsurgical treatment and that 51% of our patients had tumor in the cavernous sinus must be taken into account when comparing our results to the results reported in microsurgical series. One distinct advantage of radiosurgery *versus* microsurgery is that the normal pituitary gland appears to be more resistant to the effects of radiation than the tumor (28). Unlike the situation after fractionated radiotherapy, the risk of developing panhypopituitarism after radiosurgery appears to be low. We did not observe panhypopituitarism in any patients with preserved endocrine function prior to radiosurgery.

CHORDOMAS AND CHONDROSARCOMAS

Stereotactic radiosurgery was performed on seven patients with chordomas and three patients with chondrosarcomas involving the clivus, cavernous sinus, and middle cranial fossa. The age of the patients ranged from 7 to 69 years (mean, 38 years). There were seven males and three females. All 10 patients had neurologic deficits at the time of radiosurgery. Seven patients had microsurgical resection prior to radiosurgery, and one patient also required a shunt. The maximum dose delivered to the tumor varied from 22.3 to 40 Gy (mean, 34.5 Gy), and the margin dose varied from 11.7 to 20 Gy (mean, 18 Gy). The average number of isocenters required to treat such tumors was three. The volume of tumor irradiated varied from 1.0 to 8.0 ml (mean, 4.0 ml). In all but one patient, the 50% isodose line was prescribed to the tumor margin.

Follow-up was available in all 10 patients over a range of 9 to 57 months (mean, 27 months) (Table 8.9). The tumor volume within the margin isodose decreased or disappeared in five patients and remained stable in the other five (Fig. 8.6). However, there was delayed new tumor growth remote from the radiosurgical site in four patients, all of whom required additional treatment. Four patients had improvement in, and six remained stable in regard to pre-existing neurologic deficits (Table 8.10). One patient with a chordoma developed decreased visual acuity in the right eye and a right third nerve palsy 24 months after radiosurgery. MRI disclosed tumor growth anterior to the radiosurgical site. One 71-year-old woman with a chondrosarcoma died 41 months after radiosurgery. This patient's tumor was located in the right cavernous sinus and infratemporal fossa area and had metastasized to the right frontoparietal area 18 months after radiosurgery. The metastatic tumor was resected, and she received fractionated radiotherapy. Eighteen months later, she developed hydrocephalus and required a shunt. Over the subsequent 5 months, she developed dysphagia and poor nutrition. Follow-up CT and MRI showed no progression of the skull base tumor or recurrence of the metastasis prior to her death shortly after gastrostomy placement.

TABLE 8.9

Tumor Imaging Changes after Radiosurgery for Chordomas and Chondrosarcomas[a]

Tumor Volume	No. of Patients
Decreased	5
Unchanged	5
Increased (local)	0
Increased (remote)	4

[a]$n = 10$. Mean follow-up, 27 months (range, 9 to 57 months).

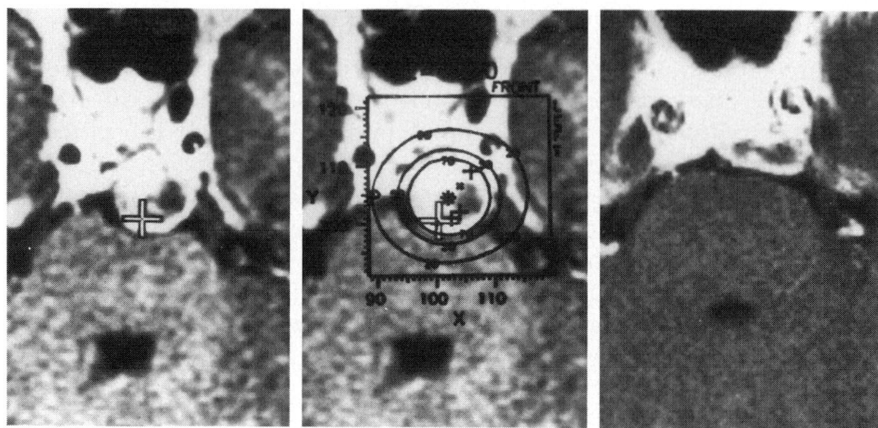

FIG. 8.6 **(Left)** Clivus-based mass presumed to be chordoma that is distorting the brainstem. Patient refused microsurgery. **(Center)** Isodose plan for stereotactic radiosurgery. **(Right)** Decreased tumor volume 1 year after radiosurgery. Note the decrease in mass effect on the brainstem.

TABLE 8.10
Neurologic Status after Radiosurgery for Chordomas and Chondrosarcomas[a]

Deficit prior to Radiosurgery[b]	No. of Patients
Improved	4
Unchanged	6
Worse	0

No Deficit prior to Radiosurgery[c]	No. of Patients
Preservation of normal function	9
New deficit	1

[a]Mean follow-up, 27 months (range, 9 to 57 months).
[b]$n = 10$.
[c]$n = 10$.

Radiosurgery achieved acceptable *local* tumor control in this small group of patients, six of whom were reported previously (15). Four of the patients with cranial nerve palsies had improvement in extraocular motor function (abducens nerve in four; oculomotor nerve in one) after radiosurgery. As also reported in microsurgical series (22) and radiation therapy series (1), tumor growth remote from the treated site remains problematic in these patients. Chordomas and chondrosarcomas are often locally invasive, and the full extent of tumor invasion may not be visualized by any imaging study. Remote tumor growth occurred in four patients in our series and was responsible for the one new neurologic deficit. Lanzino *et al.* reported that they were able to achieve gross total resection in 17 of 31 patients with chordomas or chrondrosarcomas; they detected no tumor recurrences during a median follow-up of 24 months. The complication rate reported by these authors testifies to the difficulty of attempting radical resection. One patient died from pulmonary embolism; one had significant disability related to thalamic perforator occlusion and hemorrhage; eight had CSF leaks; five required shunts; six had major medical complications; and three had either permanent endocrine dysfunction, hemiparesis, or quadriparesis (16).

CRANIOPHARYNGIOMAS

Stereotactic radiosurgery was performed for the solid component of a craniopharyngioma in seven patients. The age of the patients varied from 9 to 65 years (mean, 18 years). Five patients were female, and two were male. All of the patients had panhypopituitarism, and five had neurologic deficits at the time of radiosurgery. The solid portion of the tumor was primarily located within the sella in two patients, in the parasellar area in two patients, and in the suprasellar area in three patients. Microsurgical resection had been performed in five patients (gross total resection in two, subtotal resection in three). Fractionated radiotherapy was administered in one patient prior to radiosurgery. The maximum radiation dose delivered to the tumor varied from 26.7 to 45 Gy (mean, 33.3 Gy). The margin dose varied from 15 to 22.5 Gy (mean, 18.5 Gy). The average number of isocenters used to treat each tumor was two. The volume of tumor within the prescribed margin isodose varied from 0.5 to 2.4 ml (mean, 1.0 ml). The margin isodose was 50% in four patients; 60% in two; and 70% in one.

Four of the seven patients had follow-up between 12 and 69 months (mean, 48 months) (Table 8.11). During this time, the solid portion of the tumor decreased in two patients, remained stable in one, and increased in one. The patient whose tumor increased in size had had two prior craniotomies and one previous transsphenoidal resection prior to radiosurgery for a residual tumor within the cavernous sinus. She re-

TABLE 8.11

Tumor Imaging Changes after Radiosurgery for Craniopharyngiomas[a]

Tumor Volume	No. of Patients
Decreased	2
Unchanged	1
Increased	1

[a]n = 4. Mean follow-up, 48 months (range, 12 to 69 months).

TABLE 8.12

Neurologic Status after Radiosurgery for Craniopharyngiomas[a]

Deficit prior to Radiosurgery[b]	No. of Patients
Improved	0
Unchanged	2
Worse	1

No Deficit prior to Radiosurgery[c]	No. of Patients
Preservation of normal function	3
New deficit	1

[a] $n = 4$. Mean follow-up, 48 months (range, 12 to 69 months).
[b] $n = 10$.
[c] $n = 10$.

ceived 16 Gy to the tumor margin at the 60% isodose line. Fifteen months later, although she remained clinically stable, she had imaging evidence of cystic tumor growth, and a fourth microsurgical procedure was planned.

One of three patients with a pre-existing neurologic deficit became worse, and the other two remained stable (Table 8.12). A 65-year-old woman had 20/25 vision in both eyes and bitemporal hemianopsia at the time of radiosurgery. She had had fluctuating visual problems over the 3 years prior to radiosurgery due to the cystic portion of the tumor. She had intracavitary irradiation of the cyst 27 months prior to radiosurgery and stereotactic aspiration of the cyst 1 and 2 months prior to radiosurgery. At the time of radiosurgery, she had 20 Gy delivered at the 70% isodose line to the margin of the solid portion of the tumor. Despite the fact that the tumor appeared to be getting smaller on CT scan, her vision began to deteriorate 6 months after radiosurgery, and by 11 months, she was completely blind. This decline in vision was most likely related to either traction on the chiasm from shrinkage of the cyst or to adverse effects of radiation.

One additional patient developed a new neurologic deficit. This patient became mildly hemiparetic and dysmetric 51 months after radiosurgery. Although the solid portion of the tumor remained stable, he developed a small new cyst on the left side of the suprasellar cistern. Since he had previously undergone three craniotomies, fractionated radiotherapy, intracavitary irradiation, and cyst aspiration, he was simply observed and has remained stable at 66 months.

The number of craniopharyngioma patients with extended follow-up in this group is too small for the authors to fully analyze the role of stereotactic radiosurgery in the management of the solid portion of a craniopharyngioma. Tumor control was achieved in three of four patients. One patient became worse, either as a consequence of radiation-induced optic neuropathy or as a consequence of traction on the optic chiasm from tumor shrinkage, and one patient became worse due to the development of a new cyst. Results indicate that stereotactic radiosurgery can be utilized best in patients with small residual craniopharyngiomas located 3 to 5 mm in distance from the optic chiasm. The significant difficulty and morbidity associated with attempting gross total microsurgical resection of craniopharyngiomas warrants consideration of other treatment options such as radiosurgery in selected patients. (2, 12).

METASTATIC CANCER

Stereotactic radiosurgery was performed on seven patients with metastatic tumors to the anterior skull base. The ages of the patients ranged from 34 to 70 years (mean, 50 years). Six of the patients were men, and one was a woman. One patient had a tumor in the nasopharynx; one had tumor in the sella; one had a tumor in the clivus; and four had tumors in the cavernous sinus. The histology of these tumors included two cases of mucoepidermoid carcinoma and one case each of adeno cystic carcinoma, squamous cell carcinoma, melanoma, renal cell carcinoma, and colon carcinoma. Five of the seven patients had microsurgical resection of their tumors prior to radiosurgery, and five underwent fractionated radiotherapy. The maximum dose delivered to the tumor varied from 28 to 36 Gy (mean, 31.2 Gy). The margin doses varied from 14 to 20 Gy (mean, 16.4 Gy). The mean number of isocenters used to shape the final isodose margin was 3.7. The volume of tumor enclosed within the prescribed isodose ranged from 0.5 to 6.6 ml (mean, 3.0 ml). Six tumors were treated at the 50% isodose, and one was treated at the 70% isodose.

Follow-up was available in five patients over 4 to 16 months (mean, 7 months) (Table 8.13). One patient with metastatic adenoid cystic carcinoma to the cavernous sinus had a decreased incidence of tumor volume and of facial paresthesias at 5-month follow-up. A patient with metastatic squamous cell carcinoma to the clivus remained neurologically stable, with no change in tumor size on a 12-month follow-up MRI scan.

The three other patients died. One patient with metastic colon carcinoma to the cavernous sinus had a large increase in size of the local tumor plus extension into the posterior fossa 7 months after radiosurgery. He developed multiple new cranial nerve palsies and died 2 months later. One patient with metastatic renal cell carcinoma to the sella did well for 15 months after radiosurgery before experiencing a sudden decrease in his vision to 20/400 in one eye and hand motion-only vision in the other eye. No imaging studies were obtained to de-

TABLE 8.13
*Tumor Imaging Changes after Radiosurgery for Metastatic Tumors
to the Anterior Skull Base[a]*

Tumor Volume	No. of Patients
Decreased	1
Unchanged	3
Increased	1

[a] $n = 5$. Mean follow-up, 7 months (range, 4 to 16 months).

termine whether this change in vision was due to tumor growth, radiation, or apoplexy. He died 2 months later. The fifth patient had a metastatic mucoepidermoid carcinoma to the cavernous sinus and remained neurologically stable with right sixth and seventh nerve palsies until he died 16 months later.

The value of stereotactic radiosurgery in providing local control of intracranial metastatic lesions has been established (17). Despite the small number of patients in this series, this efficacy appears to apply to lesions of the anterior skull base as well. Tumor progression associated with neurologic deterioration was documented in only one of five patients.

CONCLUSIONS

Stereotactic radiosurgery is an increasingly safe and usually effective method of preventing growth of small- to moderate-sized primary tumors of the anterior skull base. Tumor growth control is obtained in more than 90% of patients with skull base tumors having benign histology. Neurologic function is maintained in most patients. The risk of temporary or permanent injury to critical neural and vascular structures is significantly lower than the risk associated with microsurgery.

The optic nerves, chiasm, and tracts are structures that appear most sensitive to the radiation doses used during radiosurgery of anterior skull base tumors. The incidence of injury to the optic apparatus is low when the dose to the nerve is less than 8 to 9 Gy (27). The incidence of injury to motor nerves, such as the oculomotor, trochlear, trigeminal, and abducens nerves, is extremely low at the doses used in clinical radiosurgery (27). To date no cases of delayed carotid injuries have been reported. Microsurgical complications (*e.g.*, CSF leak, wound infection, and meningitis) do not occur after radiosurgery.

Additional attractive features of radiosurgery are a relatively low, hospital-based cost and a rapid return of the patient of work. In the report of our experience with the first 207 patients treated with the Gamma Knife at the University of Pittsburgh, the average length of hospital stay was 2.24 days for a patient undergoing stereotactic radiosurgery for a skull base tumor and 11.44 days for a patient undergoing craniotomy for the same lesion. The total hospital charges were 30 to 70% lower for patients having radiosurgery (19). The average hospital stay and cost of radiosurgery are even lower now, because most radiosurgery patients are released from the hospital on the same day as their procedure. Patients are usually able to return to a full preoperative functional level and employment within 3 to 5 days.

There are patients in certain clinical situations in which microsurgery clearly is required. These include patients experiencing rapidly progressive visual deterioration or who have endocrine-active pituitary tumors. A more rapid reduction in endocrine dysfunction is best achieved by microsurgical tumor excision. In patients in whom a tumor recurs despite "gross total removal," and in cases in which tumor is left behind to preserve critical nerve and vessel integrity, stereotactic radiosurgery is a very effective alternative to additional microsurgical operations. Stereotactic radiosurgery may also be the primary treatment of choice in patients who are unable or unwilling to accept the risk:benefit ratio of microsurgery.

REFERENCES

1. Austin-Seymour M, Munzenrider J, Goitein M, *et al.:* Fractionated proton radiation therapy of chordomas and low-grade chondrosarcoma of the base of the skull. **J Neurosurg** 70:13–17, 1989.
2. Baskin DS, Wilson CB: Surgical management of craniopharyngiomas: A review of 74 cases. **J Neurosurg** 65:22–27, 1986.
3. Burch W: A survey of results with transsphenoidal surgery in Cushing's disease. **N Engl J Med** 308:103–104, 1983.
4. Davis DH, Laws ER Jr, Ilstrue DM, *et al.:* Results of surgical treatment for growth-hormone-secreting pituitary adenomas. **J Neurosurg** 79:70–75, 1993.
5. DeMonte F, Smith HK, Al-Mefty O: Outcome of aggressive removal of cavernous sinus meningiomas. **J Neurosurg** 81:245–251, 1994.
6. Dolenc VV, Kregar T, Ferluga M, *et al.:* Treatment of tumors invading the cavernous sinus, in Dolenc VV (ed): *The Cavernous Sinus: Multidisciplinary Approach to Vascular and Tumorous Lesions.* Wien, Springer-Verlag, 1987, pp 377–391.
7. Duma CM, Lunsford LD, Kondziolka D, *et al.:* Stereotactic radiosurgery of cavernous sinus meningiomas as an addition or alternative to microsurgery. **Neurosurgery** 32:699–705, 1993.
8. Flickinger JC: An integrated logistic formula for prediction of complications from radiosurgery. **Int J Radiat Oncol Biol Phys** 17:879–885, 1989.
9. Flickinger JC, Lunsford LD, Deutsch M: Repeat megavoltage irradiation of pituitary and suprasellar tumors. **Int J Radiat Oncol Biol Phys** 17:171–175, 1989.
10. Flickinger JC, Lunsford LD, Wu A, *et al.:* Treatment planning for gamma knife radiosurgery with multiple isocenters. **Int J Radiat Oncol Biol Phys** 18:1495–1501, 1990.

11. Flickinger JC, Maitz A, Kaland A, *et al.:* Treatment volume shaping with selective beam blocking using the Leksell Gamma Knife. **Int J Radiat Oncol Biol Phys** 19:783–789, 1990.
12. Hoffman JH, Desilva M, Humphreys RP, *et al.:* Aggressive surgical management of craniopharyngiomas in children. **J Neurosurg** 76:47–52, 1992.
13. Kawage T, Toya S, Shiobara R, *et al.:* Skull base approaches for meningiomas invading the cavernous sinus, in Dolenc VV (ed): *The Cavernous Sinus: Multidisciplinary Approach to Vascular and Tumorous Lesions.* Wien, Springer-Verlag, 1987, pp 346–354.
14. Kondziolka D, Dempsey PK, Lunsford LD, *et al.:* A comparison between magnetic resonance imaging and computed tomography for stereotactic coordinate determination. **Neurosurgery** 30:402–407, 1992.
15. Kondziolka D, Lunsford LD, Flickinger JC: The role of radiosurgery in the management of chordoma and chondrosarcoma of the cranial base. **Neurosurgery** 29:38–46, 1991.
16. Lanzino G, Sekhar LN, Hirsch WL, *et al.:* Chordomas and chondrosarcomas involving the cavernous sinus: Review of surgical treatment and outcome in 31 patients. **Surg Neurology** 40:354–371, 1993.
17. Loeffler JS, Alexander E III: Radiosurgery for the treatment of intracranial metastases, in Alexander E III, Loeffler JS, Lunsford LD (ed): *Stereotactic Radiosurgery.* New York, McGraw-Hill, 1993, pp 197–206.
18. Lunsford LD, Flickinger JC, Coffey RJ: Stereotactic Gamma Knife radiosurgery: Initial North American experience in 207 patients. **Arch Neurol** 47:169–175, 1990.
19. Lunsford LD, Flickinger JC, Lindner G, *et al.:* Stereotactic radiosurgery of the brain using the first United States 201 source cobalt-60 Gamma Knife. **Neurosurgery** 24:152–159, 1989.
20. Mampalam, TJ, Tyrrell JB, Wilson CB: Transsphenoidal microsurgery for Cushing's disease. A report of 216 cases. **Ann Intern Med** 109:487–493, 1988.
21. Origitano TC, Al-Mefty O, Leonetti JP, *et al.:* Vascular considerations and complications in cranial base surgery. **Neurosurgery** 35:351–363, 1994.
22. Raffel C, Wright DC, Gutin PH, *et al.:* Cranial chordomas: Clinical presentation and results of operative and radiation therapy in 26 patients. **Neurosurgery** 17:703–710, 1985.
23. Ram Z, Nieman LK, Cutler GB Jr, *et al.:* Early repeat surgery for persistent Cushing's disease. **J Neurosurg** 80:37–45, 1994.
24. Sekhar LN, Sen SN, Jho HD, *et al.:* Surgical treatment of intracavernous neoplasms: A four year experience. **Neurosurgery** 24:18–30, 1989.
25. Tindall, GT, Herring CJ, Clark RV, *et al.:* Cushing's disease: Results of transsphenoidal microsurgery with emphasis on surgical failures. **J Neurosurg** 72:363–369, 1990.
26. Tindall GT, Oyesiku NM, Watts NB, *et al.:* Transsphenoidal adenomectomy for growth hormone-secreting pituitary adenomas in acromegaly: Outcome analysis and determinants of failure. **J Neurosurg** 78:205–215, 1993.
27. Tishler RB, Loeffler JS, Lunsford LD, *et al.:* Tolerance of cranial nerves of the cavernous sinus to radiosurgery. **Int J Radiat Oncol Biol Phys** 27:215–221, 1993.
28. Woodruff KH, Lyman JT, Lawrence JH, *et al.:* Delayed sequelae of pituitary irradiation. **Hum Pathol** 15:48–54, 1984.
29. Wu A, Lindner G, Maitz AH, *et al.:* Physics of Gamma Knife approach on convergent beams in stereotactic radiosurgery. **Int J Radiat Oncol Biol Phys** 18:1495–1501, 1990.

9

Techniques of Carotid Reconstruction

TAKANORI FUKUSHIMA, M.D., D.M.Sc.

The cavernous sinus has been recognized as an elusive operative site due to the neurovascular anatomic complexity and difficulty in controlling bleeding. This is why the cavernous sinus has been designated as "the last no man's land" in neurosurgery. In the early 1980s, however, Dolenc revitalized Parkinson's direct operative method (19–21), introducing his innovative operative technique of using a combined epidural subdural approach (2, 3). After learning the Dolenc technique, the author elaborated on practical microsurgical anatomy around the cavernous sinus and established the concept of multiple triangular operative corridors to the cavernous sinus in 1986 (5, 6).

For the past 10 years, the author has used the direct operative approach to the various cavernous sinus lesions in 305 cases, including 180 cases of neoplastic lesions and 125 cases of vascular lesions (Table 9.1).

Regarding various cavernous sinus lesions, the most difficult issue has been the management of tumors engulfing the internal carotid artery (ICA) and repair of intracavernous giant aneurysms. To avoid ischemic complications by sacrificing the ICA, in October 1986 the author performed a C6 petrous carotid to C3 siphon saphenous vein interposition graft in a patient with a giant cavernous aneurysm (5). This operative technique of cavernous carotid reconstuction was designated later as the "Fukushima bypass" (24).

Since the initial experience of 1986, the author has performed the cavernous carotid replacement operation in 35 cases, including 29 cases of vascular and 6 cases of neoplastic lesions (Table 9.2). Also, this cavernous carotid reconstruction technique (skull base bypass I) has been applied to other intrapetrous or infratemporal lesions, developing a cervical carotid to C6 petrous carotid bypass (skull base bypass II) (15) or cervical carotid to C3 siphon saphenous bypass (skull base bypass III). This chapter deals with the detailed description of the surgical technique of the Fukushima skull base bypass procedures and the operative results.

TABLE 9.1
Direct Surgery for Cavernous Sinus Lesions[a]

Neoplastic[b]		Vascular[c]		No. of Patients
Meningioma	91	C_2 paraclinoid giant aneurysm		35
Neurinoma	23	C_{2-3} regular ophthalmic aneurysm		19
Pituitary adenoma	26	C_3 siphon aneurysm		
		Regular		14
Chordoma	10	Giant		4
Cavernous hemangioma	3	C_4 intracavernous		
		Regular		5
Epidermoid cyst	5	Giant		33
Dermoid cyst	3	Primitive trigeminal aneurysm		2
Chondroma	1	Meningohypophyseal aneurysm		1
Granuloma	1	CCF		12
Malignant tumors	17			

[a]Data taken from cases from 1984 to 1994.
[b]$n = 180$.
[c]$n = 125$.

TABLE 9.2
Cavernous Carotid Bypass

Intracavernous giant aneurysms	28 cases
Siphon stenosis	1
Cavernous meningiomas	3
Malignant tumors	3
Total	35 cases

CLINICAL MATERIAL

Between 1986 and 1994, skull base bypass I (C6 to C3) was performed in 35 patients, who comprised 28 cases of intracavernous giant aneurysms, 1 case of severe siphon stenosis presenting with ischemic symptoms, 3 cases of cavernous sinus meningiomas presenting with ophthalmoplegia, and 3 cases for en bloc resection of malignant tumors. Skull base bypass II (cervical ICA to C6) was performed in four cases of high cervical infratemporal chemodectomas. Skull base bypass III (cervical ICA to C3) was utilized in two cases of posterior cavernous and petrous aneurysms. Of these 41 cases, 32 were females and 9 were males, ranging in age from 23 to 84 years (mean, 58 years). The most frequent presenting symptom in 28 cases of giant intracavernous aneurysms was diplopia. Nine patients presented with single oculomotor nerve weakness, and seven patients presented with abducens nerve palsy. One patient presenting with abducens nerve palsy showed a giant intracavernous aneurysm associated with carotid cavernous fistula (CCF).

Trigeminal pain was the major presenting symptom in four patients, and seven patients had a combination of multiple cavernous cranial nerve neuropathies. One patient, a 50-year-old woman, presented with an acute carotid system stroke due to kinking and occlusion of the C3 segment, caused by compression from the giant cavernous aneurysm.

Microsurgical Anatomy of the Cavernous Sinus

In achieving successful operative results in direct cavernous sinus surgery, one cannot overemphasize the importance of the individual surgeon's knowledge of the detailed surgical anatomy of this region. A clear understanding of cavernous carotid segments and multiple entry points into the cavernous sinus is fundamental to performing successful cavernous sinus surgery.

The cavernous sinus is located at the covergence of the anterior base, middle fossa, sphenoid ridge, and petroclival ridge, which the author designates as the "four corners of the cranial base." Figure 9.1 illustrates the carotid segments and nomenclature of Fischer (4), slightly

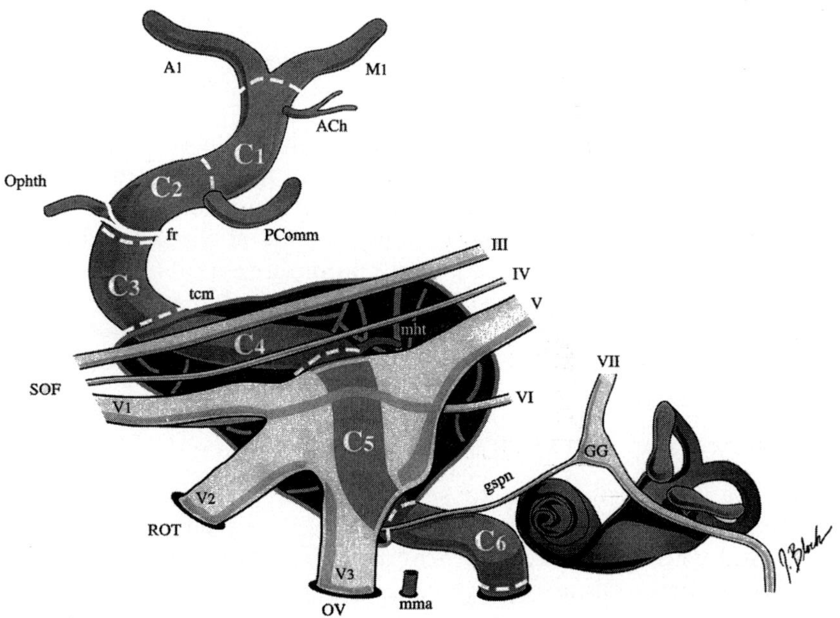

FIG. 9.1 Carotid segments and nomenclature. Segmental nomenclature of the intracranial internal carotid artery. *C1,* ICA bifurcation to the posterior communicating artery; *C2,* P Comm to Perneczky's fibrous dural ring, *C3,* Perneczky's ring to the carotid-oculomotor membrane (siphon segment); *C4,* carotid-oculomotor membrane to the meningohypophyseal trunk (intracavernous segment); *C5,* meningohypophyseal trunk to crossing of the lateral trigeminal complex (usually includes the foramen lacerum); *C6,* intrapetrous segment.

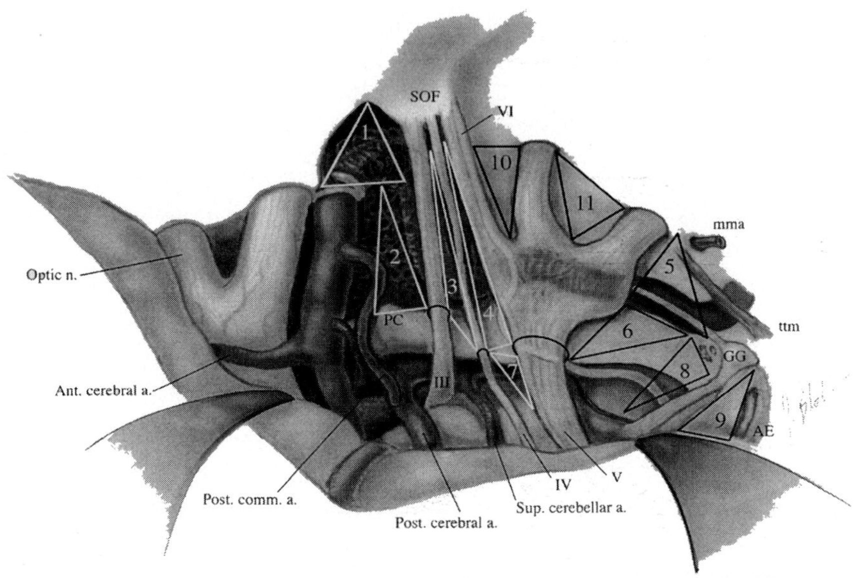

FIG. 9.2 Cavernous sinus triangles.

modified by the author; the C6 petrous carotid segment has been designated by the author. The C3 carotid segment represents the epidural clinoidal siphon portion, and only the C4 horizontal and C5 ascending segments are the true intracavernous portions of the carotid artery. Figure 9.2 illustrates various special triangular corridors around the cavernous sinus, as viewed from above the cranial base.

The basic construct of the cavernous triangular areas and nomenclature were established by the author in 1986 (5, 6). Safe entry into the cavernous sinus will be achieved by using 11 triangles as follows.

ANTEROMEDIAL TRIANGLE

This is an epidural space exposed by the removal of the anterior clinoid process, defined by the lateral border of the extradural optic nerve, the medial wall of the superior orbital fissure dura, and the dural fibrous ring surrounding the internal carotid artery as it courses intradurally. This area is the most important triangle for cavernous sinus surgery, as introduced by Dolenc (2, 3).

MEDIAL TRIANGLE

This space is designated by the siphon angle, lateral wall of the intradural internal carotid artery, posterior clinoid process, and the porus oculomotorius. By incising the dura of this triangle, the horizontal segment of the cavernous carotid artery will be exposed. The medial triangle approach was well described by Hakuba *et al.* (8, 9).

SUPERIOR TRIANGLE

This triangle is bounded by the third and the fourth cranial nerves, with its posterior margin the crest of dura between the porus oculomotorius and the trochlear nerve (5). This space is most suitable for exposure of the C4–C5 junction and the meningophypophyseal trunk.

LATERAL TRIANGLE

This is a rather narrow space delineated by the fourth cranial nerve and the trigeminal first branch. It is the original triangle described by Parkinson for entry into the cavernous sinus (19, 20).

POSTEROLATERAL TRIANGLE

This important triangle is defined by the foramen spinosum, the posterior border of the trigeminal third branch, and the cochlear apex. The greater superficial petrosal nerve runs over this triangle from the geniculate ganglion. Careful removal of the bone in this triangle exposes the C6 petrous segment of the carotid artery. Drilling of this area for exposure of the petrous carotid artery was first described by Glasscock in 1969 (7) and later by Paullus *et al.* (22).

POSTEROMEDIAL TRIANGLE

This triangle designates the anterior portion of the petrous bone bounded by the porus trigeminus, the posterior border of the proximal portion of the trigeminal third branch, and the petrous carotid artery. Drilling of this space was initially described by Kawase *et al.* (12).

POSTEROINFERIOR TRIANGLE

This area is bounded by the fourth cranial nerve to posterior clinoid process and the medial porus trigeminus. An incision in this area carried down from the petroclival ligament to Gruber's ligament will expose the sixth cranial nerve in Dorello's canal.

PREMEATAL TRIANGLE

The premeatal triangle provides a precise location of the safe area of drilling anterior to the medial lip of the internal acoustic meatus. The space is designated by the geniculate ganglion, cochlea, the carotid genu, internal acoustic meatus, and the petrous ridge. Important in identifying this triangle is a clear understanding of the basal turn of the cochlea and its anatomic relationship to the C6 carotid genu.

POSTMEATAL TRIANGLE

The postmeatal triangle defines the volume of bone that lies between the superior semicircular canal (arcuate eminence) and the internal acoustic canal. This area of bone can be completely removed by a middle fossa approach. The combination of posteromedial triangle, premeatal triangle, and postmeatal triangle forms the so-called "middle fossa rhomboid complex," defined by the four points in the middle fossa: the porus trigeminus; the intersection of the greater superficial petrosal nerve and the trigeminal third branch; the geniculate ganglion; and the intersection of the arcuate eminence with the petrous ridge (1) (Fig. 9.3A).

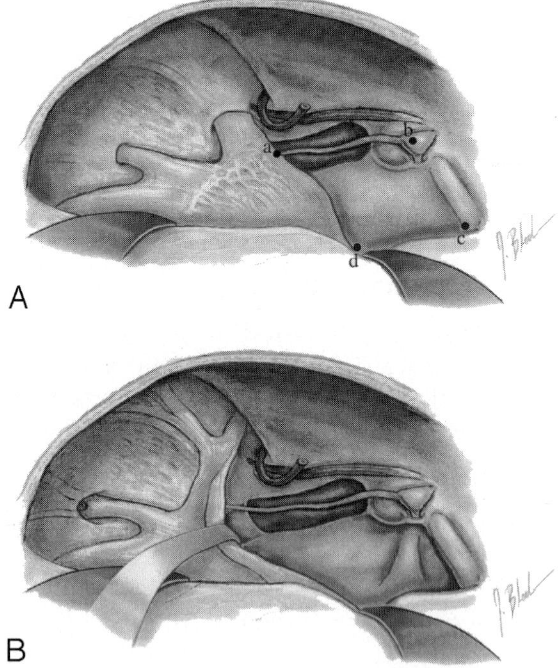

FIG. 9.3 (A) Extradural middle fossa exposure of the rhomboid area (*a-b-c-d*) between the greater superficial petrosal nerve, the accurate eminence, and the trigeminal petrous ridge corner. (B) Skeletonization of the foramen ovale and anterior translocation of the gasserian ganglion for wider exposure of the C6 petrous carotid segment.

ANTEROLATERAL TRIANGLE

This is the area between the opthalmic and maxillary divisions of the trigeminal nerve, extending anteriorly to a line from the superior orbital fissure to the foramen rotundum. This triangle is used for exposing the superior orbital vein, originally described by Mullan (16).

LATERALMOST TRIANGLE

This is the space between the foramen rotundum and the foramen ovale. Drilling of this bone deeply toward the infratemporal area will expose the Eustachian tube. This triangle is used to make a lateral access to the intracavernous tumors.

OPERATIVE TECHNIQUE

SKULL BASE BYPASS I (C6 PETROUS CAROTID TO C3 SIPHON SAPHENOUS VEIN GRAFT)

This bypass is indicated for the trapping of intracavernous fusiform or giant aneurysms and CCF, for replacement of cavernous carotid stenosis, and for radical resection of vessel-engulfing tumors. The surgery is performed through a routine frontotemporal pterional craniotomy. After the sphenoid ridge is drilled flat by means of a high-powered air drill, the epidural dissection is advanced to expose the frontal base and the anterior middle fossa. With careful use of various sizes of diamond drills with continuous irrigation and cooling, the extradural optic canal dura is exposed, and the anterior clinoid process is carefully drilled away, detached from the optic strut, and removed. Then the superior orbital fissure, the foramen rotundum, and the foramen ovale are identified in the middle cranial fossa. The petrous carotid is exposed by drilling the posterolateral triangle of Glasscock medial to the foramen spinosum and the tensor tympani muscle. Drilling the Glasscock triangle should be started just posterior to the foramen ovale and medial to the middle meningeal artery, thereby exposing the tensor tympani muscle and carefully skeletonizing the petrous carotid artery. The greater superficial petrosal nerve is sacrificed in this area; however, the geniculate ganglion is preserved intact, using anatomic landmarks and facial nerve monitoring. At the proximal genu of the C6 petrous carotid artery, the cochlea is extremely close, and drilling should be stopped without going further, to the proximal carotid canal. Exposure of the petrous carotid artery is facilitated by the skeletonization of the peripheral branch of the trigeminal third division and anterior translocation of the gasserian ganglion (Fig. 9.3 **A** and **B**).

The dura over the optic nerve is incised to expose the optic nerve

widely and to dissect the ophthalmic artery. The optic nerve is gently
retracted medially, and the fibrous ring of the C-2–C-3 junction is excised to mobilize the carotid siphon segment. Bleeding from the cavernous sinus is controlled by packing small pieces of Surgicel. In the
earlier series of cavernous bypasses, the frontal and temporal lobes
were both retracted, sacrificing the temporal tip veins to make a direct
saphenous vein interposition graft between the petrous carotid and the
siphon segment, as illustrated in Figure 9.4A.

However, in the latter half of the bypass series, a keyhole extradural
procedure has been developed to maintain the temporal tip veins. In

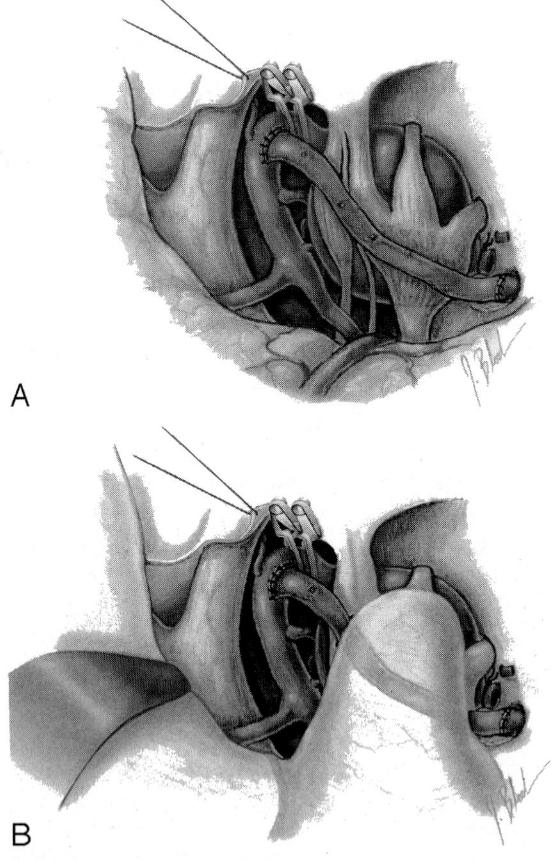

FIG. 9.4 **(A)** Illustration of Fukushima cavernous bypass. A saphenous vein is anastomosed from C6 petrous to C3 paraophthalmic area while the giant aneurysm is isolated. **(B)** Extradural keyhole technique for Fukushima bypass to protect the temporal
lobe.

this extradural procedure, the dura of the temporal lobe is maintained, and the small epidural subtemporal approach is performed to expose the petrous carotid segment. The saphenous vein is passed through a small dural incision from the subtemporal to the clinoidal area under the temporal lobe. After occluding the proximal carotid artery by packing a small cottonoid into the carotid canal, the carotid artery is ligated under the gasserian ganglion at the C6–C5 junction. Then, the petrous carotid is incised, and an end-to-end anastomosis is performed with the saphenous vein, using 8-0 monofilament nylon interrupted sutures. At the distal anastomosis area, only the C2 and C3 segments of the carotid artery are exposed with a small dural incision, and the double clip is applied to the siphon to trap the aneurysm. The distal portion of the saphenous vein is anastomosed to the paraophthalmic area with an end-to-side anastomosis technique (Fig. 9.4**B**).

In most cases the lengths of the saphenous vein were 2 to 3 inches, harvested from the upper thigh. Any branches of the saphenous vein need to be coagulated or ligated. Before the temporary occlusion of the carotid artery, 5000 units of heparin is administered, and the standard barbiturate cerebral protection procedure is undertaken. In case of poor backflow from the distal carotid artery, a moderate hypothermia technique of 32 to 34° C is used. Before completing the last suture, intraluminal blood or air is flushed away from heparinized saline. With the removal of all temporary ligatures, the saphenous vein graft connects the proximal C6 carotid artery directly to the intradural carotid artery, eliminating the pathology and replacing the cavernous carotid with a new artery. The drilled area is packed with pieces of pericranial and muscle graft or, occasionally, with abdominal fat grafting. The watertight dural closure is then achieved. After surgery, low-dose heparin administration is used for 1 day and then replaced by aspirin therapy.

Clinical examples of five patients with intracavernous giant aneurysms treated with this skull base bypass I technique are presented in Figures 9.5–9.7. One patient with a recurrent petroclival cavernous sinus meningioma who presented with ophthalmoplegia is illustrated in Figure 9.8; this patient had total removal of the mass by means of a cavernous carotid bypass.

SKULL BASE BYPASS II (HIGH-CERVICAL TO C6 PETROUS CAROTID BYPASS)

This type of bypass surgery is indicated for radical resection of high-cervical and infratemporal tumors encasing the ICA, repair of high-cervical carotid aneurysms, and treatment of any occlusive ICA lesions in this segment. Surgery is performed through a combined high-cervical

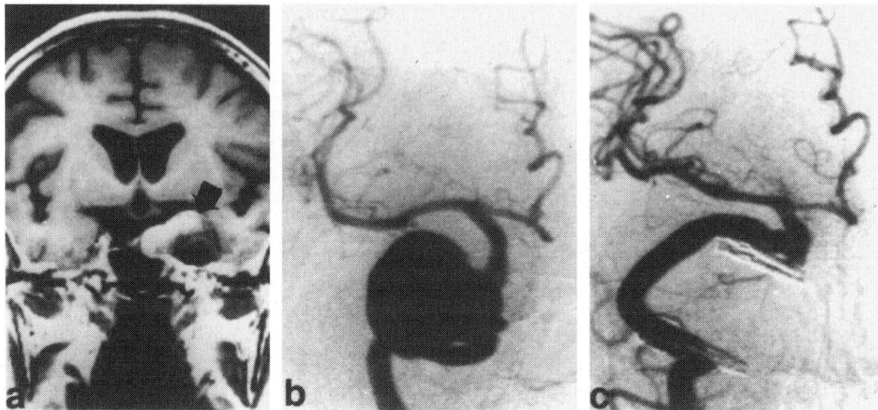

FIG. 9.5 Right oculomotor nerve palsy, in a 76-year-old woman. (a) Coronal MRI shows a half-thrombosed giant aneurysm. (b) Preoperative A-P carotid angiogram. (c) Postoperative angiogram after bypass surgery.

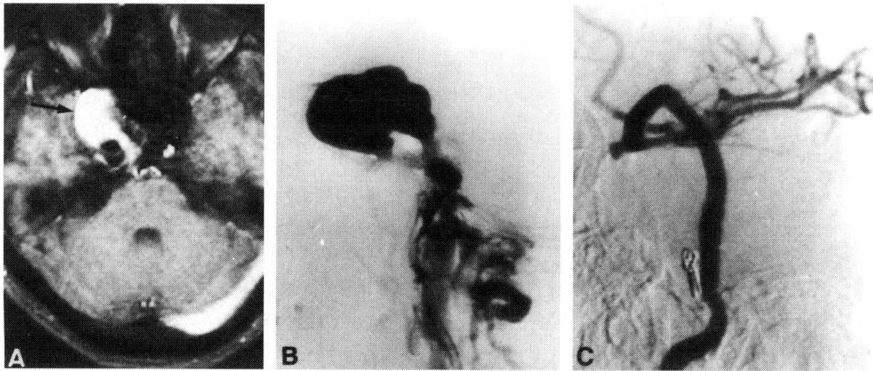

FIG. 9.6 Left abducens palsy in a 45-year-old man. (A) Preoperative axial MRI shows a giant cavernous aneurysm. (B) Preoperative left carotid angiogram (lateral view) demonstrates a huge aneurysm with CCF. (C) Postoperative angiogram shows patent bypass with excellent result.

incision and small extradural subtemporal exposure. In neoplastic cases, the tumor is resected either through a high-cervical, tunnel-operative approach or through a combined high-cervical–extradural subtemporal exposure. After elimination of the lesion, a saphenous vein of appropriate length is anastomosed end-to-end to the ICA in the neck, and then a disposable chest trocar tube is inserted from the neck through the submandibular pterygoid fossa up to the subtemporal epidural area. The other end of the saphenous vein is then inserted into

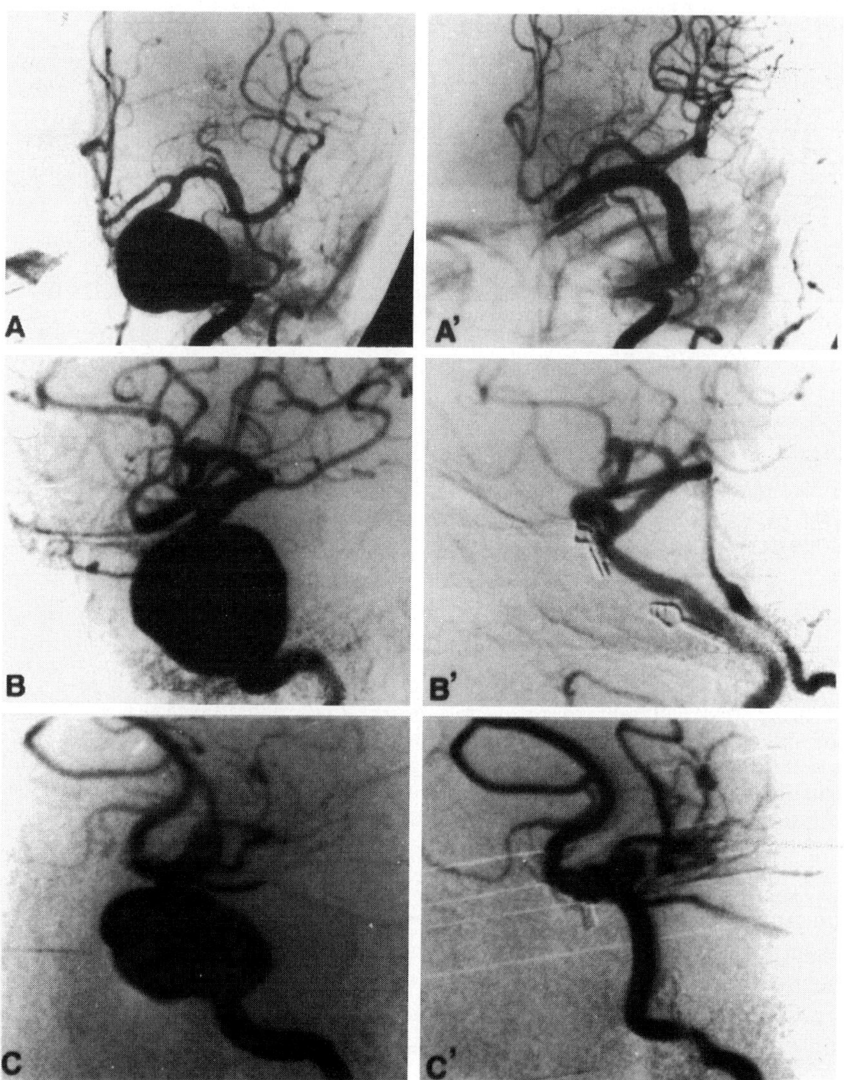

FIG. 9.7 Three examples of various sizes of cavernous giant aneurysm (*left*). (**A**) Oculomotor nerve palsy in a 52-year-old woman. (**A**) shows postoperative angiogram. (**B**) Oculomotor nerve palsy in a 66-year-old woman. (**C**) Oculomotor palsy in an 84-year-old man. Surgical results were excellent in all cases.

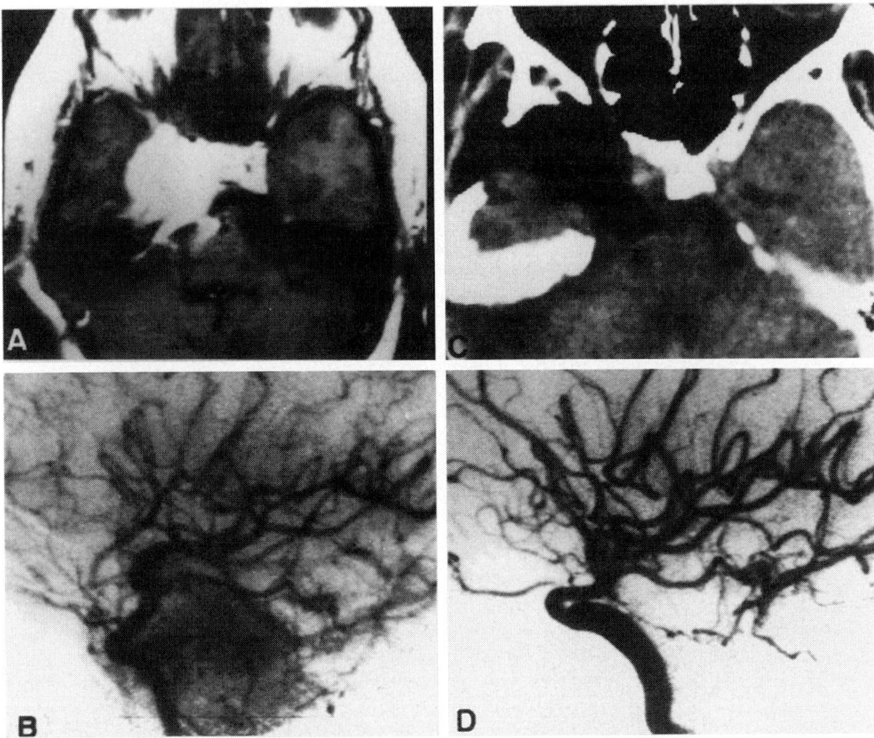

FIG. 9.8 Total ophthalmoplegia due to a recurrent petroclival-cavernous sinus meningioma in a 32-year-old woman. (A) Enhanced CT scan shows a large recurrent mass in the left cavernous sinus. (B) Preoperative angiogram demonstrates tumor stain and mild stenosis of the C4 segment. (C) Postoperative CT shows radical total resection. (D) Postoperative angiogram shows excellent bypass.

the tube from the neck, and the vein is suctioned in the subtemporal direction through the tube. Once the vein is passed through the tube, the latter is removed. The distal end of the saphenous graft is connected extradurally to the C6 petrous carotid segment with end-to-end anastomosis (15). An example of this bypass is illustrated in Figure 9.9.

SKULL BASE BYPASS III (HIGH-CERVICAL TO C3 SAPHENOUS VEIN GRAFT

This bypass is indicated for cavernous sinus lesions that involve the petrous carotid artery. In such cases, a saphenous vein is anastomosed from the high-cervical carotid to the C3 siphon segment with a long saphenous vein graft. Through a standard frontotemporal craniotomy,

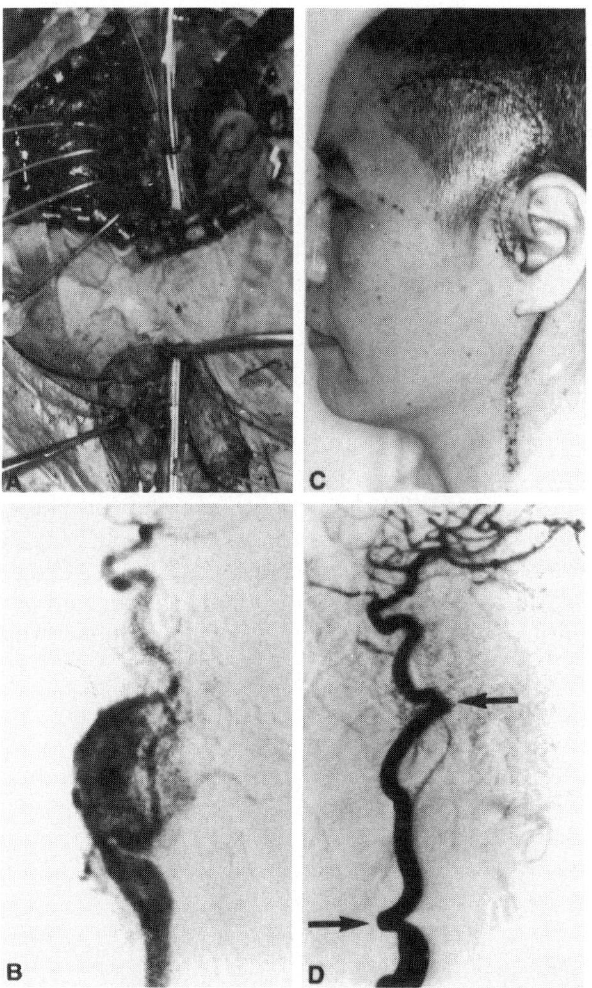

FIG. 9.9 An infratemporal chemodectoma in a 45-year-old woman. (**A**) Combined high-cervical and subtemporal exposure (*left*). (**B**) Preoperative angiogram showing a heavy stain of the tumor, extending from high-cervical area to infratemporal fossa. (**C**) Immediate postoperative incision. (**D**) Postoperative carotid angiogram demonstrates direct reconstruction of the high-cervical and infratemporal carotid artery with total resection of tumor.

the C2 and C3 junction is exposed by opening the anteromedial cavernous triangle and the excision of the fibrous carotid ring. Then the high-cervical carotid is exposed by a routine neck procedure. The long saphenous vein is anastomosed first at the neck carotid artery and then past it, using a chest trocar technique through the submandibular pterygoid route to the temporal base. The distal end of the saphenous vein is passed under the temporal lobe to the siphon area. A summary of these three skull base bypass techniques is illustrated in Figure 9.10.

OPERATIVE RESULTS

In a total of 41 bypass operations, there was no operative mortality. There were four patients who had postoperative stroke complications. Of these four, there were two patients with acute bypass occlusion, one hemiplegic, and one who had permanent hemiparesis. Of the aforementioned patients, there were two who suffered from embolic stroke with hemiparesis. Except for these four patients, the other 37 patients had favorable operative results. Because of the heat from the drill or from ophthalmic artery involvement, two patients had visual loss following surgery. Most patients with giant aneurysm improved with lessened oculomotor deficits after bypass surgery, and only three patients had persistent diplopia. In early cases, two patients had complications of deafness due to damage to the cochlea from drilling. Seventy percent of the patients had either digital subtraction angiography (DSA) or magnetic resonance (MR) angiography as follow-up control, and of these, there were three patients with asymptomatic late occlusion of the bypass.

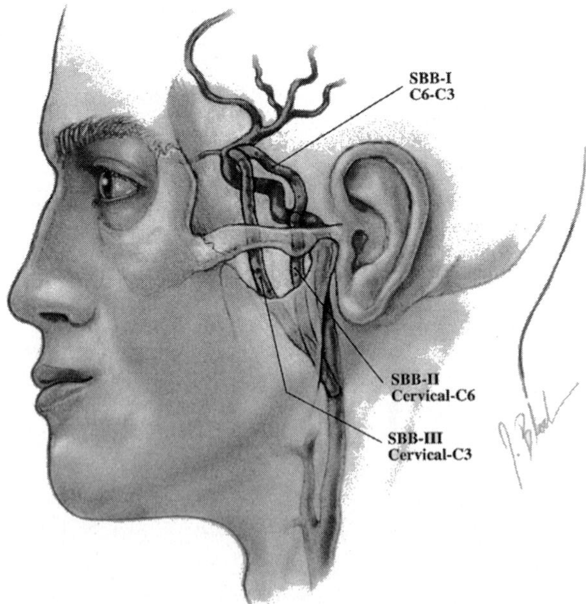

FIG. 9.10 Summary illustration of Fukushima skull base bypasses I to III.

DISCUSSION

The optimal treatment of intracavernous giant aneurysms has been controversial. There are many alternative operative procedures available, such as carotid ligation with or without superficial temporal artery-middle cerebral artery (STA-MCA) bypass or endovascular balloon occlusion. Indication of direct operative management should be determined by the severity of the symptoms, age, or medical condition of the patient. The skull base cavernous bypass establishes an immediate high flow with physiologic hemodynamics. The short length of the saphenous vein graft reduces the risk of delayed thrombosis, as compared to the degree of risk in long vein grafting. The cavernous bypass provides the definite advantage of avoiding any surgical manipulation of the cranial nerves in the cavernous sinus. This skull base bypass technique provides excellent reconstruction of the ICA while eliminating lesions of vascular or neoplastic pathology.

Conventional carotid ligation can be used as an alternative to a direct surgical approach in cases with difficult ICA aneurysms. However, it should be noted that there are significant risks for ischemic complications related to using proximal carotid ligation. Previously literature documented mortality and morbidity of carotid ligation to be in the range of 10 to 30% (13, 14, 17, 18, 23). Even with the modern technique of endovascular balloon occlusion, reports by experts demonstrated that there was 5% mortality and an additional 10% morbidity when using the interventional catheter technique (11). A Japanese multicenter study in 1985 (10) demonstrated that a carotid ligation procedure had risks of 25% ischemic complications, and there was no difference between abrupt occlusion and gradual occlusion. Also, the report demonstrated that the ischemic complication rate was the same in the group of carotid ligation with or without extracranial-intracranial (EC-IC) bypass. All available alternative treatments, modalities, and involved risks have to be discussed with the patient and his/her family before making any decision about the management of cavernous carotid lesions.

REFERENCES

1. Day JD, Fukushima T, Giannotta SL: Microanatomical study of the extradural middle fossa approach to the petroclival and posterior cavernous sinus region: Description of the rhomboid construct. **Neurosurgery** 34:1006–1009, 1994.
2. Dolenc V: Direct microsurgical repair of intracavernous vascular lesions. **J Neurosurg** 58:824–831, 1983.
3. Dolenc V: A combined epi- and subdural direct approach to carotid-opthalmic artery aneurysms. **J Neurosurg** 62:667–672, 1985.

4. Fischer E: Die Lageabweichungen der vorderen Hirnarterie in Gefassbild. **Zentralbl Neurochir** 3:300–312, 1938.
5. Fukushima T: Direct operative approach to the vascular lesions in the cavernous sinus: summary of 27 cases. **Mt Fuji Workshop Cerbrovasc Dis** 6:169–189, 1988.
6. Fukushima T, Day JD, Tung H: Intracavernous carotid artery aneurysm, in Apuzzo MLJ (ed): *Brain Surgery: Complication, Avoidance, and Management.* New York, Churchill Livingstone, 1992, vol 1, part 3, chap. 30.
7. Glasscock ME: Exposure of the intrapetrous portion of the carotid artery, in Hamberger CA, Wersall J (eds): *Disorders of the Skull Base Region: Proceedings of the Tenth Nobel Symposium.* Stockholm, Almqvist & Wiksell, 1969, pp 135–143.
8. Hakuba A, Matsuoka Y, Suzuki T, *et al.:* Direct approaches to vascular lesions in the cavernous sinus via the medial triangle, in Dolenc VV (ed): *The Cavernous Sinus.* Wien, Springer-Verlag, 1987, pp 272–284.
9. Hakuba A, Nishimura S, Shirakata S, *et al.:* Surgical approaches to the cavernous sinus: Report of 19 cases. **Neurol Med Chir (Tokyo)** 22:295–308, 1982.
10. Hashi K, Nin K: Incidence of ischemic complications after carotid ligation combined with EC-IC bypass: A multicenter study. **Cereb Revasc Stroke**: 570–577, 1985.
11. Higashida RT, Halbach VV, Dowd CF, *et al.:* Intracranial aneurysms: Interventional neurovascular treatment with detachable balloons—Results in 215 cases. **Radiology** 178:663–670, 1991.
12. Kawase T, Toya S, Shiobara R, *et al.:* Transpetrosal approach for aneurysms of the lower basilar artery. **J Neurosurg** 63:857–861, 1985.
13. Landolt AM, Millikan CHL: Pathogenesis of cerebral infarction secondary to mechanical carotid artery occlusion. **Stroke** 1:52–62, 1970.
14. Miller JD, Jawad K, Jennett B: Safety of carotid ligation and its role in the management of intracranial aneurysms. **J Neurol Neurosurg Psychiatry** 40:64–72, 1977.
15. Miyazaki S, Fukushima T, Fujimake T: Resection of high-cervical paraganglioma with cervical-to-petrous internal carotid artery saphenous vein bypass. Report of two cases. **J Neurosurg** 73:141–146, 1990.
16. Mullan S: Treatment of carotid-cavernous fistulas by cavernous sinus occlusion. **J Neurosurg** 50:131–144, 1979.
17. Nishioka H: Report on the cooperative study of intracranial aneurysms and subarachnoid hemorrhage: Section VIII, Part I. Results of the treatment of intracranial aneurysms by occlusion of the carotid artery in the neck. **J Neurosurg** 25:660–682, 1966.
18. Odom GL, Tindall GT: Carotid ligation in the treatment of certain intracranial aneurysms. **Clin Neurosurg** 15:101–116, 1968.
19. Parkinson D: A surgical approach to the cavernous portion of the carotid artery: Anatomical studies and case report. **J Neurosurg** 23:474–483, 1965.
20. Parkinson D: Transcavernous repair of carotid-cavernous fistula: Case report. **J Neurosurg** 26:420–424, 1967.
21. Parkinson D: Carotid cavernous fistula: Direct repair with preservation of the carotid artery. Technical note. **J Neurosurg** 38:99–106, 1973.
22. Paullus WS, Pait TG, Rhoton AL Jr: Microsurgical exposure of the petrous portion of the carotid artery. **J Neurosurg** 47:713–726, 1977.
23. Roski RA, Spetzler RF, Nulsen FE: Late complications of carotid ligation in the treatment of intracranial aneurysms. **J Neurosurg** 54:583–587, 1981.
24. Spetzler RF, Fukushima T, Martin N, *et al.:* Petrous carotid-to-intradural carotid saphenous vein graft for intracavernous giant aneurysm, tumor, and occlusive cerebrovascular disease. **J Neurosurg** 73:496–501, 1990.

10

Is Carotid Artery Reconstruction Mandatory?

CHANDRANATH SEN, M.D., AND DAVID SEGAL, M.D.

With the great strides made in recent years in the management of a variety of lesions at the base of the skull, the issue of "the proper way of managing the internal carotid artery (ICA)" has aroused a great deal of interest. This discussion has further been fueled by similar progress in interventional techniques, microsurgical techniques, and sophisticated ways of assessing the arterial collateral circulation of the brain. Faced with a wide armamentarium of treatment options available to the surgeon, the "right" choice may be a difficult decision. To simplify the matter, this decision process may be divided into smaller questions: What is the nature of the lesion, neoplastic or vascular, and what are the treatment options? What portion of the artery is involved by the tumor? Is the tumor benign or malignant, and what is the natural history and survival rate for such a tumor? Can the tumor be dissected off of the ICA? If the involved artery were successfully managed, what is the likelihood of being able to resect the remaining tumor that may extend into the other regions of the skull base? If in answering the preceding questions it appears that the only impediment to the successful treatment of the lesion is the ICA, the issue now remains as to whether to sacrifice the artery and excise it with the tumor or, in the case of an aneurysm, to occlude the parent vessel. If this is the course of action chosen, then is immediate reconstruction or revascularization necessary, as the patient may be left without a carotid artery? In attempting to answer the latter questions it is necessary to understand: (*a*) the consequences and risks of sacrificing a carotid artery without revascularization, (*b*) the options for revascularization, and (*c*) the risks of revascularization. The following discussion will be based on the assumption that the lesion involves the upper cervical, petrous, or intracavernous ICA on one side. Further distally, the smaller branches and perforating vessels come into play with a different set of problems.

CONSEQUENCES AND RISKS OF SACRIFICING THE ICA ON ONE SIDE

Although such problems as development of *de novo* intracranial aneurysms (8) and systemic hypertension have been reported as a

long-term consequence of ICA ligation (35), the immediate risk is that
of ischemic neurologic deficits. Carotid ligation has been used extensively for the treatment of the unclippable aneurysms and also during
the resection of tumors both malignant and benign. Nishioka, reporting on a large series of patients undergoing carotid ligation, found
about a 30% incidence of strokes: of which, 79% occurred in the first 48
hours and 95% occurred in the first 7 days (23). These strokes may be
attributed to either an embolic or hypoperfusion cause.

In the normal patient the cerebral blood flow (CBF) is maintained as
constant through a wide range of systemic blood pressures. After
carotid ligation, the ipsilateral cerebrovascular bed undergoes vasodi-
lation to maintain a constant blood flow. Sengupta et al. showed that
the vasodilatory response to hypoxia is reduced and that the autoreg-
ulatory curve is shifted to the right after unilateral carotid ligation.
This makes the patient more vulnerable to such changes (33). This altered state can continue for an indefinite length of time, leaving patients vulnerable even in the most vigilant intensive care setting. Emboli originating from the blind stump of the ligated ICA and from the
surface of intraluminal balloons have been attributed to a proportion
of these strokes. The risk of carotid ligation in a certain patient can be
determined, to some extent; however, there are no absolutely reliable
tests.

Preoperative Testing for Carotid Ligation

Since the description by Rudolph Matas in 1911 (17), there have been
several modifications and refinements for testing of the collateral reserve of the cerebral circulation. Most of the these combine the use of
a period of temporary occlusion of the ICA by an intraluminal balloon
with measurement of the CBF at that instant. About 5% of patients develop neurologic deficits immediately upon interruption of the ICA
flow, indicating poor collaterals. Another 10 to 20% can suffer a stroke
even if they did not develop deficits at the time of the balloon test occlusion (BTO) (9, 11). Detection of this latter group of patients has been
the aim of the BTO in its present state. The assessment of angiographic
collaterals (13, 34), as well as the use of provocative hypotension, have
not been reliable (15). The measurement of carotid stump pressure (38)
and the monitoring of EEG (16, 21) have also been reported, but present, some type of CBF measurement during the BTO seems to be the
most prevalent method. Cerebral blood flow and its regulation is a dynamic process. One of the shortcomings of the BTO is that the CBF
measurement is static, taken at a single point in time. Fluctuations of
CBF occur upon ligation of a carotid artery until a steady state is

reached by opening of collateral channels (3). This may not be evident in a single CBF measurement.

The two types of CBF measurement widely used are stable Xenon CT (XE CT) CBF and CBF with single photon emission computer tomography (SPECT). The Xenon CT method provides quantitative data and can be used to compare one study with another. If an acetazolamide challenge is utilized, quantitative measurement is much more useful (14). However, the most important drawback of the Xe CT method is the need to perform inflation of the intraluminal balloon twice, once in the angiogram suite when the clinical evaluation of the patient is being carried out and the second time in the CT suite for the CBF study. The patient is transported from one suite to another with the intra-arterial catheter in place. The second balloon inflation is carried out with relatively less control of the location of the balloon and the degree of its inflation (5). The SPECT method, on the other hand, provides comparative information of the CBF in one hemisphere as compared to the other. It can detect a difference of greater than 10% between the hemispheres (19). The balloon inflation is carried out only once in the angiography suite under more stringent control (25, 43).

The patients can thus be divided into those who fail the clinical test and develop transient neurologic deficits on inflation of the balloon and those who remain neurologically normal. Of these latter patients, CBF values of less than 20 ml/100 g/min are classified as "high-risk," those with CBF values between 20 and 35 ml/100 g/min are "moderate-risk." Those who remain above 35 ml/100 g/min are "low-risk" (18, 43). Several authors have shown examples of low-risk patients, who have suffered strokes upon carotid ligation (24, 27, 29) (Table 10.1). Hence, it appears that there is no patient with absolutely no risk of stroke on carotid ligation; only the degree of risk varies. Moreover, there is no

TABLE 10.1
BTO Studies

Study	Patients	Fail BTO	Abnormal CBF	Normal CBF	Complications/ Ligation
deVries *et al.,* 1990 (Xe CT)	114	11	13	90	1/23 normal CBF 4/5 abnormal CBF
Peterman *et al.,* 1990 (SPECT)	17	0	2	15	1/5
Monsein *et al.,* 1991 (SPECT)	11	0	5	6	0/2
Matthews *et al.,* 1992 (SPECT)	42	8	9	25	0/13
Origitano *et al.,* 1994 (SPECT and Xe CT)	100	7			4/18
Sekhar *et al.,* 1993 (Xe CT)	39			39	8/39

method in existence, of determining which particular patients are at high risk and which are not.

CASE STUDIES

Patient 1. A 14-year-old girl was diagnosed by needle biopsy as having a malignant schwannoma involving the right orbit. After treatment with external irradiation and chemotherapy the tumor continued to grow, leading to marked proptosis and pain (Fig. 10.1A). Because of the tumor extension into the anterior cavernous sinus around the ICA, it was decided to excise the artery, along with the orbit and the contents of the cavernous sinus. She passed the BTO with no changes on CBF seen on stable Xe CT and, consequently, underwent permanent balloon occlusion of the ICA in the upper cervical and the intracavernous segment without any difficulty. The operation was performed the next day as planned and was tolerated well by the patient (Fig. 10.1B).

About 24 hours after the operation, the patient was found to be hemiplegic in the intensive care unit. An emergency arteriogram showed filling of the right anterior and middle cerebral arteries through the anterior (ACoA) and posterior (PCoA) communicating arteries. There was no suggestion of embolic occlusions. Xe CT CBF showed hypoperfusion in the entire right MCA distribution (Fig. 10.1C). Therapeutic hypertension was instituted with dopamine until normalization of the CBF in the ischemic territory was seen (Fig. 10.1D). The patient was maintained at this level of blood pressure control for 3 days but remained hemiplegic. Although she remained free of the tumor for the 3 years of follow-up, MRI scans showed infarcts in the right hemisphere in the border zone distribution (Fig. 10.1E).

COMMENTS. En bloc resection of the orbit and cavernous sinus was the only treatment option in this patient. Although permanent intravascular balloons are known to be associated with embolic complications, this was not the situation in this case, as shown by arteriogram and CBF studies. Hypoperfusion in the entire MCA distribution was documented, even though the patient tolerated the preoperative BTO. Medical treatment did not succeed in rectifying the situation, and she was left with a profound neurologic deficit.

Patient 2. This 66-year-old man was seen with a recurrent squamous cell cancer at the skull base involving the petrous segment of the ICA. The arteriogram showed good collaterals, and BTO was tolerated without changes in the postocclusion SPECT studies (Fig. 10.2A). Temporary occlusion of the ICA was also performed in the operating room in the normotensive as well as hypotensive states without any changes in the somatosensory evoked potentials. Resection of the tumor along

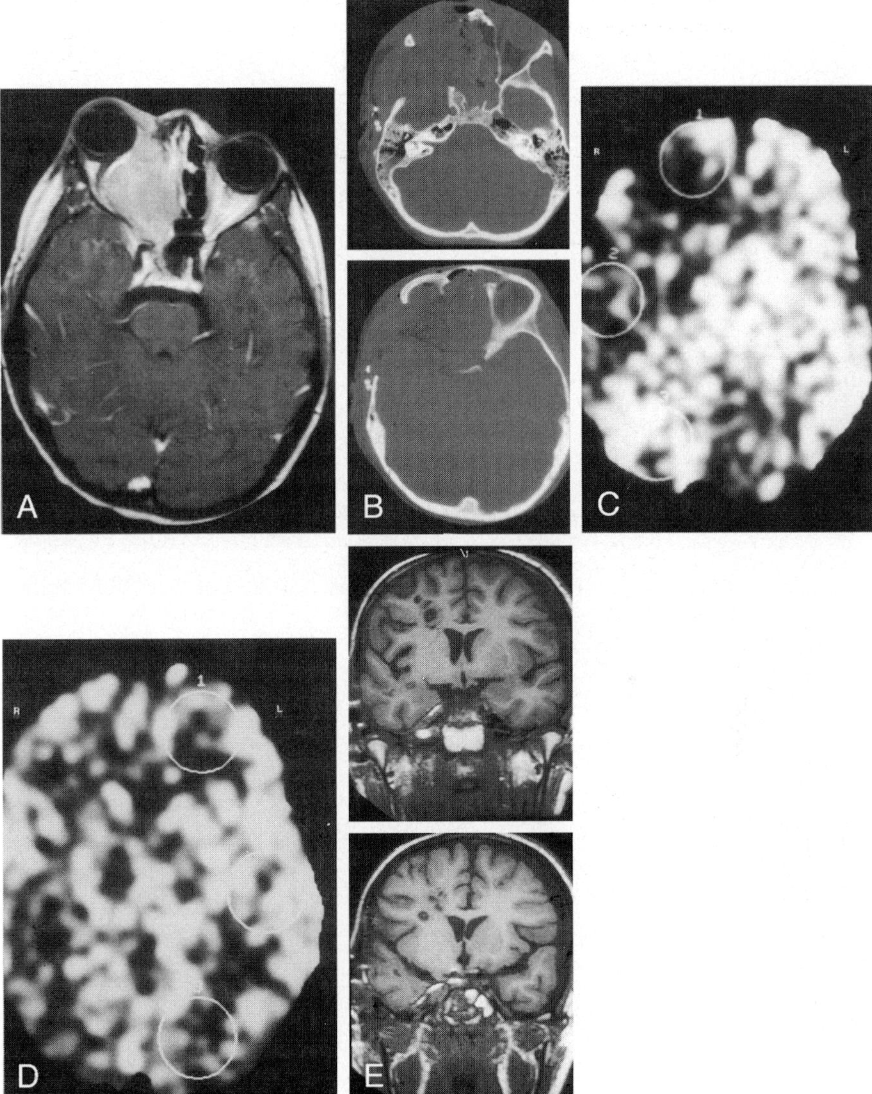

FIG. 10.1 (A) Case 1. Preoperative MRI with gadolinium, indicating that tumor in the orbit is pushing against anterior portion of intracavernous ICA. (B) Postoperative CT scan, showing extent of bony resection of anterior and middle fossa. (C) Xe CT CBF obtained when the patient was hemiplegic. Note hypoperfusion of frontal and temporal lobes (*darker shades*) in a normotensive state. (D) Xe CT CBF obtained immediately after that in C after therapeutic elevation of blood pressure. Note improvement in CBF. (E) MRI scan obtained 3 weeks after surgery, showing border zone areas of infarction.

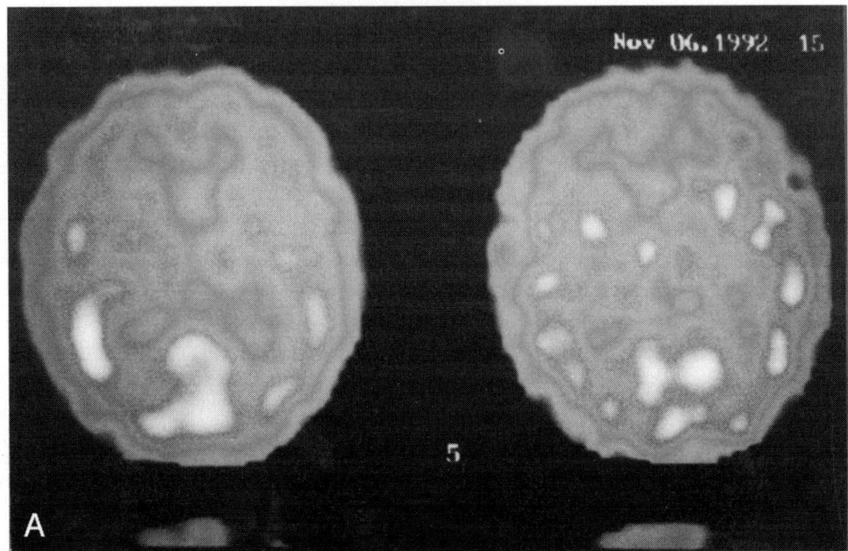

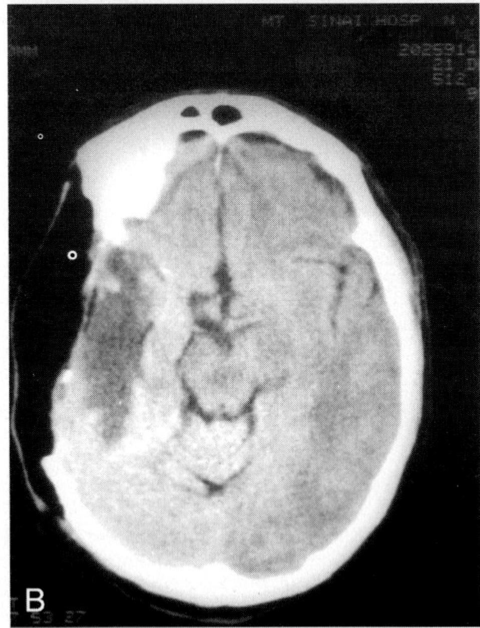

FIG. 10.2 (**A**) Case 2. Preoperative SPECT obtained at time of BTO, showing no asymmetry in CBF. (**B**) Late CT scan, showing right temporal lobe infarct.

with the ICA was subsequently performed by ligating ICA in the neck and in the supraclinoid segment immediately proximal to the origin of the PCoA. The surgical defect was reconstructed with a microvascular rectus abdominis free flap. The postoperative course in the intensive care unit was complicated by problems related to the free flap, which required revision. During this time the patient remained confused and agitated. A routine CT scan 5 days after the operation showed an infarct in the distribution of the MCA (Fig. 10.2**B**).

COMMENTS. The stroke could be attributed to an embolic or hypoperfusion basis, although measures to prevent emboli were taken (no "dead space" in the ICA was left, and the patient was on low molecular weight dextran, routinely used at microvascular flaps). No grossly apparent periods of hypotension were identified, although brief periods could have occurred during the problems with the free flap.

OPTIONS FOR REVASCULARIZATION

Several methods of revascularization have been described that may be suitable in different circumstances. They have their own advantages and drawbacks. The neurosurgeon must be well versed in these methods to make the best choice for the situation at hand (Table 10.2). Cerebral revascularization may be broadly divided into (*a*) superficial temporal artery (STA) or occipital artery to middle cerebral artery (MCA) bypass, (*b*) long vein grafts from the external carotid or subclavian artery to the MCA, and (*c*) short vein grafts from the internal carotid, in the petrous segment to the supraclinoid ICA.

TABLE 10.2

Pros and Cons of Revascularization Techniques

	Advantages	Disadvantages
STA-MCA[a] Bypass	95% patency	No immediate high-flow volume
	No ICA flow interruption	STA may be small or nonexistent from prior surgery
	Long-term patency excellent	
ECA-MCA vein graft	Immediate high-flow volume	Patency rates 50–60%
	No ICA interruption	Late occlusions
		Subject to extrinsic compression
ICA-ICA vein graft	Short graft, large-to-large vessel	ICA flow interruption of 2 hr.
	Patency rate 80–90%	Anastomosis at depth
		Potential graft occlusion

[a]STA-MCA, superficial temporal artery to middle cerebral artery; ECA to MCA, external carotid artery to middle cerebral artery; ICA to ICA, internal carotid artery to internal carotid artery.

Superficial Temporal Artery or Occipital Artery to MCA Bypass. Described initially by Yasargil as a treatment for occlusive cerebrovascular disease (45), it now plays an important role in prophylactic revascularization in preparation for ICA sacrifice (6). The bypass consists of anastomosing the anterior, the posterior, or both branches of the STA to branches of the middle cerebral artery in the sylvian fissure. Many favorable features make it a popular choice; it involves one suture line; it is a relatively straightforward procedure, because the anastomosis is performed on the surface and there is a close size match between the donor and recipient vessels; it has low morbidity; and it has a high patency rate (95%) (12, 46). Although the bypass has been shown to provide sufficient collateral flow to permit carotid artery sacrifice in giant aneurysm surgery, it may not always be enough (maximum flow, 40 ml/min) to substitute for the acute loss of carotid flow, which can be 300 ml/min (26, 41). A more common problem may be the absence of a suitable-sized STA, either naturally or because of previous surgery (31). Nevertheless, the STA or occipital artery may be an important source of potential collateral and should be preserved wherever potential injury to the ICA or MCA exists.

Long Vein Grafts from Cervical Arteries to the MCA within the Fissure. This operation utilizes a length of the greater saphenous vein to bring blood supply from the cervical external carotid artery or the subclavian artery (36). Usually a length of 15 to 20 cm of vein may be necessary. The distal end is anastomosed to the proximal MCA in the fissure distal to the origin of the lenticulostriate branches. This provides an immediate high-flow conduit approximating the ICA flow; flow in the MCA branch is interrupted only during the distal anastomosis, and only the downstream area of the MCA branch is subjected to the temporary period of ischemia. The difficulties in this procedure arise from the mismatch between the MCA and the vein. This may cause kinking of the MCA branch when the flow is resumed. Also the vein becomes turgid under arterial pressure. The other pitfall results from the vein being tunnelled for a long distance, making it vulnerable to external compression and torsion with neck movements. The overall patency rate of such grafts is lower than that of the STA-MCA bypass (approx 60%). Other types of long vein grafts have also been shown to bring in blood supply from other sources, such as one of the branches of the ECA on the same or opposite side to the MCA branches (36, 39).

Short Vein Grafts from the Petrous ICA to the Supraclinoid ICA. This technique was described as bypassing a tumor-encased portion of the intracavernous ICA, using a short segment of vein connecting the ICA in the petrous segment to that in the supraclinoid segment

(28). There are several advantages and drawbacks to this type of bypass. The advantages include the following: the bypass consists of an anastomosis of a relatively large size vein and artery; it provides a high rate of blood flow at the outset; both anastomoses are performed intracranially at the site of the pathology; and the surgeon avoids having to move from one site to another, *e.g.,* from neck to head (31). The disadvantages are: it requires temporary cessation of all blood flow through the ICA for the duration of the anastomosis; it is technically difficult because of the need to expose the intrapetrous ICA and because the anastomosis is carried out at a significant depth; and it has a patency rate of 80 to 90% (32). The temporary clamping of the ICA can pose a serious stroke risk in patients with marginal or inadequate collaterals, as indicated by BTO failures and those patients who have a CBF of less than 20 ml/100 g/min (31).

Choice of Revascularization

This decision is based on several factors: (*a*) results of BTO and the CBF studies; (*b*) the surgeon's experience; (*c*) the age of the patient; (*d*) the location and type of pathology and (*e*) prior operations that may influence the availability of suitable donor and recipient vessels.

Although it is this author's view that whenever ICA sacrifice is deemed necessary, a revascularization procedure of some type should be considered (27); a preoperative BTO with SPECT or stable Xe CT is an important test to give to help formulate a treatment plan. A large group of patients undergoing BTO and stable Xe CT CBF was reviewed by Tarr *et al.* They found a 3.7% incidence of complications (temporary and permanent) from this test. The majority of them were due to subintimal dissection (43). However, in our review of 56 consecutive patients subjected to the BTO but using the SPECT to measure CBF, there were no complications (27). This difference is most likely attributable to the need for the patient to be moved from the angiography suite to the CT suite for the Xe CT study. When the intraluminal balloon is inflated for the second time, but without a means of absolutely confirming the position of the balloon or the degree of inflation leading to intimal injury. In this respect the SPECT offers a distinct advantage (22, 25).

"High-Risk" Patients and Those That Clinically Fail the BTO. In high-risk patients, the indications for carotid sacrifice must be carefully reviewed. One may elect to either totally avoid operation on such a patient or plan a more conservative operation avoiding manipulation of the ICA. If ICA sacrifice is still considered necessary, *e.g.,* in cases of bilateral aneurysms or in patients with contralateral occlusive disease or in tumors involving more than one of the major vessels, a revascularization must be considered as an initial step in the treatment process (30). This may consist of a STA-MCA bypass or a vein graft from the cervical vessels to the MCA to be done as a first step (1, 26, 42). The BTO is then repeated to reassess the collateral status. These steps are usually enough to raise the CBF sufficiently so as to tolerate ICA sacrifice or, at least, to allow tolerance of temporary occlusion to perform a larger bypass at the time of definitive treatment of the lesion.

"Moderate-Risk" Patient Treated by Xe CT and Those That Show Low Flow on SPECT. This group of patients usually tolerates temporary interruption of flow without suffering a stroke (20). A long vein graft from the external or cervical internal carotid to the supraclinoid ICA or a short vein graft from the petrous to the supraclinoid ICA is usually selected in these cases (31). If an ICA-to-ICA vein graft is chosen, the flow interruption lasts for the entire duration of the anastomosis at both ends of the vessel; this interruption can last from 90 to 120 minutes. This occlusion time can be reduced almost by half by using the external carotid as the donor and the MCA as the recipient. In such a situation, the intracranial anastomosis is performed first. Next, a temporary clip is placed across the vein immediately proximal to the anastomosis, and all the clips on the MCA or supraclinoid ICA are released so that flow to the brain resumes. The patient is then fully heparinized, and the cervical anastomosis can then be performed under less duress.

"Low-risk" Patients and Those Who Have No Asymmetry of Flow by SPECT. Although in this group any of the above-described methods of revascularization may be chosen, the direct ICA-to-ICA vein graft is preferred, bypassing the diseased segment (32, 44), whether it is the intracavernous or the petrous segment. The vascular anastomosis is performed before tumor removal is undertaken.

The age of the patient and underlying atherosclerotic vascular disease should be considered in decision making. The collateral circulation may be impaired in such patients, giving them poor tolerance to manipulation of the vessels (4, 23). While performing the bypass, the surgeon must be particularly careful to select a disease-free segment of the vessel for donor and recipient sites; otherwise-graft occlusion or embolic complications will produce a poor outcome (10, 40). The surgeon must select the procedure with which he/she is most familiar. This is a technically exacting operation, requiring meticulous attention at every step. In most instances complications result in loss of the graft and even a stroke. Prior operations may limit the choices of donor and recipient sites available, and this must be considered in view of the results of the BTO. Prior irradiation may render the intracranial or extracranial vessels more vulnerable to surgical manipulation in that they may rupture or thrombose easily.

CASE STUDIES

Patient 3. A 41-year-old woman presented with progressive visual loss in the right eye and a new onset of visual field deficit in the opposite eye. An aneurysm arose from the anterior genu of the intracavernous ICA (Fig. 10.3A). The preoperative BTO showed a relative decrease in CBF in the right cerebral hemisphere on SPECT (Fig. 10.3B). The aneurysm was approached through a frontotemporal crainotomy with a zygomatic osteotomy. The anterior clinoid process was drilled away to expose the neck of the aneurysm. Proximal control of the artery was obtained in the petrous segment. After temporary trapping of the proximal and distal ICA, the broad aneurysm neck was reconstructed with several clips. Intraoperative arteriography, however, revealed the artery to be occluded. The aneurysm was trapped, and a saphenous vein bypass was performed from the petrous to supraclinoid segment under barbiturate coma (Fig. 10.3C and **D**). The patient sustained no additional deficits, and the vein graft has been patent over 1 year of follow-up.

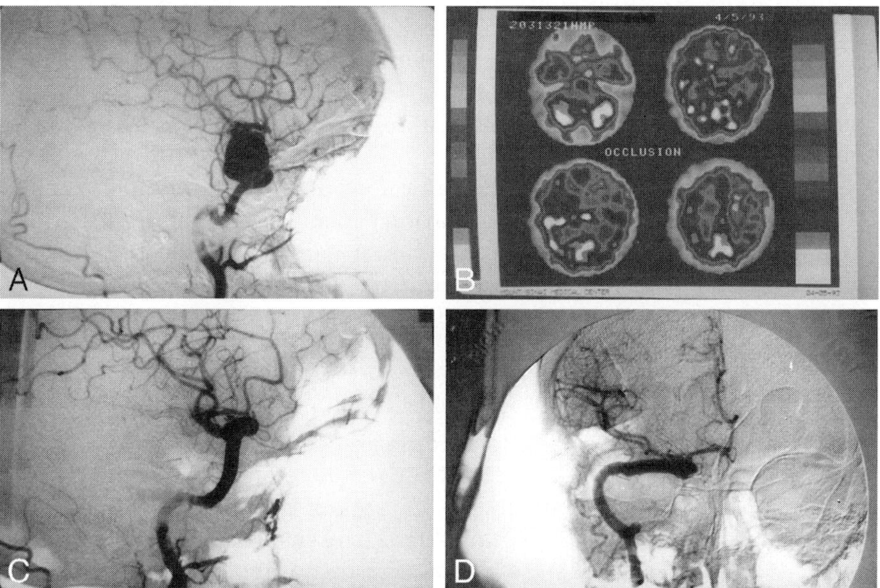

FIG. 10.3 (**A**) Case 3. Right carotid arteriogram, showing aneurysm arising from anterior genu of intracavernous ICA. (**B**) Preoperative SPECT at time of BTO showing areas of hypoperfusion of right hemisphere (*viewer's right*) in *lighter shades.* (**C** and **D**) Lateral and AP arteriogram, showing saphenous vein bypass graft from petrous to supraclinoid segment, with elimination of the aneurysm.

COMMENTS. An intraoperative arteriogram was crucial in this case to determine whether the ICA has been occluded by the aneurysm clips. Although the intraoperative evoked potentials did not change, a bypass was performed, based on the preoperative SPECT study. The short vein graft was performed, because both the proximal and distal portions of the ICA were in the operative field. The status of the vein graft was also confirmed with an intraoperative arteriogram, which allows detection of subtle problems that may subsequently lead to graft occlusion.

Patient 4. A 74-year-old woman was found to have a large intracavernous ICA aneurysm (Fig. 10.4**A** and **B**), causing total ophthalmoplegia and severe face pain on the right side of her face. She tolerated the BTO but the SPECT could not be performed for technical reasons. At surgery the aneurysm was opened and the thrombus evacuated after the ICA had been trapped in the neck and intracranially, proximal to the PCoA. After emerging from anesthesia without any new deficits, the patient developed acute onset of left hemiplegia a day later, while seated at bedside in the intensive care unit. An arteriogram performed immediately showed slow flow in the right hemisphere (Fig. 10.4**C** and 10.4**D**). No hemorrhage was seen on the CT. She underwent an emergency saphenous vein bypass from the cervical ICA to the M2 segment (Fig. 10.4**E** and **F**). Postoperative CT scans did not show an infarct, and the hemiplegia improved (Fig. 10.4**G**) but never resolved completely.

COMMENTS. The patient had a profound neurologic deficit that occurred 24 hours after the ICA ligation, even though the ligature had been performed so as not to leave a stagnant column of blood that could be the source of an embolism. The arteriogram confirmed slow flow, and the emergency bypass procedure prevented the patient from suffering a devastating stroke.

RISKS OF REVASCULARIZATION

The most significant risk is thrombosis of the graft and resultant stroke. There are several factors that influence graft survival. These have been reviewed extensively by many authors (32, 40). These factors include the technique of harvesting and preparation of the vein or the donor vessel, the diameter of the vein (or radial artery, if used), the flow rate, and the anastomotic sites (suture line stenosis and intimal flap are detrimental), and, if the graft is passed through a long tunnel in the tissues, it may be subjected to extrinsic compression. Many of these factors can be controlled by the surgeon and need meticulous attention. Occasionally, a patient in a hypercoagulable state may be en-

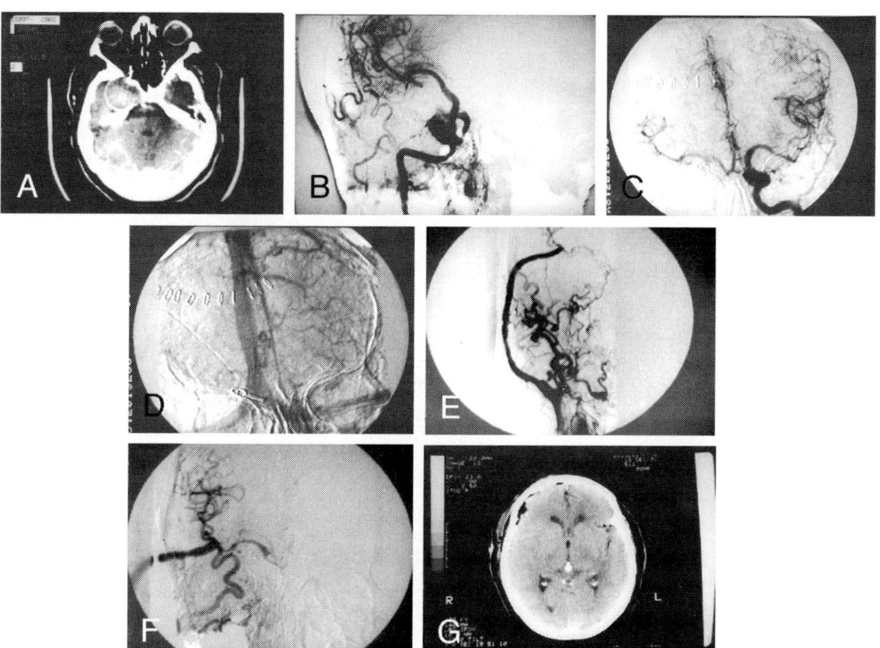

FIG. 10.4 (A) Case 4. Preoperative CT scan, showing partially thrombosed aneurysmal mass in right middle cranial fossa. (B) Only middle cerebral artery fills through the right carotid arteriogram. As seen in this anteroposterior projection, the aneurysm arose from the intracavernous ICA. (C). Anteroposterior projection of left carotid artery injection at time when patient was hemiplegic, indicating that right MCA fills through anterior cerebral artery. The flow is slower on right side, as compared to left. (D). AP projection of venous phase of left carotid injection, showing a delayed venous phase on right hemisphere (*viewer's left*), as compared to left hemisphere. (E and F). Anteroposterior projection after revascularization, showing vein graft from cervical ICA to middle cerebral artery. (G) CT scan obtained 3 weeks later shows no infarct.

countered. This condition can be caused by a malignancy and can be detected preoperatively by a hematologic work-up which includes measuring serum levels of antithrombin III and proteins C and S.

The vein is usually harvested from the upper thigh because of its large diameter and few tributaries. It is left *in situ* after the adventitia has been infiltrated with papaverine (3 mg/ml) to present spasm. Overdistension is avoided after the vein is harvested. The anastomosis is carried out, ensuring a proper intimal bite, with every suture properly compensating for the mismatch of the sizes of the vessels. The patient is fully heparinized throughout the period of temporary occlusion, after which a lower dose of heparin is continued for about 24 hours (32).

Although the rate of graft patency has been reported as ranging from 66 to 96% (7, 42), performing an intraoperative arteriogram is extremely beneficial (27). Potential problems that may compromise the graft patency can be detected and remedied early before any irreversible problems can develop. An arteriogram is much more reliable than a microdoppler probe for this purpose.

Although embolic problems have not been encountered in the author's experience, they are prevented by attention to technique and heparinization. All of the vein grafts were performed with the patient under mild hypothermia (32° C) and by using barbiturate burst suppression of the electroencephalogram (2). Somatosensory evoked responses are monitored in all cases and can help detect ischemic problems, although they may not be as sensitive when under the effect of the barbiturates. The drawback of the barbiturates stems from the slow awakening of the patient, which limits neurologic evaluation. Laser doppler flowmetry with a probe left on the brain may be useful in monitoring the patient during the early postoperative period when he/she is most susceptible to graft occlusion. The hypothermia and barbiturates may provide brain protection from ischemia during the period of temporary occlusion (37).

Whether graft occlusion in a particular case will lead to a stroke depends on the results of the preoperative BTO. It should be noted, however, that the BTO provides information only about the result of occluding the upper cervical, petrous, and intracavernous ICA. It does not take into account the collateral blood supply that is being brought in by the ophthalmic (OA) and the PCoAs when the ICA proximal to these branches is being occluded. If, when the graft occlusion occurs there is also loss of the OA and/or the PCoA, a patient may suffer a stroke even if they tolerated the BTO.

Management of Graft Occlusion

A patient who develops a neurologic deficit in the postoperative period should have immediate arteriography. If the graft is found to be occluded, the patient should be immediately returned to the operating room, and a new bypass should be performed to avert a catastrophe. This management strategy has been adopted also in patients who suffered inadvertent carotid occlusion after manipulation to dissect tumor from the vessel. In the two patients who had graft occlusion and successful revascularization within 12 hours, both had no hemiparesis and showed only border zone area infarctions. In the two patients in whom the graft could not be successfully revised, both suffered large infarctions; one died from massive stroke, and the other remains hemiparetic. Of the two patients who suffered inadvertent carotid occlusion, one was treated medically but died of complications from the stroke; the other was treated with an occipital-to-MCA bypass and showed significant improvement. More importantly, none of the revascularized patients suffered a hemorrhage. It thus appears that revascularization within a reasonable time in such patients who have a symptomatic carotid or graft occlusion in a monitored situation can limit the seriousness of their stroke. They also have a better clinical outcome, as was seen in this limited, small group of patients. This seemed to hold even though they had a profound neurologic deficit at the time of detection.

In a series of 12 cases of vein graft reconstruction performed in the past 3 years by the author, there were two instances of graft occlusion and three strokes. One of the graft occlusions were asymptomatic while the other resulted in a stroke. This symptomatic occlusion occurred in a patient with a malignant tumor and was attributed to a documented hypercoagulable state because the vein graft occluded despite three attempts at revision. In the three patients with strokes, one was the patient with graft occlusion just discussed; another had a stroke due to occlusion of the anterior choroidal artery by a malpositioned aneurysm clip during treatment of a giant aneurysm. The third patient with a stroke suffered occlusion of the MCA branch, where the vein graft was anastomosed. Thus, the majority of the graft-related problems seem to be technical in origin and can be prevented by meticulous attention to the graft's performance; this was also evident in a larger series of patients on whom the authors reported (32). Intraoperative neurophysiologic monitoring is invaluable in these operations. Intraoperative arteriography is an important tool for detecting technical errors in the operating room so that they can be attended to immediately and perhaps irreversible neurologic deficits can be avoided.

CASE STUDY

Patient 5. A 39-year-old woman was evaluated for progressive III nerve and total VIth nerve palsy (Fig. 10.5A). She also had numbness on the left side of her face. The preoperative BTO showed a decrease in CBF in the left hemisphere on the stable Xe CT (Fig. 10.5B). The tumor, a meningioma, was resected in two stages. At the first stage a saphenous vein bypass was performed from the petrous to the supraclinoid segment, and the hyperostotic bone, as well as the extradural portion of the tumor, was removed. The vascular reconstruction was performed with the patient under barbiturate coma. The next day the patient was found to be hemiplegic, and the graft was occluded. Her CBF at this time showed blood flows in the left MCA distribution to be between 11 and 18

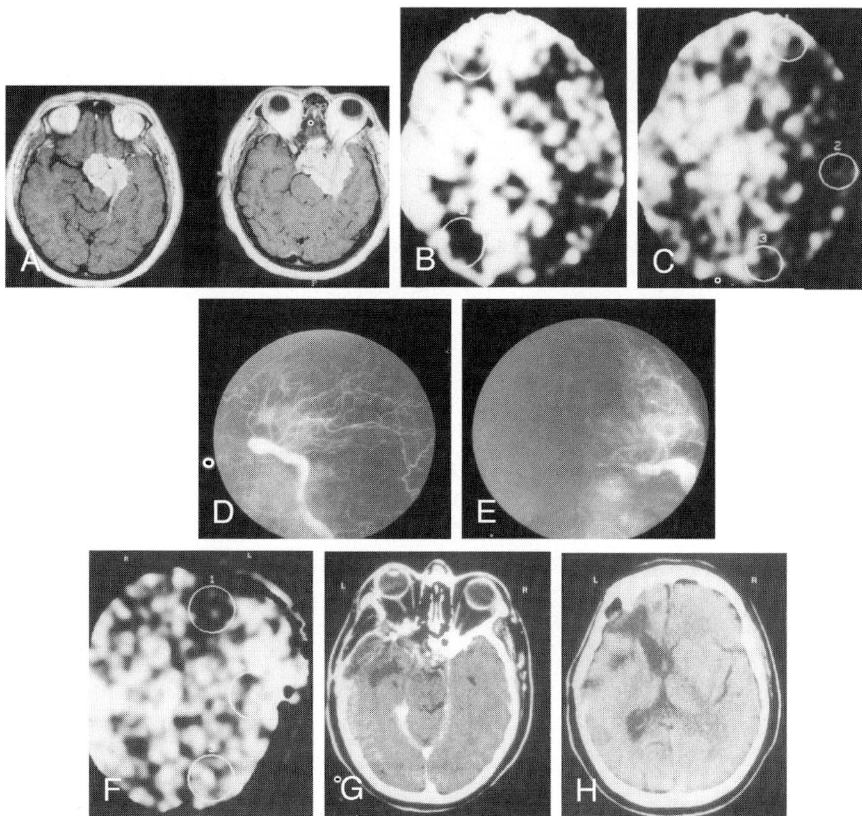

FIG. 10.5 (A) Case 5. Preoperative MRI scan of the large meningioma encasing the left ICA. (B) Xe CT CBF at the time of the preoperative BTO, indicating the areas of hypoperfusion (*darker shades*) in the left hemisphere (*viewer's right*). (C) Xe CT CBF at the time of graft occlusion, indicating the hypoperfusion of the left hemisphere as predicted by the BTO. (D and E) Lateral and anteroposterior arteriogram of the of the vein graft filling the middle cerebral artery. (F) Xe CT CBF immediately after the revascularization, showing the hyperemia in the left hemisphere. (G) CT scan after intravenous contrast obtained 3 years after the operation, showing the area of tumor resection. (H) CT scan, showing the areas of infarction in the left hemisphere.

ml/100 g/min (Fig. 10.5C). She was returned to the operating room, and a new vein was harvested. A cervical ICA-to-M2 segment bypass was performed (Fig. 10.5D and E). Postoperatively she was kept heavily sedated until the hyperemia seen on the postrevascularization Xe CT subsided (Fig. 10.5F). The remaining tumor was resected after 1 month (Fig. 10.5G). She recovered the strength on her right side, as well as her speech, completely, and she returned to work as a cook (Fig. 10.5**H**). The tumor has not recurred in the 3 1/2 years of follow-up.

COMMENTS. In view of her young age, the size of the tumor, and the partial loss of extraocular motility, the authors believed that resecting the ICA, which was surrounded and narrowed by the tumor, would provide the best chance for cure. Although the patient was hemiplegic at the time of graft occlusion, the CBF indicated low flow, but it was not "zero." Successful revision of the graft allowed the patient to recover her right side function and speech completely, although some border zone infarcts are seen on the CT scan. Despite the complication of graft occlusion, prompt intervention perhaps saved her from a poor neurologic outcome.

CONCLUSIONS

The risks and benefits of carotid artery sacrifice should be carefully weighed in every patient individually. The balloon test occlusion with CBF measurement is an important part of the decision process and can guide the surgeon regarding the treatment options most suitable in a particular situation. Although a patient may tolerate temporary occlusion with no CBF disturbance, there is a small risk of stroke on carotid sacrifice. Once the patient suffers a stroke, there is little that can be done. Therefore, if carotid sacrifice is deemed necessary in a patient, some type of revascularization should be considered. Revascularization should be performed with meticulous attention to detail, because it is not without risk. Intraoperative neurophysiologic monitoring and intraoperative arteriography are important adjuncts in such operations.

REFERENCES

1. Ausman J, Pearce J, De Los Reyes R, *et al.:* Treatment of a high extracranial carotid artery aneurysm with CCA-MCA bypass and carotid ligation. **J Neurosurg** 58:421–424, 1983.
2. Batjer H, Frankfurt A, Purdy P, *et al.:* Use of etomidate, temporary arterial occlusion, and intraoperative angiography in surgical treatment of large and giant cerebral aneurysms. **J Neurosurg** 68:234–240, 1988.
3. Bederson J, Schwartz A, Guarino L, *et al.:* Predictive value of laser doppler flowmetry in determining stroke size after middle cerebral artery occlusion. **Stroke** 25:270, 1994.
4. Brackett C: The complication of carotid artery ligation in the neck. **J Neurosurg** 10:91–106, 1953.
5. de Vries EJ, Sekhar LN, Horton JA, *et al.:* A new method to predict safe resection of the internal carotid artery. **Laryngoscope** 100:85–88, 1990.
6. deJong T, Tullekin C, Ramos L: Place of the extra-intracranial-bypass in aneurysm surgery. **Clin Neurol Neurosurg** 91:221–228, 1989.

7. Diaz F, Pearce J, Ausman J: Complications of cerebral revascularization with autogenous vein grafts. **Neurosurgery** 17:271–276, 1985.

8. Dyste G, Beck D: De novo aneurysm formation following carotid ligation: Case report and review of literature. **Neurosurgery** 24:88–92, 1989.

9. Eskridge J: The challenge of carotid occlusion. **AJNR** 12:1053–1054, 1991.

10. Heros R: Thromboembolic complications after combined internal carotid ligation and extra-to-intracranial bypass. **Surg Neurol** 21:75–79, 1984.

11. Horton J, Jungreis C, Pistoia F: *Balloon Test Occlusion*. New York, Raven Press, 1993.

12. Jack C, Sundt TM Jr, Fode N, *et al:* Superficial temporal-middle cerebral artery bypass: Clinical pre-and postoperative angiographic correlation. **J Neurosurg** 69: 46–51, 1988.

13. Jawad K, Miller J, Wyper DJ, *et al.:* Measurement of CBF and carotid artery pressure compared with cerebral angiography in assessing collateral blood supply after carotid ligation. **J Neurosurg** 46:185–196, 1977.

14. Johnson D, Stringer WA, Marks MP, *et al.:* Stable Xenon CT cerebral blood flow imaging: Rationale for and role in clinical decision making. **AJNR** 12:201–213, 1991.

15. Komiyama M, Khosla V, Tamura K, *et al.:* A provocative internal carotid artery balloon occlusion test with 99mTc-HM-PAO CBF mapping—report of three cases. **Neurol Med Chir (Tokyo)** 32:747–752, 1992.

16. Leech P, Miller J, Fitch W, *et al.:* Cerebral blood flow, internal carotid artery pressure, and the EEG as a guide to the safety of carotid ligation. **J Neurol Neurosurg Psychiatry** 37:854–862, 1974.

17. Matas R: Testing the efficiency of the collatral circulation as a preliminary to the occlusion of the great surgical arteries. **Ann Surg** 53:1–43, 1911.

17a. Mathews D, Walker B, and Purdy P: Brain flow SPECT in temporary balloon occlusion of carotid and intracerebral arteries. **J Nucl Med** 34:1239–1243, 1993.

18. Miller J, Jawad K, Jennet B: Safety of carotid ligation and its role in the management of intracranial aneurysms. **J Neurol Neurosurg Psychiatry** 40:64–72, 1977.

19. Monsein LH, Jeffrey PJ, van Heerden BB, *et al.:* Assessing adequacy of collateral circulation during balloon test occlusion of the internal carotid artery with [99mTc]-HMPAO SPECT. **AJNR** 12:104–1051, 1991.

20. Morawetz R, DeGirolami U, Ojemann R, *et al.:* Cerebral blood flow determined by hydrogen clearance during middle cerebral artery occlusion in unanesthetized monkeys. **Stroke** 9:143–149, 1978.

21. Morioka R, Matsushima K, Fuji K, *et al.:* Balloon test occlusion of the internal carotid artery with monitoring of compressed spectral arrays (CSAs) of electroencephalogram. **Acta Neurochir (Wien)** 101:29–34, 1989.

22. Neirinckx R, Canning L, Piper I: Technetium-99m HM PAO stereoisomers as potential agents for imaging regional cerebral blood flow: Human volunteer studies. **J Nucl Med** 28:191–202, 1987.

23. Nishioka H: Report on the cooperative study of intracranial aneurysms and subarachanoid hemorrhage: Section VII, Part I. **J Neurosurg** 25:574–592, 1966.

24. Origitano T, Al-Mefty O, Leonetti J, *et al.:* Vascular considerations and complications in cranial base surgery. **Neurosurgery** 35:351–362, 1994.

25. Peterman S, Taylor AJ, Hoffman JJ: Improved detection of cerebral hypoperfusion with internal carotid balloon test occlusion and [99mTc]-HMPAO cerebral perfusion SPECT imaging. **AJNR** 12:1035–1041, 1991.

26. Sampson D., Neuwelt E, Beyer C, *et al.:* Failure of extracranial-intracranial bypass in acute middle cerebral artery occlusion: Case report. **Neurosurgery** 6:185–188, 1980.

27. Segal D, Sen C, Bederson JB, *et al.:* The predictive value of balloon test occlusion of the internal carotid artery. **Skull Base Surgery**, in press, 1995.
28. Sekhar L, Burgess J, Akin O.: Anatomical study of the cavernous sinus emphasizing operative approaches and related vascular and neural reconstruction. **Neurosurgery** 21:806–816, 1987.
29. Sekhar L, Patel S: Permanent occlusion of the internal carotid artery during skull-base and vascular surgery: Is it really safe? **Am J Otol** 14:421–422, 1993.
30. Sekhar L, Schramm VL Jr, Jones NF, *et al.:* Operative exposure and management of the petrous and upper cervical internal carotid artery. **Neurosurgery** 19:967–982, 1986.
31. Sekhar LN, Sen C, Jho HD: Saphenous vein graft bypass of the cavernous internal carotid artery. **J Neurosurg** 72:35–41, 1990.
32. Sen C, Sekhar LN: Direct vein graft reconstruction of the cavernous, petrous, and upper cervical internal carotid artery: Lessons learned from 30 cases. **Neurosurgery** 30:732–743, 1992.
33. Sengupta D, Murray H, Jennett B: Effect of carotid ligation on cerebral blood flow in baboons 1. Response to hypoxia and hemorrhagic hypertension. **J Neurol Neurosurg Psychiatry** 37:578–584, 1974.
34. Small J, Holmes J, Connolly R: The prognosis and role of surgery in spontaneous intracranial hemorrhage. **Br J Med** 2:1072–1075, 1953.
35. Spetzler R: Revascularization and aneurysm surgery: Current status. **Neurosurgery** 16:111–116, 1985.
36. Spetzler R, Rhodes R, Roski R, *et al.:* Subclavian to middle cerebral artery saphenous vein bypass graft. **J Neurosurg** 53:465–469, 1980.
37. Spetzler R, Selman W, Roski R, *et al.:* Cerebral revascularization during barbiturate coma in primates and humans. **Surg Neurol** 17:111–115, 1982.
38. Steed DL, Webster MW, DeVries EJ, *et al.:* Clinical observations on the effect of carotid artery occlusion on cerebral blood flow mapped by xenon computed tomography and its correlation with carotid artery back pressure. **J Vasc Surg** 11:38–44, 1990.
39. Story J, Brown W, Eidelberg E, *et al.:* Cerebral revascularization: Common carotid to distal middle cerebral artery bypass. **Neurosurgery** 2:131–134, 1978.
40. Sundt TM III, Sundt TM Jr: Principles of preparation of vein bypass grafts to maximize patency. **J Neurosurg** 66:172–180, 1987.
41. Sundt TM Jr, Piepgras DG: Surgical approach to giant intracranial aneurysms. **J Neurosurg** 51:731–742, 1979.
42. Sundt TM, Piepgras DG, Marsh W, *et al.:* Saphenous vein bypass grafts for giant aneurysms and intracranial occlusive disease. **J Neurosurg** 65:439–450, 1986.
43. Tarr RW, Jungreis CA, Horton JA, *et al.:* Complications of preoperative balloon test occlusion of the internal carotid arteries: Experience in 300 cases. **Skull Base Surg** 1:240–244, 1991.
44. Urken M, Biller H, Haimov M: Intratemporal carotid artery bypass in resection of a base of skull tumor. **Laryngoscope** 95:1472–1477, 1985.
45. Yasargil M: *Microsurgery, Applied to Neurosurgery.* Stuttgart, Germany, Georg Thieme, 1969.
46. Yonekawa Y, Yasargil M: *Extra-intracranial Arterial Anastomosis: Clinical and Technical Aspects. Results 1–47–78.* Wien, Springer Verlag, 1976.

11

The Cavernous Carotid Artery: Preservation is the Best Means of Reconstruction

ALFRED P. BOWLES, JR., M.D., AND OSSAMA AL-MEFTY, M.D.

The cavernous sinus has previously been an elusive site for surgical intervention, despite the pioneering of Parkinson almost 20 years ago (29, 30). Interest in the surgical therapy for lesions involving the cavernous sinus has rekindled in the last 10 years, and the enthusiasm for safe surgery is continuing to gain popularity. The main risk in cavernous sinus surgery is injury to the carotid artery, and certainly this fear has contributed to the avoidance of surgery in the cavernous sinus. However, with improved neuroanatomic knowledge, imaging, and surgical techniques, direct surgery in the cavernous sinus has been accomplished without irreparable damage to the carotid artery. Cavernous sinus surgery now focuses on the carotid artery with extensive clinical and radiographic analysis to assess cerebral blood flow and techniques to repair or reconstruct the carotid artery.

The majority of operations that require direct surgery in the cavernous sinus have been for tumors and, to ensure the best potential surgical outcome, a number of strategies have been recommended that involve internal carotid artery (ICA) sacrifice with and without cerebral revascularization. ICA bypass may involve a direct vein graft with reconstruction from the petrous ICA to supraclinoid or intracavernous ICA, bypass from the superficial temporal artery (STA) to the middle cerebral artery (MCA), or grafts from the common carotid artery or external carotid artery to branches of the MCA. Manipulation of the carotid artery, however, is not without potential for complications. Carotid excision without revascularization may result in immediate stroke or long-term risks involving contralateral aneurysm formation and reduced cerebrovascular reserve. Disadvantages of direct vein graft reconstruction include 2-hour ICA flow interruption, potential graft thrombosis (which may lead to stroke), and consistently high complication rates from long grafts (extracranial-to-intracranial (EC-IC)) attended by late occlusions and by patency rates ranging from 50 to 60% (3, 16, 35).

In this chapter, we will review the advantages and disadvantages of carotid resection with cerebral revascularization for tumors of the cavernous sinus. Oncologic effects achieved with carotid resection will be addressed, and the benefits from preserving the carotid artery will be summarized.

TUMORS INVOLVING THE CAVERNOUS SINUS

Tumors that involve the cavernous sinus may originate within or outside the walls of the cavernous sinus and extend secondarily into the cavernous sinus. Tumors may be benign (meningiomas, neurilemomas), malignant yet locally confined (chordomas, chondrosarcomas, esthesioneuroblastomas), nasopharyngeal carcinomas, or metastatic. As reported by Dolenc, over 90% of all tumors involving the cavernous sinus are meningiomas (12).

Indications for operating on cavernous sinus include progression of tumor growth, defined radiographically and symptomatically, and generally with progression of cranial nerve deficits. The authors encourage operating with earlier onset of symptoms, because pre-existing cranial nerve deficits rarely improve (8). The possibility of total resection or subtotal resection should be strongly considered also, and this consideration as well is based in part on the presumed pathology of the tumor.

Meningiomas

Meningiomas are by far the most common tumor involved in the cavernous sinus and, technically, are the most difficult to remove. The difficulties are related to the potential for encasement of the carotid artery and cranial nerves and involvement of adjacent areas, including dura, bone, and sinuses (Fig. 11.1). The biology of meningiomas is not currently understood, and the rate of tumor growth is not predictable. Tumors may remain quiescent, grow slowly and steadily, or grow very rapidly. As shown in Figure 11.2, the residual cavernous sinus meningioma has remained unchanged for more than 6 years. By contrast, Figure 11.3 shows that rapid and extensive regrowth occurred within 6 months.

Other Benign Tumors

The other benign tumors that involve the cavernous sinus include neurilemomas, cavernous hemangiomas, juvenile angiofibromas, craniopharyngiomas, and pituitary adenomas. In contrast to the meningiomas, these tumors are easier to remove with the definable dissection planes around the carotid artery and cranial nerves, and complete excision should always be attempted.

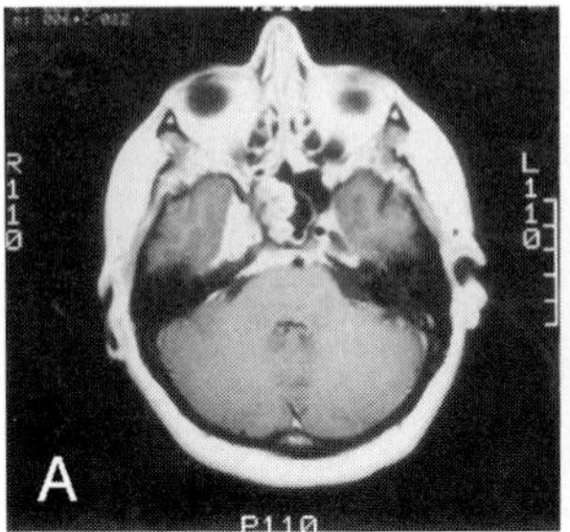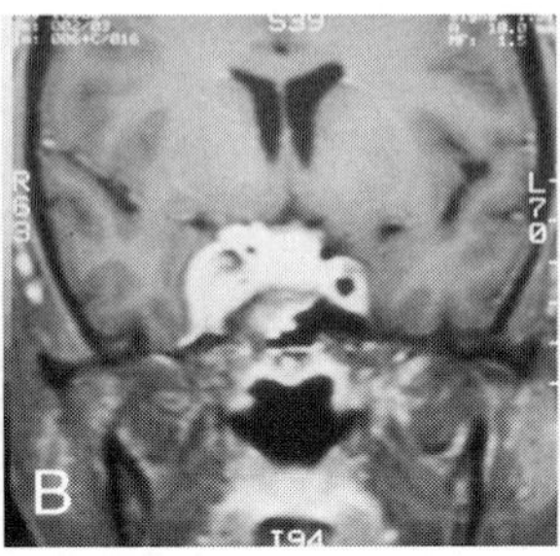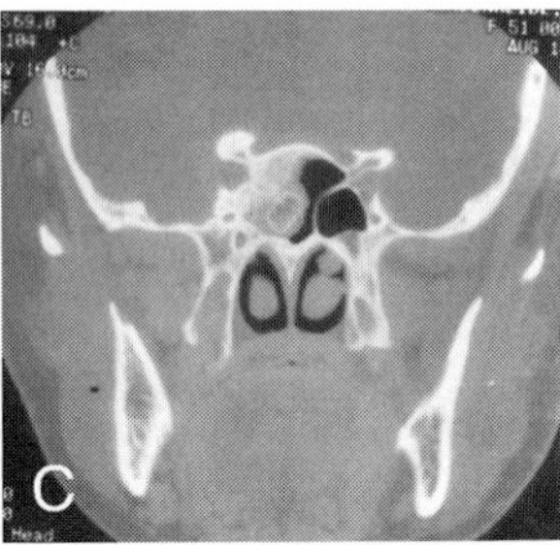

FIG. 11.1 Magnetic resonance imaging (MRI) and CT imaging of patient with a large clinoid meningioma with extension into the cavernous sinus and sphenoid sinus. Gadolinium-enhanced T_1-weighted axial MRI (**A**) shows the extensive expansion of the cavernous sinus on the right by tumor, with narrowing of the lumen of the carotid artery. The tumor is also shown to extend into the sphenoid sinus. Enhanced T_1-weighted coronal image (**B**) demonstrates the tumor elevating and completely surrounding the carotid artery. Coronal CT (**C**) also shows the extension of the tumor from the clinoid process into the sphenoid sinus.

Chordomas and Chondrosarcomas

Chordomas and chondrosarcomas can be slow growing and are locally invasive, with an aversive tumor biology. However, when chordomas and chondrosarcomas involve the cavernous sinus, the dissection planes can be readily developed, and aggressive removal can be achieved.

Carcinomas

Indications for operative removal of carcinomas involving the cavernous sinus are controversial. Surgical intervention should always impact on the tumor biology if resection is desired. Lower-grade malignancies, such as the adenoid cystic carcinoma, may be surgically approached and easily removed without sacrifice or neurovascular structures. On the other hand, in cases involving a high-grade carcinoma (*e.g.*, squamous cell carcinoma), the overall poor outcome from the spread of disease raises doubt about the merit of the local control potentially offered by cavernous sinus surgery.

REVASCULARIZATION

Tumors that more frequently involve the cavernous sinus are meningiomas; in a certain number of cases, including both meningiomas and some malignant tumors, involvement in the cavernous sinus is so extensive that the carotid artery and cranial nerves are surrounded and encased by tumor (Figs. 11.1 and 11.4). The tumor may be so severely adherent to the carotid artery (21) that safe and successful tumor re-

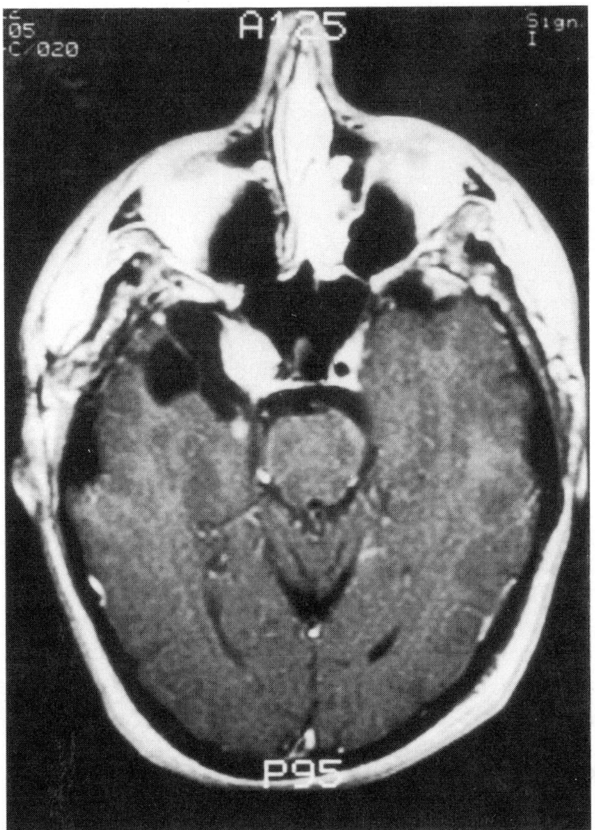

FIG. 11.2 Enhanced axial MRI of a patient with a residual meningioma of the cavernous sinus. The more accessible tumor from the sphenoid wing was removed 6 years earlier; however, there has been no evidence of regrowth.

moval becomes problematic. A suggested solution is for the surgeon to sacrifice the carotid artery, with reconstruction or revascularization to restore cerebrovascular reserve. Excision of the vessel would remove tumor from the carotid artery and also provide greater access to the sella, sphenoid sinus, and petrous apex, theoretically permitting safe and more aggressive tumor removal. This rationale is the main base of support for carotid resection.

Elective ligation of the internal carotid artery was first described by Moore and Baker and, in the 88 patients analyzed, neurologic morbidity was 45% and mortality was 31% (26). Since then, reports continue to show stroke rates at least as high as 20% with carotid ligation (3, 18, 20).

Following permanent occlusion of the ICA, stroke may occur because of decreased flow to the brain or embolic occlusion. The normal cerebral blood flow to the brain is 55 ml/100 g/min. However, patients may not become symptomatic until the cerebral blood flow drops below 20 ml/100 g/min. A permanent stroke will occur when the cerebral blood flow is diminished to 10 to 15 ml/100 g/min for a prolonged period of time (9). To assess the need for revascularization with ligation, the balloon test occlusion (BTO) with internal carotid artery occluded xenon CT cerebral blood flow (Xe CT CBF), developed from the Matas test, is currently being used by several groups (14, 18, 23, 28). With the BTO Xe CBF, patients are segregated into four risk groups. Patients in group IV (failure of clinical BTO) develop neurologic deficits within 15 minutes of occlusion of the ICA by the inflated balloon catheter. Patients in group IV are at high risk and definitely are not able to tolerate carotid artery occlusion, either permanently or temporarily. Extracranial-intracranial (EC-IC) procedures have been considered in treating this group when the need for temporary or permanent occlusion is anticipated (23, 33, 35). Nonoperative measures also have been considered for this high-risk group (23, 35). Patients who tolerate or pass the clinical BTO for 15 minutes but have the ICA occlusion Xe CT

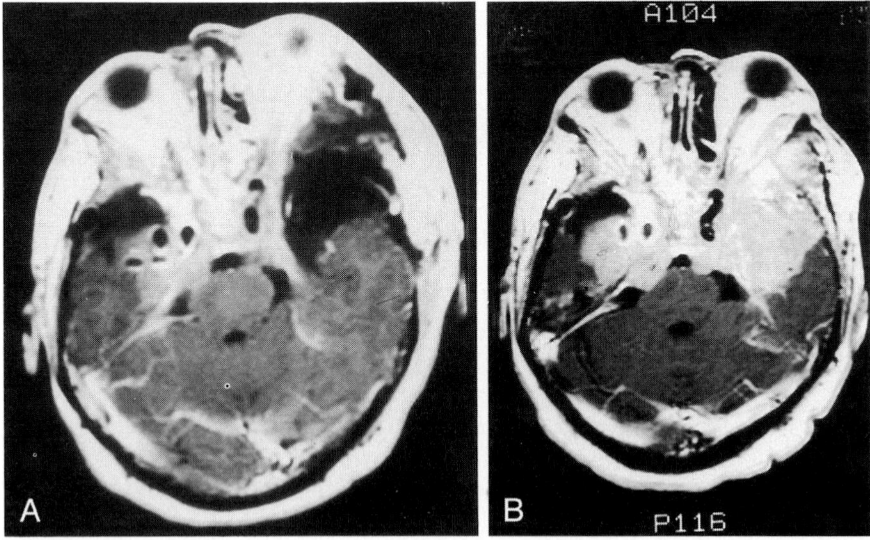

FIG. 11.3 By contrast, MRIs are compared in a patient who had a rapidly growing meningioma. The MRI obtained in the immediate postoperative period after subtotal resection is shown (**A**). However, within a period of 6 months, extensive regrowth occurred, involving both cavernous sinuses and cerebral hemispheres (**B**).

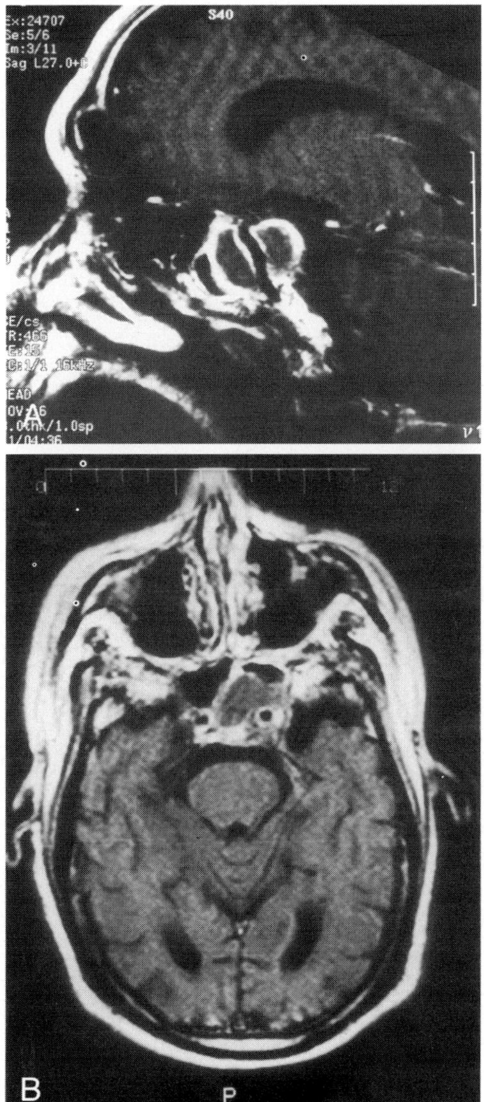

Fig. 11.4 Gadolinium-enhanced magnetic resonance imaging (MRI) of a patient with a large juxtaseller meningioma, in which the tumor completely surrounds the carotid artery in the cavernous sinus. (**A**) sagittal view. (**B**) axial view.

CBF values ≤30 ml/100 g/min (group III) are at low risk for stroke with temporary occlusion but at greater risk for stroke with permanent occlusion (3, 23, 32, 35). Temporary occlusion in this group should be supported with hypertension and preocclusion barbiturates or etomidate. Revascularization procedures have also been advocated when permanent ICA sacrifice is required (3, 23, 32, 35). In group I or II, there is either no hemispheric difference with CBF or a mild decrease with CBF values >30 ml/100 g/min. These patients are at low-risk and should tolerate carotid ligation, without revascularization. Exceptions to this rule are for very young patients, because ICA sacrifice may lead to *de novo* aneurysm formation or delayed ischemia defects over the course of their lifetime. For these reasons, some surgeons have advocated reconstructing the carotid artery in the younger patients when carotid resection is anticipated. Revascularization also has been strongly considered in treating cases of current or eventual bilateral tumor involvement of the cavernous sinus (3, 23, 28).

A number of revascularization procedures have been recently utilized and developed when the carotid artery has been either damaged or resected with tumor. Superficial temporal artery STA-MCA branch anastomosis and several long and short venous shunt venous grafts have been used. Venous grafts include STA-MCA venous grafts, external carotid artery (ECA) or common carotid artery (CCA)-to-MCA venous grafts, extracranial ICA-to-intracranial ICA long grafts, and direct vein grafts from the petrous ICA to the supraclinoid or intracavernous ICA (4, 7, 11, 15, 19, 37–40).

The most frequently performed bypass is the STA-MCA, which is the safest and, technically, the easiest procedure to perform, with patency rates approaching 90% (19, 28, 35). There is generally only temporary occlusion of the MCA without ICA flow interruption. Although blood flow improves immediately after anastomosis, the flow volume is low and does not match the previous flow volume from the occluded carotid artery or the MCA. Theoretically, such low flow volumes would still be able to protect some of the cells from permanent ischemic dysfunction and may allow enough time for sufficient collateral development. Nevertheless, a number of ischemic failures have been reported, despite patent anastomosis (10, 16).

Although long venous grafts from the extracranial-to-intracranial ICA or MCA provide immediate high flow volume; patency rates are low (50 to 60%) with late occlusion. The risk of hyperperfusion breakthrough with intracerebral hematoma has been reported (40), and this graft may also be in the way when one is working in the posterior cavernous sinus. The effectiveness of EC-IC bypasses has been analyzed and summarized in various reports (10, 13, 16, 37, 40, 41). EC-IC bypass surgery has been shown by the EC-IC Bypass Study Group to be ineffective in preventing stroke (13) while other reports have shown overall ischemic complications to be as high as 25% (10, 16).

In series of 50 or more patients, reconstruction of the carotid artery with a short interposed vein graft from the petrous carotid artery to the supraclinoid artery has been performed in patients since 1986 (23, 28, 32–35, 37, 38). One advantage is anastomosis from a large vessel to another large vessel with an immediate high volume of flow. Reported overall patency rates have been from 80 to 90% (28, 35). The major disadvantage is the minimum requirement of a 90- to 120-minute period of carotid occlusion. This period of temporary occlusion may not be tolerated by patients with compromised collateral flow, even with pharmacologic and homeostatic manipulation to provide additional cerebral protection during temporary occlusion. When patients are able to tolerate temporary occlusion, then the need for the short-vein graft becomes controversial. The use of intraluminal shunts to maintain cerebral blood flow while the ICA is temporarily occluded has been suggested from cadaver studies (3). However, the procedure has been described as technically difficult and clinically limited (17). Graft occlusion generally occurs reasonably early, yet the potential for late occlusion exists. The length of follow-up is currently inadequate to assess late occlusion. Bypass grafts that re-establish high flows may also create a hemorrhagic infarct; as with all grafts, thrombosis with distal emboli is a potential threat. Direct vein graft reconstruction of the carotid artery in the cavernous sinus has been performed and reported on by several investigators with follow-up as long as 18 months. Although the technical aspects of the procedure had been improved, a number of ischemic complications have occurred. In a series of patients treated by Sekhar *et al.*, four of five patients with insufficient collateral circulation developed postoperative ischemic deficits but recovered on follow-up (32). Another patient with temporary neurologic deficits developed an infarction demonstrated by computerized tomography (CT). In another series, of 23 patients who underwent direct-vein graft carotid reconstruction, 3 patients developed graft occlusion (34). All three remained neurologically normal, which raises a question of the need for the graft in the first place. In one patient, who eventually died, dissection of the distal ICA occurred secondary to improper suturing technique. In two other patients with compromised collateral circulation, strokes developed, presumably from temporary occlusion of the ICA. Failure of the direct vein bypass graft from occlusions, either with or without stroke, occurred in 26% of cases, with an immediate mortality rate of 4%. In another report, 30 patients underwent reconstruction, and 7 of them suffered graft occlusion, with one death secondary to a massive hemispheric infarction (35).

ONCOLOGIC EFFECTS OF CAROTID RESECTION

The premise that complete tumor removal can be achieved in the cavernous sinus with carotid resection holds true for some investigators, and the supposed provision of an opportunity for complete tumor removal outweighs the risk of carotid resection with revascularization. However, whether complete tumor removal in the cavernous sinus can be achieved is the question at hand. Carotid resection may be irrelevant when complete tumor removal is not possible.

The majority of tumors that involve the cavernous sinus are meningiomas, and in some cases tumors may circumferentially surround and encase the carotid artery. It has been pointed out by Al-Mefty that many benign tumors provide a plane of dissection from the carotid adventitia despite encasement and adherence (2; Al-Mefty, personal communication 1993). Only in a minority of cases does the tumor adhere severely to the vessel wall and is not separated by an intact arachnoid membrane (anterior clinoidal meningioma, grade I) (1).

Although the tumor biology of meningiomas is not known, the extent of tumor resection correlates favorably with decreased risk of recurrence and increased longevity (8, 22, 24, 25, 36). Theoretically, in meningiomas complete tumor removal will provide patient cure. When tumor involvement in the cavernous sinus is extensive and involves the carotid artery, tumor is deposited throughout and generally involves dura, bone, and sinuses (Figs. 11.1, 11.5 and 11.6). Even with carotid resection, tumor deposits remain on the cranial nerves, occasionally with interdigitation (Fig. 11.5). Tumor can be found infiltrating the walls of the cavernous sinus and may unpredictably involve the skull bone (Fig. 11.6). Only with en bloc resection of the cavernous sinus can complete tumor removal and oncologic cure be achieved (8, 31). Carotid resection alone or with cranial nerve resection will not suffice. However, en bloc resection of the cavernous sinus will produce unacceptable rates of morbidity and mortality.

In the cavernous sinus, following the plane of dissection from the carotid adventitia with extensive dissection of dural sheaths, aggressive tumor removal can be achieved in the cavernous sinus without carotid resection (Figs. 11.7–11.9). In a report given by DeMonte and colleagues, 41 patients with benign meningiomas underwent aggressive surgery and were followed-up for more than 5 years (8). The 5-year recurrence rate was 6%. This rate compares favorably with recurrence

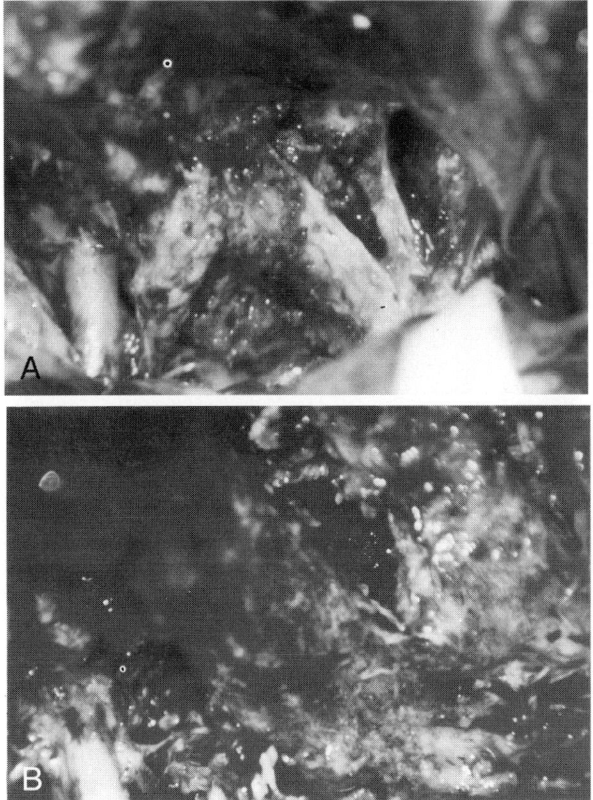

FIG. 11.5 Operative photographs depicting the surgeon's view through the microscope during the removal of a meningioma in two patients. Despite extensive piecemeal removal of tumor, tumor deposits remain adherent to the lateral and medial walls of the cavernous sinus, the third cranial nerve with interdigitation along V_1, V_2, and V_3 (**A**). In another patient, tumor remains encased around the trigeminal nerve (**B**).

rates of 20 to 50% for medial sphenoid wing meningiomas reported in the literature (6, 24, 25, 36) and also with the recurrence/progression probability of 3% at 5 years for totally resected convexity meningiomas (25). In the report by DeMonte *et al.*, complete tumor removal was achieved in 76% of patients, as judged by the surgeon and follow-up images. The morbidity from ischemic complications was 7%. By comparison, carotid resection with direct-vein reconstruction permitted a gross total removal in 13 of 17 patients (76%); however, meningioma recurrence was 18%, with a mean follow-up of 18 months (34). From the total of 30 patients, including nonmeningioma patients, the ischemic complications rate was 13%. One patient died from massive tumor recurrence after apparent gross total resection had been achieved with carotid resection and bypass, and another patient suffered an ICA dissection with graft occlusion and subsequently died from massive cerebral infarction. (35).

Aggressive tumor resection in the cavernous sinus can be achieved with carotid resection and revascularization, as defined in reports by Sen et al. and Sekhar *et al.* (34, 35). However, extensive tumor resection also can be achieved at least equally without carotid resection, as shown in a report by DeMonte and colleagues (8). The percentages of patients in whom gross total resection was achieved were comparable between the two groups (carotid resection *versus* carotid preservation) and from the report in which the carotid artery was preserved, recurrence rates were lower with longer follow-up. Whether the difference in recurrence rates is statistically significant cannot be defined; although both methods were effective, it would appear that carotid resection with reconstruction did not provide greater oncologic benefit. Likewise, the rate of ischemic complications from carotid reconstruction is significant.

In patients with malignant tumors that are locally invasive (chordomas, chondrosarcomas), a dissection plane between adventitia and tumor can be readily developed, and aggressive resection can be achieved. Carotid resection with revascularization would not improve tumor removal; because of the tumor biology, adjuvant radiotherapy is required. Although not commonly found extending into the cavernous si-

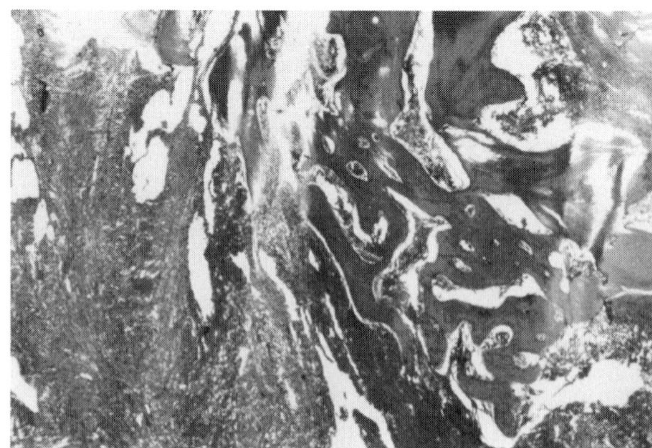

FIG. 11.6 Photomicrograph of a meningioma specimen with invasion of tumor into bone. H & E stain.

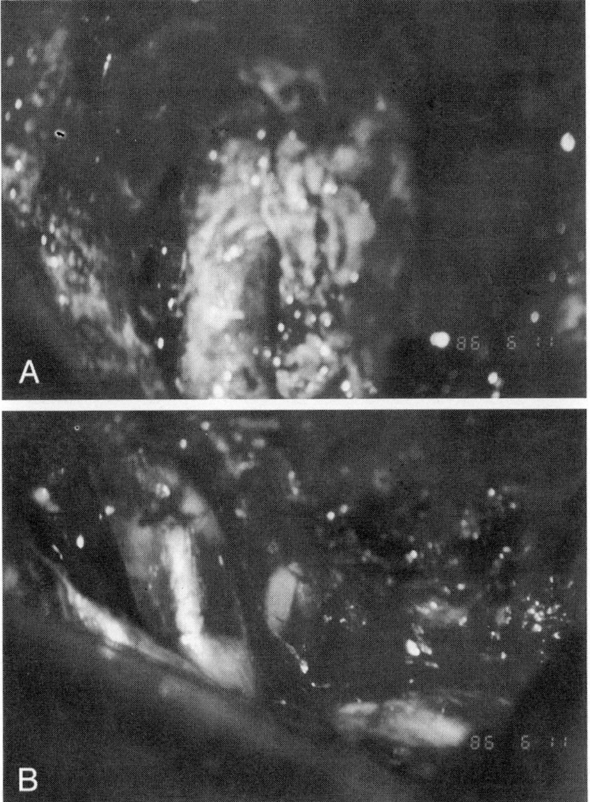

FIG. 11.7 Operative photograph depicting the surgeon's view during the resection of a meningioma. The tumor is shown as encasing the optic nerve and carotid artery (**A**). A plane of dissection between the carotid adventitia and optic nerve was developed, and artery and nerve was dissected free of tumor (**B**).

nus, adenoid cystic carcinoma can be easily removed without sacrifice of neurovascular structures. Patients with more aggressive carcinomas (anaplastic carcinomas, squamous cell carcinomas), ultimately die within 1 to 2 years. Tumors are widespread, without defined margins and with a potential for metastasis. Heroic local control may not change the systemic manifestations of the disease.

PRESERVATION OF THE CAROTID ARTERY

Regarding tumor surgery in the cavernous sinus with tumors inextricably involved with the ICA, some groups of researchers have assumed that when resection of a carotid artery can be achieved safely,

CLINICAL NEUROSURGERY

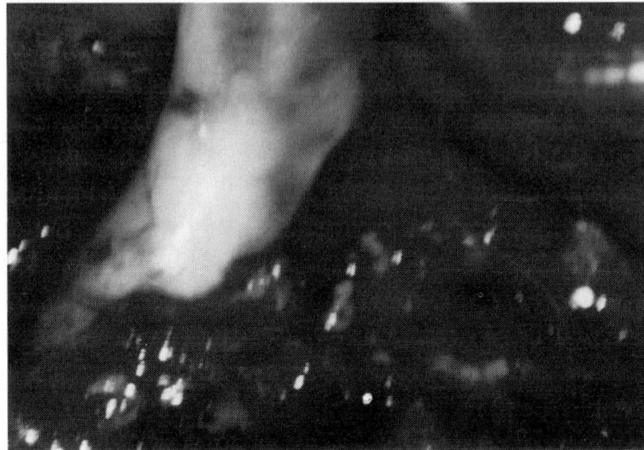

FIG. 11.8 Operative photograph of the view during the removal of an invading skull base meningioma. A dissection place between the carotid adventitia and tumor was developed, and the tumor, which circumferentially surrounded the carotid artery, was dissected free.

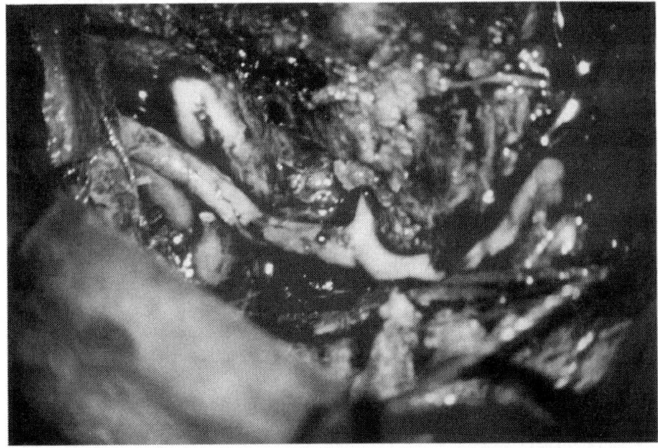

FIG. 11.9 Operative photograph of the surgeon's view during a resection of a meningioma. The totally engulfed right optic nerve and A-1 and M-1 segments have been dissected free. Tumor still engulfs a portion of the internal carotid artery; however, a plane of dissection between the carotid adventitia and tumor has been developed. (Reproduced with permission from Al-Mefty O (ed): *Surgery of the Cranial Base.* Boston, Kluwer Academic Publishers, 1989.)

more aggressive tumor removal will result, with possible cure. However, the significance of carotid artery involvement in patients with cranial base tumors has not been clearly defined for all conditions, and tumors that appear adherent to the carotid artery may be safely dissected from the carotid adventitia and completely removed. With the consideration of carotid resection and revascularization for cavernous sinus surgery, there are three issues of importance: (*a*) risks associated with carotid ligation; (*b*) risks associated with revascularization; and (*c*) ultimate feasibility of treating the tumor in question.

The overall ischemic risks associated with carotid ligation, with or without vascular assessment, exceed 20% (3, 18, 20, 26). However, at present, there are several weaknesses involved with all preoperative vascular assessments. As reviewed by Origitano and colleagues, BTO Xe CBF assesses only single temporal effects, fails to predict cerebral vascular reactivity, and only defines those patients who absolutely cannot tolerate occlusion (28). Therefore, we cannot rely on preoperative vascular assessments for adequate prediction of the need for revascularization. Without an adequate assessment of vascular need, appropriate utilization of revascularization procedures is limited.

To assume that one can resect the carotid artery and then reroute blood to the brain or can reconstruct the carotid artery and then expect the modified anatomic construct to function as well as its predecessor is overly optimistic. When the carotid artery is resectioned, no matter what revascularization technique is used, the surgically modified result will never function the same as its predecessor, despite adequate flows and patency. With carotid reconstruction, several graft occlusions have been reported, and ischemic complications from diminished flow and distal emboli are significant. Even for patients who underwent successful carotid reconstruction, follow-up has not been long enough to determine ultimate outcome.

Theoretically, surgical cure for meningiomas involving the cavernous sins cannot be achieved without complete tumor removal, including microscopic tumor deposits. Tumor deposits may involve dura and sinus walls and/or the carotid artery. The tumor may unpredictably involve bone with interdigitation of cranial nerves. Carotid resection does not improve oncologic removal, because tumor will always be left behind. Certainly, the amount of tumor that can be removed from the cavernous sinus with or without carotid resection is comparable (8, 35).

"A carotid artery is a terrible thing to lose" (28). One should not take the carotid artery for granted and should remember the importance of its presence. The authors certainly emphasize carotid preservation and do not recommend or perform carotid artery resection with tumor. When the dissection plane between the carotid adventitia and tumor cannot be established, a thin layer of tumor is left on the carotid to prevent injury. When the carotid artery is damaged, the authors recommend temporary occlusion with hypothermia, hypertension with barbiturates, or etomidate with direct repair by suture, clip graft, or both. When this is not possible, immediate EC-IC bypass or direct vein graft is carried out. Prophylactic anastomosis is also considered for high-risk patients. In patients with very poor collateral blood flow (i.e., failure of clinical BTO), who are at significant risk for carotid injury with surgery, a prophylactic EC-IC bypass is strongly considered. Preferably, a STA-MCA bypass is placed and allowed to mature adequately by creating the anastomosis several weeks before surgery in the cavernous sinus is performed.

The authors' experience, combined with a review of the literature on the impact of carotid artery sacrifice on tumor biology, leads them to take the position of strict carotid artery preservation. One should attempt to preserve the carotid artery at all times.

As understanding of tumor biology for both benign and malignant tumors grows, eventual cures will result. Defined cures will come from pharmacologic, biologic, and immunologic manipulation and not from more extensive and excessive surgery.

ACKNOWLEDGMENT

The authors thank Niki Lorenz for secretarial assistance and Lucia Griffin for editorial assistance in preparing this manuscript.

REFERENCES

1. Al-Mefty O: Clinoidal meningiomas. **J Neurosurg** 73:840–849, 1990.
2. Al-Mefty O: Direct vein graft reconstruction of the cavernous, petrous, and upper cervical internal carotid artery: Lessons learned from 30 cases (Editorial comment on article by Sen et al., **Neurosurgery** 1992; 30:732–743). **Neurosurgery** 30:742–743, 1992.
3. Al-Mefty O, Khalil N, Elwany MN, *et al.,* Shunt bypass graft of the cavernous carotid artery: An anatomical and technical study. **Neurosurgery** 27:721–728, 1990.
4. Ausman JI, Pearce JE, de los Reyes RA, *et al.:* Treatment of high extracranial carotid artery aneurysm with CCA-MCA bypass and carotid ligation: Case report. **J Neurosurg** 58:421–424, 1983.
5. Bonnal J, Thibaut A, Brotchi J, *et al.:* Invading meningiomas of the sphenoid ridge. **J Neurosurg** 53:587–599, 1980.
6. Chan RC, Thompson GB: Morbidity, mortality, and quality of life following surgery for intracranial meningiomas. A retrospective study in 257 cases. **J Neurosurg** 60:52–60, 1984.
7. Collice M, Arena O, Fontana RA: Superficial temporal artery to proximal middle cerebral artery anastomosis: Clinical and angiographic long-term results. **Neurosurgery** 19:992–997, 1986.
8. DeMonte F, Smith HK, Al-Mefty O: Outcome of aggressive removal of cavernous sinus meningiomas. **J Neurosurg** 81:245–251, 1994.

9. deVries E, Sekhar LN, Horton JA, *et al.:* A new method to predict safe resection of the carotid artery. **Laryngoscope** 100:85–88, 1990.

10. Diaz FG, Ausman JF, Pearce J: Ischemic complications after combined internal carotid artery occlusion and extracranial-intracranial anastomosis. **Neurosurgery** 1982; 10:563–570.

11. Diaz FG, Pearce J, Ausman JI: Complications of cerebral revascularization and autogenous vein grafts. **Neurosurgery** 17:271–276, 1985.

12. Dolenc VV: *Anatomy and Surgery of the Cavernous Sinus.* Vienna, Springer-Verlag, 1989.

13. The EC/IC Bypass Study Group: Failure of extracranial/intracranial arterial bypass to reduce the risk of ischemic stroke. Results of an international randomized trial. **N Engl J Med** 313:1191–1200, 1985.

14. Erba SM, Horton JA, Latchaw RE, *et al.:* Balloon test occlusion of the internal carotid artery with Xenon/CT cerebral blood flow mapping. **AJNR** 1988; 9:533–538.

15. Fitzpatrick BC, Spetzler RF, Biller JL, *et al.:* Cervical to petrous internal carotid artery bypass procedure. Technical note. **J Neurosurg** 1993; 79:138–141.

16. Hashik N: Incidence of ischemic complications after carotid ligation with EC-IC bypass: A multicenter study, in Spetzler RF, *et al* (eds): *Cerebral Revascularization for Stroke.* New York, Thieme-Stratton, 1985, pp 570–577.

17. Hori T, Ikawa E, Takenobu A, *et al.:* The use of an intraluminal shunt for bypass grafts of the cavernous internal carotid artery. **J Neurosurg** 75:661–663, 1991.

18. Horton JA, Jungreis EA, Pistoia F: Balloon test occlusion, in Sekhar LN, Janecka IP (eds): *Surgery of Cranial Base Tumors.* New York, Raven Press, 1993, pp 33–36.

19. Jack CR, Sundt TM Jr, Fode NC, *et al.:* Superficial temporal-middle cerebral artery bypass: Clinical pre and postoperative angiographic correlation. **J Neurosurg** 1988; 69:46–51.

20. Jeffreys RV, Holmes AE: Common carotid ligation for treatment of ruptured posterior communicating aneurysms. J Neurol Neurosurg Psychiatry 1971; 34:576–579.

21. Kotapek MJ, Kalia KK, Martinez AJ, *et al.:* Infiltration of the carotid artery by cavernous sinus meningioma. **J Neurosurg** 81:252–255, 1994.

22. Lesoin F, Jomin M: Direct microsurgical approach to intracavernous tumors. **Surg Neurol** 28:17–22, 1987.

23. Linskey ME, Sekhar LN, Sen C: Cerebral revascularization and cranial base surgery, in Sekhar LN, Janecki IP (eds): *Surgery of Cranial Base Tumors.* New York, Raven Press, 1993, pp 45–68.

24. Marks SM, Whitwell HL, Lye RH: Recurrence of meningiomas after operation. **Surg Neurol** 1986; 25:436–440.

25. Mirimanoff RO, Dosoretz DE, Linggood RM, *et al.:* Meningioma: Analysis of recurrence and progression following neurosurgical resection. **J Neurosurg** 1985; 62:18–24.

26. Moore O, Baker HW: Carotid artery ligation and surgery of head and neck. **Cancer** 8:712–725, 1955.

27. Nornes H, Wikeby P: Cerebral arterial blood flow and aneurysm surgery: Part I. Local arterial flow dynamics. **J Neurosurg** 47:810–818, 1977.

28. Origitano TC, Al-Mefty O, Leonetti JP, *et al.:* Vascular considerations and complications in cranial base surgery. **Neurosurgery** 35:351–362, 1994.

29. Parkinson D: A surgical approach to the cavernous portion of the carotid artery. Anatomical studies and case report. **J Neurosurg** 1965;23:474–483.

30. Parkinson D: Carotid cavernous fistula: Direct repair with preservation of carotid artery. Technical note. **J Neurosurg** 1973; 68:99–106.
31. Sekhar LN, Burgess J, Akin O: Anatomical study of the cavernous sinus emphasizing operative approaches and related vascular and neural reconstruction. **Neurosurgery** 1987; 21:806–816.
32. Sekhar LN, Sen CN, Jho HD: Saphenous vein graft bypass of the cavernous internal carotid artery. **J Neurosurg** 72:35–41, 1990.
33. Sekhar LN, Sen CH, Jho HD, *et al.:* Surgical treatment of intracavernous neoplasms: A four-year experience. **Neurosurgery** 24:18–30, 1989.
34. Sekhar LN, Sen CN, Lanzino G, *et al.:* Carotid and cranial nerve reconstruction after removal of cavernous sinus lesions. **Keio J Med** 40:187–193; 1991.
35. Sen C, Sekhar LN: Direct vein graft reconstruction of the cavernous, petrous and upper cervical internal carotid artery: Lessons learned from 30 cases. **Neurosurgery** 30:732–743; 1992.
36. Simpson D: The recurrence of intracranial meningiomas after surgery and treatment. **J Neurol Neurosurg Psychiatry** 20:22–39; 1957.
37. Spetzler RF, Carter LP: Revascularization and aneurysm surgery: Current status. **Neurosurgery** 16:111–115, 1985.
38. Spetzler RF, Fukushima T, Martin N, *et al.:* Petrous carotid-to-intradural carotid saphenous vein graft for intracavernous giant aneurysm, tumor, and occlusive cerebral vascular disease. **J Neurosurg** 73:496–501, 1990.
39. Sundt TM, Piepgras DG, Houser OW, *et al.:* Interposition saphenous vein grafts for advanced occlusive disease and large aneurysms in the posterior circulation. **J Neurosurg** 56:205–215, 1982.
40. Sundt TM Jr, Piepgras DG, Marsh WR, *et al.:* Saphenous vein bypass grafts for giant aneurysms and intracranial occlusive disease. **J Neurosurg** 65:439–450; 1986.
41. Whisnant JP, Sundt TM Jr, Fode NC: Long-term mortality and stroke mortality and stroke morbidity after superficial temporal artery-middle cerebral artery bypass operation. **Mayo Clin Proc** 60:241–246; 1985.

12

Intra-operative Neurophysiologic Monitoring in Neurosurgery: Benefits, Efficacy, and Cost-Effectiveness

AAGE R. MØLLER, Ph.D.

In economic terms, the benefits of intra-operative monitoring have usually been estimated on the basis of the savings in cost for caring for individuals with permanent neurologic deficits compared with the cost of implementing intra-operative monitoring. While the latter can be estimated with considerable accuracy, the former is more difficult to estimate. Usually, the value of reducing human suffering has not been included at all in estimates of the cost:benefit ratio of intra-operative monitoring, because it has not been possible to estimate the cost of human suffering in economic terms.

INTRODUCTION

During the past decade or so it has become evident that monitoring the function of specific parts of the nervous system intra-operatively by using neurophysiologic methods can be a useful adjunct to operations in which neural tissue may be at risk of being injured. Experience gained during the past decade has revealed that the proper use of such neurophysiologic intra-operative recordings can detect surgically induced injuries to neural tissue before these injuries lead to permanent postoperative neurologic deficits. Such intra-operative monitoring permits specific surgical manipulations that cause a change in the recorded potentials to be reversed before the injury progresses to a level which would result in a permanent neurologic deficit.

The introduction of intra-operative neurophysiologic monitoring has also brought other advantages to the modern neurosurgical operating room, *e.g.,* the possibility of identifying neural tissue that is not directly visible in the operative field, and in some cases it has been possible to use neurophysiologic techniques to guide the surgeon in the operation or ensure that the therapeutic goal of the operation has been achieved before the operation is terminated.

Intra-operative neurophysiologic monitoring mainly makes use of state-of-the-art neurophysiologic methods to monitor a variety of different systems that have been described extensively (1–4, 6–8) and will not be repeated here. Intra-operative neurophysiologic monitoring requires that those people who are responsible for such monitoring have sufficient background in neurophysiology and specific training.

BASIS OF INTRA-OPERATIVE NEUROPHYSIOLOGIC MONITORING

The basis of intra-operative neurophysiological monitoring in reducing the risk of postoperative neurologic deficits is the assumption that: (*a*) some recorded neuroelectric potentials will change as a result of neural injury and that these changes can be detected before the injury has reached a level which would result in permanent neurologic deficits and (*b*) that such injuries can be reversed by proper surgical intervention.

The most useful sign that a surgical manipulation has caused a change in neural function is a decrease in neural conduction velocity in a peripheral nerve or a fiber tract in the brain, which usually can be detected as an increase in the latency of the recorded neuroelectric potentials, such as the compound action potentials (CAP) from a nerve, or of the sensory evoked potentials. A change in the amplitude of such potentials is also a sign of impaired neural function. The occurrence of muscle activity as a result of surgical manipulation of the respective motor nerve may also be a sign of neural injury. By observing the manner in which the recorded neuroelectric potentials vary as a result of surgical manipulations, it is possible to detect when surgical manipulations have caused a change in the function of specific neural tissue; and by informing the surgeon about such changes promptly, it is often possible to identify which manipulation caused the change, making it possible to reverse the change before a permanent neurologic deficit results. The use of such changes in recorded neuroelectric potentials for the purpose of reducing the risk of permanent neurologic deficits is based on the general knowledge that neural conduction and synaptic transmission cease before permanent injury to a nerve cell occurs. There is thus a margin between a measurable change in nerve cell function and a cell injury that leads to a permanent neurologic deficit.

While methods for detecting such changes in neurologic function are relatively well described, much less attention has been devoted to defining how to reverse the cause of such changes so that an injury does not progress to a level that will result in a permanent neurologic deficit. It has, however, been established that it is important that the surgeon be informed as soon as possible after a change in neural function has occurred. For this reason neurophysiologic methods that are in practical use at present for intra-operative monitoring are usually designed to facilitate obtaining an interpretable wave form in as short a time as possible.

The question of how large a change in evoked potentials or how much muscle activity can be tolerated is the subject of constant debate. Some investigators (4) have taken the position that any change in the evoked potentials that is larger than the small changes that normally occur should be reported to the surgeon so that he or she has the opportunity to reverse the surgical manipulation that caused the change as quickly as possible or to wait and see if the change progresses. Then, if it does progress the surgeon knows which manipulation caused the change and can appropriately reverse the manipulation. If the surgeon is not informed immediately when changes occur, he or she may not know what caused the problem when the change reaches a level at which reversal is required.

HOW CAN INTRA-OPERATIVE MONITORING BENEFIT THE PATIENT?

The most obvious way in which intra-operative neurophysiologic monitoring can benefit the patient is by reducing the risk of postoperative neurologic deficits that may result from surgical manipulations.

In some operations it is possible to use recorded neuroelectric potentials to improve the outcome of an operation. For instance, it may be possible to do a total resection of a tumor because such monitoring makes it possible to protect the function of the nerves that are embedded in the tumor. When monitoring facial function during operations to remove acoustic tumors, it may be possible to remove all of the tumor from the facial nerve without injuring the nerve, whereas without monitoring surgeons may fear injuring the facial nerve and therefore choose to leave some tumor tissue behind. For operations to relieve hemifacial spasm intra-operative monitoring has greatly contributed to the current higher cure rate. The possibility of identifying the location of an injury, such as a neuroma of a peripheral nerve, may improve the outcome of operations on peripheral nerves to alleviate pain or spasm.

HOW CAN INTRA-OPERATIVE MONITORING BENEFIT THE SURGEON?

The surgeon naturally benefits from a reduction in the frequency of postoperative neurologic deficits, but there are other ways that a surgeon can benefit from intra-operative neurophysiologic monitoring. Intra-operative monitoring often gives an increased feeling of security because the surgeon knows that he or she will be warned if neural tissue is being surgically manipulated. It may also help to reduce the total time of an operation, because such monitoring makes it possible to proceed quickly inasmuch as it provides awareness to the surgeon of the location of specific nerves, such as cranial nerves that are embedded in tumors, before the nerves can actually be seen.

Intra-operative recording of neuroelectric potentials can also help to clarify the anatomy in cases in which the anatomy is distorted by natural variations, disease processes, or previous operations.

In operations in which neurophysiologic monitoring is used to help identify specific neural structures and thus avoid injuring neural tissue, the help a surgeon can receive from monitoring depends on the particular surgeon's experience in the particular type of operation. Monitoring may provide the very experienced surgeon with few advantages, except in a few cases in which problems arise. The experienced surgeon, however, may from time to time appreciate having a way to confirm the anatomy. The advantages of intra-operative monitoring are thus greater for less experienced surgeons or for surgeons in training who may also improve their surgical techniques as a result of the information obtained from monitoring. However, surgeons on all levels of experience can benefit from being alerted when neural tissue is being manipulated and from being informed about the degree to which the manipulation has caused changes in neural function.

OTHER ADVANTAGES OF INTRA-OPERATIVE MONITORING

In addition to reducing the risk of postoperative neurologic deficit and guiding the surgeon in the operation, intra-operative neurophysiologic monitoring can also provide an aid in teaching good surgical techniques to residents and surgeons with moderate experience, and it can provide a better understanding of why specific steps in an operation may cause neural injury. Intra-operative neurophysiologic monitoring can contribute to developing safer surgical techniques, because it can identify precisely which surgical step may have caused an injury to a peripheral nerve or to brain structures. The development of better surgical methods that bear a lesser risk of causing injury represents one of the long-term benefits of intra-operative monitoring.

IMPLEMENTATION OF INTRA-OPERATIVE MONITORING

Recording of neuroelectric activity evoked by controlled stimulation of the nervous system either by applying electrical impulses to nerves of the brain or by applying various kinds of sensory stimuli (evoked potentials) is important in monitoring as is recording of electromyographic (EMG) potentials.

The techniques used for intra-operative neurophysiologic monitoring have been described in a number of books and book chapters, some of which are listed below (1–4, 6–8). Intra-operative neurophysiologic monitoring essentially makes use of relatively standard methods of recording and stimulating specific parts of the nervous system that have been in use in the clinical neurophysiology laboratory for many years. Although there are advantages to having specialized equipment available for intra-operative monitoring, the recordings that are done in the operating room are rather similar to those done in the clinical testing laboratory or in the physiology laboratory, and thus equipment designed for use in the laboratory can also be used in the operating room. However, modifications that satisfy the special requirements of intra-operative monitoring, such as the necessity to interpret results instantaneously, are important.

It has been claimed that the operating room is a hostile environment with regard to electrical interference and that it is difficult to make recordings of sensory evoked potentials and other neuroelectric potentials because of such electrical interference. Experience gained over more than a decade of working in the operating room has shown that this is not at all the case and that it is indeed possible to obtain high-quality recordings in the operating room on a routine basis, provided that a few important factors are considered. These factors are outlined in detail in some of the books and book chapters listed below and will not be discussed further here (2–4, 6, 8).

It is very important to focus on the selection and training of the people who are to interpret the recorded neuroelectric potentials rather than on the choice of equipment. The people who do such monitoring must have a good background in and knowledge of physiology as well as anatomy. In addition, they must have specialized training in working in the operating room. They must know in general how the specific operation they are to monitor is carried out. These people must also be able to relate the results of monitoring in a way that is understood by surgeons, not all of whom are physiologists.

Communication between the neurophysiologist who is responsible for the monitoring and the surgeon is important to consider. The kind of changes in the recorded potentials that should be reported to the surgeon has been extensively discussed. Some have claimed that only changes that are indicative of a noticeable risk of permanent postoperative neurologic deficits should be reported. Others, like ourselves, believe that the results of monitoring should be regarded as information and not as a warning of an imminent disaster. Information about changes in the recorded neuroelectric potentials that are just slightly larger than the normal small variations that regularly occur provides the knowledge to the surgeon that his or her surgical manipulation has affected specific neural tissue to such an extent that its function has changed noticeably.

This gives the surgeon the option to continue and disregard the changes for the time being or to correct the problem immediately so that he or she does not need to worry about it later. Immediately alerting the surgeon of changes in the recorded neuroelectric potentials is also critical for identifying the step in the operation that caused the problem, which in turn is a prerequisite for correcting the problem later.

For intra-operative monitoring to be utilized to its optimal value, it is important that the information the neurophysiologist obtains from such recordings be conveyed to the surgeon in the most explicit way. Not all surgeons are experts in neurophysiology, and it is therefore not feasible to provide the surgeon only with raw data, such as giving changes in latency values in milliseconds regarding the prolongation of specific components of, *e.g.*, sensory evoked potentials. The surgeon may not know what this information means, or he or she may be too occupied with the operation itself to shift attention to interpreting physiologic data. It is best for the neurophysiologist to inform the surgeon about what the change in the recorded potentials means and to suggest what to do and/or what the consequences of not doing anything would be. This is a demanding task for the neurophysiologist that requires not only a thorough knowledge of neurophysiology and pathophysiology but also a considerable knowledge about the specific operation being monitored. In addition, it requires a good working relationship with the surgeon and that the surgeon have confidence in the neurophysiologist responsible for the monitoring.

These requirements are even more important in operations in which the results of monitoring are being used to guide the surgeon during the operation. For a surgeon to act on information provided by neurophysiologic monitoring requires confidence in the monitoring team. A surgeon who is used to being guided by his or her own vision may be told by the neurophysiologist that the location of the pathology of a peripheral nerve is at a certain location, but the surgeon sees no visual indication for pathology at that point. Or the surgeon may be informed by the neurophysiologist that he or she is operating very close to a specific nerve that is not visible.

Another operation in which such interaction is important is during microvascular decompression procedures to relieve a hemifacial spasm, in which the neurophysiologist may be able to tell the surgeon which specific blood vessel is being compressed and thus is causing the spasm (4). Will a surgeon ignore moving a blood vessel off the facial nerve when no physiologic signs are present of that particular blood vessel contributing to the patient's spasm? Or will the surgeon continue to search for offending vessels when there is no vessel to be seen but electrophysiologic signs indicate that there is a blood vessel in close contact with the facial nerve somewhere along the nerve's course and that this contact is causing the patient's symptoms? Experience at our institution shows that such reliance on the results of electrophysiologic recordings is beneficial and that a reduction in failure to achieve anticipated therapeutical goals of operations can be obtained if surgeons take this opportunity for such guidance.

WHAT ARE THE MEDICOLEGAL AND MEDICOECONOMIC ASPECTS OF INTRA-OPERATIVE MONITORING?

Because economic matters are *considered* in decisions on whether or not intra-operative monitoring should be done during a specific operation, it is important to also *consider* savings in the costs that are associated with a reduction in the occurrence of postoperative neurologic deficits that can be ascribed to the use of intra-operative monitoring.

While it is relatively easy to obtain an estimate of the cost in economic terms of intra-operative monitoring as an addition to specific operations, it is much more difficult to estimate the cost savings that may result from using intra-operative monitoring. The savings associated with intra-operative monitoring that has been considered so far has consisted mainly of costs for medical care of the patient as a result of permanent postoperative neurologic deficits.

Despite considerable effort, it has been difficult to assess the economic gains from intra-operative monitoring with respect to saving costs for care of individuals with postoperative neurologic deficits. It has not been possible to use the conventional methods of double-blind tests to assess the reduction of postoperative neurologic deficits attributed to intra-operative monitoring. It has not even been possible to use methods that imply randomized selection of patients in whom monitoring is going to be done, because surgeons who are now used to intra-operative monitoring have been reluctant to deprive any of their patients of the benefits they believe are provided by it. Estimates of the improvements derived from the use of intra-operative monitoring with regard to lowering the risk of postoperative permanent neurologic deficits have, therefore, mainly been based on historical data, which have been obtained by comparing the frequency of deficits before the introduction of intra-operative monitoring with data on the occurrence rate of such deficits after monitoring was instituted. Such methods have been criticized on the basis of the claim that other improvements in operative methods have been introduced since the introduction of intra-operative monitoring, and that these other improvements must also have contributed to the decrease in the occurrence of postoperative complications.

When estimating the costs of postoperative permanent neurologic deficits, it has been the cost of care of the individual person who has suffered the deficit that has been considered. The reduction in the probability of postoperative permanent neurologic deficits not only represents a gain in the form of a reduction in the cost of health care, but it also represents a reduction in human suffering. Although attempts have been made to evaluate the former in economic terms, little attention has been directed to the economic value of the latter, and human suffering has not been considered when the economic basis for implementation of intra-operative monitoring has been discussed.

A severe permanent neurologic deficit affects not only the individual who suffers the deficit but also at least one or more relatives in one way or another. Because of the problems in evaluating human suffering in economic terms, it is not usually considered when the economic feasibility of implementing intra-operative monitoring is discussed. However, it does not seem reasonable to ignore the value of that component of neurologic deficits when estimates of the feasibility of monitoring are considered just because it may be difficult to estimate the costs.

It may be possible to obtain an economic estimation of human suffering due to the results of permanent postoperative neurologic deficit by using the economic compensation that is awarded to a person by a court of law for human suffering that results from accidents and from malpractice. If the money awarded to patients for human suffering in such circumstances is used as a guideline for estimating the gain from intra-operative monitoring, then the economic consequences of human suffering from permanent postoperative neurologic deficits may become enormous. When the economic basis for implementation of neurophysiologic monitoring is estimated without considering a reasonble economic value for the reduction of human suffering, the gain—in economic terms—of intra-operative monitoring may be considerably underestimated, and it might have been economically feasible to have used intra-operative monitoring in many more operations than what seemed to be justified on the basis of past and still present estimations of economic feasibility.

It has not been possible to obtain quantitative assessments of other benefits of intra-operative monitoring that have contributed to the development of better surgical methods and to education in general. Also difficult to evaluate in economic terms is the gain from the (recognized) advantage of intra-operative monitoring in aiding the surgeon throughout the operation, which provides the surgeon with an increased feeling of security and which may make it possible to carry out the operation in less time than would be required without intra-operative monitoring. Such an economic evaluation in this regard seems beyond our ability.

The medicolegal aspects of intra-operative monitoring are complex. National organizations such as the National Institutes of Health recognize only a few types of intra-operative monitoring as a valuable adjunct to specific operations (5), but many other forms of intra-operative monitoring are now recognized informally as being beneficial.

As could be expected for an emerging field, all of these questions are heavily debated and so far lack definite solutions. The rapid growth of the use of intra-operative neurophysiologic monitoring throughout the past decade has shown that it is regarded to be valuable for patient care as an adjunct to many operations and that it may be regarded as a part of the ongoing development of surgical disciplines.

CONCLUSIONS

Intra-operative neurophysiologic monitoring is now a well established adjunct to many different kinds of operations in which neural tissue is being manipulated. Its main benefit is to reduce the incidence of permanent postoperative neurologic deficits, but there are also other advantages in using intra-operative monitoring, *e.g.,* it helps to identify neural tissue that is not directly visible; in some cases it can identify the anatomic location of a pathology; and in a few operations it ensures that the therapeutic goal of the operation has been achieved before the operation is completed. The value of the techniques involved in intra-operative neurophysiologic monitoring differs from operation to operation, and surgeons with different degrees of experience in a particular operation may benefit by different degrees from the use of intra-operative monitoring.

REFERENCES

1. Desmedt JE (ed): *Neuromonitoring in Surgery.* Amsterdam, Elsevier Science Publishers, 1989.
2. Kartush JM, Bouchard KR (eds): *Neuromonitoring in Otology and Head and Neck Surgery.* New York, Raven Press, 1992.
3. Loftus CM, Traynelis VC (eds): *Intraoperative Monitoring Techniques in Neurosurgery.* New York, McGraw Hill, 1994.
4. Møller AR: *Evoked Potentials in Intraoperative Monitoring.* Baltimore, Williams & Wilkins, 1988.
5. National Institutes of Health (NIH): Consensus Development Conference (held December 11–13, 1991). **Consens Statement** 9(4):1–24, 1991.
6. Nuwer MR: *Evoked Potential Monitoring in the Operating Room.* New York, Raven Press, 1986.
7. Schramm J, Møller AR (eds): *Intraoperative Neurophysiologic Monitoring in Neurosurgery.* Heidelberg, Springer-Verlag, 1991.
8. Yingling CD: Intraoperative monitoring in skull base surgery, in Jackler RK, Brackmann D (eds): *Neurotology.* St. Louis, Mosby Year Book, 1994, pp 967–1002.

13

Neurophysiologic Monitoring during Cranial Base Surgery: Is it Necessary?

LALIGAM N. SEKHAR, M.D., F.A.C.S., GHASSAN BEJJANI, M.D.,
PETER NORA, M.D., AND PEDRO L. VERA, Ph.D.

The use of intraoperative monitoring of evoked potentials to reduce postoperative permanent deficits is based on the assumption that changes in recordable electrical impulses occur as a result of injury, and that the injury is still reversible at the time of detection if proper surgical intervention occurs.

Aage R. Møller (19)

For evoked potentials to predict postoperative neurological deficits accurately, the following criteria must logically be fulfilled: the pathway monitored must fall within the vascular territory of the vessel at risk and the blood flow at some point must fall below the ischemic threshold for synaptic activity.

Friedman, W.A. *et al.* (8)

For neurophysiologic monitoring during cranial base surgery (CBS) to gain wide acceptance, it must be reliable and easy to use. Very importantly, changes in monitored activity must allow the surgeon to modify his behavior in time to avert permanent neurologic deficits. Neurophysiologic monitoring may also have other benefits: the identification of structures whose anatomy is altered by pathology and the acceleration of the surgeon's learning curve by his improved understanding of mechanisms of intraoperative injury. In this chapter, we will review our personal experience with neurophysiologic monitoring during CBS and also the existing evidence of its benefits as recorded in the literature.

PATHOGENESIS OF NEUROLOGIC DEFICITS AFTER CBS

Following CBS, permanent neurologic deficits may result from injury to the cerebral hemispheres, to the brainstem, or to the cranial nerves. Such injuries may result from direct manipulation, or the aftereffects of such manipulation (*e.g.*, edema). They may also be the result of vascular occlusion, arterial or venous. Neurophysiologic monitoring may be used to detect problems in any one of the three groups of structures. However, we do not have modalities available to conveniently monitor the most important system of all, namely, the motor pathway. The neurophysiologist and the surgeon, therefore, rely on adjacent pathways to help detect changes.

MONITORING TECHNIQUES

The human element is more important during neurophysiologic monitoring than that of equipment. The monitoring technique must be reliable, must be appropriate to the operation, and must not unduly interfere with the anesthetic technique or the operation itself.

In our center, a clinical neurophysiologist or a neurologist supervises properly trained technicians, who perform the basic functions. We use the NEURONET monitoring system (Computational Diagnostics Inc., Pittsburgh, PA), which allows multiple modalities to be monitored simultaneously, such as the electroencephalogram (EEG), somatosensory evoked potentials (SSEP), brainstem auditory evoked potentials (BAEP), and cranial nerve (CN) monitoring and stimulation. The NEURONET system also allows the networking of multiple monitoring stations (operating rooms), and a central site, allowing the clinical neurophysiologist to monitor patients in several rooms at the same time.

Changes in anesthetic technique significantly influence evoked potentials and the ability to monitor CN function. Therefore, the anesthesiologist and the neurophysiologist need to carefully discuss the patient's need with each other and with the surgeon.

Conversely, the neurosurgeon must understand the limitations of monitoring modalities being used and the physiologic basis of the various techniques available. Any significant changes in the monitoring parameters must be immediately conveyed to the surgeon, who is expected to alter the operative technique, in an effort to reverse the changes. Similarly, the surgeon must warn the anesthesiologist and the neurophysiologist about impending maneuvers that may alter the evoked potentials or other electrical parameters. Examples are temporary vascular occlusion or the retraction of the brainstem.

Before intraoperative monitoring is started, a preoperative test of the modality (*e.g.,* SSEP) is performed, if possible, to obtain a baseline for further comparison. During the operation, neurophysiologic monitoring is started at the beginning of the procedure (in some cases, even before the patient is anesthetized), and is continued until the end of the procedure. It would be ideal to continue monitoring of the EEG and evoked potentials until the patient is awake. However, this requires a monitoring setup in the recovery rooms and intensive care units, which we do not have at present.

In the next section, we will consider the utility of individual monitoring modalities and any available evidence regarding their efficacy.

EEG

The oldest of monitoring modalities, the EEG is widely used during carotid endarterectomy operations to determine the need for shunt insertion. Both the raw signal and the compressed spectral array are used in neuromonitoring. The EEG is adversely affected at the same cerebral blood flow thresholds as the SSEP. However, it is less sensitive to ischemia to deep structures.

During CBS and cerebrovascular surgery, the authors use EEG primarily to achieve barbiturate- or etomidate-induced burst suppression during prolonged vascular occlusion, for example, during the performance of a vein graft to bypass an artery encased by a tumor or for an unclippable aneurysm. The use of mild hypothermia, induced hypertension, and barbiturate coma allow the surgeon to extend the ischemic time without infarction to about 2 hours, depending on the neuronal population and the vascular territory. In most instances, the period of continuous ischemia required during the vein graft procedures is under 60 minutes.

There are no randomized controlled trials that prove the efficacy of such burst suppression in preventing stroke. In our current experience at the George Washington University Medical Center with 32 vein grafts performed with brain protection as described, only two patients sustained disabling strokes, both of which were caused by occlusion of perforating arteries and were unrelated to the vein grafting procedure (Fig. 13.1 **A** and **B** and Fig. 13.2).

SSEP

The SSEP monitors the sensory pathway from the upper or the lower extremity to the somatosensory cortex. The N_{20} wave of the median nerve SSEP indicates the arrival of the electrical impulse in the somatosensory cortex. Experimental and human studies have shown that the SSEP is altered by cerebral ischemia at or below a cerebral blood flow threshold of 15 to 20 ml/100 g/min. The SSEP is also apparently affected by direct retraction of the brainstem or injury to the brainstem. These are the basis of monitoring SSEPs in CBS, wherein the brainstem or the carotid vascular territory is at risk.

In studies involving SSEP monitoring during aneurysm surgery, previous investigators have monitored the central conduction time (time in-

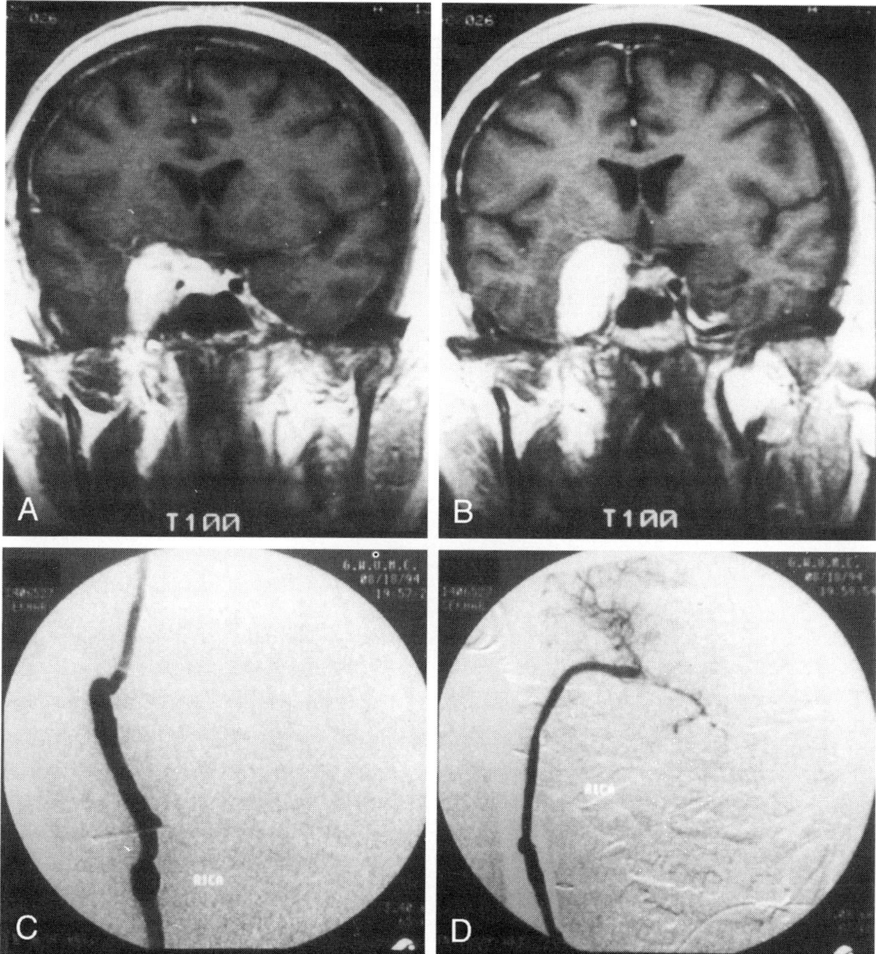

FIG. 13.1 (**A** and **B**) A tumor encasing and narrowing the internal carotid artery (ICA) is shown. (**C** and **D**) A saphenous vein graft has been placed from the ICA in the neck to the M_2 segment of the middle cerebral artery, bypassing the invaded intracavernous ICA. The tumor was totally resected during a subsequent operation.

terval between the arrival of impulse at the upper cervical area (C_2) and the arrival of impulse in the somatosensory cortex), the amplitude of the N_{20} wave, the latency of the N_{20} wave, as compared to the baseline value (23, 36). A number of nonrandomized, noncontrolled studies have established the value of median nerve SSEP monitoring for middle cerebral artery aneurysms. When the surgeon takes appropriate corrective action when SSEPs change, neurologic deficits may be averted (7, 24, 29).

For anterior cerebral artery aneurysms, potentials evoked by peroneal or posterior tibial nerve stimulation need to be monitored, which is technically more difficult to do. However, for posterior circulation aneurysms, the use of SSEP monitoring alone may be misleading; during surgery for basilar tip aneurysms especially, neurologic deficits may occur despite the presence of normal SSEPs, presumably because the pathway is not supplied by the perforating vessels (7, 17, 29).

Manninen *et al.* found that the use of combined modality monitoring by SSEP and BAEP was much more useful for posterior circulation aneurysm surgery than was either modality used alone (18). In a large study from the University Hospital, London, Ontario, Canada, monitoring with these two modalities was used in 52 patients who had temporary occlusion of an artery and 21 patients who underwent permanent occlusion. When both modalities were counted, a false-negative result (occurrence of a neurologic deficit with no change in either mon-

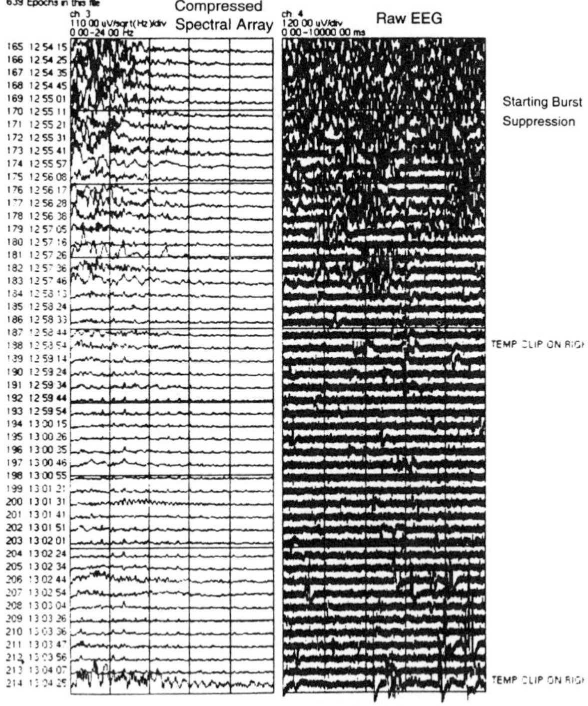

FIG. 13.2. Electroencephalographic burst suppression, with the use of intravenous sodium thiopental to protect the brain during the operation. Frequently, the patient's blood pressure is raised 20 to 40 torr, and the patient is cooled to about 34°C during the procedure, which are additional means of protecting the brain from ischemia.

itored modality) occurred in only 20%; however, with SSEP alone, false-negatives occurred in 47%, and with BAEP alone, the occurrence rate was 60%. However, every patient who exhibited a permanent change in SSEP or BAEP developed a permanent neurologic deficit. In the author's institution, they have found that the combination of intraoperative neurophysiologic monitoring of SSEP and BAEP with intra-operative angiography helps to achieve an optimal outcome after aneurysm surgery, including the surgery of giant aneurysms and involving the placement of vein grafts (3).

There has been only one published report concerning the monitoring of SSEPs during CBS. Gentili *et al.* reported the monitoring of SSEP and BAEP in a group of 12 patients undergoing CBS (9). Significant changes in potentials were noted in five patients. In three patients, the evoked potentials recovered in response to corrective action consisting of the release of the retractor or stopping tumor removal near the brainstem. No permanent deficits were noted in these patients. Two patients with permanent evoked potential alterations developed permanent neurologic deficits. One with permanent BAEP change developed loss of hearing. One patient with BAEP and SSEP change exhibited brainstem dysfunction.

In a recent study performed in our institution, SSEP monitoring was performed in 109 CBS operations in 88 patients. SSEP changes were reported to the surgeon, and corrective action was taken whenever possible. SSEP changes observed were classified as shown in Table 13.1. The SSEP changes were correlated with neurologic deficits at 24 hours postoperatively.

In this table, classification of SSEP changes observed at surgery used in our study are shown (Bejjani G, Nora P, Vera PL, *et al.* unpublished data).

In Table 13.2, the percentage of patients in each category who developed a permanent postoperative deficit is shown. There was excellent statistical correlation of the SSEP change and the neurologic deficit. The rank correlation was .83 (*P*< .05).

TABLE 13.1

Classification of SSEP Changes Observed at Surgery[a]

Class	SSEP Change	% of Total
I	No change in SSEP	69
II	Changes, which returned to baseline	26
III	Changes, which recovered partially	3
IV	Changes, which did not recover	2

[a]Bejjani G, Nora P, Vera PL, *et al.*, 1995, unpublished data.

TABLE 13.2
Immediate Postoperative Neurologic Deficit (Partial/Complete)

Class of SSEP Change	Total No. of Patients	% Patients in Each Category with Deficit
I	75	11
II	29	14
III	3	100
IV	2	100

Changes in surgical technique in response to SSEP monitoring may have prevented neurologic deficits in 25/109 patients, in view of the high correlation between persistent SSEP changes and permanent neurologic deficits. The use of combined modality monitoring with BAEP may further reduce the incidence of false negatives. However, by the very nature of what is monitored by SSEP, or BAEP, it is unlikely that false negatives can be eliminated totally. Some illustrative examples are shown in Figures 13.3 through 13.8.

BAEP

BAEP monitoring has been used mostly for the preservation of hearing during acoustic neuroma and other posterior fossa operations. Its use for the monitoring of brainstem function seems to be underutilized. Because of the partial cross over of the central auditory pathway, even with unilateral auditory stimulation, both sides of the brainstem can be monitored to some extent. This is of particular importance during CBS. Because of the considerable amount of work being done through the ipsilateral petrous temporal bone, it may be impractical to place click electrodes in the ipsilateral ear. In fact, because of the predominance of the cross over, performing BAEP from the contralateral ear, with observation of wave V, and of the III-V interval, can be quite useful for monitoring brainstem function. We have routinely used contralateral BAEP for the monitoring of brainstem functions during CBS, wherein the brainstem is at risk. This technique complements SSEP monitoring, Gentili *et al.* and Manninen *et al.* have noted (9, 18).

Motor Evoked Potentials

Since the prevention of motor deficits is one of the major goals of neuromonitoring, motor evoked potentials would seem to be an ideal monitoring technique, if available. However, despite some early studies that showed promise, this technique has not been practically useful as yet because of the difficulty of obtaining motor evoked potentials repeatedly, and safely, in the operating room setting.

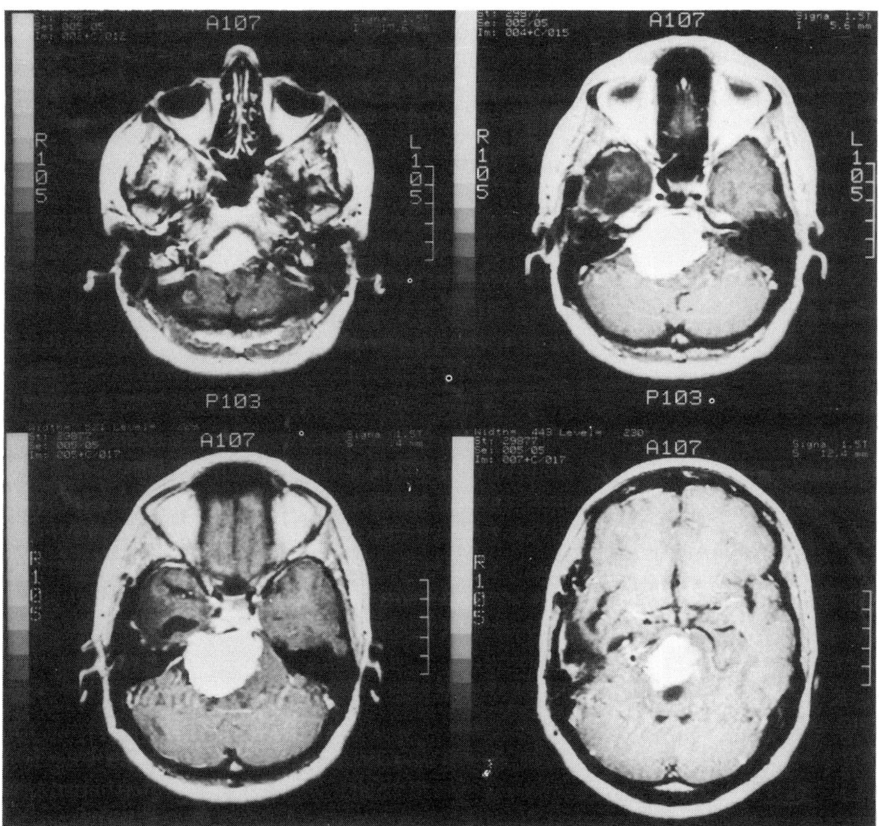

FIG. 13.3 (A–D) Patient, previously operated on for a large petroclival meningioma invading the brainstem, is shown in these enhanced magnetic resonance imaging scans.

Cranial Nerve Monitoring

OPTIC NERVE

Monitoring of visual evoked responses (VER) during operations in the anterior of the middle cranial fossae has not been practical or reliable. Pattern reversal evoked potentials cannot be used during operations, since they require visual fixation. Therefore, light-emitting diode goggles or strobe flashes have been used for evoking electrical responses during operations. However, such devices frequently become dislodged by the scalp flaps, especially when orbital osteotomies are used during CBS. The senior author LNS evaluated the use of contact lenses impregnated with a light-emitting diode to evoke VER. However, the correlation between VERs and the operative results was poor.

A similarly poor result was obtained even after the placement of a wick electrode on the exposed optic nerve for the recording of optic nerve action potentials (research performed with Dr. Aage Moller). These results are echoed in recent reports from Cedzich *et al.*, Feinsod *et al.*, Strauss *et al.* and Wilson *et al.*, although some early reports were enthusiastic (2, 5, 35, 37).

In contrast to this result, however, VER monitoring may have been a major application during operations on basilar bifurcation and posterior cerebral artery aneurysms, as well as on upper clival tumors that encase these arteries. The effects of occlusion of the posterior cerebral

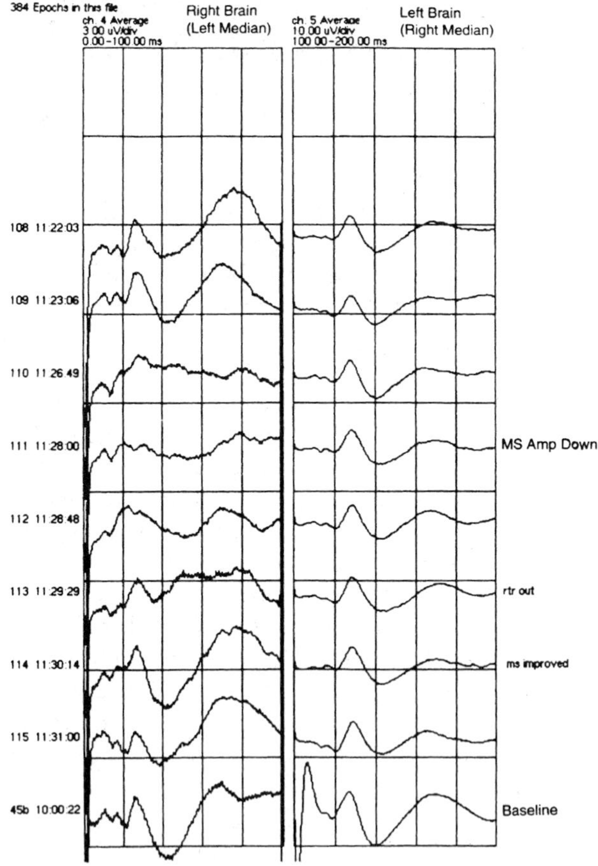

FIG. 13.4 During the resection of this patient's tumor by a partial labyrinthectomy petrosal approach, the SSEPs deteriorated bilaterally. The retractor placed on the brain was released, with recovery of potentials. This patient's tumor was resected subtotally, leaving a remnant on the brainstem. She recovered without major neurologic deficits.

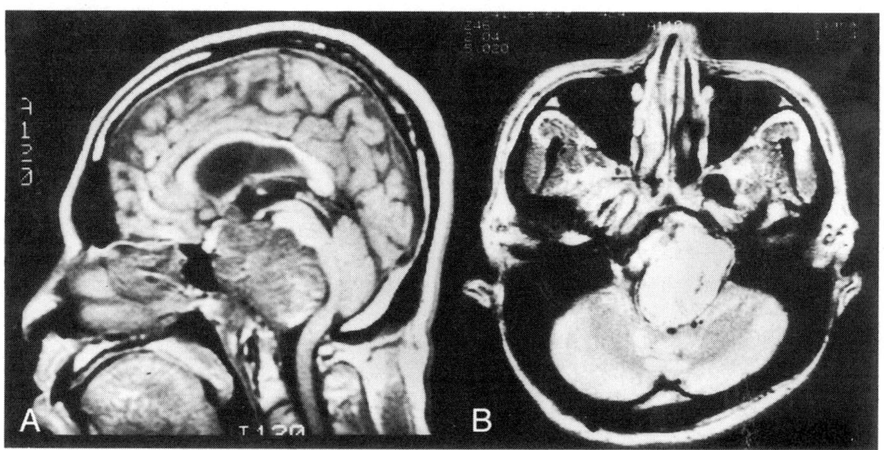

FIG. 13.5(**A** and **B**) MRI scan of patient with an extensive clivus chordoma, severely compressing the brainstem, which was removed subtotally by a petrosal and transpetrous approach.

arteries on the occipital cortex appear to be readily detected by intraoperative VER monitoring. Although the function of perforating vessels issuing from the PCA is not directly monitored, this technique has considerable potential, which needs further study.

MONITORING OF CNs III, V, AND VI

Monitoring of the motor portions of CNs III, V, and VI may be performed by the insertion of needle electrodes into the orbit in the vicinity of these nerves (30). Electromyographic (EMG) ring electrodes may also be implanted more specifically around the extra-ocular muscles by an ophthalmologist at the beginning of the operation, thus improving the precision of this monitoring technique (31).

EMG monitoring of these nerves can be used to detect the location of CNs passing through the tumor and to detect damage to these nerves during the removal of the tumor. However, in the authors' experience, the value of monitoring these nerves is not the same as that of facial nerve monitoring during the resection of acoustic neuromas. There has been no controlled study to date that proves the efficacy of neuromonitoring of CNs III, V and VI.

FACIAL NERVE MONITORING

Monitoring of CN VII during CBS has now become a widely accepted practice because of its ease, reliability, and generally perceived usefulness during various kinds of operations. Most centers currently use EMG electrodes implanted in the facial muscles, in combination with monopolar stimulation of the nerve in the operative field. During operations, the monopolar stimulator is used to localize the nerve or to confirm its physiologic integrity. Observation of spontaneous EMG activity and its acoustic display over loudspeakers helps the surgeon to avoid injury to the nerve during dissection (21, 27, 33).

During acoustic neuroma surgery, the surgeon first stimulates the areas of capsule to ensure the absence of the facial nerve and then quickly debulks the tumor. With large and giant tumors, the monopolar stimulator is then utilized to identify the facial nerve at the brain-

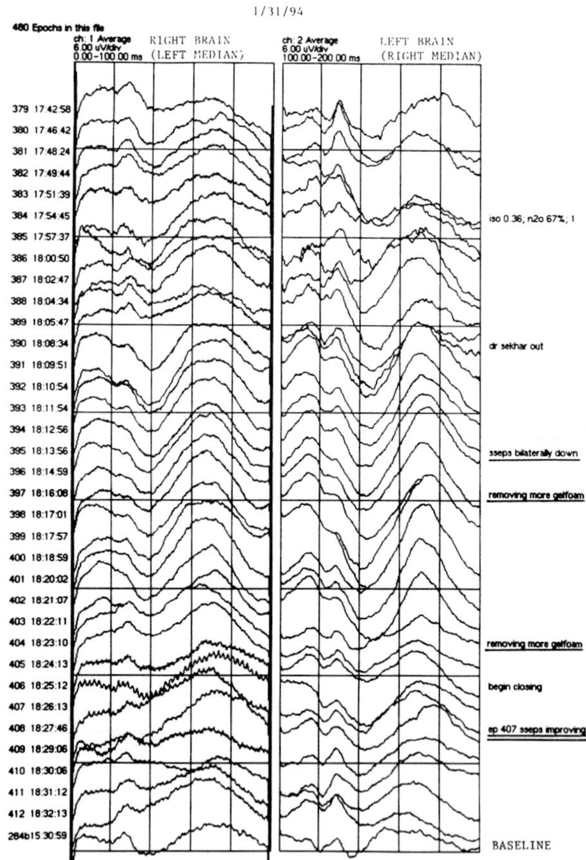

FIG. 13.6. Although mostly unaltered during the operation to remove the tumor, the SSEPs deteriorated dramatically while the surgeon was closing up. Gelfoam, which had been placed in the epidural space to stop venous bleeding, had swelled up, causing brainstem compression. Removal of the Gelfoam resulted in dramatic recovery of the potentials. The patient awoke from anesthesia without major neurologic deficits.

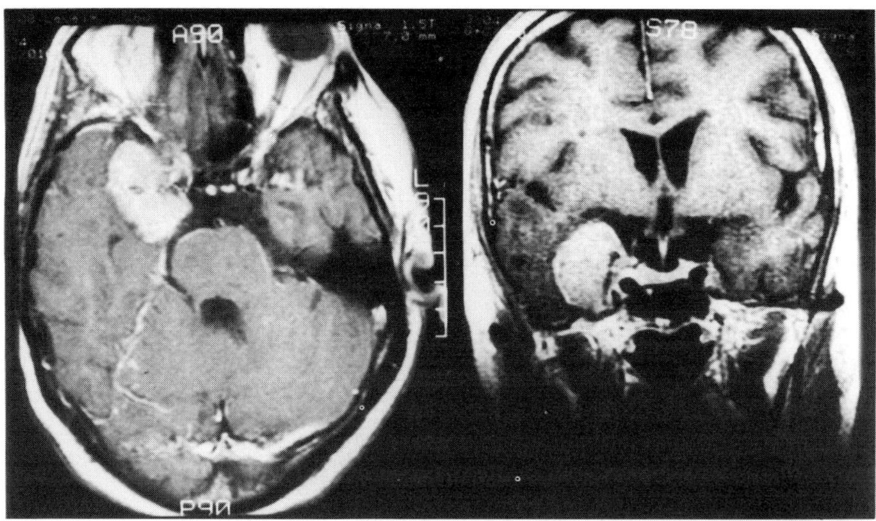

FIG. 13.7 An elderly patient with a medial sphenoid wing meningioma, who represents the major false-negative of SSEP monitoring in the group of 104 operations reported here.

stem and laterally in the internal auditory canal. The surgeon then proceeds with tumor resection in a piecemeal fashion and with tumor dissection from the facial nerve. The dissection of CN VII is greatly aided by listening to the spontaneous EMG activity of two types. *Non-repetitive* discharges, also described as *bursts,* are brief in duration, and are thought to be caused by the single firing of motor units in a relatively synchronous pattern, usually due to local manipulation of the nerve, or the indirect manipulation of the nerve (Fig. 13.9). These are not a cause for concern. However, *repetitive* grouped motor-unit discharges, also described as *trains,* are thought to represent prolonged depolarization of the axons, resulting in repetitive firing of single or multiple motor units. These may also be called *injury potentials.* They may occur because of mechanical, thermal, or chemical injury to the nerve during dissection and during bipolar coagulation. When these injury potentials are noted, the surgeon must stop his activity and use a different strategy of nerve dissection. The senior author (LNS) generally prefers to use fairly sharp dissection of the nerve from the tumor capsule and prefers dissection *perpendicular* to the nerve or *parallel* dissection, although both techniques are important. Near the end of dissection, stimulation at a medium current intensity (0.3 to 0.6 mA) may be necessary to distinguish pieces of thickened arachnoid membrane or small pieces of tumor from thinned fascicles of the facial nerve, to enable the complete resection of the tumor. At the end of the operation, stimulation of the nerve at the brainstem at decreasing current intensity allows the surgeon to obtain a prognosis for facial recovery (Fig. 13.10). If the facial muscles produce at least 500 μV of contraction when stimulated at the brainstem at thresholds below 0.3 mA,

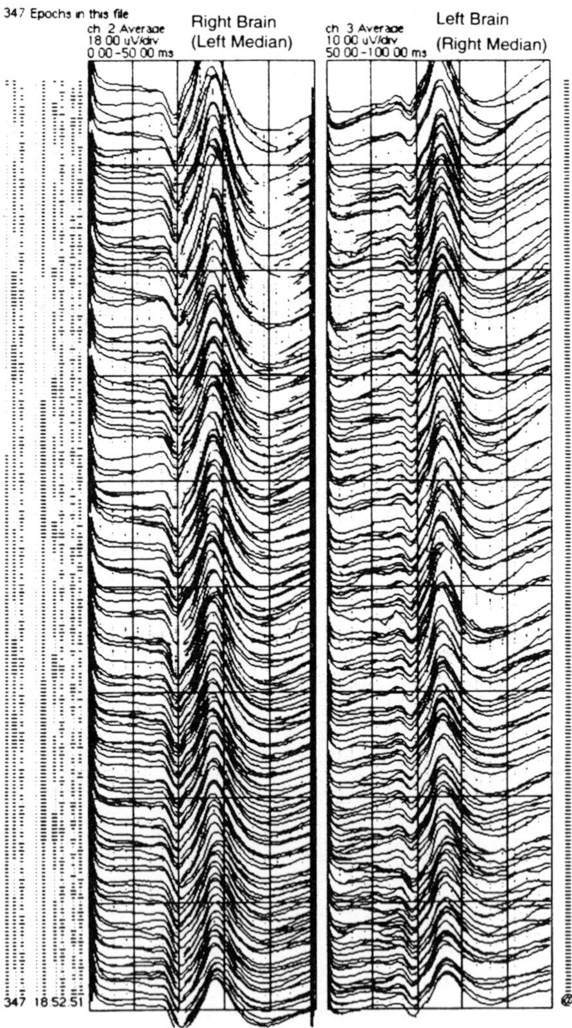

FIG. 13.8 During the operation to remove the tumor, SSEPs were bilaterally unchanged. However, the patient awoke with right hemiplegia. Postoperative computed tomographic scan revealed an infarct in the internal capsule, which was undetected by median SSEPs.

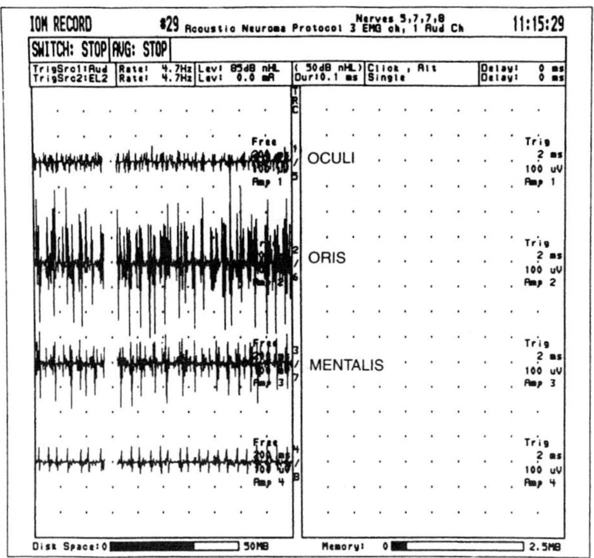

Spontaneous Facial Nerve Discharge

FIG. 13.9 Spontaneous facial EMG activity observed during the removal of a recurrent acoustic neuroma. The patient had undergone a partial tumor resection at another center previously and presented with House grade IV facial weakness. Complete tumor resection was achieved, and facial nerve function improved to House grade III.

an excellent facial function (House grade I or II) is usually obtained, immediately after the operation (1). When the facial nerve does not stimulate successfully even at a current intensity of 2.0 mA, the surgeon must evaluate the nerve carefully under very high magnification to see whether reconstruction by direct suture, or with a nerve graft, will be required.

Although no randomized studies of facial nerve outcome after acoustic neuroma surgery have been performed with and without neuromonitoring, three studies have compared the results with historical controls, in operations performed by the same group of surgeons within a short time period after the inception of monitoring. Harner *et al.* matched pairs of patients undergoing acoustic neuroma excision with and without monitoring on the basis of tumor size, the most recent year of operation, and the patient's age (10). A significant improvement in anatomic preservation of the facial nerve was noted, especially in patients with large tumors (71% in the monitored group *versus* 41% in the unmonitored group). The percent of patients with some preserved hearing improved from 13% in the unmonitored group to 22% in the monitored group. When facial nerve function was graded and assessed a percentage value 3 months after the operation, and 1 year after the operation, a statistically significant difference was found, using the Wilcoxon rank-sum test, a nonparametric test for data that do not have a normal distribution (Table 13.3).

Niparko *et al.* (Table 13.4) compared 29 patients who had acoustic neuroma excised by the translabyrinthine approach with neuromonitoring with a control group of 75 patients operated on with the same approach. They found a significant improvement in the results, at 1 year after the operation, and mainly in tumors larger than 2.0 cm.

Kwartler *et al.* compared a group of monitored translabyrinthine acoustic neuroma operations ($n = 89$) with a group of unmonitored operations ($n = 155$), using the same technique (13). Results of facial function were evaluated immediately after the operation, at discharge, and at follow-up. It was found that the results were significantly better for the whole group immediately after the operation and at discharge, but at follow-up the results did not achieve statistical significance. When

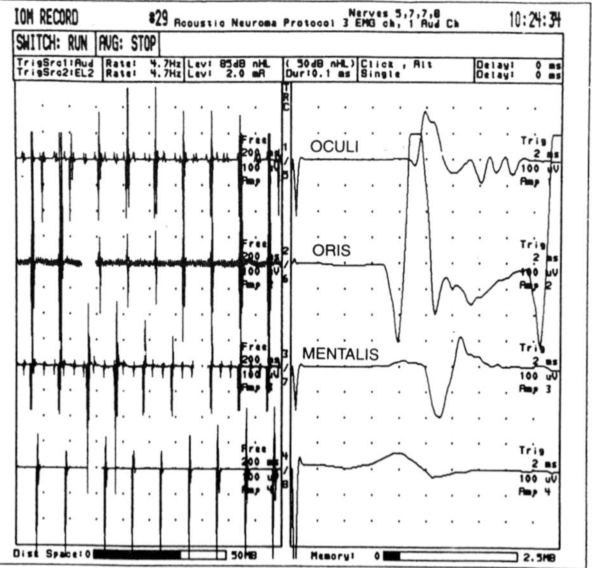

Evoked Facial Nerve Discharge

FIG. 13.10 In the patient described in Figure 13.9, facial nerve stimulation near the brainstem at a decreasing current intensity allowed the surgeon to determine the threshold for stimulation to be 1 mA. Even though the nerve was markedly attenuated, it was shown to be anatomically intact. This was confirmed by improved facial function immediately after the operation.

TABLE 13.3

Postoperative Facial Nerve Function after the Excision of Acoustic Neuromas with (n = 72) and without (n = 69) Facial Nerve Monitoring[a]

Facial Nerve Function (%)	House Grade	At 3 Months		At 1 yr	
		Monitored (%)	Unmonitored (%)	Monitored (%)	Unmonitored (%)
100	I	46	20	45	27
76–99	II	12	25	10	29
51–75	III	4	6	15	10
26–50	IV	6	7	10	13
1–25	V	17	7	18	15
0	VI	15	35	2	6
Median		93%	58%	98%	78%

[a]Reproduced with permission from (10).

TABLE 13.4

Facial Nerve Outcome in Patients with Acoustic Neuromas Operated on by the Translabyrinthine Approach[a]

Class	House Grade	1 wk Postoperatively		1 yr Postoperatively	
		Monitored (*n* = 29) %	Unmonitored (*n* = 75) %	Monitored (*n* = 29) %	Unmonitored (*n* = 75) %
Satisfactory	I and II	69	51 (ns)	86	57(< .05)
Intermediate	III and IV	21	28 (ns)	11	36
Unsatisfactory	V and VI	10	21 (ns)	3	7
Probability of difference		Significant < .05			
Size correlation		Improved outcome in tumors >2.0 cm (P < .05)			

[a]Reproduced with permission from (25).

the tumors were broken down by size, statistically significant improvement in results was found only for tumors >2.5 cm in size immediately after the operation and at discharge. At follow-up, the results for these large tumors tended to be better but did not achieve statistical significance. Thus, in these three studies of acoustic neuroma patients, facial nerve monitoring was shown to improve the outcome, although this effect was most apparent in patients with large tumors.

In a series of 125 patients with acoustic neuromas operated on according to retrosigmoid approach by the senior author (LNS; other surgeons were Wright DC, Kamerer D, and Hirsch B), facial nerve outcome was analyzed (Table 13.5). House grade I and II function of 90% was achieved for tumors 0 to 2.9 cm, 68% for tumors 3.0 to 4.9 cm, and 22% for tumors >5.0 cm.

Although there was no control group, this quality of results could not have been achieved without the use of facial nerve monitoring.

In addition to acoustic neuroma surgery, facial nerve monitoring is extremely useful during CBS in other areas, namely, for transtemporal approaches and for transfacial approaches where the facial nerve is at risk. Monopolar facial nerve stimulation has been used by Silverstein *et al.* to predict the amount of bone overlying the facial nerve canal to guide the amount of drilling that has to be performed (32). The use of facial nerve monitoring and a modified technique of mobilization of the nerve was used by Brackmann to practically eliminate the occurrence of postoperative facial paralysis after the mobilization of the facial nerve during the infratemporal approach (14). Using the same operative technique, Leonetti *et al.* compared the immediate postoperative results between 31 unmonitored and 20 monitored patients. Normal facial function was obtained in 93% of the monitored patients and 70% of the unmonitored patients. Additionally, no patients in the monitored group developed House grade V or VI facial function, whereas this occurred in 48% of the unmonitored patients (14).

MONITORING OF THE AUDITORY NERVE

Preservation of serviceable hearing is an important goal in patients with acoustic neuromas and other lesions that distort the eighth CN, such as petroclival meningiomas. Such hearing preservation is most difficult in patients with acoustic neuromas (vestibular schwannomas) because the tumor is arising from the nerve itself, and there is usually no arachnid plane between the tumor and the cochlear nerve.

For patients with petroclival meningiomas and with other lesions not arising from the eighth CN, monitoring of the BAEPs from the ipsilateral ear is adequate. In these patients, observation of the wave form and amplitude and of the interpeak latency between waves I and III is adequate enough to recognize deleterious effects caused by ex-

TABLE 13.5
Facial Nerve Function according to Tumor Size[a, b]

CP Angle	Pre-operative	Postoperative			Follow-Up
Tumor Size (cm)	I–II	I–II (%)	III–IV (%)	V–VI (%)	< 3 months
<1.9	48	43 (90)	5 (10)		1
2.0–3.9	59	40 (68)	15 (25)	4	3
>4.0	18	4 (22)	11 (61)	3 (17)	
Total	125	87 (70)	31 (25)	7 (6)	4

[a]Wright DC, Sekhar LN, *et al.*, 1995.
[b]House-Brackmann grading system was used.

cessive retraction or direct manipulation. When these effects occur, a change of surgical technique can usually prevent permanent injury. However, if the anterior inferior cerebellar artery (AICA) is interrupted proximal to the origin of the internal auditory artery, loss of hearing is usually irreversible.

During the removal of vestibular schwannomas, BAEP monitoring has certain important limitations. In some patients, even those with

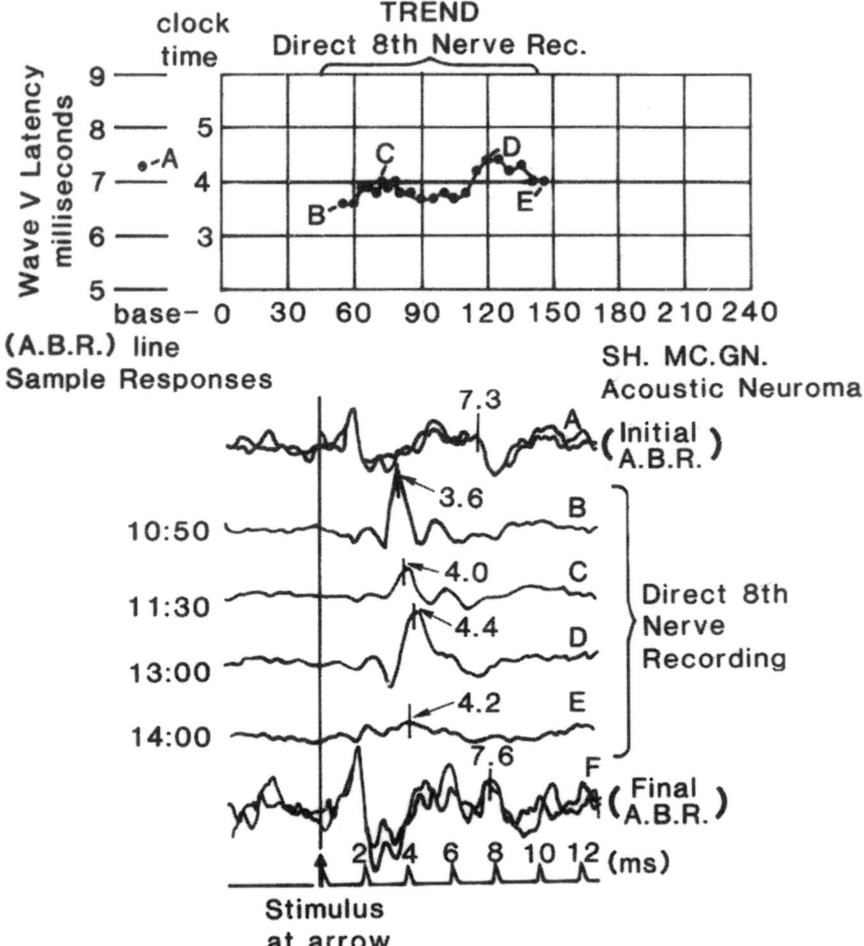

FIG. 13.11 Intra-operative monitoring of the brainstem evoked response (*A.B.R.*), and direct eighth nerve action potentials during surgery to remove a 2.4 cm acoustic neuroma (cerebellopontine angle measurement) is shown. Gardener-Robertson class I hearing was preserved in this patient postoperatively.

excellent hearing, the BAEP waves may be unrecognizable, so as to make BAEP unusable for monitoring purposes. Secondly, because of the averaging required to elicit the BAEP during the operation, a rapid feedback is not provided to the surgeon. Therefore, the surgeon may not know what event caused the deterioration of BAEP, and if he does know, it may be too late to reverse any damage.

Three types of monitoring modalities have been used to provide a rapid feedback during the removal of an acoustic neuroma. The first is the *electrocochleogram* (*ECOG*), using a transtympanic electrode (15, 26). This modality provides information rapidly about the cochlear microphonics of the hair cells of the inner ear and the compound action potential of the auditory nerve (wave N-1). The second is the potential recorded by placing a wick electrode in direct contact with the eighth CN, also termed *direct auditory nerve action potential*(20, 33). This technique provides a very rapid feedback about the status of the nerve, proximal to the tumor. However, because a healthy segment of the nerve proximal to the tumor is necessary, and the presence of the electrode does interfere with operative manipulations, this technique can only be used for small tumors. Moller *et al.* recently described a technique for recording *electrical potentials from the lateral recess of the fourth ventricle,* from the direct vicinity of the *cochlear nucleus.*(22) Using this technique, they were able to obtain reproducible recordings after the averaging of only 250 responses. Thus an interpretable response could be obtained within 15 seconds, whereas the BAEP requires about 2 minutes. The value of these cochlear nucleus potentials in monitoring the eighth CN requires further study.

The value of neuromonitoring in hearing preservation was studied in a retrospective study by Harper *et al.*, who compared 84 monitored patients with 86 historical controls matched for tumor size and pre-operative hearing status. They found that for tumors smaller than 2 cm, BAEP monitoring was associated with a higher rate of hearing preservation and with a higher rate of useful hearing preservation (11) (Table 13.6).

Many investigators have shown that loss of waves I and V of the BAEP and wave N-1 of the ECOG during acoustic neuroma surgery correlates with the loss of any useful hearing(6, 11, 15). However, the loss of wave V alone with the preservation of wave I of the BAEP during operation may still be associated with the preservation of useful hearing in a number of patients. Strauss *et al.* found that the delayed and gradual deterioration of wave V during acoustic neuroma operations may be associated with the presence of hearing in the early postoperative period but with a delayed hearing loss over a period of a few days(34). They treated such patients with low-molecular weight dextran under

TABLE 13.6
Hearing Preservation in Monitored and Unmonitored Patients

Tumor Size	Any Hearing Preserved (%)		Useful Hearing Preserved (%)	
	Monitored ($n = 86$)	Unmonitored ($n = 86$)	Monitored	Unmonitored
All tumors	37	22	20	7
<1.1	79[b]	42[b]	47[b]	21[b]
1.1–2.0	52	25	26	4
2.1–3.0	7	15	4	4
>3.1	0	0		

[a]Reproduced with permission from (11).
[b]Statistically significant, $P < .05$

TABLE 13.7
Conservation of Gardener-Robertson Class I or II Hearing in a Series of Consecutive Patients with Similar Hearing Pre-operatively[a]

CP Angle Tumor Size CM	Pre-operative Class I and II Hearing	Postoperative Class I and II	% of patients with similar hearing pre- and postoperatively
< 0.9	17	7	41
1.0–1.9	21	6	29
2.0–2.9	17	5	29
3.0–3.9	10	2	20
> 4.0	2	0	0
Total	67	20	30

[a]Wright DC, *et al.,* unpublished data.

the assumption that the pathogenesis of this early type of delayed post-operative hearing loss was microvascular ischemia. Thus, many surgeons who perform acoustic neuromas operations with the goal of hearing preservation feel that intra-operative monitoring may not only be helpful in preserving hearing but also may help the surgeon to understand the mechanisms of hearing loss during operation(15, 20, 22, 26, 32; Samii M, personal communication, 1993). An example of this phenomenon, which has been used by a number of surgeons recently, is the application of papaverine on the cochlear nerve when the N-1 wave on ECOG is lost, in order to reverse the spasm of internal auditory artery. The senior author (LNS) has routinely utilized neuromonitoring during acoustic neuroma operations. The senior author's results with attempted hearing preservation (Wright DC, Sekhar LN, Uyar Y, *et al.* 1995) are shown in Table 13.7. Since we do not have a control group of patients without neuromonitoring, its value in preservation of hearing and facial function cannot be proved on the basis of our series.

MONITORING OF CNs X, XI, AND XII

Monitoring of the motor function of the vagus nerve is made possible by the insertion of electrodes into the false vocal cords under direct laryngoscopic vision, or by the recording of the adduction of the vocal cords by a specifically designed electrical acoustic device(4, 12, 16, 28). Such monitoring may be useful during the removal of tumors involving the jugular foramen, such as paragangliomas, schwannomas, and meningiomas.

Similarly, the activity of muscles innervated by CNs XI and XII, can be monitored by EMG electrodes placed in the trapezius or sternocleidomastoid muscles or in the tongue muscles. The monitoring of these nerves is very useful during the removal of tumors involving the lower clival-foramen magnum area.

COST EFFECTIVENESS

The approximate cost for intra-operative monitoring of one patient, including both technical and professional fees, is $1800. At this price, even if one patient is prevented from having a major neurologic deficit, the hospital cost reduction alone will make it worthwhile for 50 patients to be monitored. If one counts the patient's rehabilitation costs and loss of time at work, the benefits of intra-operative neuromonitoring far outweigh the costs involved.

CONCLUSIONS

Intra-operative neurophysiologic monitoring is here to stay. Future improvements of technique will allow neurophysiologists to monitor many brain and CN functions not reliably monitored at present. It is expected that such monitoring will become a routine part of all complex neurosurgical operations, despite the current pressure to reduce the cost of health care.

REFERENCES

1. Beck DL, Atkins JS Jr, Benecke JE Jr, *et al.:* Intraoperative facial nerve monitoring: Prognostic aspects during acoustic tumor removal. **Otolaryngol Head Neck Surg** 104:780–782, 1991.
2. Cedzich C, Schramm J, Menghedoht CF, *et al.:* Factors that limit the use of flash visual evoked potentials for surgical monitoring. **Electroencephalogh Clin Neurophysiol** 71:142–145, 1988.
3. Crosby G, Riedel CJR, Vera PL, *et al.:* Intraoperative monitoring and intraoperative angiography in aneurysm surgery. Poster presented at the Congress of Neurological Surgeons, 44th Annual Meeting, Chicago, 1994.
4. DeMonte F, Warf P, Al-Mefty O: Intraoperative monitoring of the lower cranial nerves during surgery of the jugular foramen and lower clivus, in Loftus CM,

Traynelis VC (eds): *Intraoperative Monitoring Techniques in Neurosurgery*. New York, McGraw-Hill, 1944, pp 205–212.

5. Feinsod M, Auerbach E, Selhorst JB, *et al.:* Monitoring of optic nerve function during craniotomy. **J Neurosurg** 44:29–31, 1976.

6. Fischer G, Fischer C, Remond J: Hearing preservation in acoustic neurinoma surgery. **J Neurosurg** 76:910–917, 1992.

7. Friedman WA, Chadwick GM, Verhoeven FJS, *et al.:* Monitoring of somatosensory evoked potentials during surgery for middle cerebral artery aneurysms. **Neurosurgery** 29:83–88, 1991.

8. Friedman WA, Kaplan BL, Day AL, *et al.:* Evoked potentials monitoring during aneurysm operation: Observations after fifty cases. **Neurosurgery** 20:678–687, 1987.

9. Gentili F, Lougheed WM, Yamashiro K, *et al.:* Monitoring of sensory evoked potentials during surgery of skull base tumors. **Can J Neurol Sci** 12:336–340, 1985.

10. Harner SG, Daube JR, Beatty CW, *et al.:* Intraoperative monitoring of the facial nerve. **Laryngoscopy** 98:209–212, 1988.

11. Harper CM, Harner SG, Slavit DA, *et al.:* Effect of BAEP monitoring on hearing preservation during acoustic neuroma resection. **Neurology** 42:1551–1553, 1992.

12. Hvidegaard T, Vase P, Dalsgaard SC, *et al.:* Endolaryngeal devices for perioperative identification and functional testing of the recurrent nerve. **Otolaryngol Head Neck Surg** 92:292–294, 1984.

13. Kwartler JA, Lunsford WM, Atkins J, *et al.:* Facial nerve monitoring in acoustic tumor surgery. **Otolaryngol Head Neck Surg** 10:814–817, 1991.

14. Leonetti JP, Brackmann DE, Prass RL: Improved preservation of facial nerve function in the infratemporal approach to the skull base. **Otolaryngol Head Neck Surg** 101:74–78, 1989.

15. Levine RA, Ronner SF, Ojemann RG: Auditory evoked potential and other neurophysiologic monitoring techniques during tumor surgery in the cerebellopontine angle, in Loftus CM, Traynelis VC (eds): *Intraoperative Monitoring Techniques in Neurosurgery*. New York, McGraw-Hill, 1944, pp 175–190.

16. Lipton RJ, McCaffrey TV, Litchy WJ: Intraoperative electrophysiologic monitoring of laryngeal muscle during thyroid surgery. **Laryngoscope** 98:1292–1296, 1988.

17. Little JR, Lesser RP, Luders H: Electrophysiological monitoring during basilar aneurysm operation. **Neurosurgery** 20:421–427, 1987.

18. Manninen PH, Patterson S, Lam AM, *et al.:* Evoked potential monitoring during posterior fossa aneurysm surgery: A comparison of two modalities. **Can J Anaesth** 41:92–97, 1994.

19. Moller AR: Intraoperative monitoring of evoked potentials: An update, in Wilkins RH, Rengachary SS (eds): *Neurosurgery Update I*. New York, McGraw-Hill, 1990, pp 169–176.

20. Moller AR, Jannetta PJ: Monitoring auditory functions during cranial nerve microvascular decompression operations by direct recording from the eighth nerve. **J Neurosurg** 59:493–499, 1983.

21. Moller AR, Jannetta PJ: Preservation of facial function during removal of acoustic neuromas. Use of monopolar constant voltage stimulation and EMG. **J Neurosurg** 61:757–760, 1984.

22. Moller AR, Jho HD, Jannetta PJ: Preservation of hearing in operations on acoustic tumors: An alternative to recording brain stem auditory evoked potentials. **Neurosurgery** 34:688–693, 1994.

23. Momma F, Wang AD, Symon L: Effects of temporary arterial occlusion on somatosensory evoked responses in aneurysm surgery. **Surg Neurol** 27:343–352, 1987.

24. Mooij JJA, Buchthal A, Belpavlovic M: Somatosensory evoked potential monitoring of temporary middle cerebral artery occlusion during aneurysm operations. **Neurosurgery** 21:492–496, 1987.
25. Niparko JK, Kileny PR, Kemink JL, *et al.:* Neurophysiologic intraoperative monitoring. II: Facial nerve function. **Am J Otol** 10:55–61, 1989.
26. Ojemann RG, Levine RA, Montgomery WM, *et al.:* Use of intraoperative auditory evoked potentials to preserve hearing in unilateral acoustic neuroma removal. **J Neurosurg** 61:938–948, 1984.
27. Prass RL, Kinney SE, Hardy RW, *et al.:* Acoustic (loudspeaker) facial EMG monitoring. II: Use of evoked EMG activity during acoustic neuroma resection. **Otolaryngol Head Neck Surg** 97:541–551, 1987.
28. Rice DH, Cove-Wesson B: Intraoperative recurrent laryngeal nerve monitoring. **Otolaryngol Head Neck Surg** 105:372–375, 1991.
29. Schramm J, Koht A, Schmidt G, *et al.:* Surgical and electrophysiological observations during clipping of 134 aneurysms with evoked potential monitoring. **Neurosurgery** 26:61–70, 1990.
30. Sekhar LN, Moller AR: Operative management of tumors involving the cavernous sinus. **J Neurosurg** 64:879–889, 1986.
31. Sekiya T, Hatayama T, Iwabuchi T, *et al.:* Intraoperative recordings of evoked extraocular muscle activities to monitor ocular muscle function. **Neurosurgery** 32:227–235, 1993.
32. Silverstein H, Norrell H, Hyman S: Simultaneous use of CO_2 laser with continuous monitoring of eighth nerve action potential during acoustic neuroma surgery. **Otolaryngol Head Neck Surg** 92:80–84, 1984.
33. Silverstein H, Smouha E, Jones R: Routine identification of the facial nerve using electrical stimulation during otological and neurotological surgery. **Laryngoscope** 98:726–730, 1988.
34. Strauss C, Fahlbusch R, Komstock J, *et al.:* Delayed hearing loss after surgery for acoustic neurinomas: Clinical and electrophysiological observations. **Neurosurgery** 28:559–565, 1991.
35. Strauss G, Fahlbusch R, Nimsky C, *et al.:* Monitoring of visual evoked potentials during para and suprasellar procedures, in Loftus CM, Traynelis VC (eds): *Intraoperative Monitoring Techniques in Neurosurgery.* New York, McGraw-Hill, 1994, pp 135–140.
36. Symon L, Wang AD, Costa E, *et al.:* Perioperative use of somatosensory evoked potentials in aneurysm surgery. **J Neurosurg** 60:269–275, 1984.
37. Wilson CB, Kirsch WM, Neville H, *et al.:* Monitoring of visual function during parasellar surgery. **Surg Neurol** 5:323–329, 1976.

14

Intra-operative Monitoring Is Not Essential

LEONARD I. MALIS M.D., F.A.C.S.

In an era when many articles say that monitoring is an absolute requisite, and even standards promulgated by national consensus committees recommend that monitoring be routinely used for many things in operative surgery, I have completely given up the use of many types of electrophysiologic monitoring intraoperatively. I refer specifically to somatosensory evoked potential monitoring, auditory evoked response monitoring, visual evoked response monitoring, or facial nerve stimulation. I have given these up because I have found that with proper surgical techniques, monitoring produced no improvement in the end results and merely increased the length of time and cost of the surgery.

Certain types of monitoring, I always carry out. I monitor EKG, blood pressure, expiratory CO_2, blood gases, and core temperature. With the patient in the sitting position or semisitting position, I also monitor the central venous pressure, and the right atrial doppler listens for possible air embolism.

I use somatosensory evoked potentials during positioning and preparation of the patient. Older arthritic patients with some cervical stenosis are at risk for quadriplegia due to hyperextension with muscle relaxants under anesthesia. This can occur during intubation or during the positioning of the patient. The somatosensory evoked potential is recorded prior to any manipulation of the patient's neck, and latency increase in the somatosensory evoked potential must be avoided. Young patients with normal cervical spines are at risk for quadriplegia in hyperflexion with muscle relaxants under anesthesia. The cord there is stretched across the vertebral bodies, with possible compression of the anterior spinal artery, as well as the rest of the cord. This situation is different from the hyperextension injury in the cervical stenotic patient, in which the cord is compressed between the lower edge of the upper vertebral body and the anterior margin of the laminar arch of the vertebra below(6). In either case, avoiding increase in latency of the somatosensory evoked potential during anesthesia positioning and final arrangement for surgery gives the protection, and then the somatosensory evoked potential equipment may be disconnected.

I have a long experience with evoked potentials, having published my first article on somatosensory evoked potentials in 1953(7). My first article on the visual evoked potentials was published in 1956 (Fig. 14.1) and many other electrophysiologic articles were published in later years as well. From 1950 to 1967, probably two-thirds of my time was spent in the electrophysiologic laboratory, rather than in the neurosurgical operating room, with my shift to full-time surgery occurring as part of the microsurgical revolution. By 1975 I had transferred much of my electrophysiologic laboratory equipment to the operating room and had added considerable additional equipment (Fig. 14-2). This move permitted as complete a monitoring system as was feasible in that era, with reasonable computer control and recording quality quite

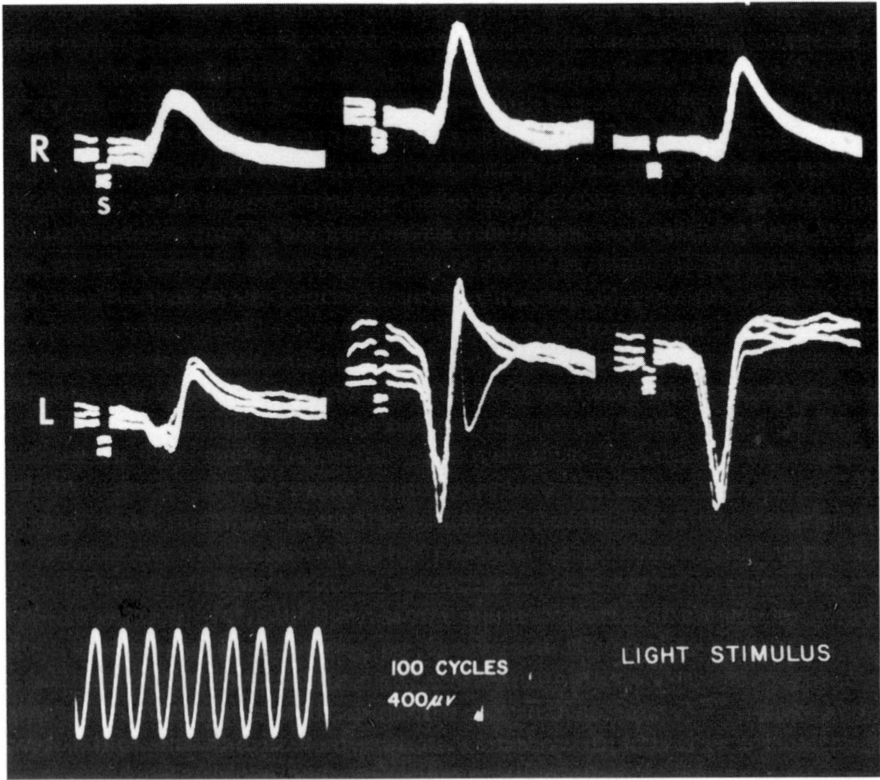

FIG.14.1 Multiple traces of direct cortical recordings of mapping of visual evoked responses. Circa 1955.

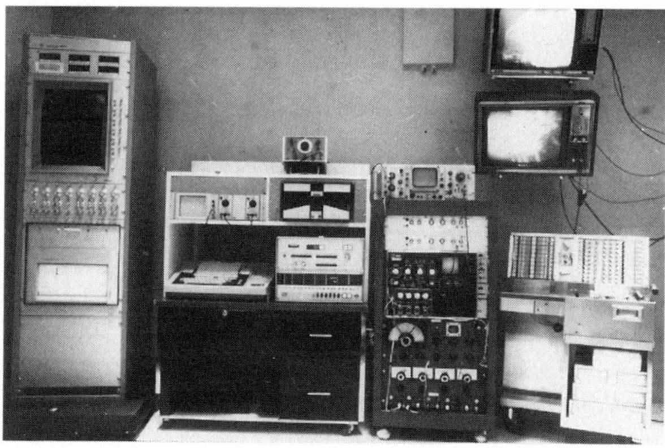

FIG.14.2 The electrophysiologic monitoring system at the author's Mount Sinai operating room in 1973.

comparable to that achieved today. As an example, a recording electrode was placed on the surface of the cerebellar retractor (Fig. 14.3) for acoustic neuroma surgery, demonstrating the difference in the recording achieved with the electrode on the brain, as compared to the electrode on the ear with brain recording providing increased amplitude and improved resolution, thus shortening the number of sweeps required for adequate tracings.

Through the years it had become increasingly obvious that the microsurgical techniques that neurosurgeons were using appeared to make the monitoring technology unnecessary. Microtechnique is a completely visual approach, subarachnoid and transfissural, and totally hemostatic. Self-retaining retractors are used with dual instrumentation and sharp anatomic division, with the principle of never being out of sight and never being out of light. The microscope provides stereoscopic vision and light through a small aperture, as well as providing magnification. Mayfield's law was followed strictly, that is to say, "Remove the tumor from the brain, not the brain from the tumor." Accordingly, it is necessary to first core and collapse all tumors, except hemangiomas. Hemangiomas are collapsed by stroking their surface with low-powered blunt bipolar coagulation so that they shrink down to a smaller size and can be removed in one piece, unlike any other tumor (3). In working in the parasagittal area, the principle that any one vein can be taken (except the vein of Labbé) but never two adjacent veins prevented postoperative complications of venous infarction.

A number of rules of perioperative care help in the handling of brain tissue (5). All patients are given dexamethasone prior to and during

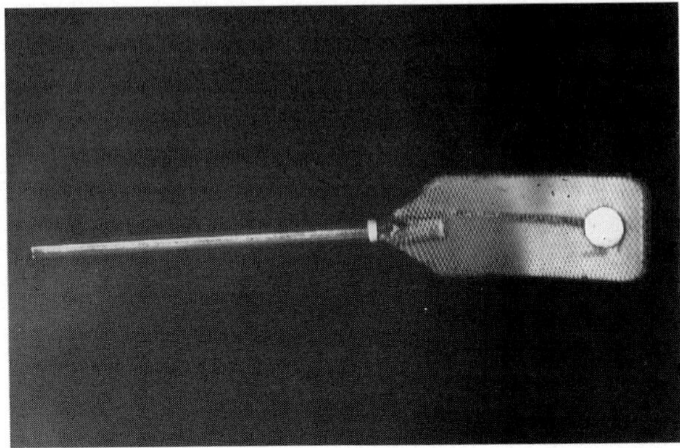

FIG.14.3 Insulated self-retaining brain retractor carrying an electrode for evoked potential direct brain recording.

the surgery. Propranolol is used in dosages of 200 mg in the 24 hours prior to surgery to prevent renin release that occurs after administration of nitroprusside, which I routinely use intraoperatively as a hypotensive agent to maintain the systolic pressure at 80 mm. This degree of hypotension makes the dissection of vessels on the surface of, or in relation to, tumors far easier since they are soft and slack, rather than tense and tight. It also makes control of any possible bleeding much easier.

I use urea for dehydration, administering 80 g during induction of anesthesia. I prefer using urea to using mannitol, because urea permits the use of much less fluid intake for the same degree of diuresis. Since dehydration is the desired result, it is essential that the anesthesiologist not attempt to replace the fluid that we so carefully had caused the patient to excrete. Essentially, 100% prevention of infection is achieved with the antibiotic protocol, which I had described in 1979 and which still remains virtually totally effective (2). All patients, except in emergencies, are stopped from taking any aspirin for 10 days prior to the surgery, and no aspirin or heparin is used in the operating room or recovery unit.

Perhaps the most important requirement for maintenance of function and good end results is the avoidance of retraction. The use of dexamethasone, dehydration, and controlled hypertension has already been mentioned. I had also stated that blood gases are monitored throughout and that adequate oxygenation and prevention of CO_2 buildup helps to prevent edema. Head positioning, nearly always above the heart level, whether the patient is supine, lateral, or semisitting, reduced venous pressure. Venous restriction by positioning with marked rotation is avoided. All patients are respirated mechanically under deep curarization. The prone position where the body is lifted with each respiratory movement is never used, even in laminectomies, for which I use the 45° oblique position.

The bone opening is always designed to permit the exposure with the least manipulation of brain. For example, in approaches to the cerebellopontine angle, I always take off the mastoid almost to the labyrinth, across the entire sigmoid sinus to the flat of the petrous (Fig. 14.4), to avoid the need for retracting or resecting cerebellum in order to achieve a straight approach to the petrous surface.

For me, one of the most important requirements is that the retractor should never press with more than 20 torr to prevent compression of venous return and subsequent subcortical necrosis. In order to ensure that this is essentially automatic, retractor blades made of stainless steel, which are thinned to a degree that permits a pressure of 20 torr but which bend backwards if that pressure is exceeded, are used throughout. These blades are securely mounted to the head so that

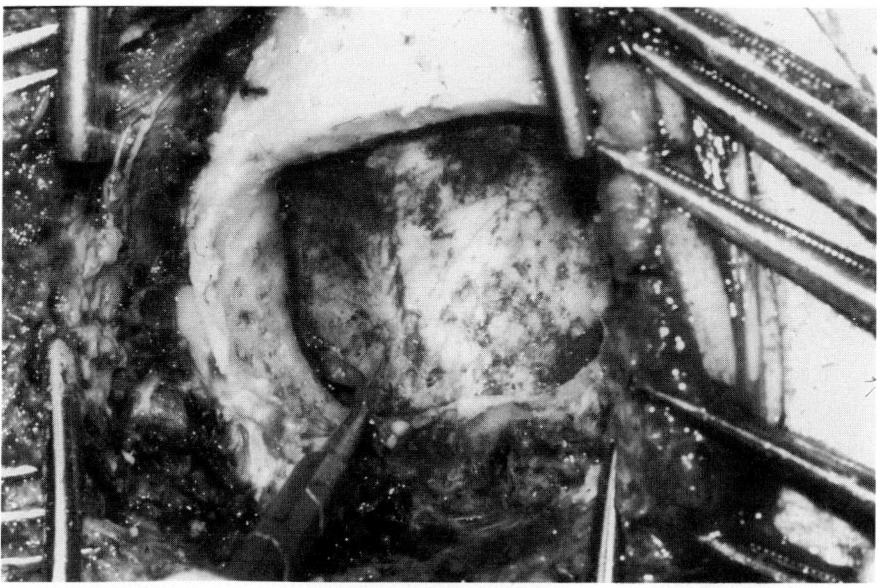

FIG.14.4 Left-sided suboccipital craniectomy with removal of mastoid process and bone removal completely across the sigmoid sinus. The dissecting instrument is seen with its tip on the flat of the petrous surface, with all of the covering bone resected. The dura has not yet been opened.

they can not be suddenly displaced by a movement of a clamp or external device and certainly are never handheld (Fig. 14.5). Wide opening of arachnoid membranes in the operative field, including opening of fissures and cisterns, permits brain structures to separate without pressure and drains cerebrospinal fluid sufficiently, supplemented by dehydration, to provide adequate exposure. I do not use spinal or ventricular drainage.

The preservation of facial nerve and auditory nerve function in the total removal of acoustic neuromas has been repeatedly cited as a reason for essential use of monitoring. In the posterior approach to these tumors, which I do with the patient in the semisitting position, coring of the tumor permits the medial capsule to be progressively drawn laterally, without retraction, thus avoiding stretching of the auditory fibers. The auditory nerve, as part of the central nervous system, has no healing or regenerative capacity, which is compounded by the fragility of the cochlear connections, which do not recover at all from injury. Retraction of the auditory nerve from lateral to medial destroys the fine cochlea attachments, no matter how much slack there is in the nerve medially.

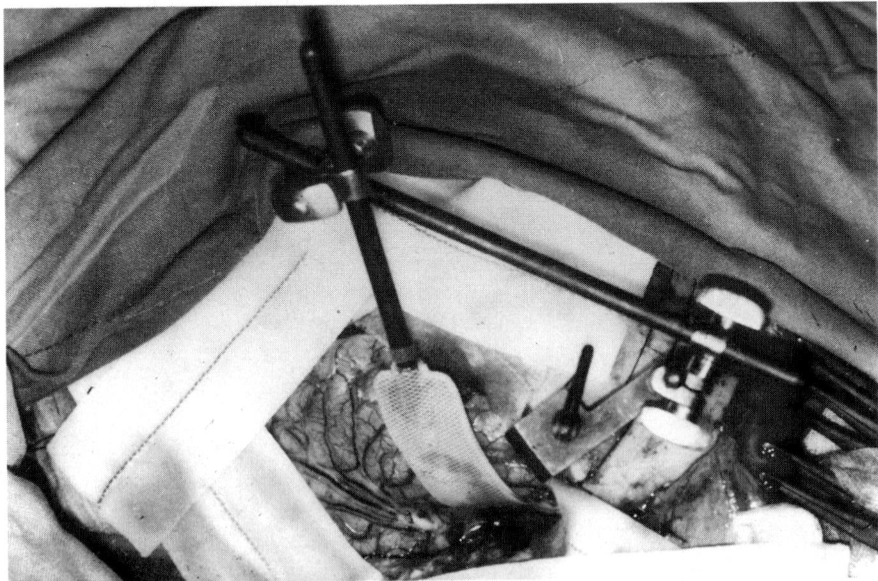

FIG.14.5 Self-retaining retractor clamped to the margin of craniotomy, supporting the right posterior frontal area from the floor of the frontal lobe. The retractor is thin so it cannot support more than a pressure of 20 torr.

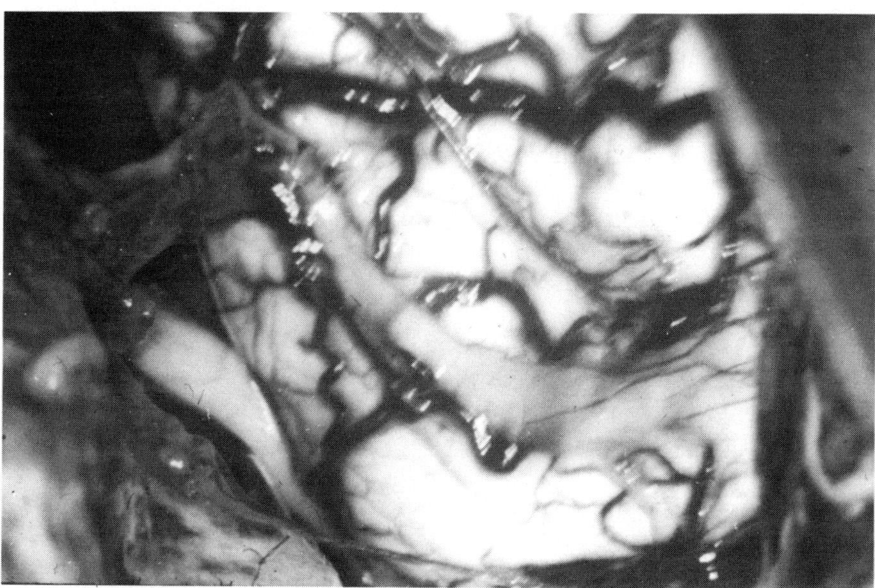

FIG.14.6 A large left acoustic neuroma has been removed. The facial nerve curves across the field from right to left, going upward and then turning downward laterally on the brainstem. The tan color of the facial nerve is obvious in the original color photograph, but in black and white it appears only as a darker area than the white of the brainstem and a darker area than the white of the sixth nerve seen to the *lower left* of the field. Photographic field diameter is 2.5 cm.

The facial nerve may be displaced by the neuroma in many directions but almost always is anterior to the tumor, which arises in 90% or more of my cases from the superior vestibular nerve. The auditory nerve tends to be displaced downward and somewhat anterior, with the inferior vestibular components posterior to it. The facial nerve is readily recognizable, because it has a tan color, as compared to the whiteness of the brainstem or the whiteness of the sixth nerve or the auditory or vestibular nerves, and color can guide one in the dissection (Fig. 14.6). After coring the tumor sufficiently, displacement of the medial capsule laterally permits the visualization of the eighth nerve just anterior to the flocculus, with the nerve emerging just above the lateral recess. The facial nerve comes up from just inferior and anterior to the lateral recess in relation to the choroid plexus and lies on the anterior surface of the eighth nerve, providing anatomical identification.

After the canal wall is drilled away, the vestibular nerves lie posteriorly, superiorly and inferiorly, while the facial nerve is anterior and enters the facial canal above the crista. The auditory nerve lies on the anterior inferior surface of the canal and enters the cochlear area inferior to the crista. Finding and following the facial nerve anatomically has for me meant just using a higher magnification if it is difficult to visualize. I usually work in this area at a magnification such that the total viewed field of the microscope is between 1.5 and 2.5 cm in diameter.

I have not found it necessary or advisable to use the facial nerve stimulator to identify the facial nerve, because its anatomic aspect, has been reasonably ascertainable. Additionally, since I keep my patients deeply curarized to maintain total control of respiration mechanically, stimulation to produce a muscle response is virtually impossible at any safe level that will not damage the delicate neural structures. In the last 500 consecutive acoustic neuroma removals (all total), the facial nerve functional saving has been 96% for tumors of 3 cm in CT diameter or less (4).

In the late 1970s I used auditory evoked response to possibly aid in hearing preservation. This too I abandoned when I found that in a consecutive series of approximately 50 patients it made no difference in the end result for preserved hearing, whether I was told the result of the evoked potential determinations or whether these were kept as a private matter for the recording physiologist (8). I have already mentioned the importance of avoiding retraction, particularly laterally to medially, because of the delicacy of the fine auditory fibers entering the cochlea.

The drilling away of the posterior wall of the internal auditory canal is done under continuous irrigation, making certain that the chalky white appearance that occurs when the bone is heated is avoided. Measurement on a bone window CT scan will show the position of the vestibule and of the jugular bulb which occasionally, though fortunately rarely, may extend upward quite high. The particular requirement is an exact measurement of the distance to the vestibule from the posterior edge of the internal auditory meatus, so that drilling in a patient who still has hearing can be limited to the maximal distance possible without entering the vestibule. This distance will be, on average, 10 mm, but in some patients it is only 7 mm, and in others it may be 12 mm. Since it is essential to remove whatever portion of tumor may lie in the distal end of the canal, the drilling should be as far as possible. If there is no hearing, this is not limited. To preserve hearing, however, the vestibule must be avoided. There may then be, approximately, a 2-mm lip of posterior canal wall, anterior to which may be a bit of tumor lying against the crista. This may be removed with the aid of a dental mirror and back-angled canal knives (Fig. 14.7). When dur-

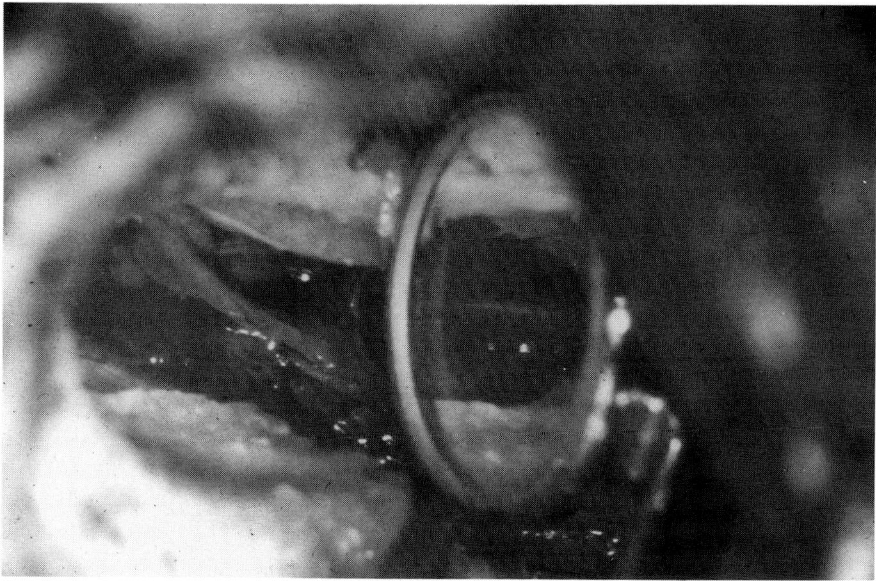

FIG.14.7 A left acoustic neuroma removal has been completed. The drilled-out posterior wall of the canal does not go all the way to the vestibule, but the dental mirror permits removal of the most distal lateral tumor and shows the crista going horizontally across the field seen in the mirror view. Photographic field diameter is 2.5 cm.

ing this part of the procedure, traction is made on the cochlear fibers, the cochlear evoked potential will drop precipitously. On the other hand, there should be no traction made. Avoidance of brainstem damage in the course of acoustic neuroma removal has been achieved both by avoidance of retraction and preservation anatomically of the branches of the anterior inferior cerebellar artery, as well as any branches of the posterior inferior cerebellar artery or superior cerebellar artery, which may be related to the tumor. When dissection of these vessels is carried out without injury, there will be no evidence of brainstem abnormality to be picked up on an evoked potential. Again, this is part of a microsurgical technique for working in the angle.

It is of interest that hearing preservation, which I have only been able to achieve in approximately half of the patients who have satisfactory hearing preoperatively, appears to be most at risk during the work in the auditory canal. I base this inference on the fact that in my series of more than 100 meningiomas of the cerebellar pontine angle, hearing preservation has been possible in more than 90% of those patients who still had satisfactory hearing, and in these cases the tumors, as a rule, did not enter the internal auditory canal. I personally believe that the greater loss occurring in the acoustic neuroma patients is due to the intermingling of blood supply between the acoustic neuroma and the auditory and facial nerves, as compared to the meningioma patient, in whom the blood supply is mainly of dural origin and does not involve the cochlear nerve. In any case, every effort is made to spare all vascular supply leading to any neural structure.

In laminectomies for the removal of spinal cord tumors the removal of the laminar arches without putting any instrument between the laminar arch and the dura avoids cord compression and damage. A laminectomy carried out to the full width of the posterior surface, reaching to the pedicles, makes cord retraction much less necessary. I prefer to sew the dura to the muscles over the cut edges of the lamina, because this produces a wider retraction of the dura than stay sutures or clamps. I have always performed midline myelotomy for intramedullary cord tumors with razor blade sharp dissection in order to preserve the fine vessels running down the raphe from the posterior surface of the cord (Fig. 14.8). The use of laser dissection to open the

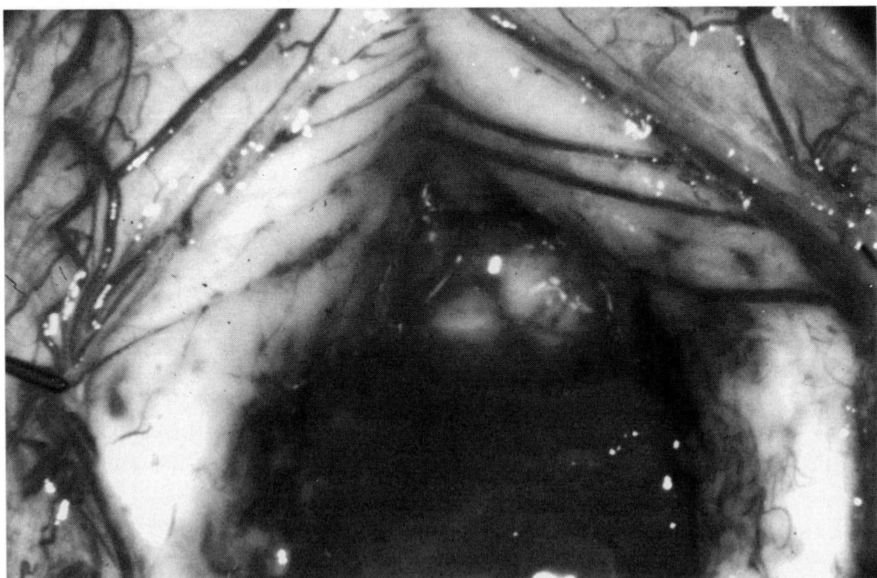

FIG.14.8 Midline myelotomy of the cervical spinal cord reveals a deep ependymoma about to be removed. At the left edge of the myelotomy, the loop of the 8-0 suture retracting the pia can be seen. Most importantly, the preservation of the vessels of the midline raphe going down through the myelotomy can be seen. Photographic field diameter is 1.5 cm.

raphe cannot preserve these microvascular connections. Microsutures from the midline pia to the dura hold the cord open without the need for retraction. Cutting of multiple dentate ligaments permits rotation of the cord, often facilitated by placing traction sutures in the dentate ligaments, which facilitates the atraumatic approach to the ventral lateral surfaces (1).

Finally, the need for meticulous hemostasis most often carried out under irrigation with the lowest possible powers of the bipolar coagulator is a requisite because, obviously, microdissection cannot be carried out with any safety in a bloody field. To summarize, I strongly believe that the use of the basic principles of meticulous microsurgical technique obviates the needs for electrophysiologic monitoring. Monitoring has the same place as training wheels on a bicycle; they are of considerable use for the learning youngster, yet perhaps are a detriment to the skilled bicyclist because of increase in time expended and in cost.

REFERENCES

1. Malis LI: Intramedullary spinal cord tumors, **Clin Neurosurg** 25:512–539, 1978.
2. Malis LI: Prevention of neurosurgical infection by intraoperative antibiotics. **Neurosurgery** 5(3):339–343, 1979.
3. Malis LI: Spinal cord tumors, in Davidoff R (ed): *Handbook of the Spinal Cord.* New York, Marcel Dekker, 1986, vol 11, pp 319–369.
4. Malis LI: Acoustic tumor, in Pillsbury HC, Goldsmith MM (eds): *Operative Challenges in Otolaryngology/Head and Neck Surgery.* Chicago, Yearbook Publishers, 1989, vol 6, pp 77–91.
5. Malis LI: Tentorial, torcular and paratorcular meningiomas, in Appuzzo M (ed): *Brain Surgery: Complication Avoidance and Management.* New York, Churchill Livingstone, 1992, vol 1, chap 13, pp 231–247.
6. Malis LI: Cervical spinal cord compression and anteroposterior diameter. **Mt Sinai J Med** 61(3):218–223, 1994.
7. Malis LI, Pribram KH, Kruger L: Action potentials of motor cortex evoked by peripheral nerve stimulation. **J Neurophysiol** 16:161–167, 1953.
8. Zappulla RA, Greenblatt ER, Kay S, et al: A quantitative assessment of the brainstem auditory evoked response during intraoperative monitoring. **Neurosurgery** 15:186–190, 1984.

III

General Scientific
Session III—Controversies
in the Management of
Cerebrovascular Malformations

15

Natural History of Giant Intracranial Aneurysms and Indications for Intervention

DANIEL L. BARROW, M.D., AND CARGILL ALLEYNE, M.D.

In 1969, Morley and Barr (59) and Bull (15) reported the first clinical series of giant intracranial aneurysms. A giant aneurysm was defined as a sac greater than 2.5 cm in largest diameter, a somewhat arbitrary designation chosen to conform to the subset of largest aneurysms in the Cooperative Study of Intracranial Aneurysms and Subarachnoid Hemorrhage (53). This simple definition of a giant aneurysm has established this lesion as a specific clinicopathologic entity justified by its unique clinical presentation, natural history, and therapeutic challenges. This distinction is only partially justified as many complex aneurysms less than 2.5 cm in size will threaten the patient with risks of hemorrhage or mass effect and present the neurosurgeon with similar technical challenges and potential for intra-operative misadventure. In general, however, these larger sacs present a distinctive clinical picture and unique therapeutic obstacles.

PATHOGENESIS

Giant aneurysms can be subdivided into saccular and fusiform aneurysms, with the saccular variety far more common. These represent two distinct etiopathologic entities. The predisposing factors leading to the development of giant saccular aneurysms are the same as those for smaller saccular aneurysms, that is, congenital or acquired defects in the vessel wall, perhaps with hypertension as a risk factor. The giant saccular aneurysm is presumed to develop from an initially smaller saccular aneurysm and undergoes progressive enlargement. Once the sac is formed, both the neck and body undergo enlargement. Hydrodynamic studies have suggested that injury to the endothelium from turbulence results in platelet aggregation and fibrin deposition (23). The intraluminal events in a giant aneurysm are dynamic, with accumulations and dissipation of platelets and fibrin-thrombus debris in an irregular fashion.

EPIDEMIOLOGY

The accumulation of a number of clinical series has allowed for determination of many epidemiologic characteristics of giant aneurysms. Some epidemiologic differences from smaller berry aneurysms seem to justify the separate clinical entity of giant aneurysms. In various clinical and autopsy series, the percentage of total aneurysms that are giant ranges from 3 to 13% (27, 41, 53, 54, 57, 59, 62, 69, 86, 89, 104), the higher number no doubt reflecting a referral bias. One of the largest series to date is a report of 1400 intracranial aneurysms from Germany, which identified 58 giant aneurysms, yielding an incidence of 4.1% (32). McCormick and Acosta-Rua (57) identified 9 giant aneurysms from a total of 191 aneurysms (4.7%) in 136 patients from a series of 1673 autopsies. The aggregate incidence of giant aneurysms from three autopsy and six large clinical series is 5.2% (Table 15.1).

Age and Gender

Giant aneurysms more commonly occur in females and usually come to clinical attention in the middle decades of life. The ratio of female:male occurrence ranges from 1:1 (62, 94) to 3:1 (40, 104). In a review of the world literature, Fox found that 60% of 693 giant aneurysms occurred in females. This predilection for females varies with aneurysm location from 73% females for internal carotid aneurysms to 52% for anterior communicating and basilar artery aneurysms (26). In a compilation of 754 patients with giant aneurysms from 14 series in which gender is identified, Anson found 461 females and 295 males (1.56:1) (5).

TABLE 15.1
Incidence of Giant Aneurysms

Author	Yr	Total No. of Aneurysms	Giant Aneurysms	% Giant Aneurysms
Stehbens[a]	1954	128	8[b]	6.2
Housepian and Pool[a]	1958	113	5	4.4
McCormick[a]	1970	191[c]	9	4.7
Morley and Barr	1969	658	28	4.3
Onuma and Suzuki	1979	1080	38	3.0
Sundt & Piepgras	1979	594	80	13.0
Pia	1980	522	19	3.6
Whittle *et al.*	1984	338	25	7.4
Hamburger *et al.*	1992	1400	58	4.1
Total		5024	264	5.2%

[a]Autopsy series.
[b]Defined as > 3 cm.
[c]Out of 136 patients.

Giant saccular aneurysms most commonly come to clinical attention during the 5th and 6th decades of life (1, 15, 22, 32, 37, 39, 59, 62, 69, 74, 80, 83, 91, 95). Anson (4) determined the age at presentation from an aggregate of 415 patients from eight clinical series (1, 15, 22, 39, 59, 74, 80, 83, 104). Ages ranged from 6 months to 76 years, with 286 (67%) presenting between ages 40 and 70 (Fig. 15.1). Fox's (26) analysis of 693 giant aneurysms reported in the world literature revealed a similar distribution, with median presentation in the 6th decade of life. This peak age at presentation is about a decade later than for nongiant berry aneurysms in adults (26).

Although more rare, giant fusiform and dolichoectatic aneurysms probably present at a slightly younger age (5, 51, 92). In three series of giant nonsaccular aneurysms, the mean age at presentation was 38, 43, and 49 years (5, 51, 92). There is a male predominance of approximately 1.5:1 for giant fusiform and dolichoectatic aneurysms (5, 51, 92).

Aneurysms are rare in children, with only 1 to 2% of all intracranial aneurysms occurring in the pediatric age group. Giant aneurysms, however, constitute a much higher proportion of aneurysms in children, are more common in males, and present less commonly with hemorrhage (3, 22, 25, 26, 48, 63, 65, 93). Fox (26) analyzed the reports of patients 19 years of age and younger and found 93 giant aneurysms among 486 aneurysms (19.9%) in this age group.

In a review of 72 cases of intracranial aneurysms in children under 5 years of age, Ferrante *et al.* (25) found that 27% had giant aneurysms. Fifty percent of the remainder had aneurysms of 1 to 2.5 cm, and only 23% of the aneurysms were less than 1 cm in size.

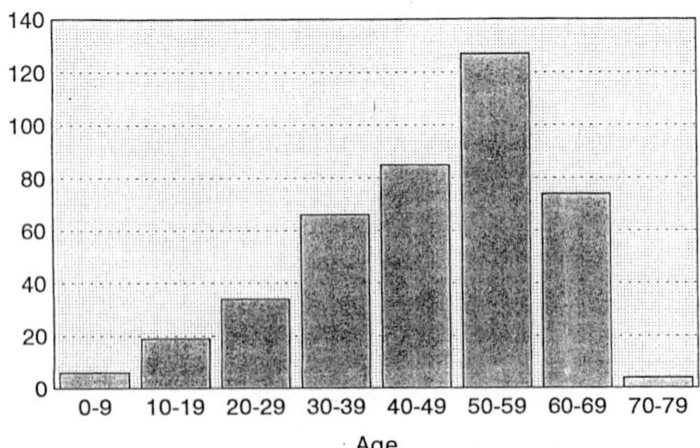

FIG 15.1 Age by decade of 415 patients with giant aneurysms. [Data compiled from (15, 22, 39, 59, 74, 80 83).]

Location

Giant aneurysms have a predilection for the same anatomic sites as smaller aneurysms, but the distribution is different (Table 15.2). The fact that giant intracranial aneurysms occur in the same locations as smaller saccular aneurysms supports the contention that giant aneurysms simply arise from small sacs. Like smaller berry aneurysms, the internal carotid artery is the most common site, but giant aneurysms occur proportionately more frequently on the vertebrobasilar system and less frequently on the anterior communicating complex (1, 26, 54, 102). In this review of the world literature, Fox (26) identified 693 giant aneurysms, with 54% on the internal carotid artery (21% on the cavernous segment and 18% on the paraclinoid segment), 23% on the vertebrobasilar system, 10% on the anterior cerebral artery/anterior communicating complex, 9% on the middle cerebral artery, and 4% located on minor or distal intracranial arteries. Anson (4) has added the results of several series published since Fox's 1983 publication, and their location frequencies are outlined in Table 15.3.

Giant fusiform and dolichoectatic aneurysms have a predilection for the vertebrobasilar circulation and the middle cerebral artery (1, 5, 34, 51, 78, 86, 92). The so-called giant serpentine aneurysms are often massive, partially thrombosed lesions, through which run a serpentine channel, and they are usually found on the middle cerebral artery (30, 31, 47, 78, 92).

It is important to note the incidence of cavernous carotid segment aneurysms in any series when considering natural history and treatment because of the distinctly different natural course of these extradural lesions, a factor that will be discussed in further detail.

Multiplicity

Whittle *et al.* (104) found that 9 (36%) of 25 patients with a giant intracranial aneurysm harbored multiple aneurysms. The additional aneurysms (one in eight patients, and two in one patient) were all less than 1.5 cm in diameter. Most other studies have reported a much lower rate of multiplicity with giant intracranial aneurysms. Multiple aneurysms were found in 12% of the cases of giant intracranial aneurysms in the Italian Cooperative Study on Giant Intracranial Aneurysms (11). Fox (26) found 38 cases of 693 in which multiple aneurysms were found (140 total). Fifteen of the 38 cases were cases that involved two giant intracranial aneurysms.

CLINICAL PRESENTATION

Giant intracranial aneurysms may come to clinical attention in a variety of ways, including via hemorrhage, as a result of their mass ef-

TABLE 15.2
Location of Giant Aneurysms[a]

Author	Yr	Total No. of Giant Aneurysms	ICA[b]	MCA	ACA-ACoA	VB
Fox (World Literature)	1983	693[c]	375	63	71	155
Whittle *et al.*	1984	25	8	11	1	5
Rosta *et al.*	1988	128	71	32	16	9
Doran	1990	13	7	0	3	3
Vorkapic *et al.*	1991	56	37	6	2	11
Symon	1992	64	30	11	7	16
Hamburger *et al.*	1992	58	25	16	8	9
Italian Cooperative	1988	130	71 (27 cavernous)	33	17	9
Total		1167	624 (53%)	156 (13%)	125 (11%)	217 (19%)

[a]Adapted from (4).
[b]ICA, internal carotid artery; MCA, middle cerebral artery, ACA-ACoA, anterior cerebral artery-anterior communicating artery; VB, vertebrobasilar artery.
[c]Includes 29 giant aneurysms on minor arteries not included in distribution.

TABLE 15.3

Twenty-Six Giant Aneurysms Managed from 1993 to mid-1994 at Emory University Hospital

Location	No. of Aneurysms (26 Total)
Internal carotid artery—extradural	5
Internal carotid artery—intradural	8
Middle cerebral artery	3
Anterior communicating artery	1
Vertebral artery-posterior inferior cerebellar artery	4
Midbasilar	3
Basilar tip	2

fects and distortion of surrounding anatomy, through thromboembolic events, or by producing seizures. Although unusual, a giant aneurysm occasionally remains clinically silent and is discovered incidentally in a patient undergoing diagnostic imaging studies for unrelated reasons.

The duration of symptoms in patients presenting with giant intracranial aneurysms is variable. A disproportionately high number of giant aneurysms have been discovered in patients with symptoms for more than 5 years (43, 53).

Hemorrhage

SUBARACHNOID HEMORRHAGE

There are very few studies in the literature that support the notion that giant intracranial aneurysms rupture infrequently (42). In fact, most studies show that subarachnoid hemorrhage is not at all uncommon and is the presenting symptom in 24 to 80% of patients (22, 32, 39, 53, 59, 62, 101).

Giant aneurysms occasionally present with a remote history of subarachnoid hemorrhage (up to 53% in some series) (66). Giant intracranial aneurysms of the cavernous portion of the internal carotid artery are less likely to present with subarachnoid hemorrhage than giant aneurysms located in other regions. They can produce a subarachnoid hemorrhage, however, if they partially extend through the dura. This feature of infrequent rupture confers an element of benignity to the natural history of intracavernous giant aneurysms. Symon and Vadja (96) have found a slightly increased incidence of basilar and carotid-ophthalmic aneurysms presenting with subarachnoid hemorrhage. The Italian Cooperative Study on Giant Intracranial Aneurysms (73) found that subarachnoid hemorrhage was more common in aneurysms of the anterior communicating artery (85% of cases) and of the internal carotid bifurcation (75% of cases).

INTRACEREBRAL HEMORRHAGE

As with other aneurysms, giant sacs may produce an intracerebral hemorrhage, either entirely or in association with subarachnoid hemorrhage. An intracerebral hemorrhage may acutely exacerbate the underlying mass effect of a giant aneurysm. This presentation is most commonly associated with middle cerebral artery aneurysms (Fig. 15.2).

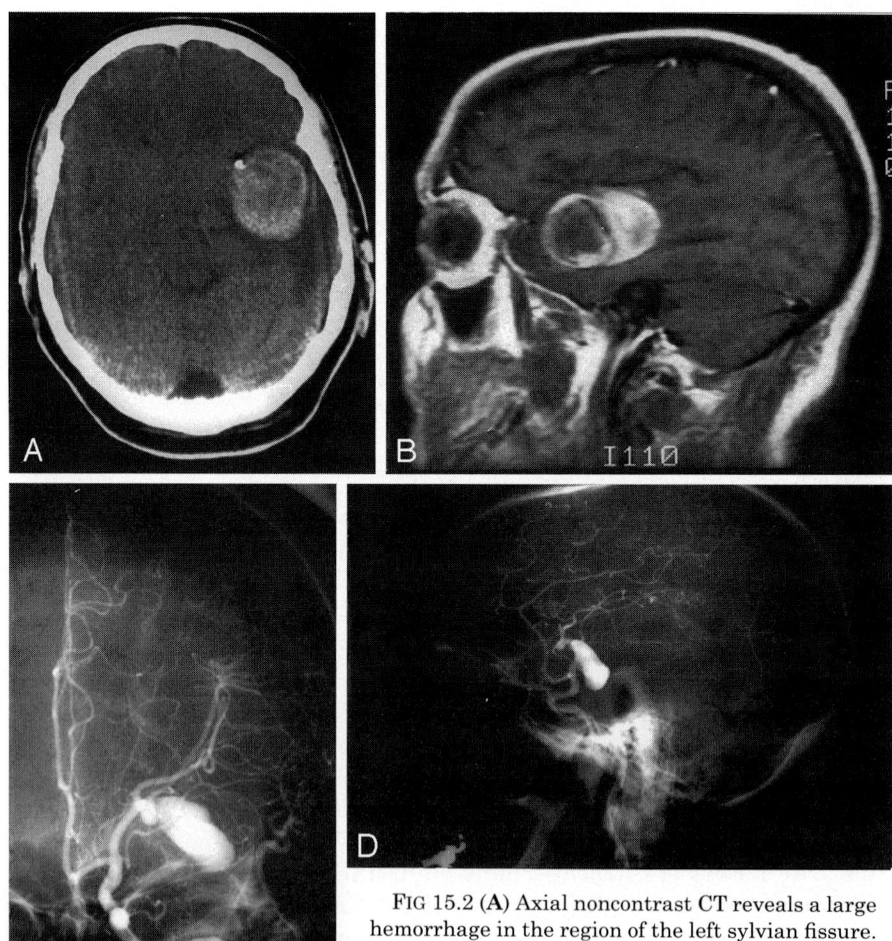

FIG 15.2 **(A)** Axial noncontrast CT reveals a large hemorrhage in the region of the left sylvian fissure. **(B)** Sagittal MRI confirms presence of partially thrombosed aneurysm with surrounding hematoma. **(C)** AP and **(D)** lateral left carotid angiograms show the patent portion of this giant middle cerebral artery aneurysm.

EPISTAXIS AND CAROTID-CAVERNOUS FISTULA

Giant intracranial aneurysms that involve the intracavernous portion of the carotid artery may potentially present with epistaxis from rupture into the sphenoid sinus. This presentation is more common with traumatic aneurysms. Giant intracavernous aneurysms also have the potential to produce a high-flow carotid fistula with rupture into the cavernous sinus, but this is more common with smaller aneurysms (59).

Mass Effect

By definition, giant intracranial aneurysms occupy more space than conventional aneurysms, and thus, are much more likely to present with symptoms of local compression. In fact, the literature is replete with reports of giant aneurysms simulating intracranial tumors, both clinically and radiographically (16, 20, 81, 82). Many of these reports have identified giant aneurysms in the posterior circulation (Fig. 15.3).

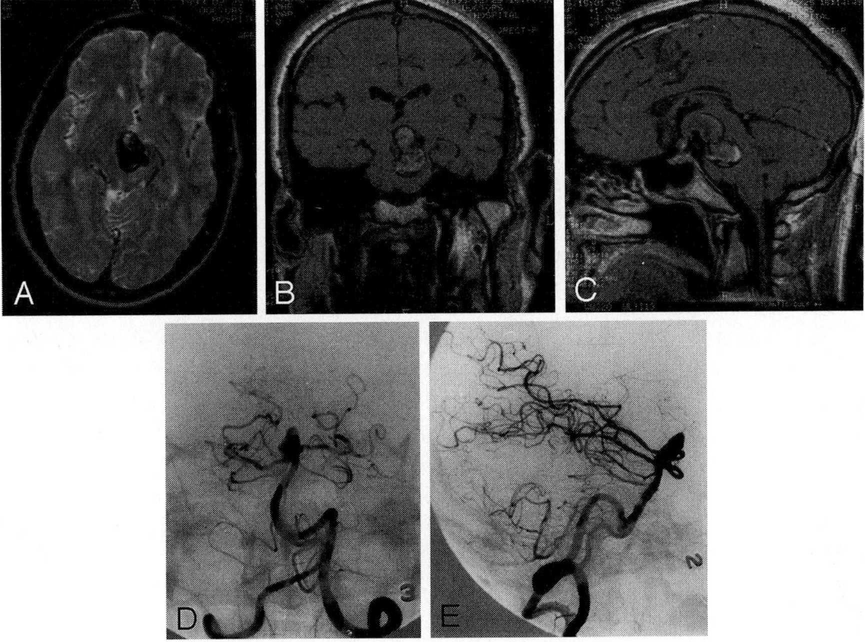

FIG 15.3 Axial (**A**) coronal (**B**), and sagittal (**C**) MRI from a 55-year-old man, who presented with a progressive left hemiparesis and right oculomotor palsy. This lesion proved to be a giant, partially thrombosed aneurysm, as seen on AP (**D**) and lateral vertebral angiography (**E**).

CRANIAL NEUROPATHY

A variety of cranial neuropathies may result from giant aneurysms. Given the unique anatomic aspects of cavernous carotid aneurysms, they are more likely to present with dysfunction of the cranial nerves traversing the cavernous sinus (III, IV, V_1, V_2 and VI). Carotid ophthalmic (paraclinoid) aneurysms are particularly prone to present with optic neuropathy. In a series of 65 carotid ophthalmic giant aneurysms reported by Vinuela *et al.* (100), compression of the optic pathways was noted in 59 cases. Cranial nerve compression, other than in the visual pathways, was seen in three cases. Visual field loss was a presenting symptom in 19 patients with giant aneurysms in a series by Peiris and Ross-Russell (67). Pain and a long history of fluctuating visual loss were sometimes present. The location of the aneurysm was the cavernous carotid in two patients, the carotid ophthalmic in two, the supraclinoid in nine, and the anterior communicating artery in six patients. The natural history of patients with untreated giant paraclinoid aneurysms presenting with visual loss is usually one of deterioration (24, 37). More rarely, giant anterior communicating artery aneurysms present with visual loss (Fig. 15.4). Patients with giant aneurysms of the vertebrobasilar system can present with lower cranial neuropathies (82). The Italian Cooperative Study on Giant Intracranial Aneurysms (11) noted that 12% of patients presented with sudden cranial neuropathies. The abruptness of onset was explained by rapid thrombosis in the aneurysmal lumen, causing acute enlargement of the sac and ischemia of the adjacent nerve.

BRAIN OR BRAINSTEM COMPRESSION AND GROWTH OF GIANT ANEURYSMS

The Italian Cooperative Study on Giant Intracranial Aneurysms noted that 39% of patients with giant aneurysms presented with the symptoms of an expanding mass lesion, with 22% presenting with hemiparesis or hemiplegia (11). Brainstem compression can result from giant vertebrobasilar aneurysms (20, 81, 82) (Fig 15.5). The compressive effects of giant intracranial aneurysms have rarely resulted in hypopituitarism, tic doulourex, obstructive hydrocephalus, and hemiathetosis, the latter from basal ganglia and midbrain compression (19, 22, 28, 63, 71, 96, 99).

Enlargement of a giant intracranial aneurysm can result from either slow progressive dilation of the aneurysmal lumen or from continued formation of thrombus in the sac. There is often continued flow between layers of thrombus that are at various stages of organization and resorption (10, 38, 76). This phenomenon may explain the continued growth and/or

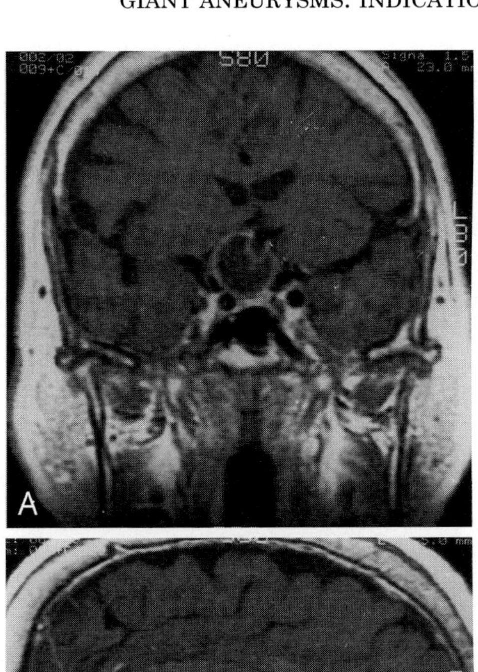

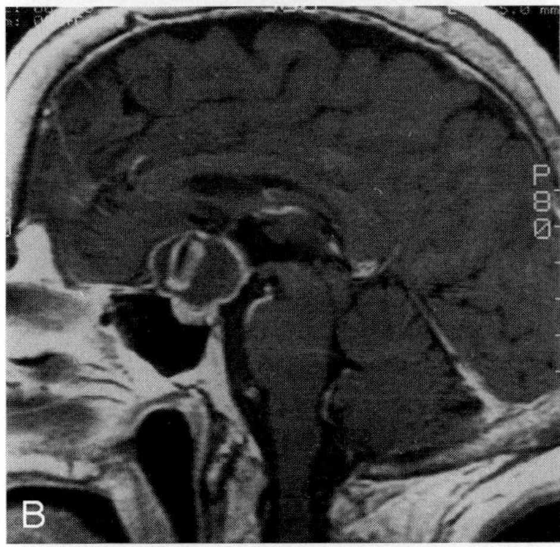

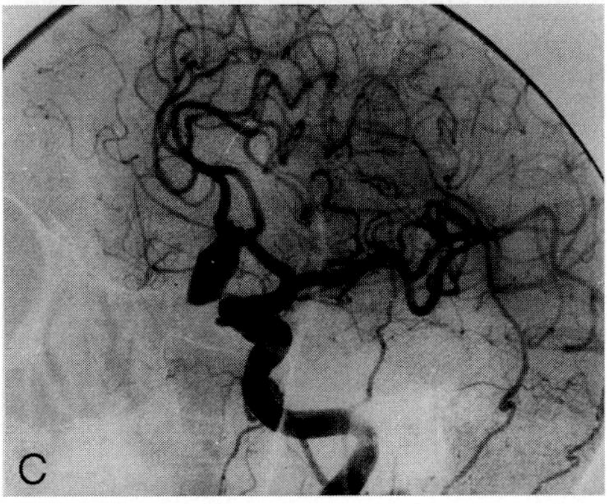

FIG 15.4 Coronal (**A**) and sagittal (**B**) MRIs of giant, partially thrombosed anterior communicating artery aneurysm. (**C**) Left anterior oblique angiogram demonstrates the portion of the aneurysm that is patent. This patient presented with a progressive bitemporal hemianopsia, from which patient completely recovered following aneurysmorrhaphy and clip ligation.

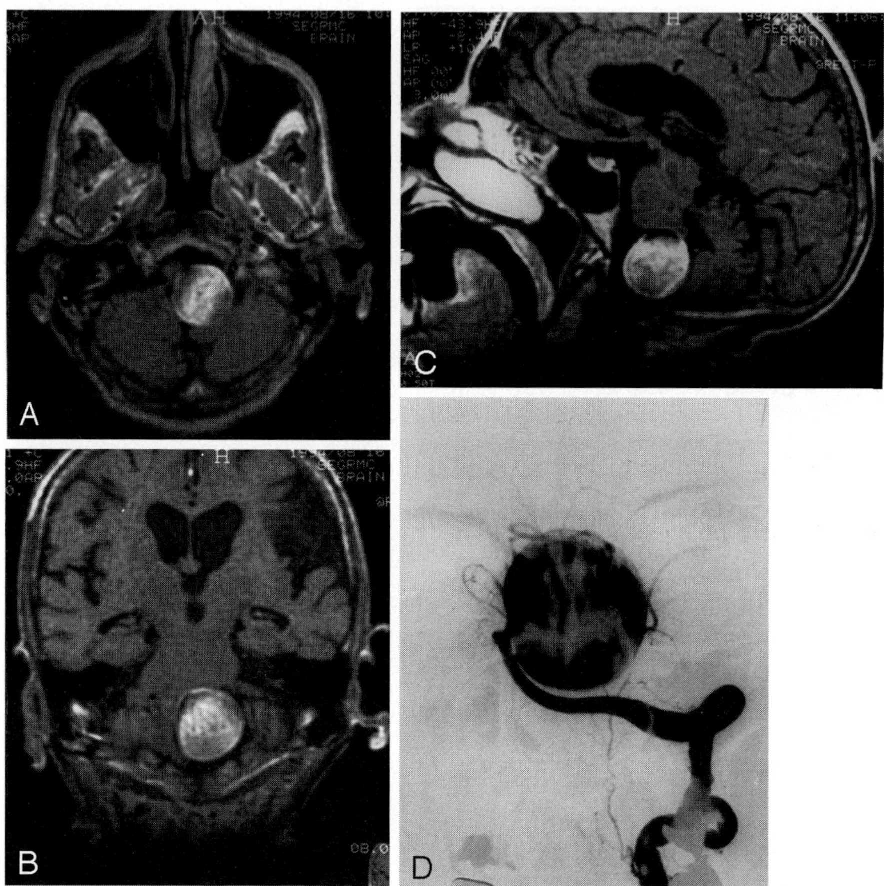

FIG 15.5 Axial (**A**), coronal (**B**), and sagittal (**C**) MRIs of a giant vertebral artery aneurysm in an 80-year-old woman, who presented with progressive lower cranial nerve dysfunction, resulting in a 60-pound weight loss due to dysphagia and hemiparesis. (**D**) AP left vertebral angiogram demonstrates the huge sac arising at the origin of the posterior inferior cerebellar artery. Despite the patient's advanced age, she was treated by clip ligation and made a rewarding recovery.

rupture of giant aneurysms that have either spontaneously occluded or that have undergone therapeutic endovascular occlusion documented by cerebral angiography (87, 88). Although it is generally believed that the formation of a giant aneurysm may take years, the review by Artmann *et al.* of 23 giant aneurysms included 3 cases with documented enlargement within 5 to 6 months, and 1 with rapid formation within 2 months (Fig. 15.6). Conversely, there are rare reports of spontaneous diminution or

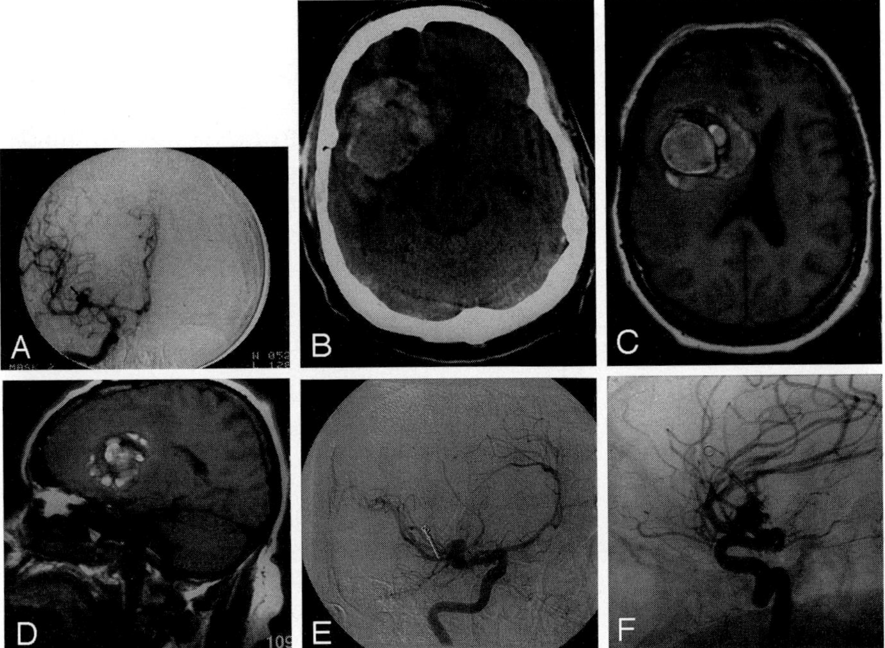

FIG 15.6 (**A**) AP right carotid angiogram shows a small middle cerebral artery aneurysm (*arrow*) in a patient who presented to an outside hospital with a subarachnoid hemorrhage. He underwent uneventful clip ligation of the aneurysm. Two years later, the patient presented with a rapidly progressive hemiparesis. (**B**) Axial CT demonstrates a large hemorrhagic mass in the region of the sylvian fissure. Axial (**C**) and sagittal (**D**) MRIs document the size of this newly formed, partially thrombosed giant aneurysm. Repeat right carotid angiography (**E** and **F**) shows that the clip has slipped off of the aneurysm and demonstrates the patent portion of the giant sac.

even disappearance of giant intracranial aneurysms (17, 59, 77). Artmann (6, 29, 61, 75) found that 70% of growing giant intracranial aneurysms were thrombosed, while in a series of giant aneurysms without enlargement, that rate is 13 to 20%.

Distal Ischemic Symptoms

Intrasaccular thrombus with organized calcification is a well-recognized source of spontaneous distal thromboembolism and of propagating thrombus in the parent artery or nutrient branches. Either of these processes can result in ischemic symptomatology, ranging from self-limited transient ischemic attacks to catastrophic infarcts. Partially thrombosed aneurysms may have an increased risk of distal ischemic symptoms, which can adversely affect the natural history. Thrombosed fusiform or dolichoectatic giant aneurysms appear to have an increased risk of thrombo-embolic stroke (60, 68, 85).

There are other mechanisms by which thrombus may affect the natural history of giant aneurysms. Studies have shown that angiogenesis is induced by the organizational process of the laminated thrombus (6, 7, 76, 87). Thus, hemorrhage from a giant aneurysm may not be simply the result of the wall withstanding the intraluminal pressure but may be secondary to rupture of these budding vessels from certain mechanical forces.

Focal Seizures

Focal seizures may rarely be the presenting symptom of giant intracranial aneurysms. Three of 22 patients in Bull's series (15), 3 of 28 patients in the series of Morley and Barr (59), and 3 of 130 in the Italian Cooperative Study of Giant Intracranial Aneurysms (11), presented with seizures. Giant aneurysms that occur on the middle cerebral artery are more prone to cause complex partial seizures. Compression of temporal lobe structures, focal cortical atrophy, and gliosis, probably resulting from minor leaks from the adventitia of the giant aneurysmal fundus, focal cerebral ischemia from a pressure effect, and transient or focal disturbance in blood flow to the temporal lobe have all been invoked to explain the etiology of these symptoms (103).

Other Rare Presentations

Intracranial hypertension without hydrocephalus has been reported in a patient with a giant carotid aneurysm. This presentation was thought to be secondary to multiple small hemorrhages that may have impaired cerebrospinal fluid vesicular transport (97). The erosive effects of giant intracranial aneurysms on bone has been manifested by the rare presentation of cerebrospinal fluid rhinorrhea from erosion of the planum sphenoidale and by hemorrhagic otitis and deafness from erosion of the petrous bone (22, 39). Massive cerebral edema associated with intra-aneurysmal thrombus and slowly progressive dementia have been described in patients with giant intracranial aneurysms (22, 36, 39).

NATURAL HISTORY

Intradural Aneurysms

As is the case with most cerebrovascular anomalies, the natural history of untreated giant aneurysms is incompletely understood. It is clear, however, that the earlier presumption of a low incidence of hemorrhage and optimistic outlook for these lesions was inaccurate. More current literature suggests that the outlook for patients harboring giant aneurysms is poor.

The natural history of giant intracranial aneurysms is dependent on several factors. The most important of these are (*a*) location of the aneurysm with respect to the subarachnoid space, *i.e.*, whether the lesion is intradural or extradural; (*b*) patho-anatomic form of the lesion, *i.e.*, saccular *versus* fusiform; (*c*) specific anatomic location on the circle of Willis; and (*d*) the presence or absence of laminated thrombus and/or artherosclerotic plaque within the fundus and neck of the aneurysm.

The prognosis for patients harboring untreated giant aneurysms is grim. In Morley and Barr's (59) original series of 28 patients, 17 had intradural aneurysms, and only 4 of these patients underwent a direct operation on their aneurysm. Of five patients who received no definitive therapy, four died. Of five patients with intradural aneurysms who had common carotid ligation, three died and one was disabled.

Peerless, *et al.* (66) followed 31 patients with giant intracranial aneurysms (25 saccular and 6 fusiform). Sixty-eighty percent of patients with saccular aneurysms were dead at 2 years. If patients presenting with subarachnoid hemorrhage were excluded, the 2-year mortality rate was 62%. Only four patients (all disabled) were alive at five years. Of the six patients with fusiform aneurysms, four were dead at 2 years, one died 3 1/2 years after diagnosis, and one remained disabled. The study of Ljunggren *et al.* (52) demonstrated a mortality or severe morbidity rate of 80% within 5 years of patients with conservatively treated symptomatic giant intracranial aneurysms.

The poor natural history of patients presenting with aneurysmal subarachnoid hemorrhage is well known, and patients with ruptured giant aneurysms do not fare any better. Pakarinen's study (64) of the population of Helsinki, Finland, provides insight into the natural history of aneurysmal subarachnoid hemorrhage from aneurysms of all sizes. This study reported a 15% mortality rate prior to hospital admission and a mortality rate of 32, 43, 56, and 60% at day 1, week 1, month 1, and month 6, respectively (64). When left untreated, 50% of patients with aneurysmal subarachnoid hemorrhage die or suffer major morbidity as a result of the initial ictus, and an additional 25 to 35% die of a subsequent hemorrhage (35). Patients with aneurysmal subarachnoid hemorrhage, who are not surgically treated and who survive the initial bleed for 6 months, remain at a higher risk for aneurysm rupture than patients with unruptured aneurysms. Winn *et al.* (106), in a 10-year evaluation of 364 such patients, calculated a rebleeding rate of 3.5% per year during the 1st decade. A second and third aneurysmal subarachnoid hemorrhage carry a mortality rate of approximately 65 and 85%, respectively. although these statistics apply to aneurysmal subarachnoid hemorrhage from aneurysms of all sizes, the outlook for bleeding giant aneurysms is every bit as bleak.

The series of Hamburger *et al.* (32) 58 patients with giant aneurysms showed that 7% of patients presenting without subarachnoid hemorrhage died, compared with 29% of patients presenting with subarachnoid hemorrhage. Only 18% of the latter group were discharged as "independent," compared with 50% of the former group. The extent of subarachnoid hemorrhage also has a direct bearing on prognosis. The Italian Cooperative Study on Giant Intracranial Aneurysms (73) found that extensive or thick cisternal deposition of blood was associated with a significantly higher mortality rate than with thin or absent depositions.

Although giant aneurysms present more commonly with mass effect or thromboembolic events, there is no evidence that they are associated with a lower rate of rupture. It is evident that the presence of thrombus in the sac does not protect against subarachnoid hemorrhage and when extensive or complete, may actually have a deleterious effect on the natural history (22, 45, 76, 84, 105).

Cavernous Segment Aneurysms

In discussing clinical manifestations, natural history, and indications for treatment of giant aneurysms, those giant sacs occurring extradurally within the cavernous sinus must be considered separately. These aneurysms occur most commonly in middle-aged females, who are often hypertensive. Approximately 21% of intracavernous aneurysms are bilateral and about 15% are giant, with intracavernous aneurysms accounting for 3 to 39% of all giant aneurysms (2, 12, 13, 46). Unlike their intradural counterparts, intracavernous aneurysms are associated with a much more benign natural history (44, 49, 50, 58, 59). Intracavernous aneurysms may come to clinical attention as an incidental finding on diagnostic imaging studies or by producing vascular or compressive symptoms. Vascular symptoms include subarachnoid hemorrhage, carotid-cavernous sinus fistulas, epistaxis, subdural hematoma, and embolic or ischemic phenomena distal to the aneurysm. Compressive symptoms result from impingement on surrounding neural structure and depend on location, size, and direction of growth of the sac.

ASYMPTOMATIC LESIONS

Earlier clinical series of intracavernous aneurysms rarely included incidentally discovered lesions. With the acceptance of cerebral angiography as a diagnostic test and the advent of noninvasive imaging studies, such as computerized tomography and magnetic resonance imaging, many of these nongiant aneurysms are now identified in the asymptomatic state. In recent series, up to 40% of intracavernous aneurysms were asymptomatic (21, 50). The vast majority of asymptomatic intracavernous aneurysms are relatively small, but on rare occasions, a sac within the cavernous sinus may reach giant proportions without producing symptoms. (Fig. 15.7).

VASCULAR SYMPTOMS

Subarachnoid Hemorrhage. Subarachnoid hemorrhage occurs only rarely with intracavernous lesions. For subarachnoid hemorrhage to occur, a portion of the sac or neck must extend through the dural ring into the subarachnoid space or extrude into the sella turcica and rupture through the diaphragma sellae. Although rare, the dural leaves of the cavernous sinus may become so thinned from expansion of an aneurysm that rupture occurs directly through the cavernous sinus wall (70). Various series (8, 21, 79, 90) report an incidence of subarachnoid hemorrhage from intracavernous aneurysms that ranged from 0 to 40%. Not all of these series report the size of the aneurysm, however. Morley and Barr (59) reported 12 giant intracavernous aneurysms in 11 patients in 1969. Only one case presented with subarachnoid hemorrhage, a 54-year-old female with an aneurysm arising from the intracavernous carotid and extending through the dural ring to the carotid bifurcation. This patient died 10 days after the hemorrhage. None of Drake's 9 giant intracavernous aneurysms bled (9). Of 37 patients with 44 intracavernous aneurysms followed by Linskey *et al.* (50), 3 experienced a subarachnoid hemorrhage, but none of these patients harbored giant aneurysms. In Meadows' series (58) of 15 patients, 8 had no surgery. Three patients presumably remained well, 3 died from 5 to 9 years after the onset of symptoms, and 2 died from 17 to 20 years after the onset. Although the cause of death was not specified, in no case was it intimated as resulting from the aneurysm (58). Thus, subarachnoid hemorrhage from purely intracavernous aneurysms is rare. Two cases of a subdural hematoma from intracavernous aneurysm rupture have been reported, one of which was 2.2 cm in size (34, 102).

Carotid-Cavernous Fistula. When an intracavernous aneurysm ruptures, it most commonly produces a carotid-cavernous sinus fistula, which is the cause of most high-flow, spontaneous carotid-cavernous fistulas (9). This presentation seems to be more common with smaller intracavernous aneurysms than with giant sacs (44, 58, 59). Since the diagnosis of an intracavernous aneurysm in this situation is usually presumptive, many series omit intracavernous aneurysms presenting

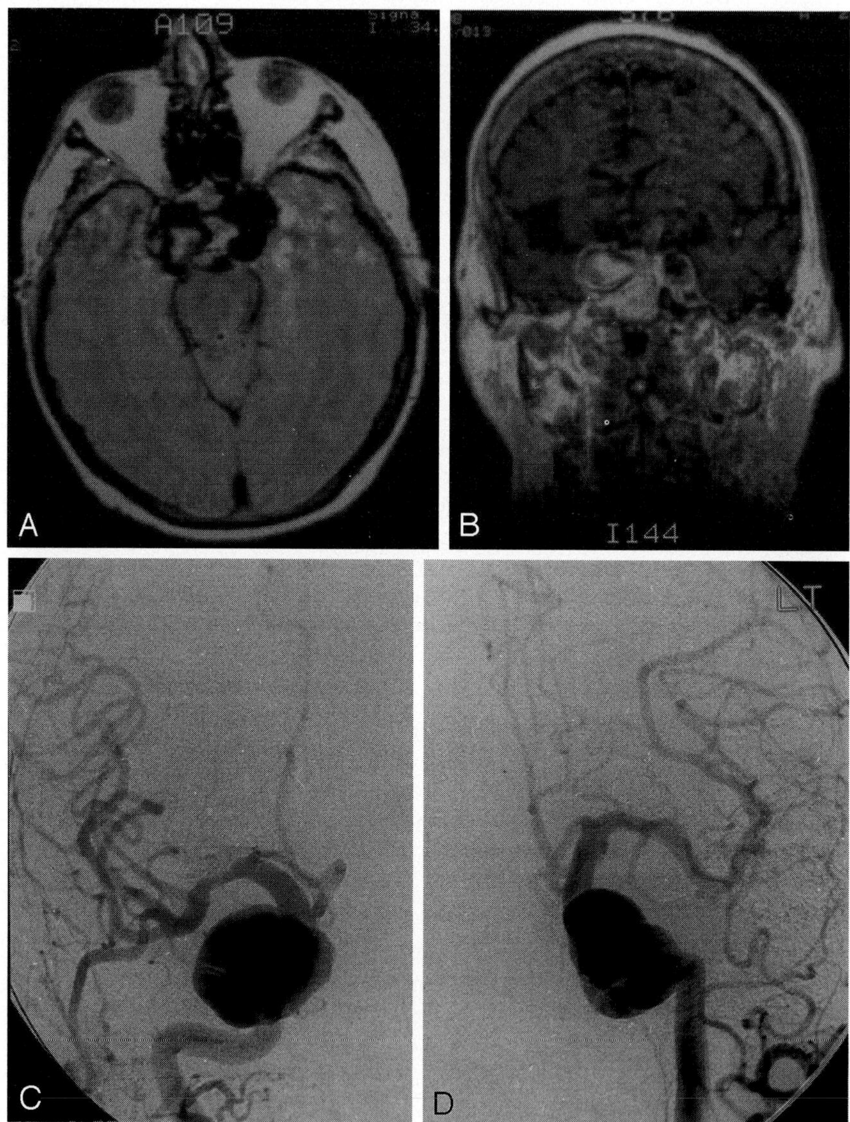

FIG 15.7 Axial (**A**) and coronal(**B**) MRIs demonstrate bilateral giant intracavernous aneurysms in a 68-year-old woman with no symptoms referable to the aneurysm. AP right (**C**) and left (**D**) carotid angiograms of the same patient.

as a carotid-cavernous fistula and, therefore, the precise incidence is probably underestimated.

Epistaxis.   The wall of the intracavernous internal carotid artery bulges into the sphenoid sinus in 71% of specimens, and bone is absent between the internal carotid artery and sphenoid mucosa in 4% (33, 72). Because of this anatomic relationship, an intracavernous aneurysm may rupture into the sphenoid sinus and produce epistaxis, which may be life-threatening. This may be a presentation of idiopathic or post-traumatic intracavernous aneurysms, although it is much more common with the latter (2, 14, 44).

Thrombo-embolism.   Spontaneous thrombosis of intracavernous aneurysms may result in occlusion of the parent internal carotid artery or in distal embolization, causing stroke. Distal vascular symptoms may be more common with giant aneurysms because of thrombus within the aneurysm (14, 50, 98). In Linskey's series (50), 2 of 37 patients had hemispheric ischemic symptoms from aneurysms between 1 and 2.5 cm in size.

Compressive Symptoms.   The vast majority of symptomatic intracavernous aneurysms cause symptoms by compressing the intracavernous cranial nerves. Usually, the abducens nerve is involved first, followed by the oculomotor and, later, the first two divisions of the trigeminal, beginning with the first division.

Lateral enlargement of an intracavernous aneurysm will usually result in a cavernous sinus syndrome, with intracavernous aneurysms accounting for about 20% of all cases of the cavernous sinus syndrome (8, 44, 55, 56, 58). In Drake's series, all 9 patients with giant intracavernous aneurysms presented with compressive symptoms, as did 10 of the 11 patients in Morley and Barr's series of giant aneurysms (22, 59).

Other, more rare compressive symptoms of intracavernous aneurysms include compression of the pituitary stalk with disinhibition of prolactin secretion (55) and deafness from posterior growth into the petrous bone (22, 55, 58).

INDICATIONS FOR TREATMENT OF GIANT INTRADURAL ANEURYSMS

As discussed earlier, the natural history of untreated giant intracranial aneurysms is dismal. Early attempts at surgical management of giant intracranial aneurysms have met with generally unsatisfactory results. As neuroradiologic methods, microsurgical techniques, knowledge of cerebral protection, and postoperative management of patients have improved, the surgical morbidity and mortality rates have decreased dramatically. Currently, results of management of giant aneurysms on the anterior circulation approach the outcomes achieved in the surgical management of smaller berry aneurysms. Those lesions involving the posterior circulation still carry a higher morbidity and mortality.

Given the extremely grave prognosis for patients harboring giant aneurysms, one could logically argue that mere presence represents an appropriate indication for treatment. It is important, however, to carefully individualize the treatment of each patient after careful consideration of the specific therapeutic goals as well as the available therapeutic options. Furthermore, appropriate clinical decision making requires consideration of a number of factors pertaining to both the patient and the individual aneurysm. After careful consideration of all of these variables, the clinician must accurately compare the risks of the natural history of the disease to the risks of the available therapeutic interventions and develop a logical therapeutic strategy.

Therapeutic Goals

The singular most important therapeutic goal is to do no harm to the patient. For an individual patient, the objective of treatment may include protection from hemorrhage, relief of mass effect, or treatment of thrombo-embolic complications. For the majority of patients with giant aneurysms, protection from hemorrhage and relief of mass effect are the two most important purposes of intervention. Therefore, the goal should be complete elimination of the aneurysm from the intracranial circulation with preservation of the parent and adjacent nutrient arteries and debulking of the giant mass. In selected patients presenting the thrombo-embolic phenomena, the therapeutic aim may be tailored more specifically to the individual patient.

Therapeutic Options

A variety of therapeutic interventions currently exist in the management of giant aneurysms. These include the following:

- No treatment
- Antiplatelet/anticoagulant therapy
- Deconstructive procedures
    Proximal parent artery occlusion
        Surgical or endovascular
        With or without bypass
    Trapping
        Surgical or endovascular
        With or without bypass
- Reconstructive procedures
    Open surgical exclusion
    Endosaccular embolization

Some of these therapeutic options are able to achieve all of the therapeutic goals listed above. Others aim specifically at achieving one or more of the objectives of intervention. As mentioned earlier, decision making requires a careful analysis of a number of factors concerning both the patient and the aneurysm itself. Patient factors that must be taken into consideration include age, health, neurologic condition, presenting symptoms, potential collateral cerebral blood flow, and psychological status of a patient with knowledge that he or she harbors a lesion that is potentially threatening to his or her neurologic health and life. Factors of the aneurysm include its size, location, configuration, presence of thrombus, and calcification, particularly within the neck.

Clearly, the durable and time-honored method for treating giant intracranial aneurysms is a reconstructive procedure that completely eliminates the aneurysm from the intracranial circulation and spares the parent nutrient vessels. This is most often achieved by direct clip ligation of the aneurysm and not only protects the patient from hemorrhage and threat of future thrombo-embolic complications but also allows for the immediate opening and decompression of the mass effect that may be present on adjacent neural structures. In selected cases, similar results may be achieved with endosaccular embolization of aneurysms, although the durability of this form of treatment in its present state of evolution is less certain and the relief of mass effect is not as immediate. It is the authors' opinion that the vast majority of intracranial aneurysms deserve surgical exploration. Angiography of giant intracranial aneurysms is often misleading, not always demonstrating an ideal surgical neck for clip placement. Modern 360° rotational digital angiographic views provide much greater detail of the angioarchitecture. However, many aneurysms that appear to have no discernible neck prove to be clippable at the time of careful surgical exploration (Fig. 15.8). Many giant aneurysms arise on intracranial arteries that are markedly distorted by the derangement of their anatomy, and a perfect intra-operative or postoperative arteriogram may not always be a reasonable goal (Fig. 15.9). However, one should always strive to completely eliminate the aneurysm and maintain adequate flow through adjacent arteries.

For those lesions that are unable to be eliminated by direct surgical techniques, consideration should be given to deconstructive procedures, such as proximal parent artery occlusion or trapping with or without a bypass procedure to augment collateral cerebral blood flow. Parent artery occlusion or trapping may be accomplished by surgical or endovascular techniques. Test occlusions of the parent artery have greatly augmented our ability to predict the patient's tolerance of sacrifice of the involved artery and to determine the availability of collateral blood flow. Balloon test occlusion, combined with methods to measure cerebral blood flow, has made these provocative tests more

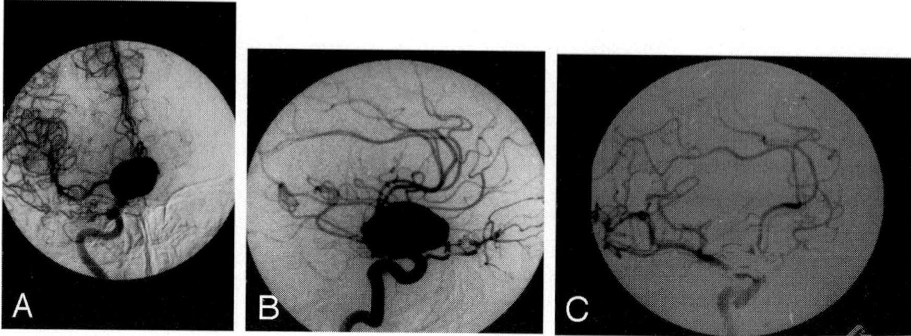

FIG 15.8 AP (**A**) and lateral right carotid (**B**) angiograms reveal a giant internal carotid artery aneurysm in a patient presenting with progressive visual loss. Despite the inability to identify a well-defined neck of the aneurysm, at the time of surgical exploration, the aneurysm was obliterated and the carotid reconstructed with multiple clips as documented on intra-operative angiography (**C**).

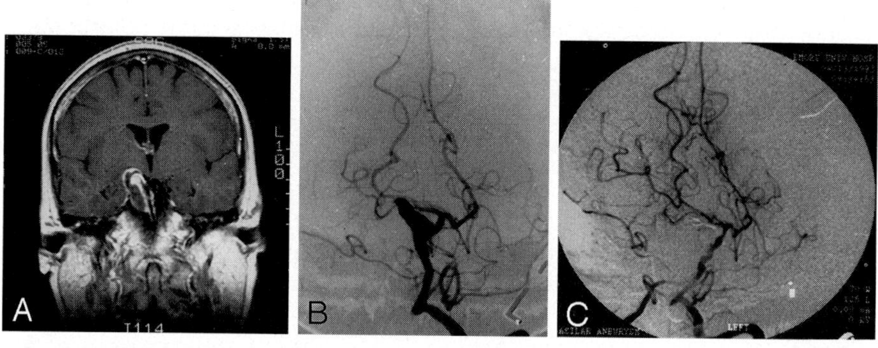

FIG 15.9 (**A**) Coronal MRI demonstrates a giant, partially thrombosed midbasilar aneurysm in a 52-year-old woman with a progressive left hemiparesis. (**B**) AP vertebral angiogram shows the patent portion of the sac and the marked abnormality of the basilar artery due to the wide-necked aneurysm. (**C**) Intra-operative AP vertebral angiogram reveals persistent irregularity of basilar artery after satisfactory clip ligation of the aneurysm.

objective. Unfortunately, no method of test occlusion has proven to be entirely reliable.

In unusual circumstances, after careful consideration of the therapeutic objectives, patient, and aneurysm factors, the decision for no treatment may be the most appropriate. Figure 15.10 shows the CT scan and angiogram of an 80-year-old woman who presented with headaches and a visual field defect. This patient had a largely thrombosed giant middle cerebral artery aneurysm with a very small portion

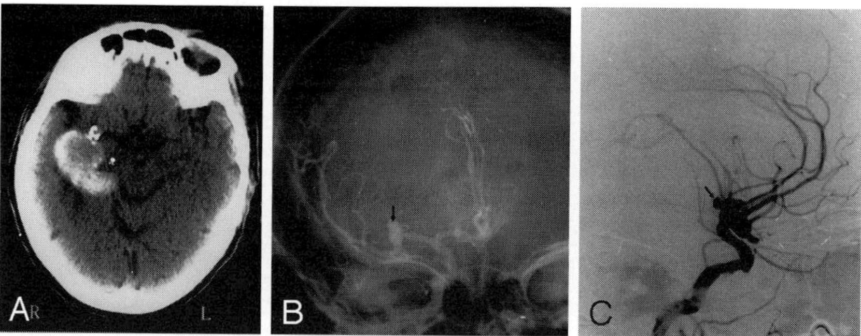

FIG 15.10 (**A**) Axial CT of an 80-year-old patient who presented with headaches and quadrantanopsia shows a large thrombotic and partially calcified lesion. AP (**B**) and lateral (**C**) angiograms demonstrate the small patent portion of the large aneurysm. Because of the patient's advanced age and minimal symptoms, no treatment was recommended.

of the sac filling angiographically. Consideration was given to both direct surgical and endovascular methods for treating the aneurysm but given the patient's age, minimal symptoms, and limited life expectancy, no specific treatment was recommended for her. In a younger patient with the same aneurysm, direct surgical treatment of the aneurysm would have been strongly recommended.

In selected instances, the judicious use of antiplatelet or anticoagulant therapy may be a reasonable option. Figure 15.11 shows the angiogram of an elderly patient who presented with a brainstem infarction believed to be due to thrombo-embolic occlusion of a brainstem perforating artery. Given the patient's advanced age, poor collateral flow, thrombo-embolic presentation, and fusiform nature of this large vertebrobasilar junction aneurysm, the patient was treated with antiplatelet therapy and has had no further symptoms. This form of treatment must be undertaken with caution, given the fact that giant aneurysms do represent a significant risk of hemorrhage.

As mentioned earlier, endosaccular obliteration of aneurysms with detachable coils is a treatment option that is in a state of evolution. Presently, the angioarchitecture of giant aneurysms does not often lend itself to techniques currently available. However, the number of reported successes is increasing, and we anticipate continued development of improved technology that will make this an important option in the management of these challenging patients (18).

Indications for Treatment of Giant Cavernous Segment Aneurysms

As with intradural giant aneurysms, decision making for giant cavernous segment aneurysm requires a careful comparison of the risks of

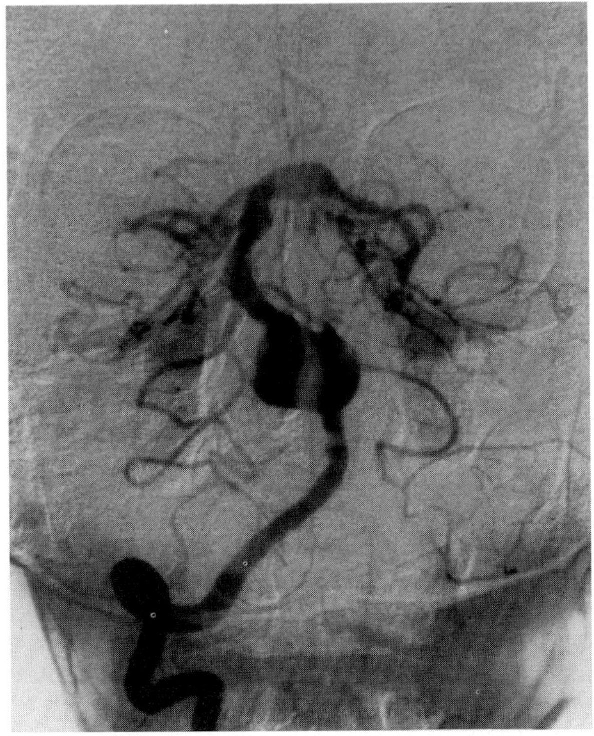

FIG 15.11 Vertebral angiogram reveals a large fusiform aneurysm of the proximal basilar artery in a 73-year-old patient, who presented with a small brainstem infarction believed to be due to a thrombo-embolic event from her aneurysm. Because of the presumed etiology of her symptoms and difficulty of surgical treatment of this aneurysm, the patient was treated with antiplatelet therapy.

the natural history and the available treatment options. As reviewed earlier, the natural history of aneurysms confined entirely to the cavernous segment of the carotid artery is distinctly more benign than that of aneurysms within the subarachnoid space. Therefore, any treatment of cavernous segment aneurysms must carry a low morbidity and mortality for intervention to be justified. Careful review of the angiogram is required to make an absolute determination that a proximal internal carotid aneurysm is truly intracavernous (70). Aneurysms are occasionally diagnosed incorrectly as intracavernous that ultimately prove to be located on the clinoidal or ophthalmic segment of the carotid. Aneurysms in these locations are associated with a more aggressive natural history and are more readily managed by direct surgical approaches.

THERAPEUTIC GOALS

Giant intracavernous aneurysms most commonly come to clinical attention by compressing the intracavernous cranial nerves. Therefore, relief of compressive cranial neuropathy is the most common goal of therapy. Occasionally, the purpose of treatment is to prevent thromboembolic events, or more rarely, to eliminate risk of recurrent epistaxis. A significant number of patients with intracavernous aneurysms require no treatment. Linskey *et al.* (49) have outlined guidelines for intervention for intracavernous aneurysms. Although this series included aneurysms of all sizes, these guidelines are applicable to giant lesions. For asymptomatic patients with intracavernous aneurysms, origin at the anterior genu of the carotid siphon and extension into the subarachnoid space indicate the need for intervention. For symptomatic patients, indications for treatment include subarachnoid hemorrhage (rare), epistaxis, progressive ophthalmoplegia or visual loss, medically intractable facial or orbital pain, and radiographic evidence of aneurysmal enlargement. The mere presence of cranial neuropathies does not necessarily warrant treatment, because as many as 40% of patients with these symptoms improve spontaneously (49).

THERAPEUTIC OPTIONS

As with intradural giant aneurysms, the treatment options for managing cavernous segment aneurysms include no treatment, anticoagulation, and deconstructive and reconstructive procedures utilizing direct surgical or endovascular techniques. In general, intervention is less aggressive due to the more benign natural history of these lesions. Therefore, patients with intracavernous aneurysms are more commonly managed without treatment or by direct methods than are those with intradural aneurysms. Once the neurosurgeon has made the decision to treat a giant intracavernous aneurysm, a number of options, both direct and indirect, are available. These include internal carotid artery sacrifice, with or without a vascular bypass graft; common carotid artery occlusion; detachable balloon or microcoil occlusion or the internal carotid artery proximal to the aneurysm; endovascular embolization of the aneurysmal sac with preservation of the internal carotid artery; a direct surgical approach to the cavernous sinus for aneurysm clipping; and cavernous internal carotid artery trapping with or without a petrosal-to-supraclinoid internal carotid artery saphenous bypass graft.

COST OF TREATMENT

Patients harboring giant intracranial aneurysms present a complex clinical challenge that frequently requires high technology diagnostic and therapeutic modalities. In most cases, a multidisciplinary approach is indicated, utilizing the skills of the neurosurgeon, the vascular neurologist, and diagnostic and interventional neuroradiologists. Those patients requiring innovative technology such as deep hypothermic circulatory arrest require the expertise of a cardiac surgeon, cardiac anesthesiologist, and specialized nurses. These patients with complex intracranial vascular pathology require the utilization of expensive technology and resources.

To determine the cost of medical and surgical management of patients harboring giant aneurysms, we reviewed the hospital charts and medical bills of all patients with giant intracranial aneurysms treated at Emory University Hospital over an 18-month period from 1993 to mid-1994. During that period of time, 26 patients were managed by the senior author. Of these 26 patients, 18 were female and 8 were male, with ages ranging from 19 to 78 years (average, 57 years). Eighteen patients presented with symptoms of mass effect, seven with hemorrhage, and one with thrombo-embolic symptoms. The locations of these 26 aneurysms are outlined in Table 15.3. Of these 26 aneurysms, 21 were saccular, and 4 were fusiform. Fifteen aneurysms were treated by clip ligation, nine utilizing standard surgical techniques, and six utilizing deep hypothermic circulatory arrest. Eight aneurysms were treated by parent vessel sacrifice, with five utilizing a bypass procedure to augment collateral cerebral blood flow, and 3 were treated without bypass. Three additional aneurysms were trapped, two utilizing a bypass procedure and one without a bypass. The outcome in these 26 patients is as follows: 8 excellent, 10 good, 3 fair, 3 poor, and 2 dead. The total cost of management of these patients ranged from $31,215 to $214,720, with an average of $82,985. The average cost for those patients treated with deep hypothermic circulatory arrest was $110,546. This compares favorably with the average cost of patients undergoing clip ligation, utilizing standard techniques, the average cost of which was $94,803. The most significant factor influencing cost of management was the presence or absence of treatment complications. The average cost of treatment for patients experiencing no complications was $60,840. In those patients experiencing a surgical complication, the average cost was $124,815. Clearly, avoidance of surgical complications is the primary method by which we can reduce the cost of managing these complex and thus expensive intracranial lesions.

SUMMARY

Giant intradural aneurysms are associated with an extremely grave natural history, yet remain potentially curable. Those aneurysms located on the intracavernous segment of the internal carotid artery are associated with a more benign natural history but frequently present with intractable cranial neuropathy requiring intervention. Proper current management requires a multidisciplinary approach through which the therapeutic goals are clearly defined. The treatment of giant intracranial aneurysms must be individualized after considering the various therapeutic options available to the multidisciplinary team. The cost of managing these complex lesions can be reduced by minimizing complications. Future advances in our ability to better manage patients with giant intracranial aneurysms will require careful assessment of outcome parameters.

REFERENCES

1. Aarabi B, Chambers J: Giant thrombosed aneurysm associated with an arteriovenous malformation. **J Neurosurg** 49:278–282, 1978.
2. Abad JM, Alvarez F, Blazquez MG: An unrecognized neurologic syndrome: A sixth nerve palsy and Horner's syndrome due to traumatic intracavernous carotid aneurysms. **Surg Neurol** 6:140–144, 1981.
3. Achslogh J: Description of a case of a giant aneurysm in a child. **Acta Neurol Belg** 70:333–347, 1970.
4. Anson JA: Giant aneurysms. Epidemiology and natural history, in Awad IA, Barrow DL (eds): *Giant Cerebral Aneurysms.* Park Ridge, IL, AANS, in press, 1995.
5. Anson JA, Spetzler RF: Characteristics and surgical treatment of fusiform and dolichoectatic aneurysms, in press, 1995.
6. Artmann H, Vonofakos D, Muller H, *et al.:* Neuroradiologic and neuropathologic findings with growing giant intracranial aneurysm. Review of the literature. **Surg Neurol** 21:391–401, 1984.
7. Austin G, Fisher S, Dickson D, *et al.:* The significance of extracellular matrix in intracranial aneurysms. **Ann Clin Lab Sci** 23:97–105, 1993.
8. Barr HWK, Blackwood W, Meadows SP: Intracavernous carotid aneurysm: A clinico-pathological report. **Brain** 94:607–622, 1971.
9. Barrow DL, Spector RH, Braun IF, *et al.:* Classification and treatment of spontaneous carotid-cavernous fistulas. **J Neurosurg** 56:248–256, 1985.
10. Batjer HH, Purdy PD: Enlarging thrombosed aneurysm of the distal basilar artery. **Neurosurgery** 26:695–699, 1990.
11. Battaglia R, Pasqualin A, Da Pian R: Italian Cooperative Study on giant intracranial aneurysms. 1: Study design and clinical data. **Acta Neurochir** [Suppl] (Wien) 42:49–52, 1988.
12. Berenstein A, Ransohoff J, Kupersmith M, *et al.:* Transvascular treatment of giant aneurysms of the cavernous carotid and vertebral arteries. **Surg Neurol** 21:3–12, 1984.
13. Blane G: History of some cases of diseases of the brain. **Trans Soc Improvement Med Chir Knowledge,** London 2:1992.
14. Brihaye J: Intracavernous carotid artery aneurysms, in Pia HW, Langmain C, Zierski J (eds): *Cerebral Aneurysm: Advances in Diagnosis and Therapy.* New York, Springer-Verlag, 1979, pp 67–78.
15. Bull J: Massive aneurysms at the base of the brain. **Brain** 92:535–570, 1969.

16. Byrd SE, Bentson JR, Winter J, *et al.:* Giant intracranial aneurysms simulating brain neoplasms on computed tomography. **J Comput Assist Tomogr** 2:303–307, 1978.
17. Carlson DH, Thomson D: Spontaneous thrombosis of a giant aneurysm in five days. **Neurology** 26:334–336, 1976.
18. Chaloupka JC, Awad IA: Therapeutic strategies and treatment options, in Awad IA, Barrow DL (eds): *Giant Cerebral Aneurysms.* Park Ridge, IL, AANS, in press, 1995.
19. Choudhury AR, al Amiri NH, al Moutaery KR, *et al.:* Giant middle cerebral aneurysm presenting as hemiathetosis in a child and its spontaneous thrombosis. **Child Nerve Syst** 7:59–61, 1991.
20. Cohen AR, Aleksic S, Budzilovich GN, *et al.:* Giant intracranial aneurysm presenting as a posterior fossa mass. **Surg Neurol** 20:160–164, 1983.
21. Dolenc V, Cerk M, Susteric J, *et al.:* Treatment of intracavernous aneurysms of the internal carotid artery and carotid cavernous fistulas by direct approach. In Dolenc VV (ed): The Cavernous Sinus, A Multidisciplinary Approach to Vascular and Tumorous Lesions. New York, Springer Verlag, 1987, pp 297–310.
22. Drake CG: Giant intracranial aneurysms: Experience with surgical treatment in 174 patients. **Clin Neurosurg** 26:12–95, 1979.
23. Ferguson GG: Physical factors in the initiation, growth and rupture of human intracranial saccular aneurysms. **J Neurosurg** 37:666–667, 1972.
24. Ferguson GG, Drake CG: Carotid-ophthalmic aneurysms: Visual abnormalities in 32 patients and the results of treatment. **Surg Neurol** 16:1–8, 1981.
25. Ferrante L, Fortuna A, Celli P, *et al.:* Intracranial arterial aneurysms in early childhood. **Surg Neurol** 29:39–56, 1988.
26. Fox JL: *Intracranial Aneurysms.* New York, Springer-Verlag, 1983.
27. Franz M, Berlit P, Tornow K: General dysplasia of the cerebral arteries with persistent primitive acoustic artery and giant aneurysm. **Eur Arch Psychiatr Neurol Sci** 238:196–198, 1989.
28. Gallagher PG, Dorsey JF, Stefanini M, *et al.:* Large intracranial aneurysm producing panhypopituitarism and frontal lobe syndrome. **Neurology** 6:829–837, 1956.
29. Golding R, Peatfield RC, Shawdon HH, *et al.:* Computer tomographic features of giant intracranial aneurysms. **Clin Radiol** 31:41–48, 1980.
30. Green KA, Anson JA, Spetzler RF: Giant serpentine middle cerebral artery aneurysm treated by extracranial-intracranial bypass. **J Neurosurg** 78:974–978, 1993.
31. Haddad GF, Haddad FS: Cerebral giant serpentine aneurysm: Case report and review of the literature. **Neurosurgery** 23:92–97, 1988.
32. Hamburger C, Schoenberger J, Lange M: Management and prognosis of intracranial giant aneurysms. A report on 58 cases. **Neurosurg Rev** 15:97–103, 1992.
33. Harris FS, Rhoton AL: Anatomy of the cavernous sinus: A microsurgical study. **J Neurosurg** 45:169–180, 1976.
34. Hayes WT, Bernhardt H, Young JM: Fusiform arteriosclerotic aneurysm of the basilar artery. **Vasc Surg** 1:171–178, 1967.
35. Heros RC: Intracranial aneurysms: A review. **Minn Med** 73:27–32, 1990.
36. Heros RC, Kolluri S: Giant intracranial aneurysms presenting with massive cerebral edema. **Neurosurgery** 15:572–577, 1984.
37. Heros RC, Nelson PB, Ojemann RG, *et al.:* Large and giant paraclinoid aneurysms: Surgical techniques, complications, and results. **Neurosurgery** 12:153–163, 1983.

38. Hirasawa T, Tsubokawa Y, Katayama Y: Growth of a giant aneurysm following complete thrombosis by detachable balloon occlusion. **Surg Neurol** 38:283–286, 1992.
39. Hosobuchi Y: Direct surgical treatment of giant intracranial aneurysms. **J Neurosurg** 51:743–756, 1979.
40. Hosobuchi Y: Giant intracranial aneurysms, in Wilkins RH, Rengachary SS (eds): *Neurosurgery.* New York, McGraw-Hill 1985, pp 1404–1414.
41. Houspian EM, Pool JL: A systematic analysis of intracranial aneurysms from the autopsy file of the Presbyterian Hospital, 1914–1956. **J Neuropathol Exp Neurol** 17:409–423, 1958.
42. Jain KK: Surgery of intracranial berry aneurysms: A review. **Can J Surg** 8:172–187, 1965.
43. Jane JA, Kassell NF, Torner JC *et al.:* The natural history of aneurysms and arteriovenous malformations. **J Neurosurg** 62:321–323, 1985.
44. Jefferson G: On the saccular aneurysms of the internal carotid artery in the cavernous sinus. **Br J Surg** 26:267–302, 1938.
45. Katayama Y, Tsubokawa T, Miyazaki S, *et al.:* Growth of totally thrombosed giant aneurysm within the posterior cranial fossa. Diagnostic and therapeutic considerations. **Neuroradiology** 33:168–170, 1991.
46. Keraver Y, Sindou M, Gaston A: Surgical occlusion of the carotid artery for treatment of giant aneurysms in the cavernous sinus. Proceedings of the International Symposium of Cavernous Sinus, June–July 1986, Ljublajana, Yugoslavia.
47. Kumabe T: Two cases of giant serpentine aneurysm. **Neurosurgery** 26:1027–1033, 1990.
48. Lansen Ta, Kasoff SS, Arguelles JH: Giant pediatric aneurysm treated with ligation of the middle cerebral artery with the Drake tourniquet and extracranial-intracranial bypass. **Neurosurgery** 25:81–85, 1989.
49. Linskey ME, Sekhar LN, Hirsch Jr WL, *et al.:* Aneurysms of the intracavernous carotid artery: Natural history and indications for treatment. **Neurosurgery** 6:933–938, 1990.
50. Linskey ME, Sekhar LN, Hirsch W Jr, *et al.:* Aneurysms of the intracavernous carotid artery: Clinical presentation, radiographic features, and pathogenesis. **Neurosurgery** 26:71–79, 1990.
51. Little JR, Louis P, Weinstein M, *et al.:* Giant fusiform aneurysms of the cerebral arteries. **Stroke** 12:183–188, 1981.
52. Ljunggren B, Brandt L, Sundbarg G, *et al.:* Early management of aneurysmal subarachnoid hemorrhage. **Neurosurgery** 11:412–418, 1982.
53. Locksley HB: Report on the Co-operative Study of Intracranial Aneurysms and Subarachnoid Hemorrhage. Section V, Part II. Natural history of subarachnoid hemorrhage, intracranial aneurysms and arteriovenous malformations. **J Neurosurg** 25:321–368, 1966.
54. Locksley HB: Report on the Co-operative Study of Intracranial Aneurysms and Subarachnoid Hemorrhage. Section V, Part I. Natural history of subarachnoid hemorrhage, intracranial aneurysms and arteriovenous malformation. **J Neurosurg** 25:219–239, 1966.
55. Lombardi G, Passerini A, Migliavacca F: Intracavernous aneurysms of the internal carotid artery. **AJR** 89:361–371, 1963.
56. Markwalder T-M, Meienberg O: Acute painful cavernous sinus syndrome in unruptured intracavernous aneurysms of the internal carotid artery. **J Clin Neuroophthalmol** 3:1983.

57. McCormick WF, Acosta-Rua GJ: The size of intracranial saccular aneurysms. An autopsy study. **J Neurosurg** 33:422–427, 1970.
58. Meadows SP: Intracavernous aneurysms of the internal carotid artery. **Arch Ophthalmol** 62:566–574, 1959.
59. Morley TP, Barr HWK: Giant intracranial aneurysms: Diagnosis, course, and management. **Clin Neurosurg** 16:73–94, 1969.
60. Nishizaki T, Tamiki N, Takeda N, *et al.:* Dolichoectatic basilar artery: A review of 23 cases. **Stroke** 17:1277–1281,1986.
61. O'Neill M, Hope T, Thomson G: Giant intracranial aneurysms: Diagnosis with special reference to computerized tomography. **Clin Radiol** 31:27–39, 1980.
62. Onuma T, Suzuki J: Surgical treatment of giant intracranial aneurysms. **J Neurosurg** 51:33–36, 1979.
63. Osenbach RK: Giant aneurysm of the distal posterior inferior cerebrellar artery in an 11-month-old child presenting with obstructive hydrocephalus. **Pediatr Neurosci** 15:309–312, 1989.
64. Pakarinen S: Incidence, aetiology, and prognosis of primary subarachnoid hemorrhage: A study based on 589 cases diagnosed in a defined urban population during a defined period. **Acta Neurol Scand** [Suppl] 29:1–128, 1967.
65. Peerless SJ, Nemoto S, Drake CG: Giant intracranial aneurysms in children and adolescents, in Edwards MSB, Hoffman H (eds): *Cerebral Vascular Disease in Children and Adolescents.* Baltimore, Williams & Wilkins, 1989, pp 255–273.
66. Peerless SJ, Wallace MD, Drake CG: Giant Intracranial Aneurysms in Youman JR (ed): *Neurological Surgery.* Philadelphia, W.B. Saunders, 1990, ed 3, pp 1742–1763.
67. Peiris JB, Ross-Russell RW: Giant aneurysms of the carotid system presenting as visual field defect. **J Neurol Neurosurg Psychiatry** 43:1053–1064, 1980.
68. Pessin MS, Chimowitz MI, Levin SR: Stroke in patients with fusiform vertebrobasilar aneurysms. **Neurology** 39:16–21, 1989.
69. Pia HW: Large and giant aneurysms. **Neurosurg Rev** 3:7–16, 1980.
70. Piepgras DG: Aneurysms of the intracavernous carotid artery: Clinical presentation, radiographic features, and pathogenesis. **Neurosurgery** 26:71–79, 1990.
71. Raymond LA, Tew J: Large suprasellar aneurysms, imitating pituitary tumor. **J Neurol Neurosurg Psychiatry** 41:83–87, 1978.
72. Renn WH, Rhoton AL: Microsurgical anatomy of the sellar region. **J Neurosurg** 43:288–298, 1975.
73. Rosta L, Battaglia R, Pasqualin A, *et al.: Italian Cooperative Study on Giant Intracranial Aneurysms.* 2: Radiological data. **Acta Neurochir** [Suppl] (Wien) 42:53–59, 1988.
74. Sarwar M, Batnitzky S, Schechter MM: Tumorous aneurysms. **Neuroradiology** 12:79–97, 1976.
75. Schubiger O, Valvanis A, Hayek J: Computed tomography in cerebral aneurysms with special emphasis on giant intracranial aneurysms. **J Comput Assist Tomogr** 4:24–32, 1980.
76. Schubiger O, Valvanis A, Wichmann W: Growth-mechanism of giant intracranial aneurysms: Demonstration by CT and MR imaging. **Neuroradiology** 29:266–271, 1987.
77. Scott RM, Ballantine HT: Spontaneous thrombosis in a giant middle cerebral artery aneurysm. **J Neurosurg** 37:361–363, 1972.
78. Segal HD, McLaurin RL: Giant serpentine aneurysm. Report of 2 cases. **J Neurosurg** 46:115–120, 1977.
79. Sindou M, Keravel Y, Debrun G, *et al.:* Intracranial giant aneurysms. Therapeutic approaches. **Neurochirurgie** 30 [Suppl]:1, 1984.

80. Sonntag VKH, Yuan RH, Stein BM: Giant intracranial aneurysms: A review of 13 cases. **Surg Neurol** 8:81–84, 1977.

81. Sorenson P, Lundorf E: Giant aneurysm of the vertebral artery simulating intracranial tumor at the foramen magnum. **Neuroradiology** 30:359, 1988.

82. Spallone A: Giant, completely thrombosed intracranial aneurysm simulating tumor of the foramen magnum. **Surg Neurol** 18:372–376, 1982.

83. Spetzler RF: The role of EC-IC in the treatment of giant intracranial aneurysms. **Neurol Res** 2:345–359, 1980.

84. Spincemaille GHJJ, Sloof JL, Hogenhuis LAH, *et al.:* Completely thrombosed giant aneurysm of the basilar trunk: A case report. **Neurosurgery** 17:968–970, 1985.

85. Steel JG, Thomas HA, Strollo PJ: Fusiform basilar artery as a cause of embolic stroke. **Stroke** 13:712–716, 1982.

86. Stehbens WE: Intracranial arterial aneurysms. **Aust Ann Med** 3:214–220, 1954.

87. Strother CM, Eldevik P, Kukuchi Y, *et al.:* Thrombus formation and structure and the evolution of mass effect in intracranial aneurysms treated by balloon embolization: Emphasis on MR findings. **AJNR** 10:787–796, 1989.

88. Strother CM, Lund S, Graves V, *et al.:* Late paraophthalmic aneurysm rupture following endovascular treatment. **J Neurosurg** 71:777–796, 1989.

89. Sundt TM, Piepgras DG: Surgical approach to giant intracranial aneurysms. **J Neurosurg** 51:731–742, 1979.

90. Sundt TM Jr, Piepgras DG, Fode NC, *et al.:* Giant intracranial aneurysms. **Clin Neurosurg** 37:116–154, 1991.

91. Suzuki J, Sato T: Direct surgical treatment of giant intracranial aneurysms. **Neurol Res** 2:305–325, 1980.

92. Suzuki S, Takahashi T, Ohkuma H, *et al.:* Management of giant serpentine aneurysms of the middle cerebral artery. Review of literature and report of a case successfully treated by STA-MCA anastomosis only. **Acta Neurochir (Wien)** 117:23–39, 1992.

93. Swamy NKS, Pope FM, Coakham HB: Giant aneurysm of internal carotid artery in a four-year-old child: A case report. **Surg Neurol** 40:138–141, 1993.

94. Symon L: Management of giant intracranial aneurysms. **Clin Neurol** 36:21–47, 1990.

95. Symon L: Surgical experiences with giant intracranial aneurysms. **Acta Neurochir (Wien)** 118:53–58, 1992.

96. Symon L, Vadja J: Surgical experience with giant intracranial aneurysms. **J Neurosurg** 61:1009–1028, 1984.

97. Trapelli F, Di Lauro L: Intracranial hypertension without hydrocephalus due to small bleedings from a giant carotid aneurysm. **J Neurosurg Sci** 29:293–295, 1985.

98. Van Dellen JR: Intracavernous traumatic aneurysms. **Surg Neurol** 13:203–207, 1980.

99. Verbalis JG, Nelson PB, Robinson AG: Reversible panhypopituitarism caused by a suprasellar aneurysm: The contribution of mass effect of pituitary dysfunction. **Neurosurgery** 10:604–611, 1982.

100. Vinuela F, Fox A, Change JK, *et al.:* Clinicoradiological spectrum of giant supraclinoid internal carotid artery aneurysms. Observations in 93 cases. **Neuroradiology** 26:93–99, 1984.

101. Vorkapic P, Czech T, Pendl G, *et al.:* Clinico-radiological spectrum of giant intracranial aneurysms. **Neurosurg Rev** 14:271–274, 1991.

102. Weir B: *Aneurysms Affecting the Nervous System.* Baltimore, Williams & Wilkins, 1987.

103. Whittle IR, Allsop JL, Halmagyi GM: Focal seizures: An unusual presentation of giant intracranial aneurysms. A report of four cases with comment on the natural history and treatment. **Surg Neurol** 24:533–540, 1985.
104. Whittle IR, Dorsch NW, Besser M: Giant intracranial aneurysms: Diagnosis, management, and outcome. **Surg Neurol** 21:218–230, 1984.
105. Whittle IR, Dorsch NW, Besser M: Spontaneous thrombosis in giant intracranial aneurysms. **J Neurol Neurosurg Psychiatry** 45:1040–1047, 1982.
106. Winn HR, Richardson AE, Jane JA: The long-term prognosis in untreated cerebral aneurysms. I: The incidence of late hemorrhage in cerebral aneurysms: A 10-year evaluation of 364 patients. **Ann Neurol** 1:358–370, 1977.

16

Surgical Management of Giant Intracranial Aneurysms: Experience with 171 Patients

MICHAEL T. LAWTON, M.D., AND ROBERT F. SPETZLER, M.D.

Honored Guest Lecture

By definition, giant intracranial aneurysms measure more than 2.5 cm in diameter (37). Their size and distinctive anatomic characteristics make these lesions difficult to manage. In one of the first large reviews of giant aneurysms in 1969, Morley and Barr (44) stated that "direct surgical attack on extracavernous giant aneurysms is seldom possible or successful, except in middle cerebral artery aneurysms." Advances in neurosurgical techniques have transformed giant aneurysms into a primarily surgical disease and have improved significantly the prognosis for patients who have them. Few neurosurgeons have acquired a large amount of experience with giant aneurysms (2, 11, 12, 21, 24, 25, 33, 45, 46, 66–68, 73). Notable are Peerless and Drake's (45) series of 305 patients and Sundt's (66) series of 315 patients. The senior author's (RFS) experience, consisting of work with 171 patients, is reviewed, and current management strategies are discussed in this chapter.

CLINICAL MATERIALS AND METHODS

Patient Population

One hundred seventy-one patients with giant intracranial aneurysms were treated between 1980 and 1994 (average age, 53 years; range, 4 to 78 years). As in most series (34, 44, 48), females predominated (111 women and 60 men). Giant aneurysms represent 3 to 5% of all cerebral aneurysms in most general neurosurgical populations (44, 48, 71); as a tertiary referral center, the authors' incidence rate was slightly higher than the norm (approximately 6%).

Patients treated early in the series (from 1980 to 1984) underwent extracranial-intracranial (EC-IC) bypass and gradual occlusion of the cervical internal carotid artery (ICA) with a Selverstone clamp. The results of treatment in these 35 patients have been described previously (65). Because the current management scheme no longer uses this approach, this report will focus on the subsequent 136 patients treated at Barrow Neurological Institute between 1985 and 1994.

Patient Presentation

Forty-nine patients (36%) exhibited symptoms and signs of mass effect and neural compression that reflected the location of the aneurysm. In the anterior circulation, giant aneurysms produced pain and dysfunction of extra-ocular movement and vision. Those in the posterior circulation produced lower cranial-nerve dysfunction, bulbar palsy, and limb weakness.

Subarachnoid hemorrhage (SAH) was the clinical presentation in 48 patients (35%), which is consistent with the range (13 to 76%) reported in other series (48). Ten patients (21%) were assessed as being Hunt-Hess (28) grade I; 15 patients (31%) were grade II; 13 patients (27%) were grade III; 7 patients (15%) were grade IV; and 3 patients (6%) were grade V. Fisher *et al.* (13) computerized tomography (CT) grades were grade I in 7 patients (15%); grade II in 8 patients (17%); grade III in 24 patients (50%); and grade IV in 9 patients (19%). Twelve patients had hemorrhaged previously.

Eleven patients (8%) presented with symptoms of distal thrombo-embolism, including transient ischemic attacks (TIAs) and stroke. Giant aneurysms were found when six patients (4%) were evaluated for seizures. The remaining 22 patients (16%) had their aneurysms diagnosed incidentally during evaluation for headaches (8 patients), syncope (5 patients), and unrelated medical problems, such as sinusitis, epistaxis, head trauma, facial shingles, confusion, contralateral stroke, chest pain, and screening magnetic resonance imaging (MRI) (9 patients).

Twelve patients were referred to this institution after being treated elsewhere. One patient with thrombo-embolic symptoms had been treated unsuccessfully with anticoagulation. Four patients had been treated surgically: one presented with TIAs after carotid ligation for a posterior communicating artery (PCoA) aneurysm; one presented with compressive symptoms from a cavernous ICA aneurysm treated with carotid ligation and EC-IC bypass; one presented with recurrent compressive symptoms from a partially clipped ICA bifurcation aneurysm; and one presented with mass effect from a paraclinoid ICA aneurysm previously encased in methylmethacrylate. Endovascular therapy had been used in seven patients. Three had their aneurysms occluded with coils and presented with residual aneurysm and mass effect; four had their aneurysms occluded proximally with balloons (two of these patients presented with TIAs, one with mass effect symptoms and one with progressive enlargement of a basilar tip aneurysm after proximal occlusion of a petrous ICA aneurysm).

Diagnostic Evaluation

High-quality, four-vessel cerebral angiography is essential in the preoperative evaluation of patients with giant aneurysms. Angiography provides detailed information about the aneurysm's location, anatomy, adjacent branch vessels, collateral circulation, and distal cerebral perfusion. Angiography only shows luminal filling, which may not represent the true size of the aneurysm. Layers of laminated thrombus frequently make giant aneurysms much larger than they appear on angiography alone. Computerized tomography (CT) scans often demonstrate a calcified, eggshell border that defines the true diameter of the aneurysm. MRIs demonstrate a signal void within a patent lumen. Alternating high- and low-signal intensity on T1-weighted images corresponds to hemosiderin and methemoglobin within the layers of thrombus. These pre-operative studies are used to determine whether the aneurysm is amenable to direct clipping and which surgical approach would optimize exposure.

Diagnostic evaluation identified 138 giant aneurysms—99 in the anterior circulation and 39 in the posterior circulation. Two patients each had two giant aneurysms. Fifty-one aneurysms were on the left side; 40 were on the right side; and 47 were in the midline. Fifteen aneurysms were giant dolichoectatic, and the remaining 123 were giant saccular. The average diameter was 3.6 cm (range, 2.5 to 12 cm).

These lesions were located as follows: petrous ICA, $n = 3$ (2%); cavernous ICA, $n = 15$ (11%); ophthalmic, $n = 13$ (9%); paraclinoid, $n = 15$ (11%); PCoA, $n = 8$ (6%); ICA bifurcation, $n = 8$ (6%); middle cerebral artery (MCA), $n = 24$ (17%); anterior cerebral artery (ACA), $n = 13$ (9%); basilar tip, $n = 24$ (17%); posterior cerebral artery (PCA), $n = 1$ (1%); superior cerebellar artery (SCA), $n = 2$ (1%); midbasilar/anterior inferior cerebellar artery (AICA), $n = 7$ (5%); vertebrobasilar junction (VBJ), $n = 3$ (2%); and vertebral/posterior inferior cerebellar artery (PICA), $n = 2$ (1%).

Most patients (68%) had a single giant aneurysm. Forty-one patients (30%) had additional aneurysms of less than 2.5 cm in diameter. Sixteen patients had a "mirror" aneurysm on the contralateral side, and 11 patients had multiple other aneurysms.

Pre-operative Management

Patients who presented with SAH were managed under the same principles and protcols that have been established for other patients with SAH (3). Blood pressure was controlled carefully to minimize the risk of rupture. Ventriculostomy with cerebrospinal fluid drainage was used to treat patients with Hunt-Hess grades IV and V, and intracranial pressure (ICP) was used to guide surgical decisions (5). ICP elevations were managed aggressively with conventional methods. Surgery was performed within 24 hours of presentation in suitable patients.

Treatment

The pterional trans-sylvian approach was used in 91 patients. A more frontal, interhemispheric approach was used in three patients with aneurysms along the ACA. The following skull base approaches were used in 43 patients (31%): subtemporal or pterional-subtemporal approach, $n = 15$; the orbitozygomatic approach, $n = 16$; the combined supratentorial-infratentorial approach, $n = 3$; the far lateral approach, $n = 7$; the far lateral-combined supratentorial-infratentorial approach, $n = 1$; and the cervical approach, $n = 1$.

Several different techniques were used to treat the aneurysms, depending on their location (Tables 16.1 and 16.2). Of the 138 treated aneurysms, 85 (62%) were clipped directly. Interestingly, the location with the highest rate of direct clipping was at the basilar apex. Twenty-seven aneurysms (20%) were trapped; 11 of these were cavernous ICA aneurysms, and only 2 were posterior circulation aneurysms (located along the distal vertebral artery). Of the 14 supraclinoid aneurysms that were not clipped directly, 7 were trapped and 6 occluded proximally. In total, 10 aneurysms (7%) were occluded proximally, and one midbasilar aneurysm was occluded distally. Aneurysm excision was used in six patients (4%), and aneurysmorrhaphy was performed in five patients (4%), three of them along the midbasilar artery and VBJ.

TABLE 16.1

Technique of Giant Aneurysm Treatment Summarized by Aneurysm Location

Location	Clipping (%)	Trapping (%)	Proximal Ligation (%)	Aneurysm-orrhaphy (%)	Excision (%)	Wrapping (%)	Total
Petrous ICA	0(0)	2(67)	0(0)	0(0)	1(33)	0(0)	3
Cavernous ICA	1(7)	11(73)	1(7)	1(7)	0(0)	1(7)	15
15 Supraclinoid ICA	30(68)	7(16)	6(14)	0(0)	0(0)	1(2)	44
MCA	13(54)	4(17)	0(0)	1(4)	4(17)	2(8)	24
ACA	11(85)	1(8)	0(0)	0(0)	1(8)	0(0)	13
Basilar apex	25(93)	0(0)	2(7)	0(0)	0(0)	0(0)	27
Midbasilar artery	3(43)	0(0)	2(29)	2(29)	0(0)	0(0)	7
Vertebral artery	2(40)	2(40)	0(0)	1(20)	0(0)	0(0)	5
Totals	85	27	11	5	6	4	138

TABLE 16.2
Surgical Adjuncts Used in the Treatment of Giant Aneurysms by Aneurysm Location

Location	Hypothermic Circulatory Arrest (%)	Revascularization (%)	Skull Base Approaches (%)	Endovascular Techniques (%)
Petrous ICA	0(0)	3(100)	1(33)	0(0)
Cavernous ICA	1(7)	12(80)	1(7)	2(13)
Supraclinoid ICA	3(7)	10(23)	1(2)	1(2)
MCA	1(4)	9(38)	3(13)	0(0)
ACA	0(0)	1(8)	3(23)	0(0)
Basilar apex	22(81)	0(0)	22(81)	0(0)
Midbasilar artery	3(43)	4(57)	7(100)	1(14)
Vertebral artery	2(40)	1(20)	5(100)	1(20)
Totals	32	40	43	5

Aneurysm wrapping with a reinforcing agent such as muslin was used in four patients (3%).

Hypothermic circulatory arrest (63) was used in 31 patients with 32 giant aneurysms. Most of these aneurysms (27, or 84%) were located along the basilar artery: basilar tip, $n = 20$; SCA, $n = 2$; midbasilar, $n = 3$; and VBJ, $n = 2$. Five anterior circulation aneurysms required circulatory arrest, one each at the cavernous ICA, paraclinoid ICA, PCoA, ICA bifurcation, and MCA. Twenty-eight aneurysms (88%) were directly clipped, 2 were proximally occluded, and 2 aneurysmorrhaphies were performed.

Forty-one bypasses were performed in 40 patients. Thirty patients had unclippable aneurysms treated with alternative techniques that involved parent vessel occlusion. One patient developed significant changes in somatosensory evoked potentials (SSEPs) during temporary parent vessel occlusion; the temporary clips were removed and a bypass was performed before aneurysm trapping was pursued any further. Poor pre-operative cerebral perfusion was the basis for revascularization in six patients. One patient had thrombo-embolic symptoms and an angiogram, demonstrating vessel incompetency and poor flow distal to the aneurysm. Four of these patients had their aneurysms treated previously with ICA sacrifice: three patients presented with ischemic symptoms or stroke, and one presented with a progressively enlarging basilar aneurysm. Another of these patients presented with an enlarging giant cavernous aneurysm and a contralateral ICA occlusion from a previous motor vehicle accident. This patient required two bypasses: revascularization of the contralateral carotid territory with an ICA-MCA saphenous graft and subsequent aneurysm trapping and petrous-to-supraclinoid ICA bypass. Neurologic deterioration occurred after direct clipping in three patients due to clip migration or inadequate distal blood flow. Although this problem usually was corrected by readjusting the clip, friable vessels in these three patients prevented optimal clip placement and necessitated a bypass.

Many revascularization techniques are available to the neurosurgeon, and the appropriate bypass was determined by the aneurysm location. Aneurysms at the skull base or along the petrous ICA ($n = 3$) were either resected and reconstructed with a saphenous vein graft ($n = 1$) or trapped proximally in the neck and distally along the petrous ICA and bypassed with a cervical-to-petrous ICA ($n = 2$) graft (14).

Cavernous ICA aneurysms typically were trapped proximally along the petrous ICA and distally along the supraclinoid ICA just before the ophthalmic artery. The petrous (C5)-to-supraclinoid (C3) carotid saphenous bypass (60) reconstituted the segment of sacrificed vessel ($n = 9$). When the petrous ICA could not be anastomosed easily, bypasses from cervical-to-supraclinoid carotid ($n = 1$) or superficial temporal artery (STA)-to-MCA ($n = 2$) were used.

Revascularization distal to giant aneurysms of the supraclinoid ICA ($n = 10$) and MCA ($n = 9$) was accomplished with a STA-MCA bypass ($n = 8$). The "double-barrel" bypass connecting two STA branches with two recipient MCA vessels augmented flow. A saphenous vein interposition graft ($n = 5$) also increased the caliber and flow of the bypass (39), which may be needed when the supraclinoid ICA is occluded surgically. Good exposure of MCA aneurysms enabled their excision and primary re-anastomosis ($n = 5$). An *in situ* bypass with the anterior temporal artery anastomosed side-to-side to the MCA distal to the aneurysm was used when extracranial vessels were injured or too small in caliber ($n = 1$) (7). The ACA territory can be revascularized with an *in situ,* side-to-side A2-A2 anastomosis distal to the aneurysm if one ACA remains intact.

Revascularization during treatment of basilar artery aneurysms ($n = 4$) was accomplished by STA-to-PCA or SCA bypass. This anastomosis was performed as a preliminary stage before treating the aneurysm with occlusion of the basilar artery during a second-stage operation. These two maneuvers altered blood flow within the aneurysm and thereby promoted thrombosis of its lumen, while maintaining adequate brainstem perfusion. Giant aneurysms of the vertebral artery or PICA treated with surgical occlusion of a vertebral artery were revascularized with an *in situ,* side-to-side PICA-to-PICA anastomosis ($n = 1$) (31). When the ipsilateral PICA is clipped proximally, it fills retrogradely from the contralateral PICA. Extracranial vessels such as the occipital artery may provide other donor vessels in case of bilateral vertebral artery involvement or variant anatomy (47).

Acute graft occlusion occurred in three patients (7%), and all occluded grafts were revised with angiographically proven patency (postoperative patency rate, 100%). Nine patients had follow-up angiograms to evaluate patency at an average 5.5 months after surgery. One patient (11%) had a late graft occlusion that was revised.

Thrombosed aneurysms were debulked in 33 patients (15). A separate surgical stage was required in 24 patients.

Endovascular techniques were used to treat five patients (4%). Selective injection of tissue plasminogen activator reopened an occluded C3-C5 bypass in one patients. Three patients had unclippable aneurysms that were proximally occluded with balloons. One of these patients had a paraclinoid aneurysm previously encased with methylmethacrylate that could not be occluded surgically. When direct exposure would have required extensive surgery, as with cavernous ICA (n = 1) or basilar artery aneurysms (n = 1), proximal occlusion was performed more simply with endovascularly placed balloons. The fifth patient failed to thrombose a vertebral artery aneurysm after proximal ligation and PICA-PICA bypass, and his aneurysm was trapped distally with endovascularly placed coils (31).

OUTCOME

Nine patients died in the peri-operative period (surgical mortality, 6.6%). Four of these patients presented with SAH and Hunt-Hess grades of IV or V. A grade III patient who had a complex MCA aneurysm clipped, using cardiac standstill, died postoperatively from a large MCA distribution infarction. One patient hemorrhaged from a contralateral aneurysm during surgery for an incidental giant aneurysm. Two patients died from postoperative hemorrhages, presumably from clip migration. One patient with multiple pre-existing medical problems developed postoperative cardiac arrhythmias, *Candida* sepsis, amphotericin-induced renal failure, and congestive heart failure and died from multisystem organ failure.

Fifteen patients were neurologically worse after treatment (treatment-associated neurologic morbidity, 11%). Three patients with Fisher grades of III and IV developed significant infarctions due to vasospasm. Three patients developed cerebral infarctions and new deficits. In two of these patients, the aneurysms were trapped and revascularized. The etiology of these infarctions was presumed to be thrombo-embolism. One patient with an occluded C3-C5 bypass developed hemiparesis that did not improve despite re-establishment of graft patency. One patient had a postoperative epidural hematoma caused by a hypocoagulable state after hypothermic circulatory arrest.

One patient had a postoperative myocardial infarction that contributed to neurlogic deterioration. Six patients developed new neurologic deficits postoperatively with no clear etiology. Three of these patients underwent hypothermic circulatory arrest (twice in one patient). Three of these patients were treated recently and are expected to improve; two patients were lost to follow-up.

Pre- and postoperative neurologic function was evaluated, using Glasglow Outcome Scale (GOS) scores (29). Of the 136 patients treated, 85% had an excellent or good outcome. Specifically, 90 patients (66%) had an excellent outcome (GOS 1); 25 patients (18%) had a good outcome (GOS 2); 9 patients (7%) had a fair outcome (GOS 3); and 3 patients (2%) had a poor outcome. The mean length of follow-up was 2.2 years.

As expected, outcome for patients who presented with SAH correlated with the Hunt-Hess grade. Patients with grades I or II had an excellent or good outcome in 92% of the cases, as compared to 43 and 33% for grade IV and V patients, respectively (Fig. 16.1). Conversely, the fair and poor outcomes and mortality rate increased as the Hunt-Hess grade increased (Fig. 16.2). As a group, the SAH patients did worse than patients with other presentations: 79% of SAH patients had an excellent or good outcome, but 13% died, as compared to 88% of the other patients, who had an excellent or good outcome and 3% who died. Excellent or good outcomes were observed in 82% of the patients with compressive symptoms, 91% of the patients with thrombo-embolic symptoms, and 95% of the patients with incidental aneurysms (Fig. 16.3).

Outcomes tended to be better in patients with giant aneurysms in the anterior circulation. Eighty-nine percent of these patients had ex-

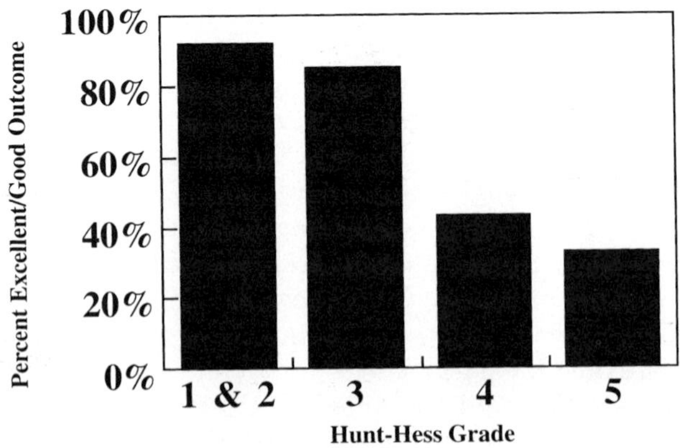

FIG. 16.1 Percent good and excellent outcomes as a function of Hunt-Hess grade.

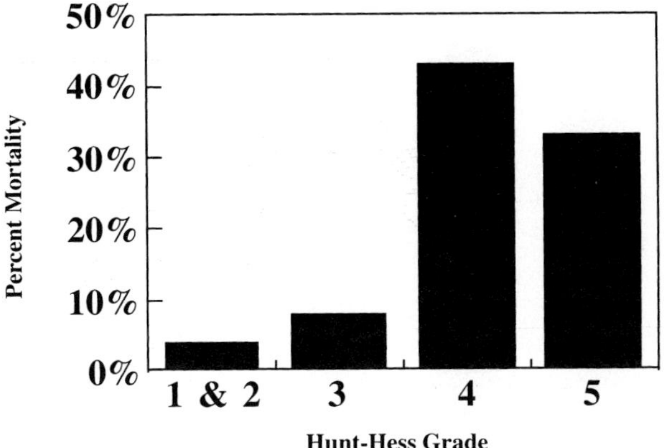

FIG. 16.2 Mortality rate as a function of Hunt-Hess grade.

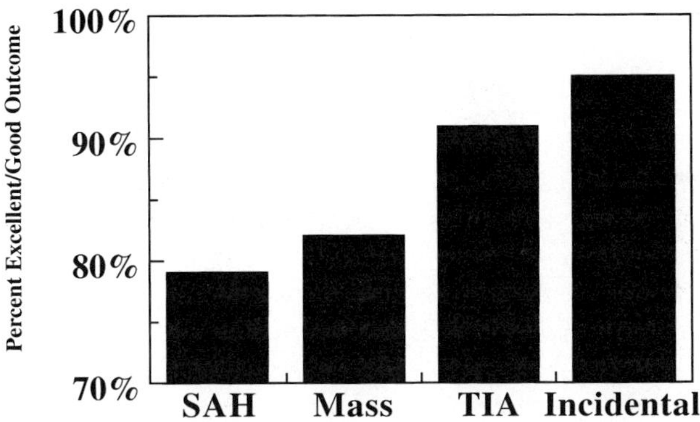

FIG. 16.3 Percent good and excellent outcomes as a function of clinical presentation.

cellent or good outcomes, as compared to 74% of the patients with posterior circulation aneurysms (Table 16.3). Interestingly, aneurysms along the supraclinoid ICA were associated with one of the highest mortality rates (16%). Patients with basilar artery aneurysms suffered the highest morbidity; fair or poor outcomes were observed in 19 and 57% of patients with basilar apex and midbasilar aneurysms, respectively.

The technique of aneurysm obliteration did not affect outcome significantly (Table 16.4). Excellent or good outcomes were associated with all techniques in 80 to 100% of the patients, except for aneurysmorrhaphy, which reflects the small sample size and the location of many of these aneurysms along the basilar artery.

TABLE 16.3
Patients' Glasgow Outcome Score by Giant Aneurysm Location

Location	Excellent/Good (%)	Fair/Poor (%)	Dead (%)	Totals
Petrous ICA	2(100)	0(0)	0(0)	2
Cavernous ICA	15(100)	0(0)	0(0)	15
Supraclinoid ICA	34(79)	2(5)	7(16)	43
MCA	23(96)	0(0)	1(4)	24
ACA	12(92)	1(8)	0(0)	13
Basilar apex	21(78)	5(19)	1(4)	27
Midbasilar artery	3(43)	4(57)	0(0)	7
Vertebral artery	5(100)	0(0)	0(0)	5
Anterior circulation	86(89)	3(3)	8(8)	97
Posterior circulation	29(74)	9(23)	1(3)	39

TABLE 16.4
Patient Outcome by Treatment Technique

Surgical Technique	Excellent/Good (%)	Fair/Poor (%)	Dead (%)	Totals
Clipping	69(82)	8(10)	7(8)	84
Trapping	24(92)	1(4)	1(4)	26
Proximal ligation	9(90)	0(0)	1(10)	10
Distal ligation	0(0)	1(100)	0(0)	1
Aneurysmorrhaphy	3(60)	2(40)	0(0)	5
Excision	6(100)	0(0)	0(0)	6
Wrapping	4(100)	0(0)	0(0)	4

The major complications of hypothermic circulatory arrest were postoperative hemorrhage and cerebral ischemia. Neurologic morbidity associated with hypothermic circulatory arrest was 13%, which is similar to 11% neurologic morbidity for the entire patient population. Twenty-three patients (74%), who were treated with hypothermic cardiac arrest, had excellent or good outcomes. Fair and poor outcomes occurred in 4 (13%) and 2 (6%) patients, respectively. Two patients died during the peri-operative period.

DISCUSSION

Prognosis of untreated patients with giant aneurysms is poor (3, 15, 16, 33). In a series of 31 patients with untreated giant aneurysms, Peerless *et al.* (46) reported a 68% mortality rate after 2 years and an 85% mortality rate after 5 years. All survivors had marked neurologic dysfunction. Michel (42) reported a 100% mortality rate at 2 years in untreated patients. SAH is the most common terminal event in patients with untreated lesions (33, 46). Seventy-five percent of Kodama and Suzuki's (33) untreated patients died of SAH during hospitalization. Studies of McCormick and Acousta-Rua (40) and by Wiebers *et al.* (72) suggest that the risk of aneurysmal rupture increases with the size of the aneurysm. Therefore, the annual risk of hemorrhage from giant aneurysms may be higher than the 1 to 3% cited for smaller aneurysms. Untreated giant aneurysms continue to enlarge, producing progressive deficits from cerebral compression. Distal thrombo-embolism also can cause stroke and contributes to the death rate.

In contrast, surgical results in large series of giant aneurysm patients reported excellent-to-good outcomes, ranging from 61 to 86%, and surgical mortality, ranging from 5 to 22% (Table 16.5). Patients in our series had excellent-to-good outcomes in 87% and surgical mortality of 5%. When these surgical results are compared with the poor outcome associated with the natural history of untreated giant aneurysms, it is apparent that surgery improves the prognosis for patients with giant aneurysms.

Therefore, the rationale for their treatment is to eliminate the risk of neurologic impairment, resulting from hemorrhage, cerebral compression, or thrombo-embolism. Consequently, the goals of surgery are to completely exclude the aneurysm from the circulation, to maintain adequate cerebral blood flow (CBF) and to decompress vital neural structures (35).

Operative Approach and Exposure

The operative approach is selected to optimize exposure of the aneurysm for complete visualization of vascular anatomy and effective clip placement. Maximizing bone removal from the skull provides flat, straight routes of access while minimizing brain retraction. Maximum

TABLE 16.5
Comparison of Outcomes in Surgical Series of Giant Intracranial Aneurysms

Author/Reference	Total No. of Patients	Outcome		
		Excellent/Good (%)	Fair/Poor (%)	Dead (%)
Sundt (66)	315	80	6	15
Peerless *et al.* (46)	305	67	22	11
Hosobuchi (25)	82	84	9	7
Ausman *et al.* (2)	62	84	11	5
Kodama and Suzuki (33)	49	61	16	22
Symon and Vajda (68)	36	86	6	8
Yasargil (73)	30	67	23	10
Heros (21)	28	82	7	5
Spetzler *et al.* (65), current series	171	87	8	5

exposure with minimum retraction is critical for safe surgery and good surgical outcomes.

The pterional trans-sylvian approach has become the standard for most neurosurgeons who treat aneurysms of the anterior circulation. This approach provides access to the ICA, its branches, and the entire circle of Willis. The sphenoid wing is drilled extensively down to the anterior clinoid process to open the sylvian fissure route. Removal of the anterior clinoid process exposes the proximal ICA. This maneuver gains proximal control of the ICA, if needed, and permits ophthalmic and paraclinoid aneurysms to be dissected.

SKULL BASE APPROACHES TO ANEURYSMS

Advances in skull base surgery have given neurosurgeons a variety of approaches to expose aneurysms at the base of the brain and to avoid retraction of vital brain structures. The orbitozygomatic-pterional approach (1, 18) enhances the exposure obtained with the pterional approach by removing the superior and lateral orbital margins, orbital roof, and anterior zygoma. This additional bone removal increases the superior limits of the angle of exposure and thereby improves the trans-sylvian access to high upper basilar artery aneurysms (PCA, basilar bifurcation, and SCA). Removing the zygoma allows the temporalis muscle to be retracted more inferiorly, improving the subtemporal access. This approach also is useful for ACA aneurysms when a lower, wider exposure is required.

The subtemporal approach and its variations (*i.e.*, the pterional-subtemporal, or "one-and-a-half") (9, 49, 50) were used originally for all upper basilar artery aneurysms (6, 7). Although this approach has been supplanted by the pterional approach, it is still useful with low-lying aneurysms of the basilar bifurcation that project posteriorly and with aneurysms of the distal PCA.

A variety of approaches can be used for giant infratentorial aneurysms. Transpetrosal approaches provides routes to the anterior brainstem and clivus by removing temporal bone (22, 26, 27). These approaches are divided into three categories, depending on the amount of bone removed: retrolabyrinthine, translabyrinthine, and transcochlear (59). The retrolabyrinthine technique removes the mastoid process and temporal bone until the posterior and superior semicircular canals are skeletonized. Hearing is preserved. The translabyrinthine technique completely removes all three semicircular canals and skeletonizes the posterior half of the internal auditory canal. Hearing is sacrificed. The transcochlear technique maximizes petrous bone resection with removal of the semicircular canals, internal auditory canal, cochlea, and tympanic portion of the temporal bone. Hearing is sacrificed, and the facial nerve is transposed. These petrosal techniques can be combined with a supratentorial-infratentorial craniotomy to increase exposure extensively from the sphenoid ridge and cavernous sinus to the foramen magnum (22, 38, 59). This combined supratentorial-infratentorial approach divides the tentorium to connect the two compartments, allowing complete visualization of vascular structures in the posterior fossa, particularly the upper and midbasilar trunk and AICA.

The inferior brainstem, inferior clivus, and upper cervical region can be exposed through the far-lateral approach, which is ideal for accessing vertebral artery, PICA, and VBJ aneurysms. The far-lateral approach removes the inferior rim of the foramen magnum, the posterior two-thirds of the occipital condyle, and the posterolateral arch of C1 to the level of the sulcus arteriosus of the vertebral artery (19, 20, 54, 61). The exposure obtained after this bony removal and dural opening requires minimal retraction of neurovascular structures.

Occasionally, a more extensive lateral exposure of the clivus is required to deal with giant aneurysms that involve the mid- and lower basilar arteries. Such an exposure can be achieved by combining the far-lateral approach with either an isolated transpetrosal approach or a combined supratentorial-infratentorial approach. This "combined-combined" approach provides a wide route to the entire length of the clivus (4).

Treatment Techniques

DIRECT ANEURYSM CLIPPING

The ideal treatment for intracranial aneurysms excludes the aneurysm completely from the circulation while preserving blood flow through the parent and branch vessels. This treatment is accomplished best by direct clip placement across the aneurysm neck (58). The feasibility of clipping is determined after careful intra-operative inspection of the aneurysm, its neck, and branch vessels.

Basic principles of aneurysm surgery are followed when dealing with giant aneurysms. First, proximal and distal vascular control is attained. Proximal control of ICA aneurysms may require removing the anterior clinoid process, exposing the petrous ICA in the carotid canal (70), or exposing the cervical ICA. Dissection of the aneurysm without temporary clipping of the parent vessel is best, but the decreased bulk of the aneurysm and the increased exposure gained by temporary clips are often invaluable.

Giant aneurysms typically have broad, complex necks that require either long clips with high closing pressures or multiple short clips.

Booster clips may be placed across the tips of a primary clip (where the closing pressure is inherently less than at the fulcrum) to eliminate persistent flow through an unoccluded neck. Tandem clips are usually short-aperture clips placed serially across the neck until the entire base has been occluded. Short clips have higher closing pressures, are less likely to slip off the neck, and can be contoured to preserve the lumen of the parent vessel. Parallel clips are applied adjacent to one another for added reinforcement. It is often safer to place a secondary parallel clip in a more optimal position on the neck, rather than to reposition the primary clip and risk tearing the aneurysm. Because the aneurysmal wall is thick with layers of organized thrombus, fibrous tissue, atherosclerotic degeneration, and calcification, clips should be placed high enough on the neck to avoid compromising the parent-vessel lumen. The neck is often fragile, and clips must be placed delicately.

Branch vessels and perforators must be preserved. These vessels are inspected after clipping to verify patency. If patency is unclear, Doppler ultrasonography is used.

INTRA-OPERATIVE CEREBRAL PROTECTION

Cerebral protection with barbiturates has become standard in the intra-operative management of aneurysm patients. Barbiturates reduce the metabolic demands of neural cells and extend the brain's tolerance to a decreased nutrient supply. Consequently, barbiturates help prevent cerebral injury from the focal ischemia associated with temporary occlusion of the parent vessel and dissection of giant aneurysms (52, 53, 56, 74). Patients receive intravenous barbiturate (thiopental) titrated to achieve electroencephalographic (EEG) burst suppression (62). Barbiturates are most effective when administered before the period of temporary ischemia (53). Intra-operative blood pressure is maintained mildly hypertensive, especially during any temporary vessel clipping, to enhance cerebral perfusion. Patients are monitored with SSEPs to determine tolerance to vessel occlusion.

HYPOTHERMIC CIRCULATORY ARREST

Hypothermic circulatory arrest is a valuable surgical adjunct to the treatment of giant aneurysms (57, 63). The size of many giant aneurysms precludes adequate visualization of the anatomy. This problem is probably most dramatic when one is dealing with giant basilar artery aneurysms because of the limitations associated with even the most elegant surgical exposures. Additional exposure can be obtained through hypothermic circulatory arrest (57, 63). During cardiac arrest the aneurysm can be collapsed to provide more working room and easier manipulation of neurovascular structures. The anatomy is defined in a bloodless surgical field without the risk of hemorrhage.

Hypothermic circulatory arrest is complex but highly effective. The success of this tool for clipping complex aneurysms is determined by five key variables: the depth of hypothermia, the duration of circulatory arrest, the use of barbiturates, the hemostasis, and the rate of rewarming after aneurysm clipping. In our experience, the mean brain temperature during standstill has been 14.6°C, and the mean duration of standstill 22.5 minutes (range, 2 to 72 minutes). The absolute maximum duration of cerebral ischemia that can be tolerated safely is unknown. Duration can be increased significantly by the use of profound hypothermia and intravenous barbiturates administered to the point of EEG burst suppression. The period of circulatory arrest should be limited to the final period of aneurysm dissection and clip application.

Meticulous attention must be given to intra-operative hemostasis, with close surveillance of the patient's clotting mechanisms. Several factors contribute to a hypocoagulable state: heparinization during cardiopulmonary bypass, red blood cell and platelet dysfunction resulting from the trauma of the bypass pump (10), platelet sequestration and slowing of the coagulation cascade due to hypothermia (6), and hemodilution of coagulation factors (43). Steps taken to treat this hypocoagulable state include heparin reversal with protamine, whole-blood and platelet transfusions, fresh frozen plasma, calcium chloride, and restoring normothermia. The patient must be rewarmed at a carefully controlled rate (0.2 to 0.5°C/min), with a mean rewarming time of 90 minutes. The potential morbidity (13%) associated with circulatory arrest stipulates that it be used only when the parent vessels and aneurysm cannot be exposed and controlled with routine surgical techniques, including such measures as the application of multiple temporary clips. However, when required, circulatory arrest provides an added measure of safety without significantly increasing the inherent morbidity or mortality associated with these lesions. The rate of direct clipping in this series (62%) exceeds the rates in other series (Drake, 39% (11); Sundt, 49% (66)). This difference is attributed to the use of hypothermic circulatory arrest.

ALTERNATIVE TECHNIQUES OF ANEURYSM OCCLUSION

Many giant aneurysms (38% in this series) are not amenable to direct clipping because of their size, the lack of a discrete neck, or the technical difficulty associated with the dissection. Alternative techniques for these unclippable aneurysms include proximal vessel occlusion, trapping, aneurysmorrhaphy, and excision of the aneurysm.

These techniques are inferior to direct clipping, because they sacrifice the parent and branch vessels. Consequently, patients are at risk for hemodynamic compromise and ischemic complications. These alternative techniques are therefore recommended only after attempts at direct clipping have failed.

Aneurysm trapping along the parent vessel completely eliminates the aneurysm from the circulation. The segment of vessel sacrificed is minimized by applying the clips as close to the aneurysm as possible. When important branch vessels are located along this segment of parent vessel and cannot be sacrificed safely (for example, along the supraclinoid ICA), it is advisable to only occlude proximally. Proximal vessel occlusion produces vascular dead space and does not prevent retrograde filling of the aneurysm, thereby making thrombo-embolism a potential complication. However, the reduced blood flow within the aneurysm can reduce the risk of rupture and promote thrombosis of the lumen.

Aneurysm excision is an alternative for MCA aneurysms, where the vessels can be reconstructed more easily (17). Primary re-anastomosis of the parent vessel is attempted but is often impossible after resection of these large lesions. When the vascular tissues around the neck are not too friable to prevent suturing, the aneurysm dome can be resected partially and the artery reconstructed with vessel wall around the neck (8). Aneurysmorrhaphy is technically difficult but has the advantage of reconstituting the parent vessel and maintaining CBF without a bypass procedure.

CEREBRAL REVASCULARIZATION

Safe treatment of unclippable giant aneurysms with trapping, proximal vessel occlusion, or excision often requires revascularization to maintain CBF and to guard against ischemic complications (58, 64). Most decisions regarding the need for revascularization can be made based on clinical (*e.g.*, TIAs and previous stroke) and angiographic information. Angiographic evidence of incompetent vessels, poor collateral circulation, and low flow distal to the aneurysm may indicate a need to revascularize. Occasionally, xenon CT-cerebral blood flow (Xe CT-CBF) studies and positron emission tomography (PET) scans are used to determine whether the region of brain in question is hypoperfused. Provocative tests, such as balloon test occlusion with Xe CT-CBF studies, have been advocated to determine a patient's tolerance to ICA occlusion (23, 36, 51, 55). These tests can confirm the need for revascularization. However, because these tests have a false-negative rate of 2 to 22% (12a, 41, 44a, 55), they do not establish definitively the safety of vessel sacrifice, nor do they address the risks of delayed ischemic deficits and *de novo* aneurysm formation.

ANEURYSM DEBULKING

Compression of neural structures by the aneurysm mass caused more than one-third of patient morbidity in this series. Therefore, after a giant aneurysm has been completely eliminated from the circulation—regardless of the technique—it is debulked to relieve mass effect on surrounding structures. If the lumen is not thrombosed, simple aspiration will debulk the aneurysm. However, the lumen is filled typically with layers of thrombus that can be resected easily. Clipped or trapped aneurysms are debulked immediately. In contrast, proximally occluded aneurysms require time for thrombotic occlusion to develop and for angiographic verification of occlusion. Debulking is then performed in a separate surgical stage. The goal of aneurysm debulking is reduction of mass effect, not necessarily complete removal of the aneurysm. An aneurysm wall that is adhered densely to the brain or cranial nerves may be left behind, because complete removal could injure these structures.

Endovascular Therapy

The role of endovascular therapy for giant aneurysms continues to evolve. Currently, several endovascular techniques are available, including intra-aneurysmal placement of detachable balloons, occlusion coils, and ethylene vinyl alcohol copolymer (16, 32, 69). The risks and efficacy of endovascular therapy are in the process of being defined. Early experience, however, suggests that the large and irregular shape of the aneurysmal base and the thrombus in the sac makes endovascular treatment of giant aneurysms difficult. Complications of treatment include TIAs, temporary ischemic deficits, and death from rupture during the procedure. Complete obliteration of the aneurysm frequently fails (69).

Giant aneurysms tend to require debulking to alleviate mass effect, and this goal cannot be accomplished with standard endovascular techiques. Therefore, endovascular techniques will contribute to the treatment of giant aneurysms, but they should remain part of a multidisciplinary management strategy.

Postoperative Management

All patients are evaluated from postoperative angiography to confirm complete elimination of the aneurysm and patency of bypass grafts. Treatment cannot be considered complete until the aneurysm is eliminated. Residual aneurysm filling is treated with direct surgical or, occasionally, with endovascular techniques until the aneurysm is obliterated. Graft occlusions are treated in an emergency to re-establish patency. Patients with SAH are managed according to established protocols with hypervolemia, hypertension, and hemodilution for 2 weeks after hemorrhage, or until the symptoms resolve (30).

SUMMARY

Patients with untreated giant intracranial aneurysms have a dismal prognosis as a result of hemorrhage, cerebral compression, and thromboembolism. Therefore, giant aneurysms should be treated. The operative approach is chosen to maximize exposure of the aneurysm. Direct clipping of the aneurysm neck, with preservation of the parent and branch vessels, is the preferred method of occlusion. Hypothermic circulatory arrest may facilitate clipping in selected patients. Alternative techniques for unclippable aneurysms can be utilized, but they compromise parent arteries and require revascularization to maintain CBF. Because mass effect is an important cause of patient morbidity, giant aneurysms are usually debulked after they have been eliminated completely from the circulation. Giant aneurysms are complex lesions that demand thorough surgical planning, individualized strategies, and a multidisciplinary effort.

REFERENCES

1. Al-Mefty O: The cranio-orbital zyomatic approach for intracranial lesions. **Contemp Neurosurg** 14(9):1–6, 1992.
2. Ausman JI, Diaz F, Sadasivan B, *et al.*: Giant intracranial aneurysm surgery: The role of microvascular reconstruction. **Surg Neurol** 34:8–15, 1990.
3. Awad IA, Carter LP, Spetzler RF, *et al.*: Clinical vasospasm after subarachnoid hemorrhage: Response to hypervolemic hemodilution and arterial hypertension. **Stroke** 18(2):365–372, 1987.
4. Baldwin HZ, Miller CG, Van Loveren HR, *et al.*: The far lateral-combined supra- and infratentorial approach. A human cadaveric prosection model for routes of access to the petroclival region and ventral brain stem. **J Neurosurg** 81:60–68, 1994.
5. Bailes JE, Spetzler RF, Hadley MN, *et al.*: Management morbidity and morality of poor-grade aneurysm patients. **J Neurosurg** 72:559–566, 1990.
6. Baumgartner WA, Silverberg GD, Ream AK, *et al.*: Reappraisal of cardiopulmonary bypass with deep hypothermia and circulatory arrest for complex neurosurgical operations. **Surgery** 94(2):242–249, 1983.
7. Bederson JB, Spetzler RF: Anastomosis of the anterior temporal artery to a secondary trunk of the middle cerebral artery for treatment of a giant M^1, segment aneurysm. **J Neurosurg** 76:863–866, 1992.
8. Bojanowski WM, Spetzler RF, Carter LP: Reconstruction of the MCA bifurcation after excision of a giant aneurysm: Technical note. **J Neurosurg** 68(6):974–977, 1988.

9. Diaz FG: Vertebrobasilar aneurysms: Surgical management. **Crit Rev Neurosurg** 2:146–158, 1992.

10. Doutremepuich C: Haemostasis defects following cardio-pulmonary by-pass based on a study of 1350 patients. **Thromb Haemost** 39:539–541, 1978 (letter).

11. Drake CG: Giant intracranial aneurysms: Experience with surgical treatment in 174 patients. **Clin Neurosurg** 26:12–96, 1979.

12. Drake CG: The treatment of aneurysms of the posterior circulation. **Clin Neurosurg** 26:96–144, 1979.

12a. Drake CG, Peerless SJ, Ferguson GG: Hunterian proximal arterial occlusion for giant aneurysms of the carotid circulation. **J Neurosurg** 81:656–665, 1994.

13. Fisher CM, Kistler JP, Davis JM: Relation of cerebral vasospasm to subarachnoid hemorrhage visualized by computerized tomographic scanning. **Neurosurgery** 6(1):1–9, 1980.

14. Fitzpatrick BC, Spetzler RF, Ballard JL, *et al.:* Cervical-to-petrous internal carotid artery bypass procedure. Technical note. **J Neurosurg** 79:138–141, 1993.

15. Greene KA, Anson JA, Spetzler RF: Giant serpentine middle cerebral artery aneurysm treated by extracranial-intracranial bypass. **J Neurosurg** 78:974–978, 1993.

16. Guglielmi G, Viñuela F, Dion J, *et al.:* Electrothrombosis of saccular aneurysms via endovascular approach. Part 2: Preliminary clinical experience. **J Neurosurg** 75:8–14, 1991.

17. Hadley MN, Spetzler RF, Martin NA, *et al.:* Middle cerebral artery aneurysm due to *Nocardia asteroides:* Case report of aneurysm excision and extracranial-intracranial bypass. **Neurosurgery** 22:923–928; 1988.

18. Hakuba A, Liu SS, Nishimura S: The orbitozygomatic infratemporal approach. A new surgical technique. **Surg Neurol** 26(3):271–276; 1986.

19. Hammon WM, Kempe LG: The posterior fossa approach to aneurysms of the vertebral and basilar arteries. **J Neurosurg** 37(3):339–347; 1972.

20. Heros RC: Lateral suboccipital approach for vertebral and vertebrobasilar artery lesions. **J Neurosurg** 64:559–562; 1986.

21. Heros RC: Management of giant paraclinoid aneurysms, in Kikuchi H, Fukushima T, Watanabe K (eds): *Intracranial Aneurysms.* Niigata, Japan, Nishimura, 1986, pp 273–282.

22. Hitselberger WE, House WF: A combined approach to the cerebellopontine angle. A suboccipital-petrosal approach. Arch Otolaryngol 84(3):49–67; 1966.

23. Horton JA, Jungreis CA, Pistoia F: Balloon test occlusion, in Sekhar LN, Janecka IP (eds): *Surgery of Cranial Base Tumors.* New York, Raven Press, 1993, pp 33–36.

24. Hosobuchi Y: Direct surgical treatment of giant intracranial aneurysms. **J Neurosurg** 51:743–756; 1979.

25. Hosobuchi Y: Giant intracranial aneurysms, in Wilkins RH, Rengachary SS (eds): *Neurosurgery.* New York, McGraw-Hill, 1985, pp 1404–1414.

26. House WF: Translabyrinthine approach, In House WF, Luetje CM (eds): *Acoustic Tumors.* Baltimore, MD, University Park Press, 1979, pp 43–87.

27. House WF, Hitselberger WE: The transcochlear approach to the skull base. **Arch Otolaryngol** 102(6):334–342, 1976.

28. Hunt WE, Hess RM: Surgical risk as related to time of intervention in the repair of intracranial aneurysms. **J Neurosurg** 28:14–20; 1968.

29. Jennett B, Bond M: Assessment of outcome after severe brain damage. **Lancet** 1:480–484; 1975.

30. Kassell NF, Peerless SJ, Durward QJ, *et al.:* Treatment of ischemic deficits from vasospasm with intravascular volume expansion and induced arterial hypertension. **Neurosurgery** 11:337–343, 1982.
31. Khayata MH, Spetzler RF, Mooy JJA, *et al.:* Combined surgical and endovascular treatment of a giant vertebral artery aneurysm in a child. Case report. **J Neurosurg** 37:304–307, 1994.
32. Knuckey NW, Haas R, Jenkins R, *et al.:* Thrombosis of difficult intracranial aneurysms by endovascular placement of platinum-Dacron microcoils. **J Neurosurg** 77(1):43–50, 1992.
33. Kodama N, Suzuki J: Surgical treatment of giant aneurysms. **Neurosurg Rev** 5:155–160; 1982.
34. Koshikawa N, Kamio M, Sekino H, *et al.:* Giant aneurysm: A case report with review of the literature (author's translation of the Japanese). **No Shinkei Geka** 8(1):79–88; 1980.
35. Lawton MT, Spetzler RF: Management strategies for giant intracranial aneurysms. **Contemp Neurosurg** 16(17):1–6; 1994.
36. Linskey ME, Sekhar LN, Sen C: Cerebral revascularization in cranial base surgery, in Sekhar LN, Janecka IP (eds): *Surgery of Cranial Base Tumors.* New York. Raven Press, 1993, pp 45–68.
37. Locksley HB: Natural history of subarachnoid hemorrhage, intracranial aneurysms and arteriovenous malformations based on 6368 cases in the cooperative study. **J Neurosurg** 25(2):219–239; 1966.
38. Malis LI: Surgical resection of tumors of the skull base, in Wilkins RH, Rengachary SS (eds): *Neurosurgery* New York, McGraw-Hill, 1985, pp 1011–1021.
39. Marano SR, Spetzler RF, Carter LP: Autogeneous saphenous vein interposition grafts for high flow augmentation of cerebral blood flow. **BNI Q** 1(4):29–33, 1985.
40. McCormick WF, Acosta-Rua GJ: The size of intracranial saccular aneurysms: An autopsy study. **J Neurosurg** 33(4):422–427, 1970.
41. McIvor NP, Willinsky RA, TerBrugge KG, *et al.:* Validity of test occlusion studies prior to internal carotid artery sacrifice. **Head Neck** 16(1):11–16; 1994.
42. Michel WF: Posterior fossa aneurysms simulating tumours. **J Neurol Neurosurg Psychiatry** 37:218–223; 1974.
43. Morgan H, Nofzinger JD, Robertson JT, *et al.:* Hemorrhagic studies with severe hemodilution in profound hypothermia and cardiac arrest. **J Surg Res** 14:459–464; 1973.
44. Morley TP, Barr HW: Giant intracranial aneurysms: Diagnosis, course and management. **Clin Neurosurg** 16:73–94; 1969.
44a. Origitano TC, Al-Mefty O, Leonetti JP, DeMonte F, and Reichman OH. Vascular considerations and complications in cranial base surgery. **Neurosurgery** 35:351–363, 1994.
45. Peerless SJ, Drake CG: Management of aneurysms of the posterior circulation, in Youmans JR (ed): *Neurological Survey. A Comprehensive Reference Guide to the Diagnosis and Management of Neurosurgical Problems.* Philadelphia, WB Saunders, 1990, vol 3, pp 1764–1806.
46. Peerless SJ, Wallace MC, Drake CG: Giant intracranial aneurysms, in Youmans JR (ed): *Neurological Surgery. A Comprehensive Reference Guide to the Diagnosis and Management of Neurological Problems.* Philadelphia, W.B. Saunders, 1990, pp 1742–1763.
47. Roski RA, Spetzler RF, Hopkins LN: Occipital artery to posterior inferior cerebellar artery bypass for vertebrobasilar ischemia. **Neurosurgery** 10:44–49, 1982.

48. Pia HW, Zierski J: Giant cerebral aneurysms. A review of clinical picture, diagnosis, and management with illustrative cases. **Neurosurg Rev** 5:117–148, 1982.

49. Sano K: Temporo-polar approach to aneurysms of the basilar artery at and around the distal bifurcation: Technical note. **Neurol Res** 2(3–4):361–367; 1980.

50. Sano K, Asano T, Tamura A: Surgical technique, in Sano K, Tamura A (eds): *Acute Aneurysm Surgery. Pathophysiology and Management*. New York, Springer-Verlag, 1987, pp 194–246.

51. Sekhar LN, Sen CN, Jho HD: Saphenous vein graft bypass of the cavernous internal carotid artery. **J Neurosurg** 72:35–41; 1990.

52. Selman WR, Spetzler RF, Roski RA, *et al.:* Regional cerebral blood flow following middle cerebral artery occlusion and barbiturate therapy in baboons. **J Cereb Blood Flow Metab** 1(Suppl 1):S214–S215, 1981.

53. Selman WR, Spetzler RF, Roski RA, *et al.:* Barbiturate coma in focal cerebral ischemia: Relationship of protection to timing of therapy. **J Neurosurg** 56:685–690, 1982.

54. Sen CN, Sekhar LN: An extreme lateral approach to intradural lesions of the cervical spine and foramen magnum. **Neurosurgery** 27:197–204; 1990.

55. Sen C, Sekhar LN: Direct vein graft reconstruction of the cavernous, petrous and upper cervical internal carotid artery: Lessons learned from 30 cases. **Neurosurgery** 30(5):732–743; 1992.

56. Shapiro HM: Barbiturates in brain ischemia. **Br J Anaesth** 57(1):82–95; 1985.

57. Solomon RA, Smith CR, Raps EC, *et al.:* Deep hypothermic circulatory arrest for the management of complex anterior and posterior circulation aneurysms. **Neurosurgery** 29:732–737; 1991.

58. Spetzler RF, Carter LP: Revascularization and aneurysm surgery: Current status. **Neurosurgery** 16:111–116, 1985.

59. Spetzler RF, Daspit CP, Pappas CTE: The combined supra- and infratentorial approach for lesions of the petrous and clival regions: Experience with 46 cases. **J Neurosurg** 76:588–599; 1992.

60. Spetzler RF, Fukushima T, Martin N, *et al.:* Petrous carotid-to-intradural carotid saphenous vein graft for intracavernous giant aneurysm, tumor, and occlusive cerebrovascular disease. **J Neurosurg** 73(4):496–501; 1990.

61. Spetzler RF, Grahm TW: The far-lateral approach to the inferior clivus and upper cervical region: Technical note. **BNI Q** 6(4):35–38, 1990.

62. Spetzler RF, Hadley MN: Protection against cerebral ischemia: The role of barbiturates. **Cerebrovasc Brain Metab Rev** 1:212–229; 1989.

63. Spetzler RF, Hadley MN, Rigamonti D, *et al.:* Aneurysms of the basilar artery treated with circulatory arrest, hypothermia, and barbiturate cerebral protection. **J Neurosurg** 68(6):868–879; 1988.

64. Spetzler RF, Schuster H, Roski RA: Elective extracranial-intracranial arterial bypass in the treatment of inoperable giant aneurysms of the internal carotid artery. **J Neurosurg** 53:22–27; 1980.

65. Spetzler RF, Selman W, Carter LP: Elective EC-IC bypass for unclippable intracranial aneurysms. **Neurol Res** 6:64–68; 1984.

66. Sundt TM Jr: Results of surgical management, in Sundt TM Jr (ed): *Surgical Techniques for Saccular and Giant Intracranial Aneurysms*. Baltimore, Williams & Wilkins, 1990, pp 19–23.

67. Sundt TM Jr, Piepgras DG: Surgical approach to giant intracranial aneurysms: Operative experience with 80 cases. **J Neurosurg** 51:731–742, 1979.

68. Symon L, Vajda J: Surgical experiences with giant intracranial aneurysms. **J Neurosurg** 61:1009–1028, 1984.

69. Taki W, Nishi S, Yamashita K, *et al.:* Selection and combination of various endovascular techniques in the treatment of giant aneurysms. **J Neurosurg** 77: 37–42; 1992.
70. Wascher TM, Spetzler RF, Zabramski JM: Improved transdural exposure and temporary occlusion of the petrous internal carotid artery for cavernous sinus surgery: Technical note. **J Neurosurg** 78(5):834–837; 1993.
71. Weir B: Special aneurysms: Saccular, in Wier B (ed): *Aneurysms Affecting the Nervous System.* Baltimore, Williams & Wilkins, 1987, pp 185–208.
72. Wiebers DO, Whisnant JP, Sundt TM Jr, *et al.:* The significance of unruptured intracranial saccular aneurysms. **J Neurosurg** 66:23–29; 1987.
73. Yasargil MG: Giant intracranial aneurysms, in Yasargil MG (ed): *Microneurosurgery II. Clinical Considerations, Surgery of the Intracranial Aneurysms and Results.* New York, Thieme-Stratton, 1984, pp 296–304.
74. Yatsu FM: Pharmacologic protection against ischemic brain damage. **Neurol Clin** 1:37–53; 1983.

17

Endovascular Management of Giant Intracranial Aneurysms

SCOTT C. STANDARD, M.D., LEE R. GUTERMAN, Ph.D., M.D.,
TAMERLA D. CHAVIS, M.D., MARY DUFFY FRONCKOWIAK, Ph.D.,
KEVIN J. GIBBONS, M.D., AND L. NELSON HOPKINS, M.D.

Within the past 2 decades, the management of giant (>25 mm) intracranial aneurysms has been dramatically impacted by advances in neurosurgical techniques. Improved instrumentation and novel neuroprotective agents have allowed the present generation of neurosurgical pioneers to address these formidable lesions. New neuro-imaging techniques provide detailed information regarding the anatomy of the aneurysm and its composition. However, giant aneurysms remain one of the most formidable lesions confronting the neurosurgeon, and their treatment represents a substantial risk to the patient.

The modern concept of aneurysm surgery is based on the development of cerebral angiography. Egas Moniz, a Portuguese neurologist, devised the technique of cerebral angiography, using direct carotid artery puncture, and demonstrated an anterior communicating artery aneurysm (68). The refinement of cerebral angiography led surgeons to become increasingly aggressive in the management of intracranial aneurysms. Craniotomy and clipping became the gold standard for the definitive treatment of giant aneurysms. Giant aneurysms considered inoperable, using craniotomy and clipping techniques, were treated by the more traditional approaches of hunterian ligation or gradual proximal arterial occlusion. In the hands of competent neurosurgeons, surgical management has proven efficacy in providing definitive protection from aneurysm rebleeding and enlargement.

Since its inception, neuro-endovascular therapy has been challenged to address the most difficult problems encountered in neurosurgery, and a variety of endovascular techniques have been developed to augment the surgical approach to the management of giant aneurysms. Endovascular treatment is in a state of evolution and is rapidly changing. Some current endovascular treatment options include parent artery occlusion or aneurysm trapping, endosaccular occlusion and, in some circumstances, endovascular reconstruction with stents (Fig. 17.1). Of these, endosaccular occlusion is the most widely used technique. Ironically, initial results indicate that those patients who are the best candidates for surgical clip ligation are also the best candidates for endosaccular occlusion, *i.e.,* those harboring smaller aneurysms with small necks.

Currently in the United States, endovascular techniques are reserved for patients with aneurysms considered to be poor surgical risks or for those in whom conventional surgical techniques have failed. Endovascular techniques are attractive to patients because they may obviate the need for craniotomy. To replace existing surgical techniques and become widely endorsed for the treatment of giant aneurysms, however, endovascular therapy must offer a reduced procedural morbidity and mortality and provide a definitive result. Wide-necked and giant aneurysms represent a major challenge to both conventional surgical and endovascular surgical techniques. The challenge of the next decade will be to find endovascular methods to reconstruct the normal arterial wall while excluding flow to the aneurysm. The "winds of change" in medicine that Dr. Richard Roski cited in his 1994 Presidential Address to the Congress of Neurosurgeons (Chapter 1 of this book) are placing increasing pressure on the economy of care. The endovascular approach may demonstrate reduced cost not only in terms of shorter hospitalizations with fewer treatment-related costs but also in terms of neurologic disability and overall cost to society.

Based on a foundation of pathophysiology, the history of neuro-endovascular treatment of giant intracranial aneurysms is reviewed. Current treatment options and research investigations are discussed.

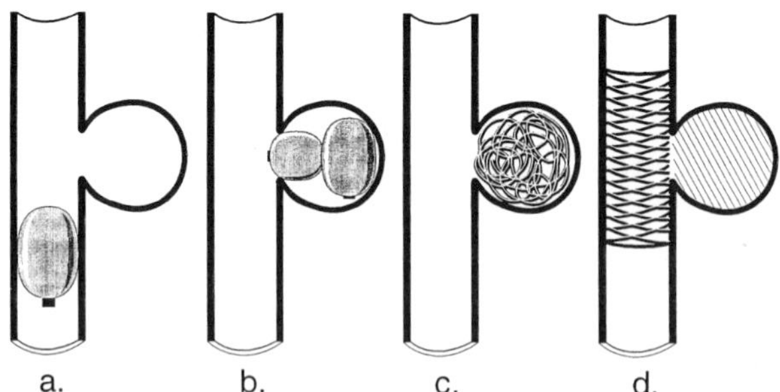

FIG. 17.1 Endovascular techniques to treat aneurysms. **(a)** Parent artery occlusion or aneurysm trapping. **(b)** Endosaccular balloon occlusion. **(c)** Endosaccular coil occlusion. **(d)** Endovascular reconstruction (stent maintains the cylindrical geometry of the parent vessel while directing blood flow away from the aneurysm).

In the present setting of health care reform, an analysis of the cost of endovascular therapy is also presented.

HEMODYNAMIC CONSIDERATIONS

The pathogenesis of giant aneurysms has been elucidated by numerous *in vitro* investigations and clinical observations. Early theories regarding congenital defects in the arterial wall are being replaced by experimental evidence suggesting that hemodynamic factors play a major role in pathogenesis (79). A better understanding of hemodynamics and pathophysiology of the arterial wall, which contribute to aneurysm formation, enlargement, thrombosis, and thrombus remodeling, may explain the success or failure of endovascular devices used to treat these lesions. Although for the neurosurgeon, the anatomy of the artery is most important, for the endovascular surgeon, the hemodynamic profile of the aneurysm is paramount.

As suggested by Ferguson (16), higher shear stresses at arterial bifurcations may initiate the development and growth of aneurysms by producing focal destruction of the internal elastic lamina of the vessel wall. His *in vitro* studies in nondistensible glass models showed that disturbed flow is present within the aneurysm cavity (Fig. 17.2). At low flow rates, flow division is seen at boundary layers at the bifurcation and the adjacent parent vessel. The streamline reattaches downstream, and laminar flow is re-established. However, Liepsch *et al.* (62) calculated flow velocities in glass and silastic lateral aneurysm models with laser Doppler anemometry and found that shear stresses at the aneurysm lips (*i.e.*, orifice) at a bifurcation are definitely below velocities required to induce endothelial disruption of the arterial wall but may be sufficient to further damage an already diseased aneurysm wall.

Strother *et al.* (82) analyzed the flow profiles in three types of canine intracranial aneurysms by using digital subtraction angiography and duplex color Doppler techniques. Aneurysms were classified as lateral wall, bifurcation, or terminal, depending on the geometric relationship of the aneurysm and its parent artery and branches (Fig. 17.3). Flow within giant aneurysms was predictable, in that there were well-defined inflow and outflow tracts.

Kerber and Heilman (53) prepared a series of glass models of human intracranial aneurysms. Their flow chamber experiments showed that, depending on the position of the aneurysm at the bifurcation, the central streamline with the highest kinetic energy ($P_{Total} = P_{Static} + P_{Kinetic}$, where pressure [$P$] = energy) may enter the aneurysm. This force may be important in the initiation and growth of human saccular aneurysms.

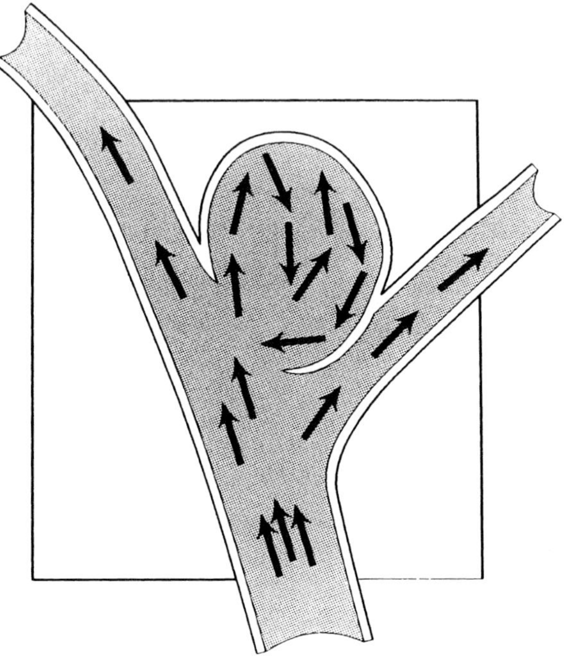

FIG. 17.2 Schematic diagram depicting disturbed flow within a giant aneurysm. Aneurysm inflow is derived from a high-energy streamline within the parent vessel. As blood enters the aneurysm, the flow is disturbed. A congruent outflow tract exits the aneurysm with preferential flow into one daughter vessel. (Reproduced with permission from Standard SC, Chavis TD, Guterman LR, *et al.:* Endovascular occlusion of aneurysms. **Neurosurg Q,** Volume 4, pages 201–219, 1994.)

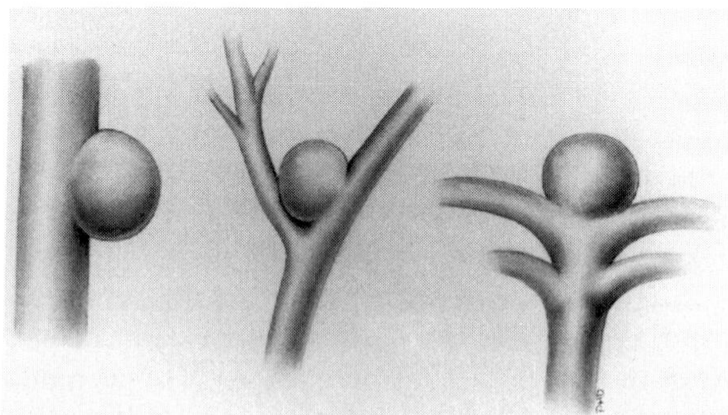

FIG. 17.3 Aneurysms are classified as lateral-wall or side-wall (*left*), bifurcation (*center*), or terminal (*right*). Aneurysm geometry has a great impact on the success or failure of endovascular therapy. (Reproduced with permission from Standard SC, Guterman LR, Chavis TD, *et al.:* Hopkins LN: Endovascular treatment of giant aneurysms, in Awad I, Barrow D (eds): *Giant Intracranial Aneurysms.* Park Forest, IL, AANS Publications, in press, 1995.)

Graves *et al.* (30) demonstrated in animal experiments, using digital subtraction angiography for follow-up studies, that the success of endosaccular aneurysm treatment depends on the shape of the aneurysm and how and which kind of occlusive material is used. Complex coil shapes, such as the "flower petal" configuration, were most stable (*i.e.,* less predisposed to migrate from their original position immediately or on a delayed basis). Filling the aneurysms with balloons or coils and deflecting the inflow tract from its usual position in the distal orifice to a midostial position resulted in reduced size or thrombosis of the aneurysm with preservation of the parent artery. They discussed different hemodynamic forces responsible for delayed changes of position and shape of occlusive material inside the aneurysms, which may allow regrowth and early recanalization.

Stagnant flow within the aneurysm cavity is commonly observed in angiographic studies of human giant aneurysms. Stagnant flow may be important in the pathophysiology of giant aneurysms, because it may promote the deposition of leukocytes and fibrin onto the aneurysm wall and may also inhibit the diffusion of oxygen and metabolites from blood to the vessel wall.

Giant aneurysms may present with hemorrhage because of structural weakness of the aneurysm wall. This phenomenon may be partially attributed to the law of La Place, which states that the wall tension (F) at the equator of an aneurysm will be higher as a function of increasing the radius of the aneurysm (14). With a larger radius (R), the force (F) tending to rupture the aneurysm will be greater, even with constant blood pressure (P), or $F = \pi R^2 P$.

Low-frequency flow fluctuations have been implicated in the production of vibration and resonance within the arterial and aneurysmal wall (80). Vibrations recorded from the adventitial surfaces of aneurysms (78) may contribute to endothelial and medial disruption.

The incomplete endovascular treatment of giant aneurysms is of questionable value, analogous in many respects to the formation of aneurysm remnants (*i.e.,* residual aneurysm neck or sac) following surgical clipping. Drake *et al.* (11, 12) and Lin *et al.* (63) reported an 8 to 25% rate of rebleeding from aneurysm remnants; however, other series, notably that of Feuerberg *et al.* (17), estimated the risk to be less than 1% per year. The risk of hemorrhage from a giant aneurysm remnant is undefined but cannot be disregarded. Alterations in flow patterns adjacent to the aneurysm orifice may actually increase the risk of rupture by changing the point of impact of the central streamline possessing the highest kinetic energy. Rupture of a giant aneurysm at the neck has been reported from even a small aneurysm remnant present after cerebral bypass and parent vessel occlusion (66). Giant aneurysm thrombosis must not be equated with cure until long-term follow-up is available and regression or stabilization of aneurysm size is seen on computerized tomography (CT) or magnetic resonance imaging (MRI) (81).

Another consideration is that giant aneurysms may grow as a result of recurrent hemorrhage from vessels of the aneurysm wall into the aneurysm cavity, as suggested by Schubiger *et al.* (75). Hecht *et al.* (35) reported the enlargement of a previously thrombosed giant aneurysm after endovascular parent vessel occlusion, presumably by this mechanism. Other authors have reported similar findings (3, 51).

ENDOSACCULAR APPROACH

Balloon Occlusion

A great deal of interest was generated by the first catheter-based treatment of an intracranial aneurysm by Luessenhop and Velasquez in 1964 (64). In 1974, Serbinenko (76) described successful endosaccular treatment of intracranial aneurysms, using latex balloons. Subsequently, Romodanov and Shcheglov (73) reported 137 endosaccular occlusions in 119 patients. Their results included recanalization of the aneurysm in three patients and four deaths, of which three were from thrombosis of the internal carotid artery (ICA).

Hieshima *et al.* (37, 39) described the use of a detachable silicone balloon affixed to a coaxial microcatheter system. The silicone balloon could be reliably detached by traction on the catheter. A self-sealing miter valve was incorporated (Fig. 17.4) to prevent premature deflation. This

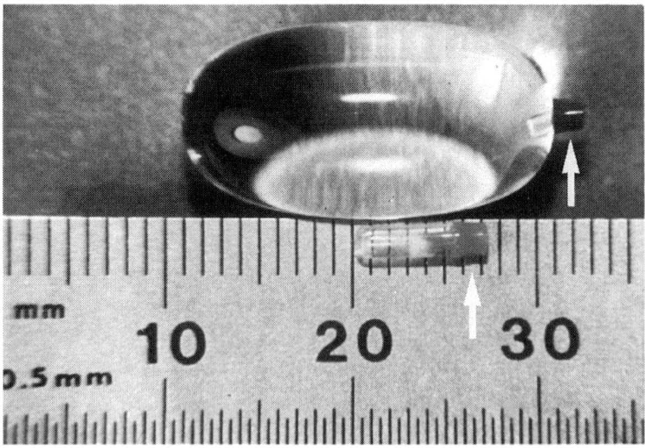

FIG. 17.4 Detachable silicone balloon (inflated, *top;* noninflated, *center*). Delivery catheter (not shown) is placed through the balloon's self-sealing miter valve (*arrows, top* and *bottom*).

device was subsequently used to treat a carotid-ophthalmic artery aneurysm with preservation of the parent vessel lumen (38). Late deflation of the balloon occurred, and bony spicules in the region of inflation caused early balloon rupture (48), which led to the development of a polymer (2-hydroxy ethyl methacrylate) that solidified within the balloon to ensure permanent inflation (28). However, this material was found incompatible with latex balloons (19, 69).

Higashida *et al.* (41) reviewed their initial experience with 25 patients with 26 inoperable aneurysms of the posterior circulation treated by detachable balloon embolization. Seventeen cases were treated with preservation of the parent artery, and nine cases required occlusion of the parent artery. Sixty percent of the patients were neurologically unchanged 2 to 43 months after the procedure. Their experience with anterior and posterior circulation aneurysms was reported the following year (40). Detachable balloon embolization with preservation of the parent artery was performed in 84 patients, who failed surgical clipping, could not tolerate general anesthesia, or had surgically difficult aneurysms. Ten deaths resulted from regrowth and rupture of the aneurysm cavity, and nine strokes occurred after balloon placement. The French experience with detachable latex balloons was similar (23).

Results from Moscow were presented at the Stonwin Lectures (56). Endosaccular aneurysm occlusion was used in 62.7% of 267 operated cases. Although technical details were not provided, balloons were shaped to conform to the aneurysm geometry. Thrombo-embolism occurred in 7.9% of cases, and postoperative mortality was 7.5%.

Currently, endosaccular balloon occlusion of giant intracranial aneurysms is rarely performed because of the risk of distal embolization of the balloon and the possibility of aneurysm recanalization and rerupture (44, 83). Recanalization is prone to occur at terminal aneurysm locations with the occurrence of the "water-hammer" effect of blood striking the balloon (36, 60). The impact of a high-energy streamline entering the aneurysm may lead to recanalization at an early stage (58).

Concerns relating to the biocompatibility of silicone implants have thus far prevented approval of the use of silicone balloons by the United States Food and Drug Administration.

Coil Occlusion

PLATINUM COILS

In 1965, Mullan *et al.* (70) reported the first series of electrically induced thrombosis in intracranial aneurysms. Hosobuchi (49) subsequently deployed metal wire for the direct thrombosis of cerebral aneurysms, using

                    CLINICAL NEUROSURGERY

a stereotaxic percutaneous approach. In 1988, Target Therapeutics (Fremont, CA) developed a series of platinum coils designed to induce thrombosis after catheter-based delivery into an aneurysm, thus providing a new approach to the treatment of intracranial aneurysms.

In 1990, Graves *et al.* (29) studied the effectiveness of simple and complex platinum coils in a vein graft aneurysm model in canines. Complex coils, such as the "flower petal" design, maintained spatial stability. Dacron threads woven into the coil mesh (Fig. 17.5) enhanced the thrombogenicity of the coils, resulting in a 40% rate of aneurysm thrombosis (30, 59); however, partial thrombosis of the parent vessel was noted in 50% of the treated vessels. Limitations of the platinum coil system were the inability to retrieve and reposition coils and to control subsequent intra-aneurysmal and intra-arterial thrombosis.

Dowd *et al.* (9) reported the clinical use of platinum coils to successfully treat three posterior inferior cerebellar artery aneurysms unsuitable for balloon occlusion. Further reports of the clinical use of thrombogenic coils followed, including the treatment of a distal vertebral artery giant aneurysm in an elderly patient (42, 61).

The results of two significant clinical series of thrombogenic coil treatment have been published. Casasco *et al.* (5) reported the French experience of 71 intracranial aneurysms treated with Dacron-fibered platinum coils. Thirty-eight aneurysms (54%) were large or giant. Com-

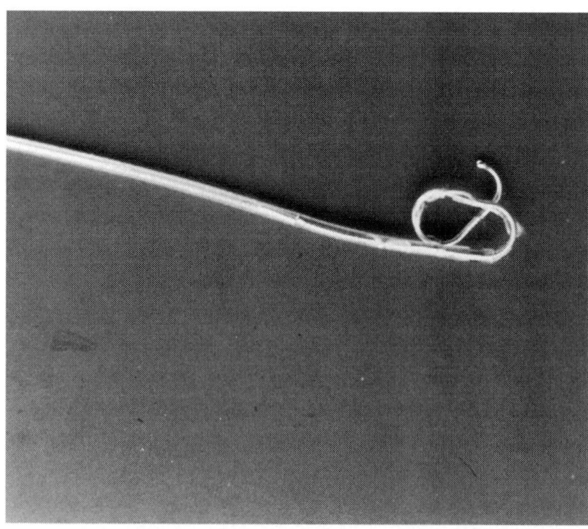

Fig. 17.5 Fibered coil emerging from Tracker microcatheter (Target Therapeutics, Fremont, CA).

plete occlusion was achieved in 85%, and more than 90% occlusion was accomplished in 15%. Two deaths occurred in patients with giant aneurysms. Four inadvertent parent vessel occlusions resulted in the death of two patients. Three patients had enlargement of the aneurysm, resulting in subarachnoid hemorrhage and death in two. Of the patients with residual necks after coil treatment, 25% of the lesions enlarged and rebled. Knuckey *et al.* (55) reported seven patients treated with endosaccular placement of thrombogenic coils. Four patients had total obliteration of the aneurysm, two had more than 90% occlusion, and one died following inadvertent carotid artery occlusion. The procedural morality and morbidity was 9%, with an overall mortality of 14%. Of greatest importance, recanalization of giant aneurysms occurred in two patients within 6 months of the procedure and necessitated the placement of additional coils.

In giant aneurysms with wide necks, coils may migrate into the lumen of the parent vessel and cause inadvertent occlusion. Occlusion in this setting is associated with increased morbidity and mortality. The aneurysm must be packed as tightly as possible to promote thrombosis but not so tightly as to risk occlusion of the parent vessel. The use of a combination of occlusive coils and detachable balloons has been reported to enhance the geometry of aneurysm packing (71); however, the future development of coils will be directed toward enhancing the thrombogenicity of the coil mass to limit the need for tight packing or making the coils softer to conform to the aneurysm cavity.

ELECTRICALLY DETACHABLE COILS

The ability of the neuroendovascular surgeon to control coil deployment and subsequent aneurysmal thrombosis is necessary to enhance the safety of endosaccular coil occlusion. Guglielmi *et al.* (33) developed a system that allows the operator to deliver a platinum coil into a desire site and detach it atraumatically by electrolysis. Any coil inadvertently deposited into the parent vessel may be withdrawn and repositioned, or exchanged for a different coil. The Guglielmi detachable coil (GDC) system consists of a standard platinum coil attached to a portion of insulated stainless steel delivery wire by a solder junction composed of a gold alloy (Fig. 17.6). The stainless steel junction adjacent to the alloy undergoes electrolysis rapidly, whereas the platinum and insulated stainless steel undergo electrolysis slowly. By generating a small direct current, the junction undergoes electrolysis, and the coil is detached without manipulation. The coil is electropositive and attracts negatively charged blood particles, which may potentiate electrothrombosis within the aneurysm.

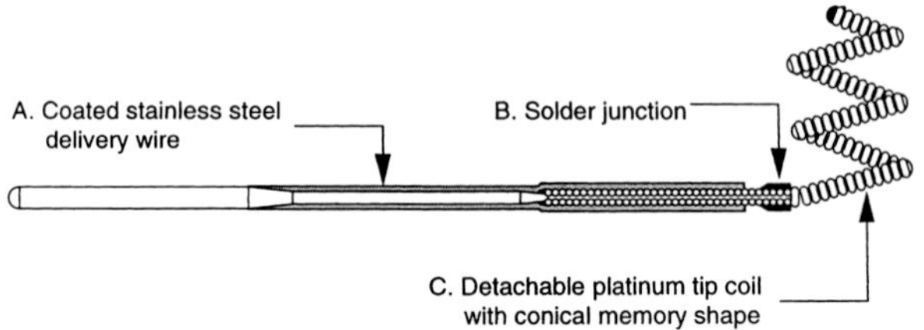

FIG. 17.6 Diagram of GDC. A coated stainless steel delivery wire is connected to a standard platinum coil by a solder junction. When a small electric current is passed through the wire, the junction undergoes electrolysis, and the coil is detached atraumatically. Typical detachment times are 3 to 8 min. (Reproduced with permission from Standard SC, Guterman LR, Chavis TD, *et al.*: Endovascular treatment of giant aneurysms, in Awad I, Barrow D: (eds) *Giant Intracranial Aneurysms.* Park Forest, IL, AANS Publications, in press, 1995.)

In a swine model, GDC treatment resulted in the successful obliteration of all aneurysms with no angiographic evidence of distal embolization (33). Histopathology showed neoendothelialization and organization of thrombus around the coil mass. Angiographic follow-up at 6 months demonstrated no recurrence of aneurysms; however, no control animals were included in the report.

In a companion report, Guglielmi *et al.* (31) published their experience with 15 high-risk patients with saccular aneurysms (including five giant and four large) treated with the GDC system. One transient deficit occurred during the procedure, but there were no permanent deficits or deaths. Two aneurysms were 100% occluded angiographically, whereas the remainder were 70 to 90% thrombosed. Long-term follow-up was not provided.

A multicenter clinical study was then completed, involving 43 aneurysms of the posterior fossa, of which 10 were giant (32). Twenty-three aneurysms were located at the basilar bifurcation, and 26 were wide-necked (>4 mm). Wide-necked aneurysms were clearly associated with a higher risk of migration of the coil mass into the parent vessel lumen; however, the procedural morbidity and mortality were quite low (4.8% and 2.4%, respectively), considering the risk factors of this subgroup of patients. There were two cases of permanent neurologic deficit related to the procedure, both in patients with wide-necked aneurysms involving the basilar bifurcation. One procedure-related death occurred in a patient with a grade V subarachnoid hemorrhage. Complete angiographic obliteration was achieved in 4 of 26 (15%) wide-necked aneurysms, with partial obliteration in the remaining aneurysms. Two patients with incomplete occlusion required operative intervention. Details of long-term observation were not provided.

Results of the United States experience with GDC treatment of intracranial aneurysms were presented in 1993 (87a). Of all treated aneurysms, 41% were large or giant aneurysms and 46% had wide necks. Of the large and giant aneurysms, 26 to 30% had complete immediate angiographic occlusion, and 50% had persistent neck remnants. At 6-month follow-up, 29% of large aneurysms and 30% of giant aneurysms had recanalized; 42% of all aneurysms containing significant thrombus recanalized.

The GDC system is satisfactory for the treatment of some giant aneurysms, particularly if the aneurysm geometry allows tight packing of the aneurysm cavity without protrusion of the coil mass into the parent vessel (34, 92). However, some aneurysms do not allow such a coil configuration, particularly bilobed aneurysms (Fig. 17.7).

Recanalization or regrowth of a previously coil-occluded aneurysm may occur in one of four ways: through (*a*) compaction or remodeling of coils, (*b*) rotation of the coil mass, (*c*) migration of coils into aneurysmal thrombus, and (*d*) entry of blood around the coil-to-aneurysm interface (Fig. 17.8).

The volume of the coil mass, even if tightly packed, is no more than 25% (I. Szikora, *in vivo* animal studies, unpublished data) to 40% (Target Therapeutics, *in vitro* glass model experimental studies, unpublished data) of the aneurysm volume and is confined to the angiographic lumen of the aneurysm. Aneurysm recanalization may occur through coil compaction or remodeling.

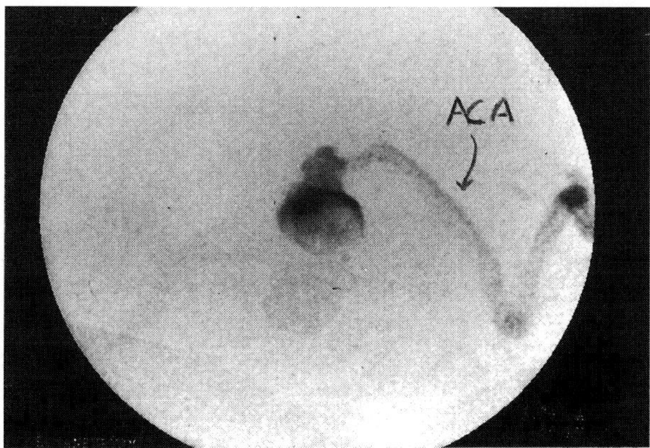

FIG. 17.7 Bilobed aneurysm (superselective angiogram, oblique projection). Body of aneurysm accepts coil mass, but second lobe does not allow aneurysm packing without parent vessel occlusion. *ACA*, anterior cerebral artery.

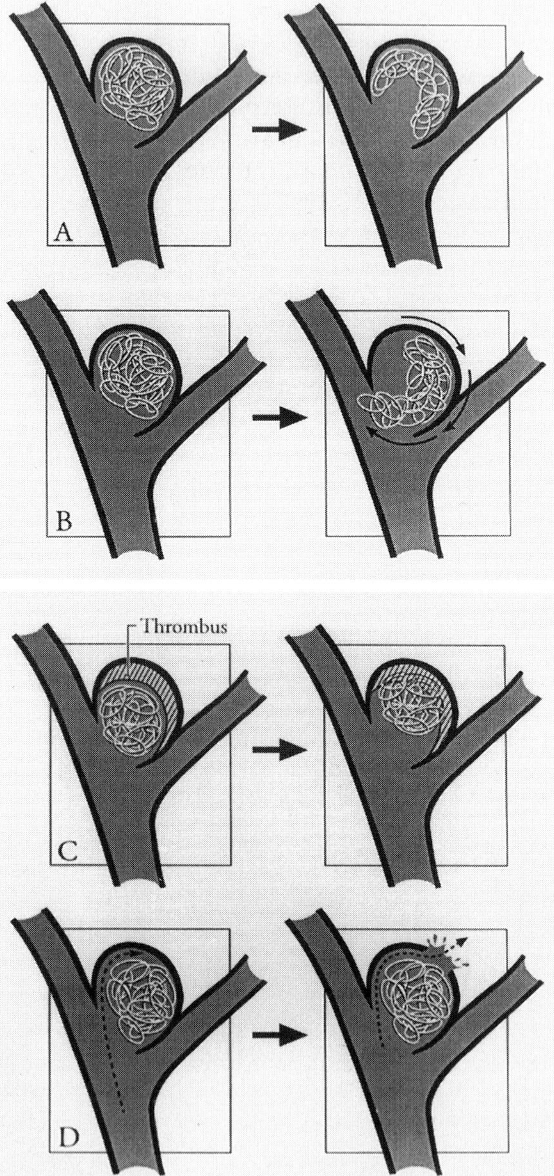

FIG. 17.8 Four mechanisms of aneurysm recanalization or regrowth after coil occlusion. (**A**) Compaction or remodeling of the coil mass. (**B**) Rotation of the coil mass in the aneurysm. (**C**) Migration of coils into aneurysmal thrombus. (**D**) Entry of blood around the wall of the aneurysm at the coil-to-aneurysm interface. (Reproduced with permission from Standard SC, Guterman LR, Chavis TD, *et al.:* Endovascular treatment of giant aneurysms, in Awad I, Barrow D (eds): *Giant Intracranial Aneurysms.* Park Forest, IL, AANS Publications, in press, 1995.)

Recanalization may also occur if the coil mass rotates within the aneurysm and assumes an undesirable configuration that may compromise the lumen of the parent vessel and may result in vessel stenosis or occlusion. The unfilled portion of the aneurysm may then be unprotected and subject to recanalization.

The coil mass may migrate into thrombus. A giant aneurysm contains both an angiographically demonstrable lumen, which contains flowing blood, and a compartment of intraluminal thrombus, which is in a constant state of balanced thrombosis and fibrinolysis. As the coil mass is displaced by inflow, it may migrate into the thrombus, resulting in recurrence of the aneurysm at the neck. The aneurysm remnant must be treated with additional coils or conventional surgery. The patient must not be considered protected from rebleeding until complete obliteration is achieved.

A final possible mechanism of recanalization is flow around the periphery of the coil mass within the aneurysm, which may be possible if no biologic bond is created between the coil mass and the aneurysm wall. Rupture could then occur at the aneurysm dome as blood enters the coil mass.

The GDC system is an important first step in the treatment of giant aneurysms with endovascular devices, but major problems exist with recanalization and regrowth. Long-term follow-up is necessary to determine the efficacy of endovascular procedures.

Neurosurgeons may also consider partial clipping of the neck of an otherwise unclippable giant aneurysm. Surgical reconstruction of the aneurysm neck may convert a wide-necked aneurysm to a small-necked aneurysm, thus enhancing the efficacy of endovascular therapy. This combined approach may then allow effective GDC coiling of the aneurysm.

PARENT ARTERY OCCLUSION

One of the earliest surgical methods of treating intracranial aneurysms was by proximal ligation. Hunter first used proximal arterial ligation to treat a popliteal aneurysm in 1784 (45). Cooper (6, 84) successfully treated an extracranial carotid artery aneurysm by proximal ligation in 1809. Treatment of giant aneurysms by proximal ligation was associated with a neurologic ischemic rate of 49% for ICA ligation and 28% for common carotid artery occlusion, as reported in the Cooperative Study of Intracranial Aneurysms and Subarachnoid Hemorrhage and other studies (72, 84, 89). Nishioka (72) reported a significant rebleeding rate of 7.8% after using surgical ICA ligation and 9.8% after common carotid artery ligation to treat intracranial anterior circulation aneurysms. The development of catheter-based balloon occlusion devices and the high rate of complications associated with surgical proximal occlusion led investigators to use balloon test occlusion of the parent artery before carotid artery sacrifice.

Gradual proximal arterial occlusion (*i.e.,* externally, by Selverstone clamp) may lead to spontaneous aneurysm thrombosis (26). Carotid artery ligation without balloon test occlusion is associated with a significant risk of neurologic complication secondary to abrupt hemodynamic change and thrombo-embolic complication (10, 22). Aneurysm trapping is effective when parent vessel occlusion is possible and collateral vessels are present distal to the site of occlusion (25). Extracranial-to-intracranial bypass procedures of the anterior fossa (22, 47) and posterior fossa (46) may prevent ischemic complications in patients who lack collateral vascular supply.

Endovascular techniques for parent vessel occlusion have been developed to perform test occlusion within a selected vascular territory with constant neurologic monitoring of changes in sensorimotor, cognitive, and cranial nerve function to determine tolerance before arterial sacrifice. The endovascular approach also offers the ability to perform occlusion within the distal petrous and cavernous portions of the carotid artery, proximal to the ophthalmic artery, to reduce the column of thrombus, which may propagate and subsequently embolize.

Berenstein *et al.* (4) treated 14 aneurysms of the cavernous carotid and vertebral artery with parent-vessel occlusion, using a double-lumen balloon catheter. Arterial sacrifice with detachable latex balloons was tolerated in all but one case. Kupersmith *et al.* (57) observed recanalization of the cavernous portion of the carotid artery through collateral vessels to the C3 and C4 portions of the artery. They suggested that proper balloon placement could successfully obliterate these potential collateral channels, particularly the capsular arteries, the inferolateral trunk, the posteroinferior hypophyseal artery, and the lateral artery of the clivus. Delayed ischemic deficit was attributed to recanalization and distal migration of thrombus. Another early series reported a similar occurrence of delayed ischemic deficit (21).

Hodes *et al.* (43) obtained excellent outcomes in 12 of 16 aneurysm cases treated by endovascular occlusion of parent vessels after tolerance to balloon test occlusion. Two patients died of procedural complications, and two patients died of other causes. Four patients experienced vessel recanalization at 3 months to 4 years after complete occlusion with coils and detachable balloons. No patient experienced growth or rerupture at a mean follow-up of 3.5 years. Aymard *et al.* (1) reported the successful treatment of a giant fusiform aneurysm of the basilar artery by use of this method.

The need for extracranial-to-intracranial bypass or surgical trapping is based on clinical intolerance to balloon occlusion. However, the risk of stroke following carotid sacrifice after a clinically tolerated test occlusion has been reported to range from 5 to 20% (7, 27). In an effort to reduce this morbidity, several investigators combined balloon test occlusion with ancillary tests to measure cerebral blood flow (CBF), such as ^{99m}Tc-hexamethylpropyleneamine oxime and xenon-133 cerebral perfusion single-photon emission computed tomography imaging (7, 15, 50). Yonas *et al.* (90) have noted that quantitative CBF measurements may increase the sensitivity of the test occlusion for ischemia. However, these measurements may exclude patients who might have tolerated carotid sacrifice without revascularization or trapping procedures.

Quantitative perfusion imaging may define a low-risk group for parent vessel sacrifice, particularly ICA sacrifice. Incorporating the use of hypotension during test occlusion may increase the sensitivity of the test for ischemia and identify an intermediate group of patients who have limited vascular reserve and are at risk for stroke (78a). The risk of vessel occlusion in this intermediate group is unknown, and revascularization procedures should be strongly considered.

Serbinenko *et al.* (77) described nine patients with giant ICA aneurysms treated with a combination of an extracranial-to-intracranial bypass procedure and an endovascular ICA occlusion. In all cases, collateral circulation had been judged insufficient by panangiography, electroencephalography, or somatosensory evoked potential monitoring during carotid artery compression. No complications or neurologic deterioration resulted after the procedure. All patients with incomplete visual deficits had improvement in visual function.

Negative balloon test occlusion may fail to predict tolerance to sacrifice of a parent vessel in a region with multiple perforating vessels (18). Test occlusion under conditions of systemic heparinization may not predict tolerance to definitive vessel occlusion either.

The late effects of carotid artery ligation are not well-defined, but *de novo* aneurysms are known to occur following carotid artery ligation (13). The risk of aneurysm formation after carotid artery ligation may warrant surveillance angiography or MRI angiography. The presence of a contralateral untreated aneurysm is a relative contraindication to vessel sacrifice.

Currently, parent artery sacrifice is used for giant aneurysms of the proximal anterior and posterior circulation that either cannot be treated by or fail treatment by neurosurgical or endosaccular means. We often employ balloon test occlusion in aneurysms that may undergo subsequent endosaccular occlusion if the neck of the aneurysm is wide and the risk of parent-vessel occlusion is high. Parent vessel sacrifice is by detachable balloon as close to the aneurysm as possible to limit the column of thrombus that may form and potentially undergo embolization, should revascularization occur. If balloon test occlusion is not tolerated or ancillary tests are abnormal, cerebral revascularization is recommended.

A new technique that offers promise for therapy of giant aneurysms is the placement of a proximal balloon for suction decompression and parent vessel control, followed by surgical dissection of the aneurysm and clip application. Mizoi and colleagues (67) reported their experience with nine paraclinoid aneurysms, using this technique. Bailes *et al.* (2) reported a case of temporary balloon occlusion of the basilar artery that facilitated aneurysm clipping. Combined endovascular and neurosurgical procedures offer the potential advantages of reduced operative time and reduced patient morbidity.

EXPERIMENTAL TECHNIQUES

A variety of novel techniques have been implemented to treat aneurysms of the intracranial circulation system. Techniques being investigated include the placement of intravascular stents and the use of rapidly solidifying prolymers. Each technique has certain theoretical advantages for the treatment of surgically inoperable giant aneurysms.

Intravascular Stents

Intravascular stents were initially developed to prevent restenosis after transluminal angioplasty in the peripheral and coronary circulation (74) and have been shown to be efficacious in stratifying flow within arteries (88). The porous nature of a stent may allow the orifices of perforating vessels adjacent to the aneurysm to remain patent after the stent is deployed.

Because of these advantages, several groups have examined intravascular stents in animal models (24, 85, 88). Geremia *et al.* reported a small series of stainless steel stents placed across the orifice of canine lateral wall aneurysms (24). Follow-up study showed aneurysm thrombosis. However, Szikora *et al.* (85) reported that, although immediate angiographic obliteration of the aneurysm was observed, a large proportion of the aneurysms were patent 2 and 4 weeks after stent placement. The specific design and biomechanical properties of stents may influence the efficiency of treatment.

High rates (30%) of parent vessel stenosis have been observed in the region of the stent, which stabilized 2 months after placement (74). Histopathologic evaluation revealed significant fibrointimal hyperplasia within the lumen of the parent vessel, resulting in vessel stenosis.

This phenomenon is postulated to occur because of damage to the myofibroblasts within the media of the vessel during balloon inflation or microcirculatory changes induced by the stent at the vessel wall. Stents made of self-expanding materials, such as nitinol, a nickel-titanium alloy, appear to elicit a less significant fibrointimal reaction than balloon-expandable tantalum stents. Nitinol stents used to treat four side-wall aneurysms with total aneurysm occlusion in three cases and a lower rate (5 to 15%) of fibrointimal hyperplasia (88).

Despite the theoretical advantage of restoring physiologic flow to the vessel, stents are impractical, in their present form, for treating most aneurysms. Although stents are attractive treatment alternatives for accomplishing luminal reconstruction in fusiform aneurysms of the carotid artery, most aneurysms occur at bifurcations with complex geometries that are unsuited to tubular stent designs. Furthermore, the currently available stents have limited flexibility and are difficult to navigate past tortuous vessels of the circle of Willis. Improvement in stent designs and compositions may eliminate the phenomenon of restenosis and provide a promising therapy for selected aneurysms.

The combination of intraluminal stents and endosaccular occlusive devices is presently being investigated. Szikora *et al.* (85) recently reported the results of the combined use of tantalum stents and GDC to treat canine side-wall aneurysms. Combining the implantation of balloon-expandable stents with tight endosaccular packing of coils resulted in complete obliteration of aneurysms. Late stenosis of the parent artery was seen due to fibrointimal hyperplasia induced by the stent. Without the stent, tightly packed coils within aneurysms with large orifices tended to bulge into the parent artery, which resulted in significant luminal stenosis, and may promote vessel occlusion.

Liquid Polymeric Adhesive

Zanetti and Sherman in 1972 (91) used polymers to obliterate several aneurysms in humans. Several centers developed experience in this technique in laboratory models. Debrun *et al.* (8) used isobutyl-cyanoacrylate in the treatment of 22 canine side-wall aneurysms. Complete obliteration of the aneurysm was accomplished in 20 of 24 treated aneurysms. The parent vessel was occluded in the remaining aneurysms. Similarly, Kerber *et al.* (52) treated 18 aneurysms with cyanoacrylate in a canine model by intravascular technique. Fifteen aneurysms were occluded, and one parent vessel was occluded. In the remaining two cases, cyanoacrylate protruded into the arterial lumen.

The advantage of polymeric occlusion of an aneurysm is that the immediate solidification of the material may prevent the phenomenon of late remodeling of the occlusive mass. However, these materials may not provide adequate resistance to the entry of blood between the polymer and the aneurysm wall, which may lead to recanalization. In wide-necked aneurysms, polymer may protrude into the lumen of the parent vessel, resulting in stenosis or occlusion of the parent vessel and adjacent perforating arteries. An additional risk is gluing the catheter into the aneurysm lumen. Furthermore, the use of cyanoacrylate has been restricted by the Food and Drug Administration because of its possible carcinogenicity.

Cellulose Acetate Polymer

Mandai *et al.* (65) presented a novel technique for the endosaccular treatment of aneurysms, using cellulose acetate polymer, a biocompatible material that is commonly used for hemodialysis membranes. When dissolved in a nonionic solvent, such as dimethyl sulfoxide, the material is easily injected through a microcatheter. On contacting an ionic solvent, such as physiologic saline, the outer surface hardens. As more material is injected, the droplet of cellulose acetate forms an expansile balloon, which conforms to the shape of the aneurysm. Since the material is nonadhesive, the microcatheter is easily detached after injection. The injected volume solidifies centripetally within 5 minutes.

This method was tested in 10 dogs with both side-wall and surgically created bifurcation aneurysms (65). Carotid occlusion was performed by temporary balloon occlusion or surgical exposure, and the polymer was delivered into the aneurysm through a microcatheter. In all cases, the aneurysms were occluded, and parent arteries were preserved. No distal emobolization of the polymer was observed on plain skull radiographs.

The technique was then utilized in seven aneurysms in six patients (54). Indications for treatment were failed surgical clipping, surgical inaccessibility, or poor operative risk. Parent artery flow was reduced by direct carotid compression for anterior circulation aneurysms or by balloon occlusion of the vertebral artery for posterior circulation aneurysms. Rates of angiographic obliteration of the aneurysm varied from 80 to 100%. There was one case of regrowth of the aneurysm after incomplete occlusion of an ophthalmic artery aneurysm. Another patient experienced a temporary deficit related to intentional carotid sacrifice for treatment of a proximal ICA aneurysm. One death occurred in a patient assessed at a poor neurologic grade.

The use of cellulose acetate, cyanoacrylate, and other rapidly solidifying materials shows promise for the treatment of intracranial giant aneurysms. Stents may prevent distal embolization of cellulose acetate polymer, as demonstrated in an experimental study (84a). More effective delivery systems will need to be developed to limit the possibility of polymer migration into the parent vessel lumen and the occurrence of distal embolization.

COST ANALYSIS

Because the field of endovascular therapy is in its infancy, the ultimate cost-effectiveness of its interventions cannot be fully assessed at this point in time. A true and detailed comparison between a gold standard technique, such as surgical clipping of aneurysms, and its endovascular counterparts is possible only when both approaches have undergone comparable development. As a result, we have chosen to delimit this cost analysis to a direct comparison of the hospitalization costs associated with single inpatient episodes of endovascular *versus* surgical aneurysm treatment. The reader should bear in mind that the cost estimates presented reflect our particular institutional setting: a large, established teaching hospital in a highly regulated health care locale in upstate New York.

The data comparing surgical *versus* endovascular (GDC) admissions for repair of giant intracranial aneurysms are summarized in the *bar graphs* in Figure. 17.9. The respective factors graphed are length of stay (LOS), cost per admission, and cost per day. Costs are further subdivided into routine and ancillary categories. Routine costs are those associated with basic inpatient care, *et al.,* bed charges, whether in an intensive care suite or in the ward, and basic nursing care. Ancillary costs are any costs incurred above and beyond this basic level of care, *e.g.,* operating and special procedures room costs, MRI scans, lab work, and radiology and cardiology services. It is generally assumed that routine costs are lower with endovascular treatment since the overall LOS, and, specifically, LOSs in the intensive care unit are reduced, compared to those of the surgical situation. This savings is purportedly offset to some extent on the ancillary side by increased capital cost outlays for angiographic *versus* surgical equipment and for the training of specialized personnel. Figure 17.9 reflects the balances between these competing cost factors in our institutional setting.

We are focusing on a particular subset of aneurysm patients in this review, those with giant intracranial aneurysms. The trends found in this small subgroup directly mimic those that we have seen throughout a comprehensive study of all intracranial aneurysm admissions, both hemorrhaging and nonhemorrhaging, that we have undertaken covering a 4-year time span at our hospital. Links to the larger study will be drawn here; however, the figures included in this review reflect only our most current cost data on the giant aneurysm patient subpopulation.

The comparative statistics in Figure 17.9 are drawn from four inpatient admissions for giant intracranial aneurysm repair in 1994—en-

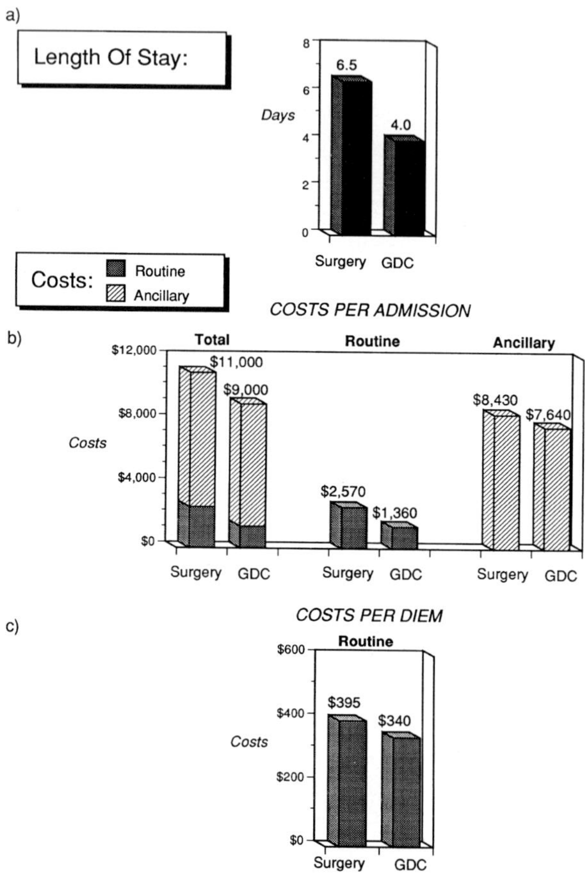

FIG. 17.9 Surgical *versus* endovascular (GDC) admissions for repair of giant intracranial aneurysms. (**a**) LOS. (**b**) Costs per admission. (**C**) Costs per day.

dovascular and surgical regimes being equally represented. As indicated by inspection of the *graphs* in Figure 17.9, this subset of data shows a definite cost advantage associated with endovascular admissions. Most significantly, the overall LOS is reduced by 40% in the endovascular treatment group, shortened, on average, by 2.5 days *versus* surgical admissions (6.5 *versus* 4.0 days) (Fig. 17.9**a**). Routine *per diem* bed costs are also cut due to the reduced need for intensive care services ($55 per day, −14%) (Fig. 17.9**c**). Taken together, this amounts to a savings of $1210 in routine costs per endovascular admission (−47%) (Fig. 17.9**b**). There is a concomitant savings of $790 in ancillary costs

(-9%). The final cost per admission for the endovascular group is $9,000 *versus* $11,000 for the surgical group, a savings of $2,000 per admission for the minimally invasive modality (-18%, Fig. 17.9**b**).

In summary, the most important factors affecting hospitalization costs for aneurysm treatment are the patient's hemorrhaging status and overall severity profile. However, given similar uncomplicated clinical conditions and considering single episodes of inpatient care, the endovascular approach shows significant cost advantages over the surgical approach. Moreover, this cost advantage is sustained throughout varied patient groupings—showing similar trends in general grouping as well as for specific patient subsets, such as the giant intracranial aneurysm subset discussed here. On average, inpatient LOS is reduced by 30 to 40% with endovascular treatment, eliminating 2 to 5+ days of inpatient care per admission. Routine *per diem* bed costs are also reduced (about -10%) due to the reduced need for intensive care services. These two factors translate into substantial savings in routine costs per admission (about 45%). In our institution, these savings average out at approximately $1000 to $2500 per admission, given bed costs of approximately $450 per day. Institutions or geographic areas with higher *per diem* bed costs may show even greater savings. The ancillary cost picture is less clear. A 9% savings in ancillary costs is shown in the giant aneurysm subgroup discussed here (Fig. 17.9**b**), yet this varies, with some subgroups showing increased ancillary costs. In general, the overall cost savings, routine plus ancillary, for endovascular *versus* surgical inpatient episodes for aneurysm treatment is approximately $1000 to $2000 (10 to 20%) per admission at our institution.

As stated earlier, these data are provisional in nature, representing a one-stage, snapshot assessment of an evolution in progress. Larger patient numbers, as well as improvements in techniques and equipment, will further reduce endovascular costs. Moreover, due to the minimally invasive nature of this alternative therapy, leading to reduced trauma and shortened recovery time, issues of patient acceptance and demand will assume very great importance in the ongoing assessment of relative value.

CONCLUSIONS

The role of endovascular therapy for the treatment of giant aneurysms is presently being defined. Results derived from the endovascular treatment of giant aneurysms must be compared to the effectiveness and safety of operative treatment and the natural history of the disease. Most reports on the results of endovascular aneurysm treatment are of patients who have failed operative intervention or in whom operative intervention was not attempted because of their poor medical condition or other factors. Thus, the results of these techniques are from a high-risk subgroup. In a recent series of 19 giant aneurysms treated by a variety of techniques, including coils, balloons, and rapidly solidifying polymers, one death resulted after aneurysm rupture during the procedure (86). However, the major cause of mortality was cardiopulmonary complications within the first 2 weeks after the procedure. At present, it may be appropriate to reserve endovascular techniques for patients with no other reasonable therapeutic option. As experience with these techniques is gained, a comparison must be undertaken in a series of patients clinically equivalent to those in surgical series.

Presently, the consensus is that endovascular therapy for giant aneurysms is efficacious for parent-vessel occlusion after balloon test occlusion to assess tolerance to sacrifice. Endosaccular occlusion is most effective if the aneurysm contains little thrombus, as determined by the size of the aneurysm seen on CT or MRI (87), as compared to the angiographic image. Small-necked aneurysms are particularly suited to coil occlusion if the aneurysm can be tightly packed. In wide-necked aneurysms, coil occlusion is possible, although the risk of parent-vessel occlusion is high. We often perform balloon test occlusion of the vessel before placing coils in wide-necked aneurysms.

Failure of endovascular therapy after complete angiographic obliteration is based on recanalization or regrowth, resulting from device migration or remodeling at the junction of the device with the inflow tract and aneurysm wall, or by migration of the device into thrombus. The effect of aneurysm remnants after balloon or coil occlusion will be determined by long-term follow-up, as emphasized by Fox *et al.* (20, 63). Whenever there is an aneurysm remnant, some risk of subsequent hemorrhage exists (66). Further device refinement will enhance the safety and effectiveness of the endovascular treatment of giant aneurysms. The use of combined endovascular and conventional surgical techniques may be an increasingly important option in the treatment of giant aneurysms.

Endosaccular packing of an aneurysm with occlusive material may not provide the ability to completely exclude the aneurysm from the circulation, and thus, will not necessarily prevent the process of regrowth. A further limitation of the currently implemented endovascular treatment of aneurysms is that fluoroscopy does not provide detailed information of aneurysm remnants due to the superimposition of occlusive materials, which may necessitate the development of new real-time imaging modalities for interventional procedure, such as intravascular ultrasound and ultrafast-sequence MRI.

ACKNOWLEDGMENTS

The authors thank Ajay K. Wakhloo, M.D., Ph.D., of the Department of Neurosurgery at SUNY-Buffalo for his review and critique of this chapter.

REFERENCES

1. Aymard A, Hodes JE, Rüfenacht DA, *et al.:* Endovascular treatment of a giant fusiform aneurysm of the entire basilar artery. **Am J Neuroradiol** 13:1143–1146, 1992.
2. Bailes JE, Deeb ZL, Wilson JA, *et al.:* Intraoperative angiography and temporary balloon occlusion of the basilar artery as an adjunct to surgical clipping: Technical note. **Neurosurgery** 30:949–953, 1992.
3. Batjer HH, Purdy PD: Enlarging thrombosed aneurysm of the distal basilar artery. **Neurosurgery** 26:695–700, 1990.
4. Berenstein A, Ransohoff J, Kupersmith M, *et al.:* Transvascular treatment of giant aneurysms of the cavernous carotid and vertebral arteries. Functional investigation and embolization. **Surg Neurol** 21:3–12, 1984.
5. Casasco AE, Aymard A, Gobin YP, *et al.:* Selective endovascular treatment of 71 intracranial aneurysms with platinum coils. **J Neurosurg** 79:3–10, 1993.
6. Cooper A: A case of aneurysm of the carotid artery. **Med Chir Trans** 1:1–110, 1809.
7. de Vries EJ, Sekhar LN, Horton JA, *et al.:* A new method to predict safe resection of the internal carotid artery. **Laryngoscope** 100:85–88, 1990.
8. Debrun GM, Varsos V, Liszczak TM, *et al.:* Obliteration of experimental aneurysms in dogs with isobutyl-cyanoacrylate. **J Neurosurg** 61:37–43, 1984.
9. Dowd CF, Halbach VV, Higashida RT, *et al.:* Endovascular coil embolization of unusual posterior inferior cerebellar artery aneurysms. **Neurosurgery** 27:954–961, 1990.
10. Drake CG: Ligation of the vertebral (unilateral or bilateral) or basilar artery in the treatment of large intracranial aneurysm. **J Neurosurg** 43:255–274, 1975.
11. Drake CG, Friedman AH, Peerless SJ: Failed aneurysm surgery. Reoperation in 115 cases. **J Neurosurg** 61:848–856, 1984.
12. Drake CG, Vanderlinden RG: The late consequences of incomplete surgical treatment of cerebral aneurysms. **J Neurosurg** 27:226–238, 1967.
13. Dyste GN, Beck DW: *De novo* aneurysm formation following carotid ligation: Case report and review of the literature. **Neurosurgery** 24:88–92, 1989.
14. Early CB, Fink LH: Some fundamental applications of the Law of La Place in neurosurgery. **Surg Neurol** 6:185–189, 1976.
15. Erba SM, Horton JA, Latchaw RE, *et al.:* Balloon test occlusion of the internal carotid artery with stable xenon/CT cerebral blood flow imaging. **Am J Neuroradiol** 9:533–538, 1988.
16. Ferguson GG: Physical factors in the initiation, growth, and rupture of human intracranial saccular aneurysms. **J Neurosurg** 37:666–677, 1972.
17. Feuerberg I, Lindquist C, Lindqvist M, *et al.:* Natural history of postoperative aneurysm rests. **J Neurosurg** 66:30–34, 1987.
18. Forsting M, Resch KM, von Kummer R, *et al.:* Balloon occlusion of a giant lower basilar aneurysm: Death due to thrombosis of the aneurysm. **Am J Neuroradiol** 12:1063–1066, 1991.
19. Forsting M, Sartor K: HEMA and latex: A dangerous combination? **Neuroradiology** 33:338–340, 1991.

20. Fox AJ, Drake CG: Endovascular therapy of intracranial aneurysms. **Am J Neuroradiol** 11:641–642, 1990.
21. Fox AJ, Viñuela F, Pelz DM, *et al.:* Use of detachable balloons for proximal artery occlusion in the treatment of unclippable cerebral aneurysms. **J Neurosurg** 66:40–46, 1987.
22. Gelber BR, Sundt TM Jr: Treatment of intracavernous and giant carotid aneurysms by combined internal carotid ligation and extra- to intracranial bypass. **J Neurosurg** 52:1–10, 1980.
23. George B, Aymard A, Gobin P, *et al.:* Endovascular treatment of intracranial aneurysms. Value and prospects based on a series of 92 cases. **Neurochirurgie** 36:273–278, 1990.
24. Geremia G, Haklin M, Brennecke L: Embolization of experimentally created aneurysms with intravascular stent devices. **Am J Neuroradiol** 15:1223–1231, 1994.
25. Gewirtz RJ, Awad IA: Giant aneurysms of the proximal anterior cerebral artery: Report of three cases. **Neurosurgery** 33:120–124, 1993.
26. Giannotta SL, McGillicuddy JE, Kindt GW: Gradual carotid artery occlusion in the treatment of inaccessible internal carotid artery aneurysms. **Neurosurgery** 5:417–421, 1979.
27. Gonzalez CF, Moret J: Balloon occlusion of the carotid artery prior to surgery for neck tumors. **Am J Neuroradiol** 11:649–652, 1990.
28. Goto K, Halbach VV, Hardin CW, *et al.:* Permanent inflation of detachable balloons with a low-viscosity, hydrophilic polymerizing system. **Radiology** 169:787–790, 1988.
29. Graves VB, Partington CR, Rüfenacht DA, *et al.:* Treatment of carotid artery aneurysms with platinum coils: An experimental study in dogs. **Am J Neuroradiol** 11:249–252, 1990.
30. Graves VB, Strother CM, Partington CR, *et al.:* Flow dynamics of lateral carotid artery aneurysms and their effects on coils and balloons: An experimental study in dogs. **Am J Neuroradiol** 13:189–196, 1992.
31. Guglielmi G, Viñuela F, Dion J, *et al.:* Electrothrombosis of saccular aneurysms via endovascular approach. Part 2: Preliminary clinical experience. **J Neurosurg** 75:8–14, 1991.
32. Guglielmi G, Viñuela F, Duckwiler G, *et al.:* Endovascular treatment of posterior circulation aneurysms by electrothrombosis using electrically detachable coils. **J Neurosurg** 77:515–524, 1992.
33. Guglielmi G, Viñuela F, Sepetka I, *et al.:* Electrothrombosis of saccular aneurysms via endovascular approach. Part 1: Electrochemical basis, technique, and experimental results. **J Neurosurg** 75:1–7, 1991.
34. Halbach V: The "current" status of aneurysm treatment? **Am J Neuroradiol** 14:799–800, 1993.
35. Hecht ST, Horton JA, Yonas H: Growth of a thrombosed giant vertebral artery aneurysm after parent artery occlusion. **Am J Neuroradiol** 12:449–451, 1991.
36. Heilman CB, Kwan ES, Wu JK: Aneurysm recurrence following endovascular balloon occlusion. **J Neurosurg** 77:260–264, 1992.
37. Hieshima GB, Grinnell VS, Mehringer CM: A detachable balloon for therapeutic transcatheter occlusion. **Radiology** 138:227–228, 1981.
38. Hieshima GB, Higashida RT, Halbach VV, *et al.:* Intravascular balloon embolization of a carotid-ophthalmic artery aneurysm with preservation of the parent vessel. **Am J Neuroradiol** 7:916–918, 1986.

39. Hieshima GB, Higashida RT, Wapenski J, et al.: Balloon embolization of a large distal basilar artery aneurysm. Case report. **J Neurosurg** 65:413–416, 1986.
40. Higashida RT, Halbach VV, Barnwell SL, et al.: Treatment of intracranial aneurysms with preservation of the parent vessel: Results of percutaneous balloon embolization in 84 patients. **Am J Neuroradiol** 11:633–640, 1990.
41. Higashida RT, Halbach VV, Cahan LD, et al.: Detachable balloon embolization therapy of posterior circulation intracranial aneurysms. **J Neurosurg** 71:512–519, 1989.
42. Higashida RT, Halbach VV, Dowd CF, et al.: Interventional neurovascular treatment of a giant intracranial aneurysm using platinum microcoils. **Surg Neurol** 35:64–68, 1991.
43. Hodes JE, Aymard A, Gobin YP, et al.: Endovascular occlusion of intracranial vessels for curative treatment of unclippable aneurysms: Report of 16 cases. **J Neurosurg** 75:694–701, 1991.
44. Hodes JE, Fox AJ, Pelz DM, et al.: Rupture of aneurysms following balloon embolization. **J Neurosurg** 72:567–571, 1990.
45. Home E: An account of Mr. Hunter's method for performing the operation for the popliteal aneurysm. **Lond Med J** 7:391–406, 1786.
46. Hopkins LN, Budny JL, Castellani D: Extracranial-intracranial arterial bypass and basilar artery ligation in the treatment of giant basilar artery aneurysms. **Neurosurgery** 13:189–194, 1983.
47. Hopkins LN, Grand W: Extracranial-intracranial arterial bypass in the treatment of aneurysms of the carotid and middle cerebral arteries. **Neurosurgery** 5:21–31, 1979.
48. Horton JA, Jungreis CA, Stratemeier PH: Sharp vascular calcifications and acute balloon rupture during emoblization. **Am J Neuroradiol** 12:1070–1073, 1991.
49. Hosobuchi Y: Electrothrombosis of carotid-cavernous fistula. **J Neurosurg** 42:76–85, 1975.
50. Jawad K, Miller JD, Wyper DJ, et al.: Measurement of CBF and carotid artery pressure compared with cerebral angiography in assessing collateral blood supply after carotid ligation. **J Neurosurg** 46:185–196, 1977.
51. Katayama Y, Tsubokawa T, Miyazaki S, et al.: Growth of totally thrombosed giant aneurysm within the posterior cranial fossa. Dignostic and therapeutic considerations. **Neuroradiology** 33:168–170, 1991.
52. Kerber CW, Cromwell LD, Zanetti PH: Experimental carotid aneurysms. Part 2: Endovascular treatment with cyanoacrylate. **Neurosurgery** 16:13–17, 1985.
53. Kerber CW, Heilman CB: Flow in experimental berry aneurysms: Method and Model. **Am J Neuroradiol** 4:374–377, 1983.
54. Kinugasa K, Mandai S, Terai Y, et al.: Direct thrombosis of aneurysms with cellulose acetate polymer. Part II: Preliminary clinical experience. **J Neurosurg** 77:501–507, 1992.
55. Knuckey NW, Haas R, Jenkins R, et al.: Thrombosis of difficult intracranial aneurysms by the endovascular placement of platinum-Dacron microcoils. **J Neurosurg** 77:43–50, 1992.
56. Konovalov AN, Serbinenko F, Filatov JM: Endovascular treatment of arterial aneurysms. **Am J Neuroradiol** 11:225, 1990 (abstr).
57. Kupersmith MJ, Berenstein A, Choi IS, et al.: Percutaneous transvascular treatment of giant carotid aneurysms: Neuro-ophthalmologic findings. **Neurology** 34:328–335, 1984.

58. Kurokawa Y, Abiko S, Okamura T, *et al.:* Direct surgery for giant aneurysm exhibiting progressive enlargement after intraaneurysmal balloon embolization. **Surg Neurol** 38:19–25, 1992.
59. Kwan ES, Heilman CB, Roth PA: Endovascular packing of carotid bifurcation aneurysm with polyester fiber-coated platinum coils in a rabbit model. **Am J Neuroradiol** 14:323–333, 1993.
60. Kwan ES, Heilman CB, Shucart WA, *et al.:* Enlargement of basilar artery aneurysms following balloon occlusion—"water-hammer effect". Report of two cases. **J Neurosurg** 75:963–968, 1991.
61. Lane B, Marks MP: Coil embolization of an acutely ruptured saccular aneurysm. **Am J Neuroradiol** 12:1067–1069, 1991.
62. Liepsch DW, Steiger HJ, Poll A, *et al.:* Hemodynamic stress in lateral saccular aneurysms. **Biorheology** 24:689–710, 1987.
63. Lin T, Fox AJ, Drake CG: Regrowth of aneurysm sacs from residual neck following aneurysm clipping. **J Neurosurg** 70:556–560, 1989.
64. Luessenhop AJ, Velasquez AC: Observations on the tolerance of intracranial arteries to catheterization. **J Neurosurg** 21:85–91, 1964.
65. Mandai S, Kinugasa K, Ohmoto T: Direct thrombosis of aneurysms with cellulose acetate polymer. Part I: Results of thrombosis in experimental aneurysms. **J Neurosurg** 77:497–500, 1992.
66. Matsuda M, Shiino A, Handa J: Rupture of previously unruptured giant carotid aneurysm after superficial temporal-middle cerebral artery bypass and internal carotid occlusion. **Neurosurgery** 16:177–184, 1985.
67. Mizoi K, Takahashi A, Yoshimoto T, *et al.:* Combined endovascular and neurosurgical approach for paraclinoid internal carotid artery aneurysms. **Neurosurgery** 33:986–992, 1993.
68. Moniz E: L'encéphalographie artérielle, son importance dans le localization des tumeurs cérébrales. **Rev Neurol** 34:72–89, 1927.
69. Monsein LH, Debrun GM, Chazaly JR: Hydroxyethyl methylacrylate and latex balloons. **Am J Neuroradiol** 11:663–664, 1990.
70. Mullan S, Raimondi AJ, Dobben G, *et al.:* Electrically induced thrombosis in intracranial aneurysms. **J Neurosurg** 22:539–547, 1965.
71. Nakahara I, Taki W, Nishi S, *et al.:* Treatment of giant anterior communicating artery aneurysm via an endovascular approach using detachable balloons and occlusive coils. **Am J Neuroradiol** 11:1195–1197, 1990.
72. Nishioka H: Report on the Cooperative Study of Intracranial Aneurysms and Subarachnoid Hemorrhage. Section VIII, Part I: Results of the treatment of intracranial aneurysms by occlusion of the carotid artery in the neck. **J Neurosurg** 25:660–682, 1966.
73. Romodanov AP, Shcheglov VI: Intravascular occlusion of saccular aneurysms of the cerebral arteries by means of a detachable balloon catheter, in Krayenbühl H, Sweet WH (eds): *Advances and Technical Standards in Neurosurgery.* New York: Springer-Verlag, vol. 2, pp 25–49, 1982.
74. Schatz RA, Baim DS, Leon M, *et al.:* Clinical experience with the Palmaz-Schatz coronary stent. Initial results of a multicenter study. **Circulation** 83:148–161, 1991.
75. Schubiger O, Valavanis A, Wichmann W: Growth-mechanism of giant intracranial aneurysms: Demonstration by CT and MR imaging. **Neuroradiology** 29:266–271, 1987.
76. Serbinenko FA: Balloon catheterization and occlusion of major cerebral vessels. **J Neurosurg** 41:125–145, 1974.

77. Serbinenko FA, Filatov JM, Spallone A, *et al.:* Management of giant intracranial ICA aneurysms with combined extracranial-intracranial anastomosis and endovascular occlusion. **J Neurosurg** 73:57–63, 1990.
78. Simkins TE, Stehbens WE: Vibrations recorded from the adventitial surface of experimental aneurysms and arteriovenous fistulas. **Vasc Surg** 8:153–165, 1974.
78a. Standard SC, Ahuja A, Guterman LR, *et al.:* Balloon test occlusion of the internal carotid artery with hypotensive challenge. Presented at the 32nd Annual Meeting of the American Society of Neuroradiology, Nashville, TN, May 1993.
79. Stehbens WE: Etiology of intracranial berry aneurysms. **J Neurosurg** 70:823–831, 1989.
80. Steiger HJ, Reulen H-J: Low frequency flow fluctuations in human saccular aneurysms. **Acta Neurochir** (Wien) 83:131–137, 1986.
81. Strother CM, Eldevik P, Kikuchi Y, *et al.:* Thrombus formation and structure and the evolution of mass effect in intracranial aneurysms treated by balloon embolization: Emphasis on MR findings. **Am J Neuroradiol** 10:787–796, 1989.
82. Strother CM, Graves VB, Rappe A: Aneurysm hemodynamics: An experimental study. **Am J Neuroradiol** 13:1089–1095, 1992.
83. Strother CM, Lunde S, Graves V, *et al.:* Late paraophthalmic aneurysm rupture following endovascular treatment. Case report. **J Neurosurg** 71:777–780, 1989.
84. Swearingen B, Heros RC: Common carotid occlusion for unclippable carotid aneurysms: An old but still effective operation. **Neurosurgery** 21:288–295, 1987.
84a. Szikora I, Guterman LR, Standard SC, *et al.:* Endovascular delivery of liquid polymer for treatment of experimental aneurysms: Prevention of distal embolization by employing stents. Presented at the American Association of Neurological Surgeons Annual Meeting, San Diego, CA, April 1994 (abstr).
85. Szikora I, Guterman LR, Wells KM, *et al.:* Combined use of stents and coils to treat experimental wide-necked carotid aneurysms: Preliminary results. **Am J Neuroradiol** 15:1091–1102, 1994.
86. Taki W, Nishi S, Yamashita K, *et al.:* Selection and combination of various endovascular techniques in the treatment of giant aneurysms. **J Neurosurg** 77:37–42, 1992.
87. Tsuruda JS, Sevick RJ, Halbach VV: Three-dimensional time-of-flight MR angiography in the evaluation of intracranial aneurysms treated by endovascular balloon occlusion. **Am J Neuroradiol** 13:1129–1136, 1992.
87a. Viñuela F: Endovascular occlusion of intracranial aneurysms using the GDC system: The USA experience. Presented at the GDC investigators meeting during the 31st Annual Meeting of the American Society of Neuroradiology, Vancouver, British Columbia, Canada, May 1993.
88. Wakhloo AK, Schellhammer F, de Vries J, *et al.:* Self-expanding and balloon-expandable stents in the treatment of carotid aneurysms: An experimental study in a canine model. **Am J Neuroradiol** 15:493–502, 1994.
89. Winn HR, Richardson AE, Jane JA: Late morbidity and mortality of common carotid ligation for posterior communicating aneurysms. A comparison to conservative treatment. **J Neurosurg** 47:727–736, 1977.
90. Yonas H, Linskey M, Johnson DW, *et al.:* Internal carotid balloon test occlusion does require quantitative CBF. **Am J Neuroradiol** 13:1147–1152, 1992, (letter).
91. Zanetti PH, Sherman FE: Experimental evaluation of a tissue adhesive as an agent for the treatment of aneurysms and arteriovenous anomalies. **J Neurosurg** 36:72–79, 1972.
92. Zubillaga AF, Guglielmi G, Viñuela F, *et al.:* Endovascular occlusion of intracranial aneurysms with electrically detachable coils: Correlation of aneurysm neck size and treatment results. **Am J Neuroradiol** 15:815–820, 1994.

18

Therapy of AVMs: A Decision Analysis

WINK S. FISHER III, M.D.

Some clinical decisions are made difficult by the shear number of choices and data that are available. An analytic tool, decision analysis (DA), allows for accounting of data from such large databases and assists in analysis of this information in medical decision-making scenarios (3, 15, 20, 21, 30, 31). DA is not meant to supplant medical decision-making but to assist in the more difficult task of deciding among many choices, especially where decisions deal with diseases that occur over very long time horizons. In addition, it may behoove all neurosurgeons to take note of the technique, because DA may become a tool used by third-party carriers as they assess the care of patients.

The decisions leading up to the therapy of arteriovenous malformations (AVMs) are certainly complex enough to consider the use of DA (1, 2, 6, 7, 10, 12–15, 22). Factors taken into account during the decision-making process of a patient harboring an AVM include such things as the age of the patient, risks associated with therapy, success rate of the therapy and, most importantly, the natural history of the disease. The complexity of the process becomes apparent when one is trying to decide whether an intact patient should undergo therapy and, if so, what type (open surgical resection, embolization, stereotaxic radioneurosurgery (SRNS) or in which combination (embolization plus open surgery *versus* embolization plus SRNS) (see Fig. 18.1 **A** and **B**).

The use of DA in the decision-making of AVMs was first introduced in 1983 by Iansek *et al.* (14). Since then, other authors have used similar techniques during analysis of the therapy of AVMs. (1, 2, 6, 7, 10, 12–15). The DA of AVMs is made feasible because (a) the natural history of AVMs is well documented (19), and (b) the risks and benefits of the therapies available for AVMs (embolization, surgery, SRNS) are also well know (11, 18, 29). By drawing on these published values, a decision tree can be formulated and a decision-making scheme analyzed. The computer model presented is an attempt to duplicate, as closely as possible, a real-life scenario of the decision making for the therapy of a patient with an AVM.

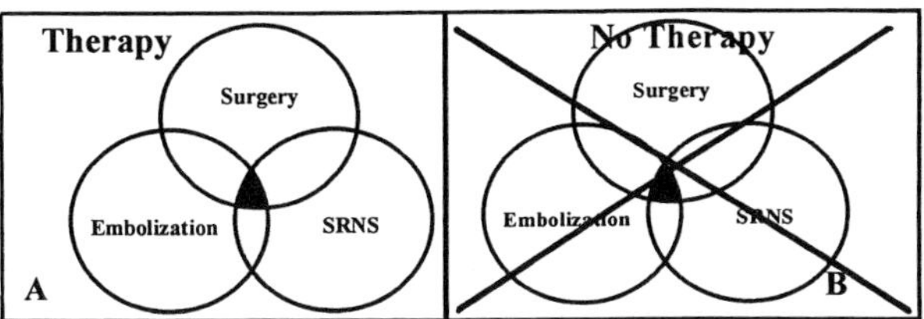

FIG.18.1 (**A**) Schematic representing the therapeutic choices available for therapy of an AVM. Some combination of all therapies may eventually prove to be worthwhile in some given cases. (**B**) However, some cases surely exist where no therapy is beneficial.

WHAT IS DECISION ANALYSIS?

DA arose from operations research and game theory in the 1950s and was applied to medicine in the 1960s (30, 31). Decision-making strategies, using DA, are becoming more frequent even in contemporary publications, many times adding a different perspective to caring for patients (1, 2, 6, 7, 12–15). Traditionally, DA has involved the use of Bayes' theorem and decision trees. More sophisticated techniques have now become available on a simple computer format, allowing for desktop evaluations with little, if any, formal training.

DA can be likened to a coin sorter that takes a mixture of coins and sorts them according to denominations. A coin sorter does this sorting by allowing coins to fall down a path according to size and weight. The path for a more valued coin, say, a quarter, can easily be recognized as a "preferred path" and be followed back to where branches ("decisions") occurred during the sorting. Similarly, DA involves many different aspects of patient care, which are introduced into a manufactured scheme called a "decision tree," and the path with the best outcome for the patient can be identified (Fig. 18.2). An analysis varying many of the deciding elements is accomplished during a sensitivity analysis. During this analysis changes in baseline values are introduced into the model to determine how "sensitive" the model is and at the same time to check whether the preferred path remains the best path. If the preferred path does not alter, despite many changes in the variables, then the validity of this path as the finest pathway is hard to discredit (20, 21).

CONSTRUCTED DECISION TREE AND TECHNIQUE (METHODS)

For those interested, an addendum describing the methods of the analysis appears at the end of this chapter. The focus of this presentation will be on the results of the analysis. Suffice to say that several steps were completed in sequence in order to accomplish and perform the analysis. These steps included: (*a*) the construction of a decision

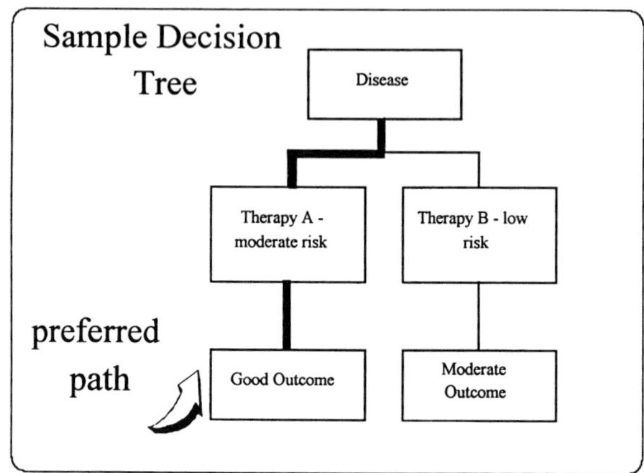

FIG.18.2 Sample decision tree. DA analyzes those choices with risk and compares outcomes as well, allowing selection of the best choice by relying on mathematical comparisons. Note in the diagram that although *Therapy A* had moderate risk, it was preferred over *Therapy B,* because of the strong value assigned to *Therapy A's* outcome.

tree, duplicating as best as possible a real-life decision-making scenario, (*b*) consolidation and summation of data from published therapeutic reports to be used in the analysis, (*c*) assignment of values to outcomes ("payoffs"), and (*d*) evaluation of the tree to determine the preferred path and performance of many sensitivity analyses.

Figure 18.3 shows a simplified decision tree used in the model presented. The tree was formulated to answer this question: "When confronted with a patient with an AVM, which therapeutic strategies should be used?" Seven potential outcomes are possible: delayed therapy followed by surgery, delayed therapy followed by SRNS, embolization followed by open surgery, embolization followed by SRNS, open surgery alone, SRNS alone, or natural history (see Fig. 18.3) The tree attempts to confront the issue of delayed therapy (that therapy delivered only after bleeding occurs during the natural history of the disease) *versus* immediate therapy (avoiding the risk of the natural history of AVMs), as well as the question of combined therapy (embolization plus surgery or embolization plus SRNS) *versus* single therapy (surgery or SRNS alone). No arm for embolization as a single therapy was designed, because the cure rate for embolization alone is known to be quite low. In addition, no arms for delayed embolization plus surgery or delayed embolization plus SRNS were designed.

Running commercially available software (DATA from TreeAge, Boston, MA) on an IBM format desktop computer, it was possible to con-

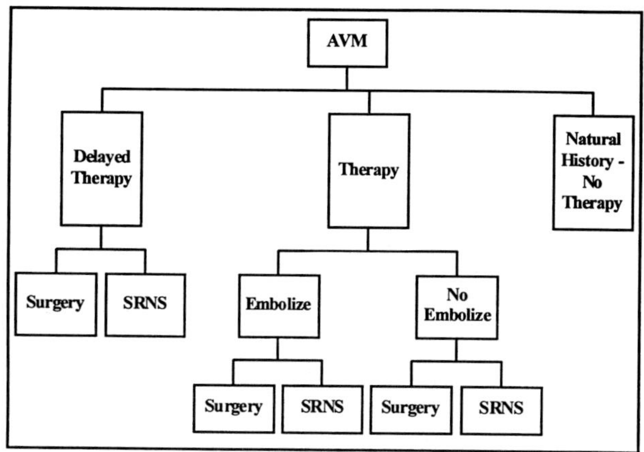

FIG.18.3 Simplified decision tree used in the model (original has 124 nodes). *Delayed therapy* implies that therapy was delivered after hemorrhage. *Embolize* implies that embolization was used with reduction of both surgical morbidity and mortality, as well as improvement in cure rates for large SRNS lesions. *Natural History* implies taking the risk of the natural history of the disease without any intervening therapy.

struct, assign variables for, and analyze all aspects of the DA tree. A technique called Markov cycling was used to allow hypothetical patients to move through a series of transition cycles (years) after exposure to various risks (natural history of the disease, surgical risks, *etc.*) and continue to run through many cycles (years) until death occurred (3, 20, 21, 30). Accounting of each cycle (year) by the computer allowed for comparison at each branch of the DA tree and identification of the preferred path. After the preferred path was identified, numerous sensitivity analyses were performed to observe how the preferred path was altered.

BASELINE VALUES USED

A hypothetical female patient 38 years of age was used in the analysis (see Fig. 18.4). This patient was assigned an American Society of Anesthesiologists (ASA) grade of 1. The baseline values for the patient's AVM were as follows: the size was 3.5 cm; is was noneloquent; and it had no deep venous drainage (2 + 0 + 0 + 0 = 2 Spetzler-Martin (Spetzler) Grade) (26).

Data for the natural history of AVMs was drawn from the work of Ondra *et al.* to represent the best baseline data. In developing natural history formulas used in the DA, a yearly rate of hemorrhage of 4%, with a combined morbidity and mortality rate of 3% (2% morbidity and 1% mortality), was used (19). This yearly mortality rate of hemorrhage

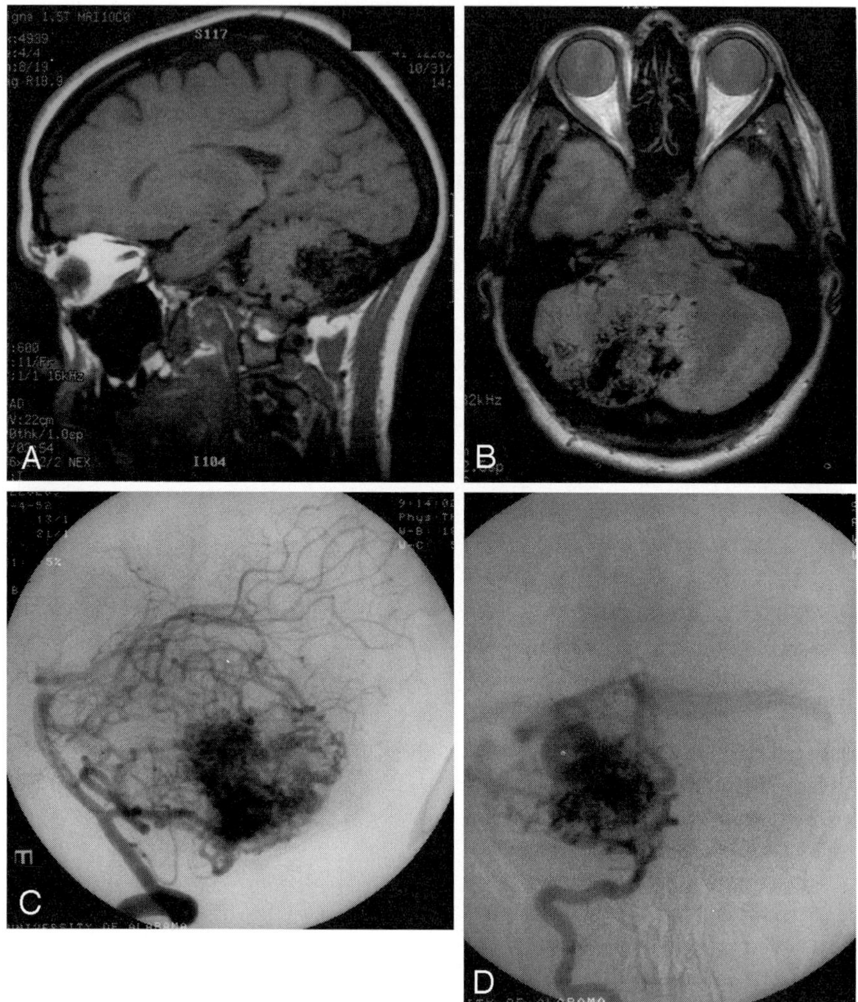

FIG.18.4 MRI and angiographic images of hypothetical cases presented. (**A**) Sagittal MRI. (**B**) Axial MRI. (**C**) lateral angiogram. (**D**) AP view of angiogram.

was added to all other causes of mortality drawn from life tables during the cycles of the model.

Surgical cure rates were drawn from the literature and found to be close to 100% (11). For purposes of the model a complete cure was assumed with each open surgical excision. Surgical morbidity and mortality values, determined according to Spetzler grades, were used as described by Heros *et al.* (Table 18.1 and 18.2) (11).

TABLE 18.1
Baseline Values Used in the Model

Variable	Baseline Value
Age	38
ASA	1
Bleed rate	4%
Bleed rate morbidity and mortality rate	2 and 1%
Surgical cure rate	100%
Surgical morbidity and mortality rate	See Table 18.2
SRNS cure rate	90% for small lesions
	50% for larger lesions
SRNS morbidity and mortality rate	2 and 1 %
Embolization cure rate	4%
Embolization morbidity and mortality rate	10 and 1%
Well state	0.95
Well-cured state	1
Disabled state	0.4
Disabled state cured	0.5
Dead state	0
Discount rate	5%
Eloquence	None
Size	3.5 cm
Venous drainage	None

TABLE 18.2.
Open Surgical Morbidity and Mortality Rates Used in the Model[a]

Spetzler Grade	Surgical Morbidity (%)	Surgical Mortality (%)
1	8	0
2	3	0
3	11	0
4	37	2.4
5	71	4.8

[a]Adapted from (11).

SRNS rates of cure are dependent on the size of the lesion and have been reported to be as high as 90% for lesions less than 3 cm and 50% for larger lesions (16, 18, 27, 28). The morbidity and mortality rates for SRNS are low and may be directly related to the natural history of the disease. However, the SRNS morbidity and SRNS mortality rates (presumed due to radiation necrosis) used in the model are 2% and 1%, respectively (16, 18, 27, 28). The time horizon for cure with SRNS was chosen as 3 years.

Embolization cure, morbidity, and mortality rates are not as well documented (4, 5, 8, 9, 23–25). Close review of the literature reveals

TABLE 18.3
Alternate Grading System Used in the Model

Author	Yr	No[a]	Cure(%)	MT(%)	MB-P(%)	MB-T
Pelz *et al.* (23)	1988	15	0(0)	0(0)	3(20)	3(20)
Benati *et al.* (4)	1989	42	0(0)	0(0)	0(0)	2(5)
Viñuela *et al.* (29)	1989	213	?	6(2.8)	26(12)	?
Berthelsen *et al.* (5)	1990	29	3(10)	2(7)	3(10)	3(10)
Fox *et al.* (9)	1990	38	0(0)	0(0)	4(10.5)	?
Purdy-1 *et al.* (24)	1990	12	?	0(0)	2(17)	4(33)
Purdy-2 *et al.* (24)	1990	39	3(8)	1(3)	2(5)	3(8)
Fournier *et al.* (8)	1991	49	7(14)	0(0)	4(8)	8(16)
Schumacher *et al.* (25)	1991	35	0(0)	0(0)	3(9)	5(14)
Total		472	13/247 (5.2)	9/472(2)	47/472(10)	28/221(13)

[a]No., number of cases reported; MT, mortality rate; Cure, cure rate (complete obliteration of the AVM); MB-P, permanent morbidity rate; MB-T, transient morbidity rate.

cure rates of 4% (4, 5, 8, 9, 23–25). Drawing on similar data, embolization morbidity and mortality rates of 10% and 1%, respectively, were used in this model (see Table 18.3). The benefit of embolization for reducing morbidity and mortality and improving cure rates of surgery or SRNS is not known or published. In designing the model presented, it was assumed that embolization improved surgical morbidity, surgical mortality, and SRNS cure rates by 25% (in lesions greater than 3 cm). A summary of baseline values used can be found in Table 18.1.

Outcomes were assigned equivalent values despite mode of therapy; a "cure" with SRNS was assigned the same value as a "cure" with surgery or a "cure" with embolization. "Disability" outcomes were rated the same despite mode of therapy, as was the value assigned to "death" for each branch of the tree. Two sequential disabilities (independent of therapy) were assigned the same value as "death", *i.e.,* a patient who suffered major morbidity from embolization and then suffered major morbidity from surgery was assigned a value equivalent to "death." Nontherapy "well" and "disability" states were valued slightly less than therapeutically treated "well" and "disability" states when the patient was cured (95 and 80%, respectively) (see Table 18.1). All values of outcomes were "discounted" for future years; *i.e.,* future years were valued less than present years by a value of 5% per year. All annual rates were converted to mean annual probabilities in the model for computational purposes (2, 3, 20, 21).

RESULTS

The baseline values (Table 18.1) were placed on the decision tree, and the model favored surgery without embolization over other modes

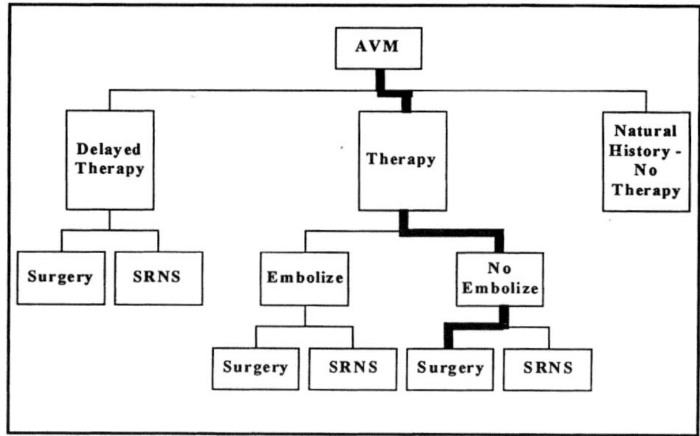

FIG.18.5 Simplified decision tree outlining the preferred path, using baseline values from the model (*heavy line*; see Fig. 18.3 for comparison). Delayed therapy, embolization, and natural history arms were not favored.

of therapy, natural history, or delayed therapy (see Fig. 18.5). When the model is altered for a smaller lesion, for example, an AVM that is 2.5 cm size, with deep venous drainage, and is in a noneloquent location (1 + 1 + 0 = 2 Spetzler grade), the model still favors open surgery.

The Spetzler grade was used as a variable in the analysis, because it easily reflected both surgical morbidity and mortality (see Table 18.2). Spetzler grade 2 and 3 patients, however, are unique in that not all grade 2 and 3 patients have lesions similar in size (because Spetzler grade 2 and 3 patients may have, depending on the AVM, lesions greater than or less than 3 cm) (see Table 18.4). The size limitations of SRNS therapy impart a certain degree of need for differentiation of the Spetzler grading system to distinguish between small and large lesions. Therefore, to compare SRNS with surgical therapy, it was necessary during the evaluation of the Spetzler grades to differentiate between lesions less than 3 cm designating them as small (s), and

TABLE 18.4
Embolization in the "Modern Era"

Size	<3 cm	<3 cm	<3 cm	>3 cm	>3 cm	>3 cm
Size <3	1	1	1			
Size > 3 <6				2	2	2
Venous drainage	0	1	1	0	1	0
Eloquence	1	0	1	0	0	1
Spetzler grade	2 (s)	2 (s)	3 (s)	2 (l)	3 (l)	3 (l)

[a]Not all Spetzler grade 2 and 3 AVMs are alike. AVMs were differentiated by size: small (s) and large (l); small = <3 cm; large = ≥3 cm.

designating those greater in size, designating them as large (l) (see Table 18.4). The following sensitivity analyses are therefore grouped according to whether the lesion was small (less than 3 cm) or large (greater than or equal to 3 cm).

A two-way sensitivity (two variables varied simultaneously) analysis was performed for age *versus* Spetzler grade (see Figures 18.6 and 18.7). This analysis divided patients into two groups: those with lesions

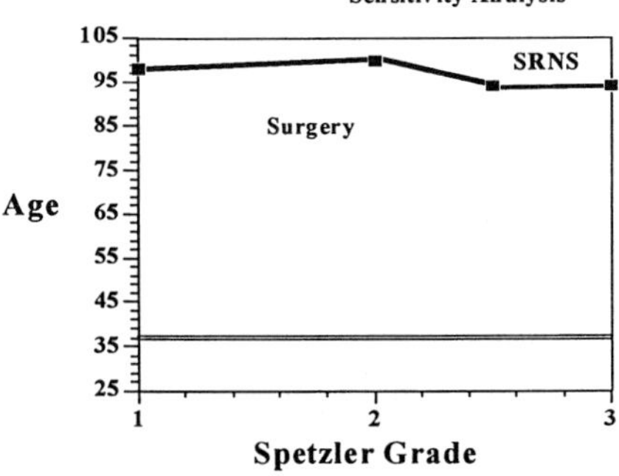

FIG.18.6 Sensitivity analysis of age *versus* Spetzler grade for small AVMs (<3 cm). The *solid line* represents the "break-even" points between surgery and SRNS (*i.e.,* a "tossup" between the two therapies). For all values *above line,* SRNS is favored; for all values *below line,* open surgery is favored. *Double line* represents the baseline age used in the model.

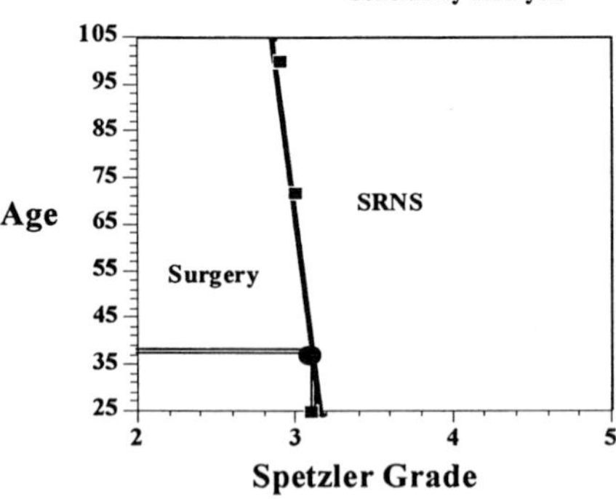

FIG.18.7 Sensitivity analysis of age *versus* Spetzler grade for large AVMs (≥3 cm). The *solid line* represents the "break-even" points between surgery and SRNS (*i.e.,* a "tossup" between the two therapies). For all values *right of line,* SRNS is favored; for all values *left of line,* open surgery is favored. *Double line* represents baseline age used in the model and its "break-even" value on the *x* axis (Spetzler grade 3).

TABLE 18.5

American Society of Anesthesiologists (ASA) Grades Used in the Model[a]

ASA Grade	Physical Status Classification	Mortality Rate[b] (%)
ASA 1	A normal healthy patient	0.06
ASA 2	A patient with a mild systemic disease (mild diabetes, controlled hypertension, anemia, chronic bronchitis, morbid obesity)	0.40
ASA 3	A patient with severe systemic disease that limits activity (angina, obstructive pulmonary disease, prior myocardial infarction)	4.30
ASA 4	A patient with an incapacitating disease that is a constant threat to life (heart failure, renal failure)	23.40
ASA 5	A moribund patient not expected to survive 24 hr (ruptured aneurysm, head trauma with increasing intracranial pressure)	50.70

[a]Reproduced with permission from (17).
[b]Note the associated mortalities.

less than 3 cm and those with lesions that were larger. These two groups were graphically displayed in Figures 18.6 and 18.7. Note that surgery is preferred in these groups for all Spetzler grades 3 or less (ASA = 1). For AVMs of a higher Spetzler grade, SRNS is preferred (despite its low cure rate, approximately 50%). Never are the natural history, embolization, or delayed therapy branches of the tree preferred.

The hypothetical baseline patient analyzed in the model is a patient who remains in an ASA 1 class despite the variance of age. Rarely do we find a patient at our institution who, if older than 55, is an ASA 1 patient (see Table 18.5); minor ongoing diseases will elevate the ASA grade to 2 (17). Sensitivity analyses were performed for all ASA classes. These analyses are summarized in Figures 18.8 and 18.9 and listed in Table 18.6. Note that for small lesions the "break-even" point between open surgery and SRNS is an ASA grade of 3, whereas with larger lesions the "break-even" point was an ASA grade of 3 to 4 for Spetzler grade 2 (1) lesions (despite the poor cure rate of SRNS with these larger lesions).

FAILURE OF THE MODEL

When does the model fail? The model does not deal with the issue of multiple AVMs or concomitant aneurysms and AVMs. There are some AVMs that are clearly best treated by SRNS. For example, small brainstem AVMs may be best treated by SRNS, even though the Spetzler grade may not be prohibitive according to the model's guidelines. Figure

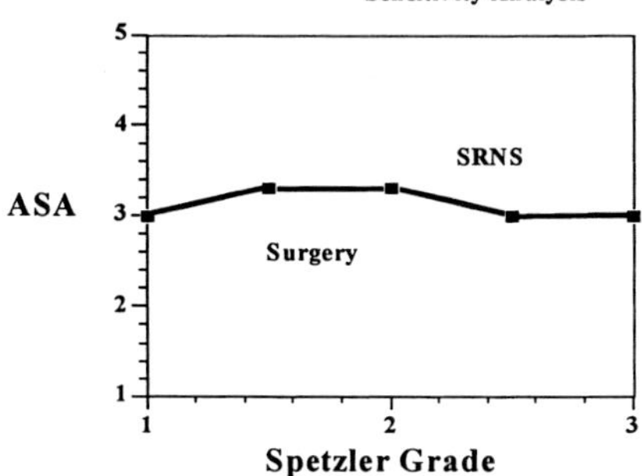

FIG.18.8 Sensitivity analysis of ASA *versus* Spetzler grade for small AVMs (<3 cm). *Solid line* represents the "break-even" points between surgery and SRNS (*i.e.,* a "tossup" between the two therapies). For all values above line, SRNS is favored; for all values below line, open surgery is favored.

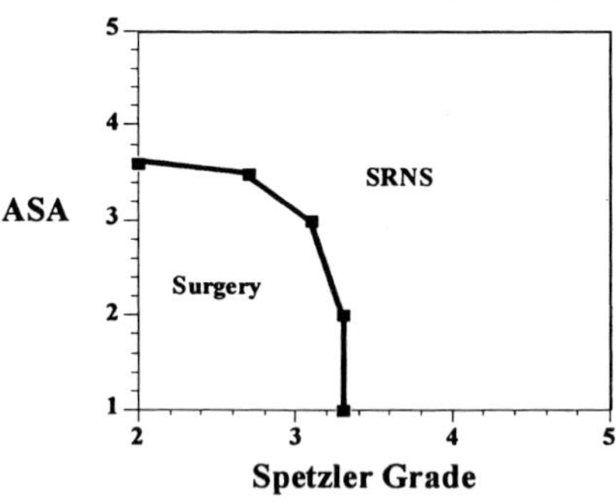

FIG.18.9 Sensitivity analysis of ASA *versus* Spetzler grade for large AVMs (≥3 cm). *Solid line* represents the "break-even" points between surgery and SRNS (*i.e.,* a "tossup" between the two therapies). For all values to *right of line,* SRNS is favored; for all values to left of line, open surgery is favored.

TABLE 18.6
Summary of Decision Sensitivity Analysis for AVMs[a]

Spetzler Grade	1	2 (s)	2 (l)	3 (s)	3 (l)	4	5
ASA1	S	S	S	S	S	R	R
ASA2	S	S	S	S	S	R	R
ASA3	R/S	R/S	S	R/S	S	R	R
ASA4	R	R	R	R	R	R	R
ASA5	R	R	R	R	R	R	R

[a]The sensitivity analysis varied ASA grades *versus* Spetzler grade. Note that open surgery was favored for all Spetzler grade 1 to 3 AVMs unless the ASA grade was sufficiently high. For large complex lesions, SRNS was favored despite low cure rate (<50%). S, open surgery favored; R, SRNS favored; *R/S*, "tossup," open surgery *versus* SRNS; (s), small lesions (AVMs <3 cm); (l), large lesions (AVMs ≥3 cm).

18.10 shows a patient who was operated on but whose operation was aborted for fear of imparting significant injury. The patient underwent SRNS with complete obliteration. These types of lesions, deep brainstem lesions (Fig. 18.10), may be lesions that only can be treated by SRNS. No large open surgical series exists for these brainstem lesions, and therefore the true risks of surgery may not be fully known, therefore making application to the model difficult.

In addition, for lesions which carry significant risk of aphasia, SRNS may be the best therapy. The Spetzler grading system may need to be modified again for these lesions by adding an additional point (1), because both physician and patient find this complication intolerable. Surgical judgment in these particular cases should prevail over any statistical model.

CONCLUSIONS AND SUMMARY

A DA tree representing the possible outcomes of a real-life scenario of decision-making with an AVM has been constructed and presented. Baseline values for a young female with a grade 2 (Spetzler) AVM were drawn from the literature, and when computed in a decision tree, favor open surgical resection. Sensitivity analysis was performed by dividing lesions into small (<3 cm) and large ($\geq$3 cm) categories. With small and large AVMs that were Spetzler grade 3 or less, open surgery was favored over SRNS, delayed therapy, embolization plus therapy, or the natural history of the disease. However, with increasing risk of anesthesia (ASA grade 3 or greater), SRNS becomes a more reasonable therapy for small AVMs (less than 3 cm.). For large AVMs (greater than 3 cm), open surgical resection is favored for Spetzler grade 2 and 3 AVMs, depending on the patient's age and anesthesia risk. However, for large and complex lesions (Spetzler grades 4 and 5), SRNS is favored despite low cure rates (50%).

At no time were natural history, delayed therapy, or embolization therapy favored. In the future, cost may be factored into the analysis as well. The complexity of that evaluation is beyond the scope of this report; however, DA is especially equipped to deal with financial analysis of such questions, because the technique has been borrowed from the business community. In the spirit of the "winds of change," techniques will continue to improve, and other modalities may be found for therapy, requiring further analysis of the therapy of AVMs. As more difficult and complex alternatives become available, DA may play an integral role in sorting these complex issues of patient care.

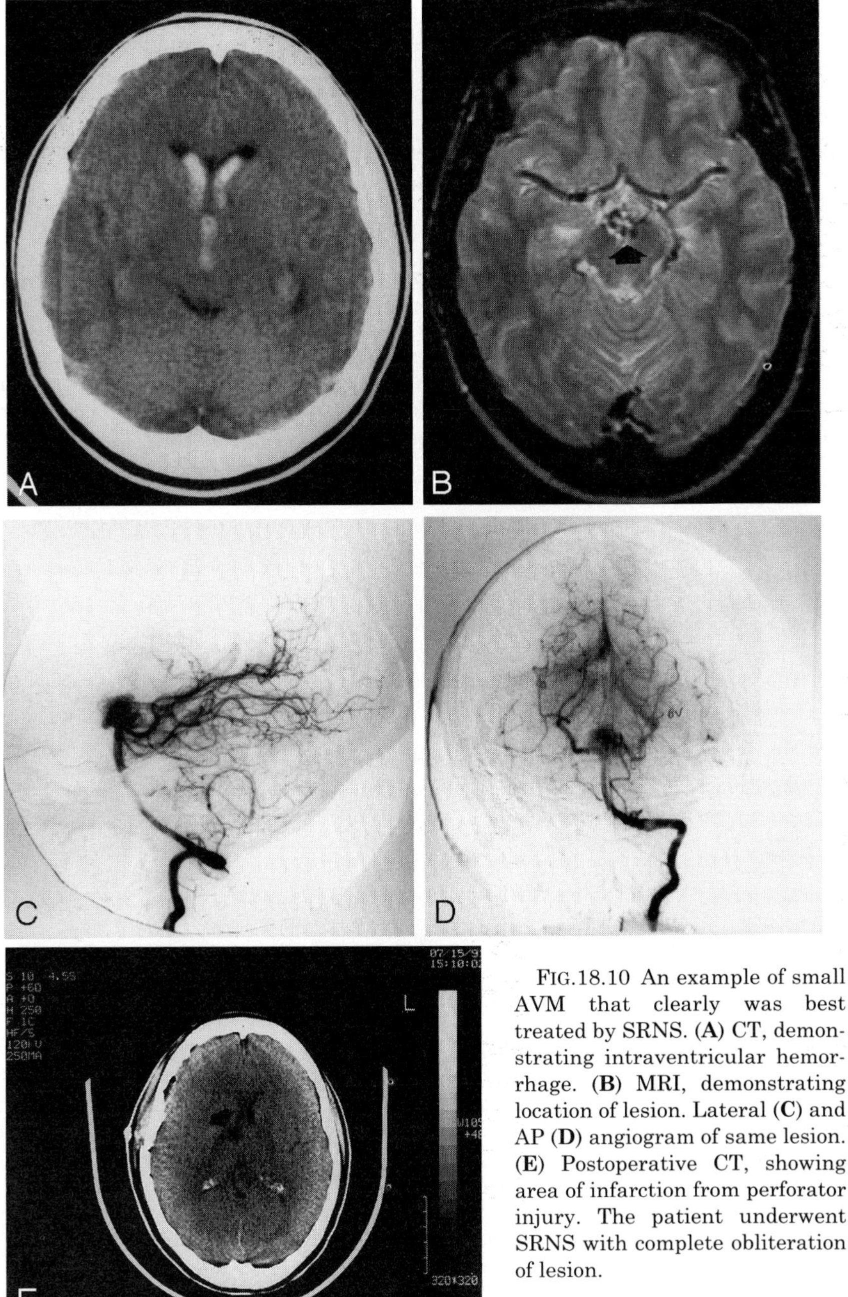

FIG.18.10 An example of small AVM that clearly was best treated by SRNS. (**A**) CT, demonstrating intraventricular hemorrhage. (**B**) MRI, demonstrating location of lesion. Lateral (**C**) and AP (**D**) angiogram of same lesion. (**E**) Postoperative CT, showing area of infarction from perforator injury. The patient underwent SRNS with complete obliteration of lesion.

REFERENCES

1. Aminoff NJ: Management of unruptured arteriovenous malformations. **Clin Neurosurg** 33:177–185, 1986.
2. Auger RG, Wiebers DO: Management of unruptured intracranial arteriovenous malformations: A decision analysis. **Neurosurgery** 30:561–569,1992.
3. Beck JR, Kassirer, Pauker SG: The Markov process in medical prognosis. **Med Decis Making** 3:419–458,1983.
4. Benati A, Beltramello A, Colombari R, *et al.:* Preoperative embolization of arteriovenous malformations with polylene threads: Techniques with wing microcatheter and pathologic results. **Am J Neuroradiol** 10:579–586, 1989.
5. Berthelsen B, Lofgren J, Svendsen P: Embolization of cerebral arteriovenous malformations with bucrylate. **Acta Radiol** 31 (Fasc 1): 13–21,1990.
6. Elstein AS, Balla JI, Iansek R: Application of decision analysis to unruptured arteriovenous malformations. **Neurosurgery** 26:545–546,1990.
7. Fisher III WS: Decision analysis: A tool of the future, an application to unruptured arteriovenous malformations. **Neurosurgery** 24: 129–134, 1989.
8. Fournier D, TerBrugge KG, Willinsky R, *et al.:* Endovascular treatment of intracerebral arteriovenous malformations: Experience in 49 cases. **J Neurosurg** 75:228–233, 1991.
9. Fox AJ, Pelz DM, Lee DH: Arteriovenous malformations of the brain: Recent results of endovascular therapy. **Radiology** 177:51–57, 1990.
10. Garretson HD: Intracranial arteriovenous malformations, in Wilkins RH, Rengachary SS (eds): **Neurosurgery.** New York, McGraw-Hill, 1985, pp 1448–1458.
11. Heros RC, Korosue K, Diebold PM: Surgical excision of cerebral arteriovenous malformations: Late results. **Neurosurgery** 26:570–578, 1990.
12. Hudgins WR: Decision analysis of the treatment of AVMs with radiosurgery. **Stereotact Funct Neurosurg** 61 (Suppl):11–19, 1993.
13. Hudgins WR: Management of unruptured intracranial arteriovenous malformations: A decision analysis. (Letter; Comment). **Neurosurgery** 33:172–173, 1993.
14. Iansek R, Elstein AS, Balla JL: Application of decision analysis to management of cerebral arteriovenous malformation. **Lancet** 1:1132–1135, 1983.
15. Koprowski CD, Longstreth WT Jr, Cebul RD: Clinical neuroepidemiology III. Decisions. **Arch Neurol** 46:223–229, 1989.
16. Lunsford LD, Kondziolka D, Flickinger JC, *et al.* Stereotactic radiosurgery for arteriovenous malformations of the brain. **J Neurosurg** 75:512–524, 1991.
17. Marx GF, Mateo CV, Orkin LR: Computer analysis of postanesthetic deaths. **Anesthesiology** 39:54–58, 1983.
18. Ogilvy CS: Radiation therapy for arteriovenous malformations: A review. **Neurosurgery** 26:725–735, 1990.
19. Ondra SL, Troupp H, George ED, *et al.:* The natural history of symptomatic arteriovenous malformations of the brain: A 24-year follow-up assessment. **J Neurosurg** 73:387–391, 1990.
20. Pauker SG, Kassirer JP: Clinical decision analysis by personal computer. **Arch Intern Med** 141:1831–1837, 1981.
21. Pauker SG, Kassirer JP: Decision analysis. **N Engl J Med** 316:250–258, 1987.
22. Pellettieri L, Carlsson CA, Grevsten S, Norlen G, *et al.:* Surgical versus conservative treatment of intracranial arteriovenous malformations: A study in surgical decision-making. **Acta Neurochir Suppl (Wien)** 29:1–86, 1979.
23. Pelz DM, Fox AJ, Viñuela F, *et al.:* Preoperative embolization of brain AVMs with isobutyl-2 cyanoacrylate. **Am J Neuroradiol** 9:757–764, 1988.

24. Purdy PD, Samson D, Batjer HH, *et al.:* Preoperative embolization of cerebral arteriovenous malformations with polyvinyl alcohol particles: Experience in 51 adults. **Am J Neuroradiol** 11:501–510, 1990.
25. Schumacher M, Horton JA: Treatment of cerebral arteriovenous malformations with PVA. Results and analysis of complications. **Neuroradiology** 33:101–105, 1991.
26. Spetzler RF, Martin NA: A proposed grading system for arteriovenous malformations. **J Neurosurg** 65:476–483, 1986.
27. Steinberg GK, Fabrikant JI, Marks MP, *et al:* Stereotactic heavy-charged-particle Bragg-peak radiation for intracranial arteriovenous malformation. **N Engl J Med** 323:96–101, 1990.
28. Steiner L, Lindquist C, Adler JR, *et al.:* Clinical outcome of radiosurgery for cerebral arteriovenous malformations. **J Neurosurg** 77:1–8, 1992.
29. Viñuela F, Dion J, Lylyk P, *et al:* Update on interventional neuroradiology. **Am J Roentgenol** 153:23–33, 1989.
30. Weinstein MC, Fineberg IEV: *Clinical Decision Analysis.* Philadelphia, W.B. Saunders, 1980.
31. Weinstein MC, Statson WB: Foundations of cost-effectiveness analysis for health and medical practices. *N Engl J Med* 296:716–721, 1977.

ADDENDUM

The techniques used in the analysis were similar to those described by other authors (See 2, 3, 7, 12, and 13). A complex decision tree (124 nodes) was devised for the analysis. Software (DATA by TreeAge Boston, MA) was used to graphically display each node in the formal decision tree and allowed manipulation of variables for multiple sensitivity analyses. A decision analysis technique called Markov cycling was used in the process to best estimate exposure of a patient to the risk of AVM hemorrhage over the duration of a normal life span. Markov cycling requires complex accounting of patient "health states." During each Markov cycle a hypothetical "patient" is allowed to move through a time cycle (in this model, 1 year), occupying one of several "health states," depending on the risks of the disease or therapy; for simplicity the health states assigned in the model were: "well," "disabled," and "dead." A patient can move in any logical direction during the cycle, but all those patients moving to the "dead" state remain. The dead state is therefore referred to as "absorptive."

As an example, in Fig. A.1 one can see the probabilities plotted for a patient after multiple Markovian cycles; this chart graphically displays the probability of each Markov state that a patient may occupy after open surgery. The logarithmic decline in the "well" state in con-

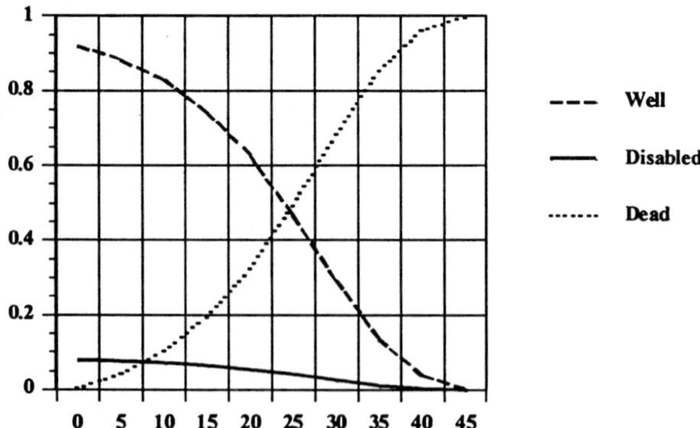

FIG.A.1 *Graph* representing the probabilities of three "health states" during a Markov cycling of the "open surgery" arm of the decision tree used in the model. Note that after surgery, approximately 90% plus patients are in the *well* state. These patients then die from natural causes over a period of time, while they are absorbed into the *dead* state. A similar cycling occurs for patients in the *disabled* state.

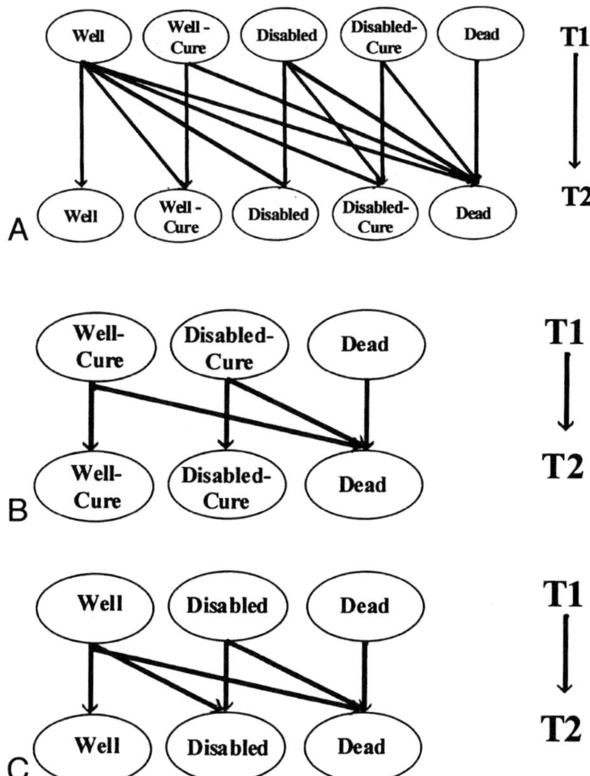

FIG.A.2 **(A)** Markov transition states for delayed therapy followed by SRNS, delayed therapy followed by surgery, embolization therapy followed by SRNS, and SRNS alone. Although the actual transitions were different for each cycle, the transition states were similar. **(B)** Markov transition states for embolization therapy, followed by surgery and open surgery alone. Again the transitions from *T1* to *T2* are different; the transition states are the same. **(C)** Natural history transition states for the model. When comparing with **B**, note that the *well* state may make a transition to *disabled* state.

junction with the logarithmic increase in the "dead" state reflects the life expectancy of the patient and underscores how the "dead" state is ultimately "absorbing." Values can be assigned to each state, and the summation of these values performed at the end of the analysis allows for comparison between therapeutic choices; a computer allows for accounting of all these iterative processes.

The seven Markov transition cycles are graphically outlined in Figure A.2. These seven branches (delayed therapy followed by surgery, delayed therapy followed by SRNS, embolization followed by open surgery, embolization followed by SRNS, open surgery alone, SRNS alone, or natural history) represent seven separate Markovian cycles. Each transition cycle had its own unique transitions that occurred (see legend for Fig. A.2.)

Initial baseline variables are listed in Table 18.1 of the original chapter. Several mathematical formulas were used during the analysis so that life tables could be better estimated and to allow for estimation of annual probabilities of specific diseases; a discounting formula was used to devalue future years of the analysis. A Gompertzian formula was used for an estimation of the mortality rate. This formula was: Mortality rate $= 1 - e^{b\_Age)}$ where $b\_Age = -0.000021383 \times e^{(0.0985 \times Age2)}$, and Age 2 = Age + stage of each Markovian cycle. Similarly, disease specific annual rates were estimated as mean annual probabilities by using the following equation: $1 - e^{(-\,annual\,rate)}$. Discounting was performed by using this formula: discount value $= 1/1.05^{stage}$.

19

Role of Embolization in the Management of Arteriovenous Malformations

TAKASHI YOSHIMOTO, M.D., AKIRA TAKAHASHI, M.D.,
HIROYUKI KINOUCHI, M.D, Ph.D., KAZUO MIZOI, M.D.,
AND HIDEFUMI JOKURA, M.D.

It is still challenging to treat brain arteriovenous malformations (AVMs) because of their vast anatomic complexity and diverse clinical presentation. Even though modern therapeutic modalities are available, including microneurosurgery, intravascular neurosurgery (21, 22), and stereotactic radiosurgery (1, 9, 11, 13, 15, 16), each modality itself raises some controversy that must be resolved. However, combining these three modalities with the participation of its respective specialist would provide the maximum clinical benefits (2, 5, 6, 8, 10). Special emphasis should be given to using these three modalities in combination, because any one of these modalities used alone cannot solve the problems associated with treatment of AVMs. We have been mainly focusing on surgical treatment of AVMs during the past several decades (23, 24). As a result of these clinical and research activities, we introduced an intravascular neurosurgical technique in 1986 (18) and gamma knife stereotactic radiosurgery in 1991 for the treatment of AVMs. Since then, we have tried to maximize clinical results, combining these three modalities. In this chapter, we will discuss our experience over the past 10 years, with special emphasis on the role of intravascular neurosurgical techniques in the context of a multidisciplinary approach.

MATERIALS AND TREATMENT METHODS

Materials Treated with Three Major Modalities

From January 1984 to April 1994, we treated 244 cases with 245 brain AVMs. There were 156 males and 88 females, and average age was 32.0 years at the time of primary treatment. Primary clinical symptoms were hemorrhage in 157 cases, seizure in 57, and miscellaneous in 30 patients. Of the total AVMs, 212 were located in the cerebrum, 25 in the cerebellum, and 8 in the brainstem. As the initial treatment, conventional neurosurgical resection was used in 50 AVMs

(20%), while embolization was used in 144 cases (59%) and gamma knife radiosurgery in 51 of them (21%) (Table 19.1). As a result of combined treatment, the final treatment was conventional neurosurgical resection in 69 AVMs (28%), embolization in 39 (15%), and gamma knife radiosurgery in 137 cases (57%). From the viewpoint of embolization therapy, among 144 AVMs that had been treated primarily with embolization, 39 AVMs (27%) received embolization only. Combined treatment following embolization was surgical resection in 19 (13%) and gamma knife radiosurgery in 86 AVMs (60%).

Indication for the Initial Treatment of AVMs

In the patient who has no history of bleeding, we choose the treatment according to the size of the nidus. If the nidus is more than 3 cm, the first choice is embolization. If the nidus is less than 3 cm, we choose gamma knife radiosurgery because the best indication for gamma knife radiosurgery are that the volume of the nidus is less than 10 ml and the diameter is less than 3 cm. The patient who has a history of bleeding is treated by embolization and/or surgery in general. When hematoma evacuation is necessary and/or the AVM is accessible, we resect the AVM surgically. In other cases, we prefer embolization first.

Role of Embolization in AVM Treatment

The role of embolization in our treatment protocol for brain AVMs is as follows (Table 19.2). First of all, a complete cure can be achieved using embolization without any adjunctive treatment. Secondly, embolization is a better preparation for radical microsurgical resection and radiosurgery. Obliteration of the difficult portions of the nidus and flow reduction in the fistulous component make surgical resection easier and result in better overall outcomes. Embolization decreases the nidus volume to less than 10 ml, the limit of gamma knife radiosurgery. Reducing the nidus volume may also decrease the total radiation dose to obtain complete obliteration of the nidus and shorten the period from stereotactic radiosurgery to a complete cure. Another reason for therapy by embolization includes the elimination of critical parts co-exist-

TABLE 19.1

Treatment of AVMs

	Initial	Final
Surgical resection	50	69
Embolization	144	39
Gamma knife	51	137

TABLE 19.2
The Role of Embolization

1. Complete cure
2. Adjuvant to surgery and radiosurgery
3. Elimination of dangerous part like AN

ing with AVMs such as aneurysms of the nidus and/or feeding arteries or varix of the draining vein (19).

Methods of Embolization

Under local anesthesia with neurolepto-anesthetics, transfemoral catheterization was performed using the standard Seldinger technique. Then, a microcatheter, including a calibrated leak balloon or minicatheter, was introduced into the target feeding artery. After the confirmation of a negative provocation test using amytal and lidocaine hydrochloride, embolization was carried out using a chemical embolization method. We developed this method in the late 1980s after experimental work. The chemical embolization method consists of two liquid embolization materials (3, 4, 17, 18). First, the liquid chemical agent of conjugated estrogen diluted with 25% ethanol (estrogen-alcohol: 20 mg estrogen diluted in 1 ml of 25% ethanol) was infused into the feeding pedicle to induce an intimal specific embolization effect. Estrogen-alcohol was usually infused slowly by infusion pump for 10 to 20 minutes for a dosage of 5 to 10 ml depending on the flow and anatomic characteristics of the feeding arterial system (12). This infusion resulted in diffuse occlusion of the vessels with a diameter of less than 100 μm, and diffuse damage in intimal cells that may prevent future recanalization. Then alcohol-soluble polymer, polyvinyl acetate (PVAC), was injected under real-time subtraction monitoring until the target vessel and the compartment of the nidus were obliterated. PVAC can be injected slowly or quickly, continuously or intermittently, and repeatedly through the same catheter. There is no possibility of the catheter becoming glued to the vessel. Moreover, we have never seen recanalization of the embolized pedicle. Other benefits of this method include less tissue reaction, no biotoxicity, and the result that the pedicle can be easily cut. The lesion embolized with this method is not hard and does not cause any difficulties for a radical resection.

RESULTS

Volume Reduction

As a result of embolization, 12 cases (8.5%) showed complete nidus obliteration at the time of discharge (2 to 3 weeks after the last embolization). In this group, there was no recanalization in the follow-up angiography. Obliteration rates are shown in Table 19.3. There were 35 cases with an obliteration rate of more than 95% (24.7%). Distribution of the Spetzler and Martin grading system comparing pre- and postembolization is presented in Table 19.4 (7, 14). Almost all of the cases showed a one-or two-grade improvement after the embolization. Fifty-five cases (39.6%) were classified as grade IV, V or VI before the embolization. Of these sixteen cases (11.5%) remained at a IV or V grade level after embolization.

The volume of nidus was compared before and after embolization in patients who received gamma knife radiosurgery following the embolization (Fig. 19.1). Among 87 cases treated with this combination, mean volume of nidus was reduced from 11.3 to 5.4 ml, and mean volume reduction rate was 51.8%. In 32 cases, the nidus volume was more than 10 ml (large group), and in 55 cases, it was less than 10 ml (small group) before the embolization. The mean nidus volume of the large group decreased from 23.3 to 11.0 ml due to the embolization. The mean volume reduction in the large group was 47.1%. In this group, 17 nidi (53.1%) were reduced to 10 ml of what is considered to be an appropriate size for gamma knife radiosurgical treatment. The mean nidus volume of the small group in pre-embolization was 4.3 ml, and it was reduced to 2.2 ml (average volume reduction, 50.3%). In this group, 28 nidi (50.9%) were larger than 4 ml before embolization. After the embolization, 47 nidi (85.5%) were reduced to within 4 ml of

TABLE 19.3
Obliteration Rates after Embolization

Complete	12	8.5%		
99%	7	4.9%	13.4%	24.7%
>95%	16	11.3%		
>90%	16	11.3%		
>70%	39	27.5%		
>50%	24	16.9%		
<50%	28	19.7%		

TABLE 19.4
Spetzler and Martin Grading System

	0	I	II	III	IV	V	VI
Pre-emb[a]		7	14	63	40	13	2
Post-emb	12	11	27	73	13	3	

[a]emb, embolization.

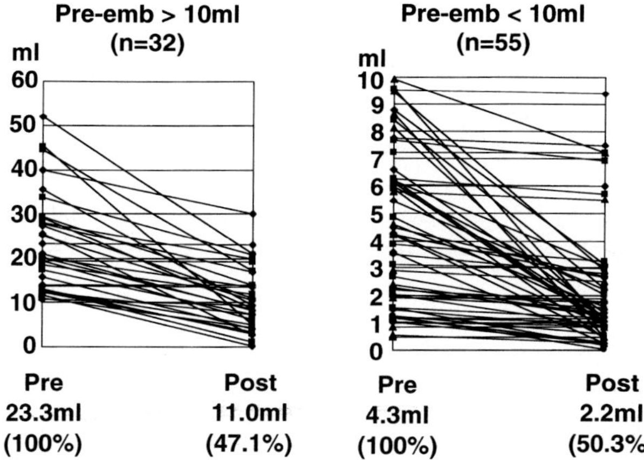

FIG.19.1 Changes of the nidus volume before and after embolization in cases that were treated by embolization initially followed by gamma knife radiosurgery.

what is considered to be the treatable size for gamma knife radiosurgery.

Complications of Embolization

Fatal hemorrhage occurred during the third embolization procedure for giant deep-seated AVMs. Morbidity was classified into major morbidity (neurologic deterioration persisting after discharge causing restriction in social life) and minor morbidity (neurologic deterioration persisting after discharge and causing no restriction in social life). Major morbidity was noted in 7 cases (5.1%) and minor morbidity in 14 cases (10.1%). The main neurologic deficits were visual field disturbances in 9 cases (43%) and sensorimotor disturbances in 8 cases (38%).

Rate of Bleeding

In 144 initially embolized cases, complete cure was achieved in 31 cases (12 cases by embolization and 19 cases by embolization followed by neurosurgical resection). Among the remaining 105 cases, 86 cases were treated with gamma knife radiosurgery, after embolization. These cases are still at risk of bleeding. Overall risk of bleeding was calculated from the period free from bleeding. Ten cases showed bleeding during the follow-up period (average, 2.7 years). The cumulative hemorrhage rate after embolization was 2.82%/year. Fatal bleeding occurred in two cases. Both cases involved giant AVMs, and the bleeding began after several embolizations. Obliteration rates of these patients were 70% and 30%, respectively.

TABLE 19.5
Outcomes according to the Final Treatment

	Good	MD[a]	SD	VD	Dead	Total
Surgical	46	14	8		1	69
resection	(67)	(20)	(12)		(1)	(100)
Embolization	30	4	1		3	38
alone	(79)	(11)	(1)		(8)	(100)

[a]MD, moderately disabled; SD, severely disabled; VD, vegetative (%).

Outcome

Outcomes according to the treatment used are shown in Table 19.5. These outcome performance states were examined just after the completion of the final treatment. In the surgical resection group, the preoperative performance states were: good, 53%; moderately disabled, 16%. Sixty-nine percent of the cases in the surgical resection group were favorable preoperatively. Following the operation, the percentage of patients in a favorable condition increased to 87% (good, 67% and moderately disabled, 20%). However, we lost one case because of an uncontrollable brain edema. Pre-embolization performance states were as follows: good, 19 (50%); moderately disabled, 10 (26%); severely disabled, 9 (24%). Following embolization, performance states were: good, 79%; moderately disabled, 11%. The percentage of patients in a favorable condition was 80%. We lost three cases due to bleeding related to embolization. These cases will be discussed below.

Follow-up Results of Embolization Combined with Gamma Knife Radiosurgery

Among 86 cases who were treated with embolization followed by gamma knife radiosurgery, we examined the angiography for 50 cases at 1 year after gamma knife radiosurgery and for 23 cases at 2 years. By 1 year after gamma knife radiosurgery, complete obliteration was obtained in 10 cases (20%), nearly complete obliteration in 6 cases (12%), size reduction in 23 cases (46%), and status was unchanged in 11 cases (22%). By 2 years, complete obliteration was confirmed in 9 cases (39%), nearly complete obliteration in 5 cases (22%), size reduction in 8 cases (35%), and status was unchanged in 1 case (4%).

REPRESENTATIVE CASES

Embolization Alone

Case 1. This is a case of complete obliteration by embolization alone. The patient, a 53-year-old female, had a past history of intracranial hemorrhage with nausea, vomiting, and monoparesis of the right leg when she was 19 years old. Since then she also had had episodes of generalized convulsion and was referred to our clinic. A carotid angiogram on admission showed a nidus in the frontoparietal cortex with feeders from the anterior cerebral artery (ACA) (Fig. 19.2). Embolizations were performed in two stages, and the AVM was completely obliterated. The nidus and drainer were completely obliterated in the angiogram 6 months after the embolization.

Neurosurgical Resection after Embolization

Case 2. A 12-year-old boy suddenly had a consciousness disturbance and became comatose. A computerized tomography scan revealed a massive intracerebral and intraventricular hemorrhage. After that included an emergent ventricular drainage and ventriculoperitoneal shunt, he recovered gradually and was referred to our practice with moderate dysphasia and right-sided hemiparesis. Angiography revealed a giant AVM located in the left basal ganglionic region extending into the thalamus fed by numerous perforators from the left posterior cerebral artery (PCA), basilar artery, left posterior communicating artery, left middle cerebral artery (MCA), and left internal carotid artery and anterior choroidal artery (Figs. 19.3 and 19.4). He received embolization in four stages. Using a 1.5-Fr progressive suppleness catheter together with a 0.010-inch hydrophilic coated guide wire, it was possible to achieve complete elimination of feeders, including their corresponding parts of nidus (Figs. 19.3 and 19.4). Spetzler and Martin's grade for this patient was improved to IV from V due to the four sessions of embolization.

He underwent surgery 14 days after the last session of the embolization. The AVM was resected by the trans-sylvian approach. The dilated feeders from the posterior communicating artery, anterior choroidal artery, and MCA were clipped. We dissected the nidus through the hematoma cavity. The medical segment of the nidus was almost completely obliterated by the embolization. The angiograms at the patient's discharge showed no nidus and no drainer (Figs. 19.3 and 19.4) Early in the postoperative course, the patient showed slight aggravation of right motor weakness and expressive aphasia that resolved within 1 month after the surgical resection. He transferred to another hospital for further rehabilitation 1½ months later with constantly improved neurologic deficits.

Case 3. This 14-year-old girl had right cerebellar hemorrhage with headache, vomiting, vertigo, and tinnitus. Angiography disclosed a giant high-flow right holohemispheric cerebellar AVM fed by a bilateral

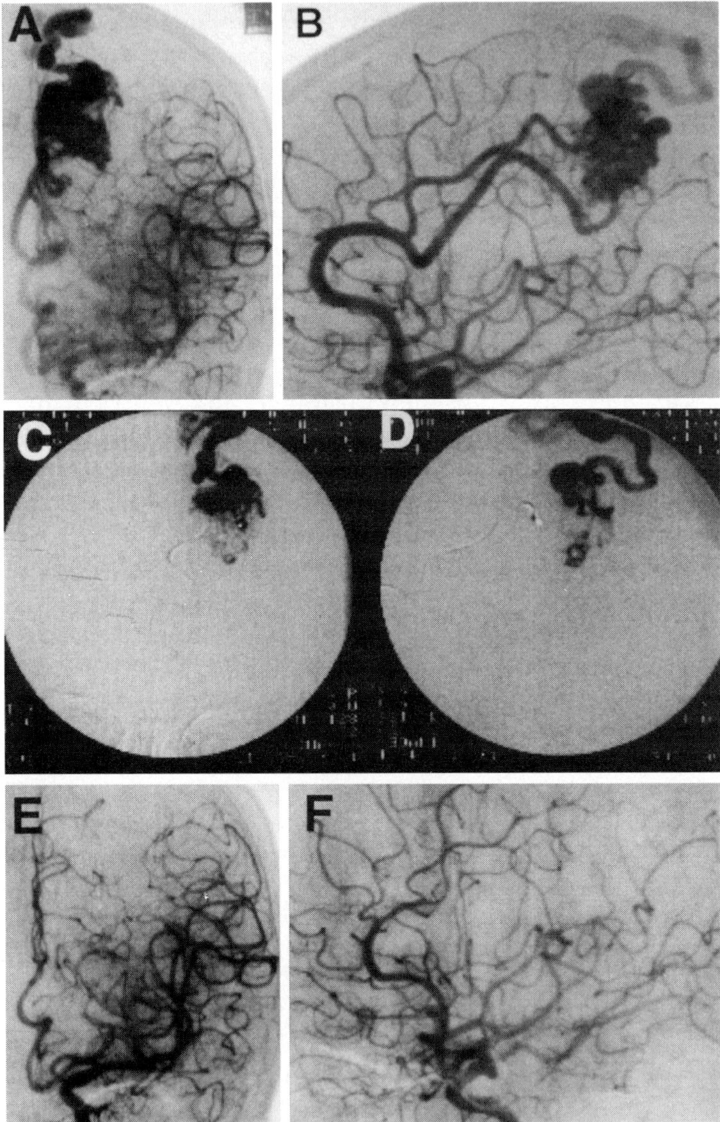

FIG.19.2 Carotid angiograms before embolization (**A** and **B**), during embolization (**C** and **D**), and 6 months after embolization (**E** and **F**). The carotid angiogram showed on admission the nidus in the frontoparietal cortex with feeders from the ACA (**A** and **B**). A superselective angiogram during embolization shows that the nidus and drainer are stained through the microcatheter (**C** and **D**). The nidus and drainer were completely obliterated on the angiogram 6 months after the embolization (**E** and **F**).

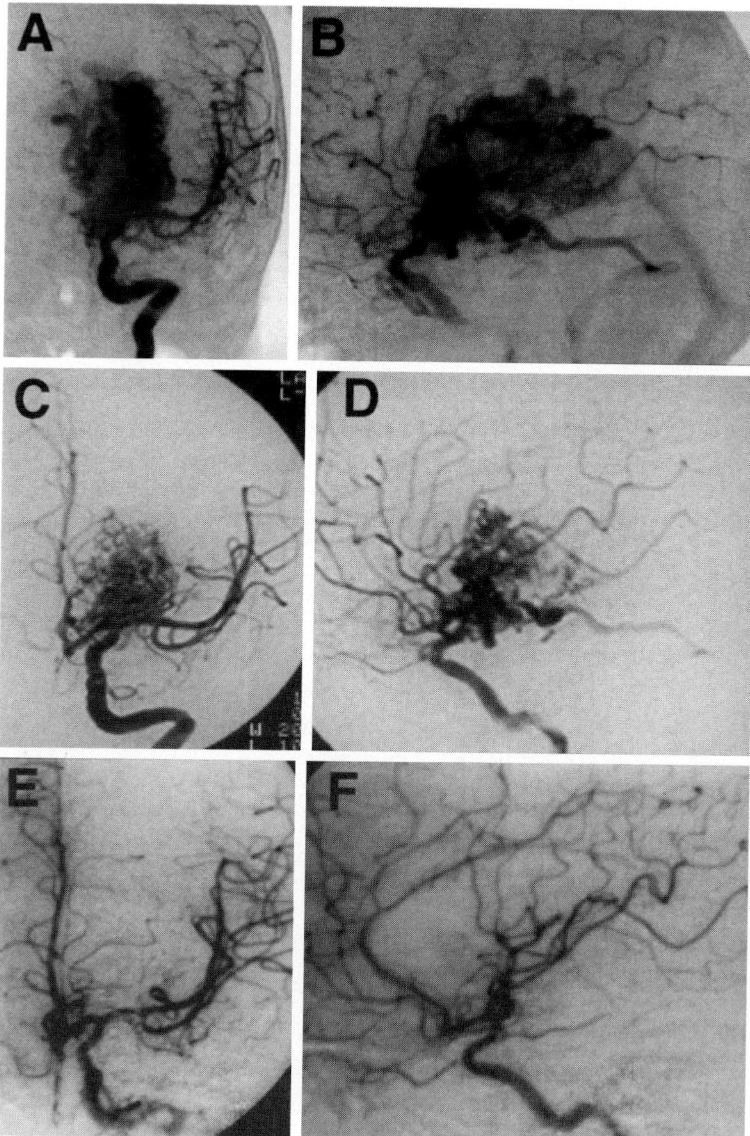

FIG.19.3 Carotid angiogram of an AVM in the left basal ganglia. The AVM was supplied by many distal branches of the major arteries, such as the anterior and posterior choroidal artery, MCA, ACA, and PCA (**A** and **B**). The feeders from the anterior circulation were obliterated partially but significantly (**C** and **D**). The AVM was completely removed by the operation (**E** and **F**).

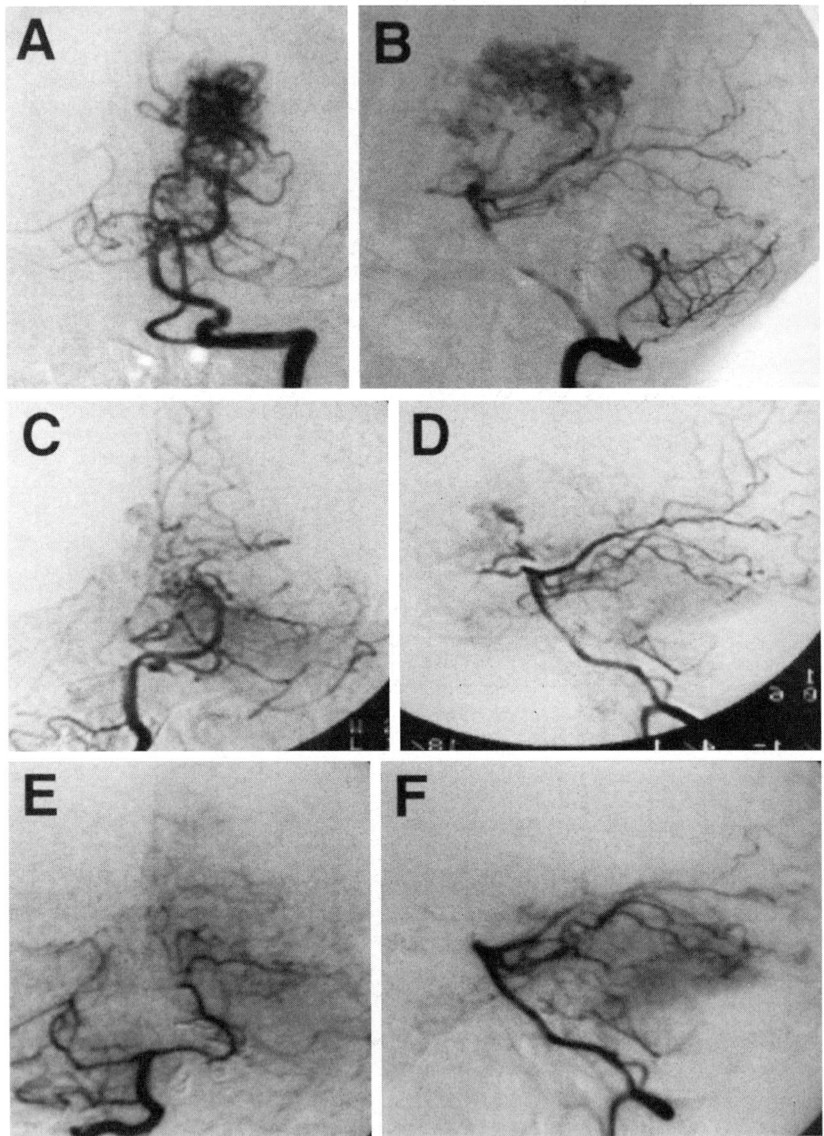

FIG.19.4 Vertebral angiogram AVM. The AVM is fed by branches of the PCA (**A** and **B**). The nidus was almost completely embolized (**C** and **D**). The AVM was totally excised (**E** and **F**).

superior cerebral artery (SCA), a right anterior inferior cerebellar artery (AICA) and right posterior inferior cerebellar artery (PICA) together with contributions from bilateral dural branches of the external carotid artery (Fig. 19.5). Embolization had been done through all of these feeders in five stages. For a portion of the extremely high-flow shunt, 5–0 silk threads were adjunctively used together with the abovementioned chemical embolization method.

Two weeks after the last embolization, surgery was undertaken with monitoring by intra-operative digital subtraction angiography (DSA). The dissection at the surface portion of the nidus was easily performed because of the embolization effect. However, during dissection of the nidus around the brachium pontis, certain difficulties were noted because many fine feeders remained unembolized, perforating through the ventral portion of the brainstem. Across the embolized nidus, it was easy to transect that portion without bleeding. Eventually, the nidus was excised with the entire right cerebellar hemisphere. The completeness of nidus resection was confirmed by intra-operative DSA.

The postoperative course was uneventful, and there was no aggravation of the pre-existing cerebellar dysfunction. Postoperative conventional angiography confirmed total resection, and she returned to normal life. She continued to attend high school.

Gamma Knife Radiosurgery after Embolization

Case 4. The initial symptom of the patient, a 30-year-old male, was a Jacksonian seizure. Neurologic findings on admission showed only slight motor weakness of his right leg. The AVM was in the left motor cortex, and feeding arteries were ACAs (Fig. 19.6). Embolization was done in two stages. The volume of AVM decreased from 26 ml to less than 3 ml, and the diameter reduced to less than 2 cm. Spetzler and Martin's grade became II from III (Fig 19.6). Three months after the embolization, he underwent gamma knife radiosurgery. Target volume was 2.7 ml using a single shot with 18 mm and two shots of 14-mm collimators. Peripheral dosage of radiation was 25 Gy. The nidus and the drainer disappeared 1 year after the gamma knife radiosurgery (Fig. 19.6). The clinical course after this treatment was uneventful.

COST EFFECTIVENESS

Average expenses during admission for treatment were compared among surgical resection alone, surgical resection following embolization, embolization alone, gamma knife radiosurgery alone, and gamma knife after embolization (Table 19.6). The cost of gamma knife radiosurgery is not comparable to the other treatment modalities because of

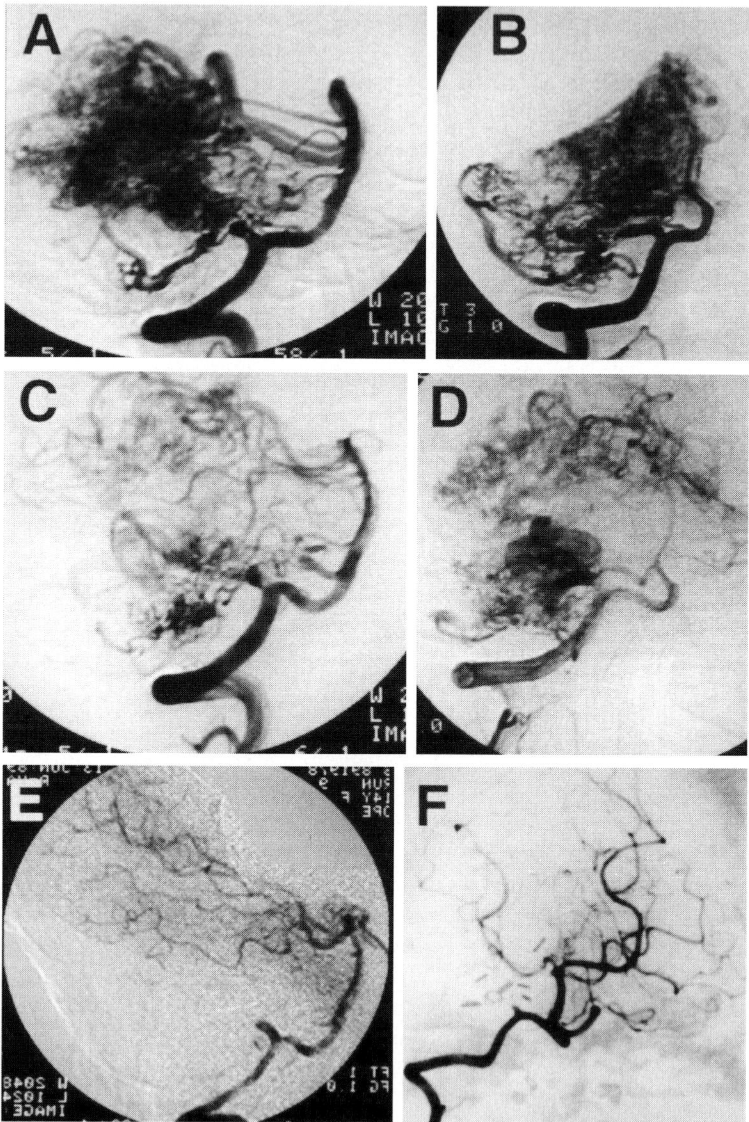

FIG.19.5 Vertebral angiograms on admission show a large, high-flow AVM (**A** and **B**). The feeders are from SCA, AICA, and PICA, contralateral SCA, and external carotid artery (**A** and **B**). After the final embolization, main feeders were obliterated, and a diffuse nidus through perforating arteries was still revealed (**C** and **D**). The AVM was excised with the entire right cerebellar hemisphere (**E** and **F**).

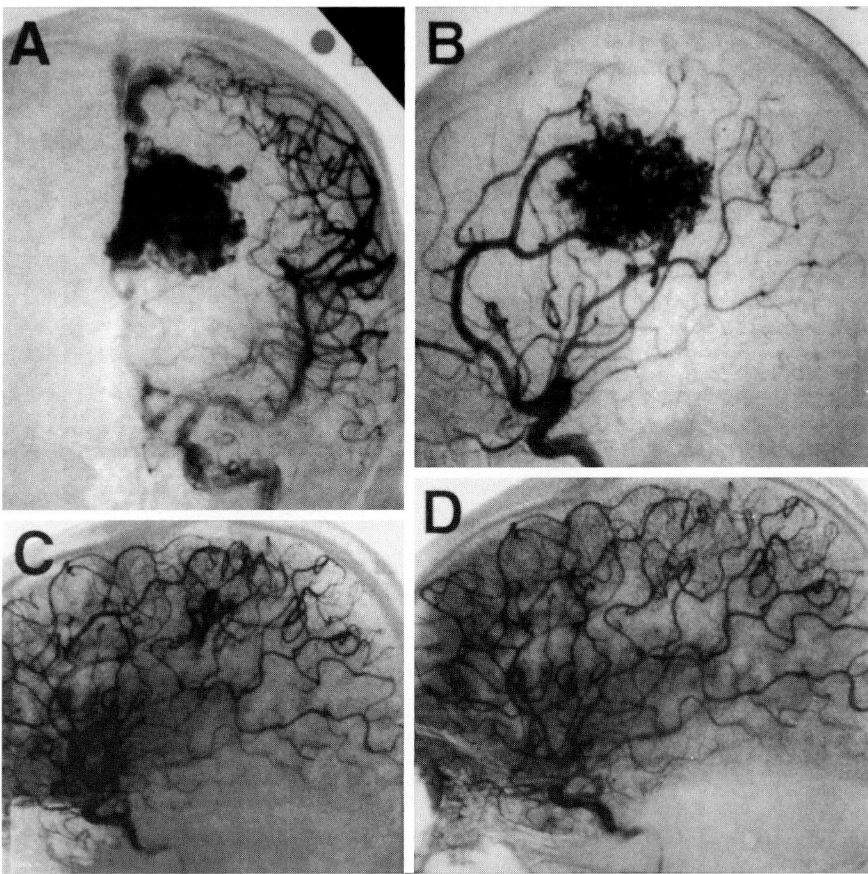

FIG.19.6 The AVM was in the left motor cortex, and feeding arteries were ACAs (**A** and **B**). The volume of AVM decreased from 26 ml to less than 3 ml, and the diameter became less than 2 cm (**C**). The nidus and the drainer disappeared 1 year after the gamma knife (**D**).

TABLE 19.6
Mean Cost according to Treatment

Treatment	Mean Cost/patient
Resection	$28,070
Embolization-resection	55,370
Embolization	36,660
Gamma knife radiosurgery	12,000
Embolization-gamma knife radiosurgery	40,070

TABLE 19.7
Cost of AVM Treatment

	1984–1986	1987–1991	1991–1994
Mean/patient	$28,070	35,679	34,780

the duration of admission. Gamma knife radiosurgery requires only 3 days' admission; however, surgical resection requires a 1 to 2 month admission period. However, the average cost for the treatment of AVMs was not significantly different among the three time periods shown in Table 19.7. Under the Japanese system, all of the cost for admission, including medical services, is covered by insurance unless the admission is extremely extended. Usually patients can return to their normal social life as soon as they are discharged from the hospital. Presently, gamma knife radiosurgery is not included in this medical insurance system.

CONCLUSIONS

For the best management of AVMs, it is essential to achieve complete elimination of abnormal arteriovenous shunting. Classically, it was considered that surgical resection of the nidus was the only way to achieve this objective. With the significant advancement and introduction of new technology, the quality of the treatment using embolization and radiosurgery improved so rapidly that it is difficult to introduce all of these achievements. However, we should utilize these three modalities, depending on the patient's condition and the anatomic condition of the lesion. Furthermore, it is better to use less invasive methods, including embolization and gamma knife radiosurgery, than to use a treatment that requires craniotomy.

One of the major drawbacks of embolization as a primary modality of treatment is the low rate of complete radioanatomic cure. We should further advance the embolization technique because it facilitates any treatment that follows.

REFERENCES

1. Colombo F, Pozza F, Chierego G, *et al.:* Linear accelerator radiosurgery of cerebral arteriovenous malformations using a linear accelerator. **Neurosurgery** 34:14–20, 1994.
2. Deruty R, Pelissou-Guyotat I, Mottolese C *et al.:* The combined management of cerebral arteriovenous malformations. Experience with 100 cases and review of the literature. **Acta Neurochir (Wien)** 123:101–112, 1993.
3. Ezura M, Takahashi A, Yoshimoto T: Successful treatment of an arteriovenous malformation by chemical embolization with estrogen followed by conventional radiotherapy. **Neurosurgery** 31:1105–1107, 1992.

4. Ezura M, Takahashi A, Yoshimoto T, *et al.:* Hydrophilic polymer-coated guided wire combined with progressive suppleness pursil catheter for safer, more definitive embolization of arteriovenous malformation. **Neuroradiology** 36:326–329, 1994.

5. Grzska U, Westphal M, Zanella F, *et al.:* A joint protocol for the neurosurgical and neuroradiologic treatment of cerebral arteriovenous malformations: Indication, technique, and results in 76 cases. Surg Neurol 40:476–484, 1993.

6. Guo WY, Wikholm G, Lindquist C, *et al.:* Combined embolization and gamma knife radiosurgery for cerebral arteriovenous malformations **Acta Radiol** 34:600–606, 1993.

7. Hamilton MG, Spetzler RF: The prospective applications of a grading system for arteriovenous malformations. **Neurosurgery** 34:2–6, 1994.

8. Jafar JJ, Cavis AJ, Berenstien A, *et al.:* The effect of embolization with N-butyl cyanoacrylater prior to surgical resection of cerebral areteriovenous malformations. **J Neurosurg** 78:60–69, 1993.

9. Lunsford LD, Kondziolka D, Flickinger JC, *et al.:* Stereotactic radiosurgery for arteriovenous malformation of the brain. **J Neurosurg** 75:512–524, 1991.

10. Marks MP, Lane B, Steinberg GK, *et al.:* Endovascular treatment of cerebral arteriovenous malformations following radiosurgery. **AJNR** 14:297–303, 1993.

11. Mizoi K, Takahashi A, Yoshimoto T, *et al.:* Surgical excision of giant cerebellar hemispheric arteriovenous malformations following preoperative embolization. Report of two cases. **J Neurosurg** 76:1008–1011, 1992.

12. Nagamine Y, Komatsu S, Fujiwara S, *et al.:* New embolization method using estrogen on microcirculation. **Surg Neurol** 20:269–275, 1984.

13. Redekop GJ, Elisevich KV, Gasper LE, *et al.:* Conventional radiation therapy of intracranial arteriovenous malformations. **J Neurosurg** 78:413–422, 1993.

14. Spetzler RF, Martin NA: A proposed grading system for arteriovenous malformations. **J Neurosurg** 65:476–483, 1986.

15. Steiner L, Lindquist C, Adler JR, *et al.:* Clinical outcome of radiosurgery for cerebral arteriovenous malformations. **J Neurosurg** 77:1–8, 1992.

16. Steiner L, Lindquist C, Cail W, *et al.:* Microsurgery and radiosurgery in brain arteriovenous malformations. **J Neurosurg** 79:647–652, 1993.

17. Sugawara T, Takahashi A, Su CC, *et al.:* Experimental investigation of a new liquid embolization method: Combined administration of estrogen-alcohol and polyvinyl acetate. **Neurol Med Chir** (Tokyo) 32:71–76, 1992.

18. Takahashi A, Suzuki J: Nonsurgical treatment of AVM: Development of new liquid embolization method. In Suzuki J (ed): *Advances in Surgery for Cerebral Stroke.* Berlin, Springer-Verlag, 1988, pp 215–224.

19. Takahashi A, Yoshimoto T: Intravascular sugery and gamma knife for arteriovenous malformations, in Yoshimoto T (ed): Neurosurgeons. Proceedings of the Japanese Congress of Neurological Surgeons, vol 14, pp 95–107, 1995.

20. Takahashi A, Yoshimoto T, Sugawara T, *et al.:* New embolization method for brain arteriovenous malformations: Combined infusion of estrogen-alcohol and polyvinyl acetate. **Neuroradiology** 33(Suppl):190–192, 1991.

21. Taki W, Yonekawa Y, Iwata H, *et al.:* A new liquid material for embolization of arteriovenous malformations. **AJNR** 11:163–168, 1990.

22. Vinuela F, Dion JE, Duckwiler G, *et al.:* Combined endovascular embolization and surgery in the management of cerebral arteriovenous malformations: Experience with 101 cases. **J Neurosurg** 75:856–864, 1991.

23. Yoshimoto T, Kayama T, Suzuki J: Treatment of cerebral arteriovenous malformations. **Neurosurg Rev** 9:279–283, 1986.

24. Yoshimoto T, Suzuki J: Surgical treatment of cerebral arteriovenous malformations. In Kikuchi H (ed): Neurosurgeons. Proceedings of the Japanese Congress of Neurological Surgeons, 1985, vol 4, pp 281–287 (English abstr).

20

Radiosurgery for Arteriovenous Malformations

WILLIAM A. FRIEDMAN, M.D.

Radiosurgery is a relatively old concept, first espoused over 40 years ago by Lars Leksell (2, 19). Recent developments in computer technology for dose planning, as well as refinements in radiation delivery systems, have led to a veritable explosion of interest in this treatment methodology. Perhaps it is equally important that increasing amounts of scientific evidence have persuaded the majority of the international neurosurgical community that radiosurgery is a viable treatment option for selected patients suffering from a variety of challenging neurosurgical disorders. In this chapter, the use of radiosurgery in the treatment of arteriovenous malformations (AVMs) will be reviewed.

GENERAL RADIOSURGICAL PARADIGM

Although the details of radiosurgical treatment techniques differ somewhat from system to system, the basic paradigm is quite similar everywhere. Below is a detailed description of a typical radiosurgical treatment at the University of Florida.

Almost all radiosurgical procedures in adults are performed on an outpatient basis. The patient reports to the neurosurgical clinic at 8:15 a.m. There, a stereotactic head ring is applied under local anesthesia. No skin shaving or preparation is required. If the treatment is for an AVM, the patient is transported to the angiography suite, where a stereotactic angiogram is performed. Subsequently, stereotactic computerized tomography (CT) scanning and/or stereotactic magnetic resonance imaging (MRI) scanning is performed. A bolus of intravenous contrast material is administered to the patient just before imaging through the lesion, to maximize resolution. Because the stereotactic angiogram is a relatively poor 3-dimensional database (4, 5, 34), we also rely on the appearance of the nidus on contrast-enhanced CT scans for treatment planning. After CT scanning, the patient is transported to outpatient radiology for postangiographic observation.

The stereotactic angiogram, stereotactic CT scan, and/or stereotactic MRI (transferred via Ethernet) are taken to radiation physics for dosimetry. The nidus of the AVM is outlined on the angiogram, which is then mounted on a digitizer board. A mouse-like device is used to identify the stereotactic fiducial markers and to trace the nidus; they simultaneously appear on the computer screen. The computer then generates anteroposterior, lateral, and vertical coordinates of the center of the lesion, as well as its demagnified diameter. Next, the computer quickly determines the position of all of the CT and/or MRI images within the stereotactic coordinate system. The angiographic target centerpoint is displayed on the CT/MRI image. Dosimetry then begins and continues until the neurosurgeon, radiation therapist, and radiation physicist are satisfied that an optimal dose plan has been developed. A final computer printout shows all of the treatment parameters in a checklist format.

Patients rest comfortably until the end of the normal radiation therapy treatment day (around 3:00 p.m.). The radiosurgical device is attached to the linear accelerator LINAC. The patient then is attached to the device and treated. The actual radiation treatment time averages approximately 20 minutes. Afterward, the head ring is removed and, after a short observation period, the patient is discharged. The radiosurgical device is disconnected from the LINAC, which is then ready for conventional usage.

RADIOSURGERY FOR AVMS—LITERATURE REVIEW

Multiple studies have demonstrated a substantial (3 to 4%/year) risk of hemorrhage, often associated with morbidity or mortality, in patients harboring AVMs (28). Refinements in microsurgical technique, as well as the development of increasingly effective endovascular treatments, render many of the lesions amenable to successful, safe, surgical cure (12, 13, 31, 33). Those AVMs not suitable for surgical removal are often considered for radiosurgical management.

Angiographic Thrombosis Rates

Radiosurgery appears to produce AVM thrombosis by inducing a pathologic process in the AVM nidus, leading to gradual thickening of the vessels until thrombosis occurs (27, 43). Several radiosurgical series have systematically evaluated this process by obtaining 1- and 2-year follow-up angiograms. Steiner has published multiple reports on gamma knife radiosurgery for AVMs (26, 38–40). He has reported 1-year occlusion rates, ranging from 33.7 to 39.5%, and 2-year occlusion rates, ranging from 79 to 86.5%. However, these results were "optimized" by retrospectively selecting patients who had received a minimum treatment dose. For example (20), in a recent report, he stated that "a large majority of patients received at least 20 to 25 Gy of radiation. . . . Of the 248 patients treated before 1984, the treatment specification placed 188 in this group." The reported thrombosis rates in that study only applied to these 188 patients (76% of his total series). Interestingly, Yamamoto and colleagues recently reported on 25 Japanese patients treated on the gamma unit in Stockholm, Sweden, but followed-up in Japan (43). The 2-year thrombosis rate in those AVMs, which were completely covered by the radiosurgical field, was 64%. One additional patient had complete thrombosis at 3-year angiography and one at 5-year angiography, for a total cure rate of 73%. In another paper (42), Yamamoto *et al.* reported angiographic cures in 6/9 (67%) children treated in Stockholm or Buenos Aires, Argentina, and followed-up in Japan.

Kemeny *et al.* reported on 52 AVM patients treated with gamma knife radiosurgery (15). They all received 2500 cGy to the 50% isodose line. At 1 year, 16 patients (31%) had complete thrombosis, and 10 patients (19%) had "almost complete" thrombosis. They found that the results in younger patients were better and in patients with relatively lateral location of AVMs. There was no difference in outcome among patients with small (<2ml), medium (2 to 3 ml), and large (>3 ml) AVMs.

Lunsford *et al.* reported on 227 AVM patients treated with gamma knife radiosurgery (23). The mean dose delivered to the AVM margin was 21.2 Gy. Multiple isocenters were used in 48% of the patients. Seventeen patients underwent 1-year angiography, which confirmed complete thrombosis in 76.5%. As indicated in that study, "this rate may be spurious since many of these patients were selected for angiography because their MR image had suggested obliteration." Among 75 patients who were followed for at least 2 years, 2-year angiography was performed in only 46 (61%). Complete obliteration was confirmed in 37/46 (80%). This thrombosis rate strongly correlated with AVM size, as follows: <1 ml, 100%; 1 to 4 ml, 85%; 4 to 10 ml, 58%. Recently, this group reported on 65 patients with AVMs less than 3 cm in diameter that were treated with radiosurgery (29). No patient had a radiation-induced complication. Only 32 patients were evaluated with post-treatment angiography. Twenty-seven (84%) had complete thrombosis.

Steinberg *et al.* (36), in a recent analysis of 86 AVMs treated with a particle-beam radiosurgical system, reported 29% 1-year thrombosis, 70% 2-year thrombosis, and 92% 3-year thrombosis rates respectively. The best results were obtained with smaller lesions and higher doses. Initially, a treatment dose of 34.6 Gy was used, but a higher-than-expected neurologic complication rate (20% for the entire series) led to the currently used dose range of 7.7 to 19.2 Gy. No patients treated who received the lower dose range of radiation had complications.

Betti *et al.* reported on the results of 66 AVMs treated with a linear accelerator radiosurgical system (3, 16). Doses of "no more than 40 Gy" were used in 80% of patients. They found a 66% 2-year thrombosis rate. The percentage of cured patients was highest when the entire malformation was included in the 75% isodose line (96%) or the maximum diameter of the lesion was less than 12 mm (81%).

Colombo, *et al.* reported on 97 AVM patients treated with a linear accelerator system (6). Doses ranging from 18.7 to 40 Gy were delivered in one or two sessions. Of 56 patients who were followed-up for longer than 1 year, 50 underwent 12-month follow-up angiography. In 26 patients (52%) complete thrombosis was demonstrated. Fifteen of 20 patients (75%) undergoing 2-year angiography had complete thrombosis. They reported a definite relationship between AVM size and thrombosis rate, as follows: lesions <15 mm in diameter had a 1-year obliteration rate of 76% and a 2-year rate of 90%. Lesions 15 to 25 mm in diameter had a 1-year thrombosis rate of 37.5% and a 2-year rate of 80%. Lesions greater than 25 mm in diameter had a 1-year thrombosis rate of 11% and 2-year rate of 40%. In a more recent report (6), Colombo and colleagues reported follow-up on 180 radiosurgically treated AVMs. The 1-year thrombosis rate was 46%; the 2-year rate was 80%.

Souhami *et al.* (32) reported on 33 AVMs treated with a linear accelerator system. The prescribed dose at isocenter varied from 50 to 55 Gy. A complete obliteration rate of 38% was seen on 1-year angiography. For patients whose AVM nidus was covered by a minimum dose of 25 Gy, the total obliteration rate was 61.5%, whereas none of the patients who had received less than 25 Gy at the edge of the nidus achieved total obliteration.

Loeffler *et al.* (22) reported on 16 AVMs treated with a linear accelerator system. The prescribed radiation dose was 15 to 25 Gy, typically to the 80 to 90% line. The total obliteration rate was 5/11 (45%) at 1 year and 8/11 (73%) at 2 years after treatment.

Complications

HEMORRHAGE

Multiple series have reported that the hemorrhage rate for AVMs treated but not yet obliterated with radiosurgery is the same as it would have been if the patients had not been treated (27). Most recently, Steiner *et al.* analyzed clinical outcomes in 247 consecutive cases of AVM treated with the gamma knife (41). No patient with angiographically proven thrombosis had a hemorrhage. The protective effect of radiosurgery against hemorrhage in incompletely obliterated lesions was evaluated, using both the person-year and the Kaplan-Meier life table methods of analysis. The person-year method showed a rebleed rate of 2 to 3%/year—very similar to that for the known natural history of the disease. The Kaplan-Meier analysis showed a risk of 3.7%/year until 5 years after radiosurgery. At that point, the risk seemed to "plateau." As discussed by the authors, this plateau, which has long been the source of controversy in radiosurgery literature, is very likely an artifact of this statistical method when applied to a relatively small group of patients. In general, most authors believe that radiosurgery provides no protective effect against hemorrhage until the AVM has undergone thrombosis. This is, in fact, the major known drawback of radiosurgery, as compared to microsurgery.

Colombo (6) recently studied the risk of hemorrhage after radiosurgery of 180 patients. In 163 totally irradiated AVMs, the bleeding rate decreased from 4.8% in the first 6 months to 0% from 12 months and upward. In subtotally irradiated AVMs, the bleeding risk increased from 4% in first 6 months to 10% from 12 to 18 months and then decreased to 5.5% from 18 to 24 months. There were no hemorrhages observed in this group after 24 months had elapsed.

Pollock *et al.* (29) recently reported on 65 patient with AVMs less than 3 cm in size. Five patients (7.7%) had a hemorrhage, all in the first year after treatment. Two of these patients died.

RADIATION-INDUCED COMPLICATIONS

Several authors have previously reported that radiosurgery can acutely exacerbate seizure activity. Others have reported nausea, vomiting, and headache occasionally occurring in patients after radiosurgical treatment (1).

Delayed radiation-induced complications have been reported by all groups performing radiosurgery. Steiner found symptomatic radiation necrosis in approximately 3% of his patients (38). Statham *et al.* described one patient who developed radiation necrosis 13 months after gamma knife radiosurgery of a 5.3-ml AVM with a dose of 25 Gy to the margin (35). Lunsford *et al.* reported that 10 patients in their series (4.4%) developed new neurologic deficits that were thought to be secondary to radiation injury (23). Symptoms were location dependent and developed between 4 and 18 months after treatment. All patients were treated with steroids, and all improved. Only two patients were reported to have residual deficits that appeared permanent. The radiation dose and isodose line treated did not correlate with this complication. As they noted, the failure of correlation of dose and complications may very well be because the dose was selected to fall below the computed 3% risk line of Flickinger *et al.* This is a mathematically derived line that prescribes lower doses for larger lesions (8, 9).

Steinberg *et al.* reported a definite correlation between lesion dose and complications (36). As indicated above, the initial treatment dose of 34.6 Gy led to a relatively high complication rate. No patients treated with the subsequently utilized lower dose range had complications. In an earlier report on 75 AVM patients treated with helium particles at a dose of 45 Gy, 7/75 patients (11%) experienced radiation-induced complications (14). Kjellberg *et al.* (16, 17), using a compilation of animal and clinical data, constructed a series of log-log lines, relating prescribed dose and lesion diameter. Their 1% isorisk line is quite similar to Flickinger's mathematically derived 3% risk line.

In Colombo's series, 9/180 patients (5%) experienced symptomatic radiation-induced complications (6). Four had (2.2%) complications that were permanent. Loeffler *et al.* reported that 1/21 AVM patients developed a similar problem, which responded well to steroids (22). Souhami *et al.* reported "severe side effects" in 2/33 patients (6%) (32). Marks and Spencer recently reviewed six radiosurgical series and found a 9% incidence of clinically significant radiation reactions (24). Seven of 23 cases received doses below Kjellberg's 1% risk line.

THE UNIVERSITY OF FLORIDA EXPERIENCE

Patient Population

Between 5/18/88 and 8/9/94, 363 patients were treated with the University of Florida radiosurgery system. Of these patients, 190 had AVMs (10, 11). There were 97 men and 93 women in the series. The mean age was 39 years (range, 7 to 70). Presenting symptoms included hemorrhage (70), seizure (75), headache/incidental (40), and progressive neurologic deficit (5). The location of these lesions is given in Table 20.1.

TABLE 20.1
AVM Location

Frontal	44
Temporal	12
Parieto-occipital	83
Basal ganglia/internal capsule	15
Thalamus	14
Brainstem	10
Cerebellum	9
Corpus callosum	3

Spetzler-Martin classification (33) is given in Table 20.2. Twenty-two patients had undergone prior surgical attempts at AVM excision. Eighteen patients had undergone at least one embolization procedure. All patients referred for radiosurgery were first screened by a cerebrovascular surgery expert. Only if he felt the patient to be a poor candidate for conventional microsurgery was radiosurgery undertaken.

The mean radiation dose to the periphery of the lesion was 1520 cGy (range, 1000 to 2500 cGy). Dose diameter (or dose volume) guidelines previously described, as well as lesion location and clinical variables, were used to select the dose. In general, the larger the lesion, the smaller the dose of radiation (see Fig. 20.1). This treatment dose, was

TABLE 20.2
Spetzler-Martin Classification of AVMs in the University of Florida Series[a]

Tumor Grade	No. of Patients
I	12
II	73
III	78
IV	27

[a]The distribution of our patients denotes both the limitations of radiosurgery and the selection criteria applied at our institution. Grade I malformations usually are treated surgically. Grade V lesions are not considered radiosurgical, because their size (>6 cm) prevents the safe delivery of an effective radiation dose. True Grade VI malformations, in our interpretation, cannot be treated by any current therapeutic modality.

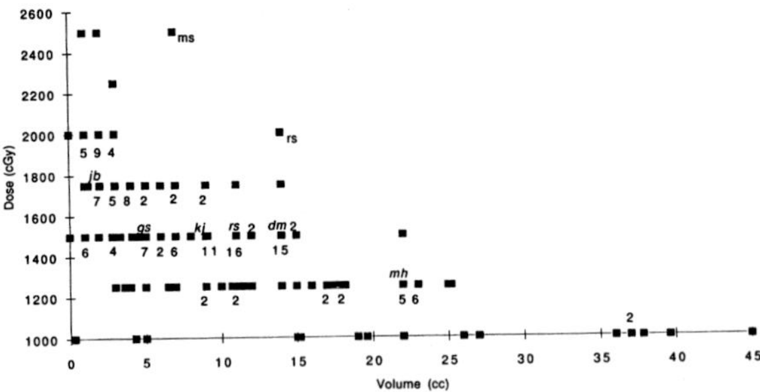

FIG. 20.1 This figure displays the dose prescribed to the periphery of every AVM *versus* that AVM's volume. Numbers displayed adjacent to *data points* indicate the number of patients treated at that particular volume and dose. In general, the larger the AVM volume, the lower the dose that can be safely prescribed. The two patients with minor, permanent neurologic complications are indicated by roman initials. They were treated early in the series and received doses that are higher than those the author uses for lesions of similar volume. The six patients (*italic initials*) with transient radiation-induced complications are indicated with italicized initials. They received doses that have been safely used in other patients.

almost always delivered to the 80% isodose line (range, 70 to 90%). One hundred fifty-eight patients were treated with one isocenter, 21 patients with two isocenters, 9 patients with three isocenters, 1 patient with four isocenters, and 1 patient with five isocenters. Less than half of the patients treated with a single isocenter had a "spherical" treatment plan. Various treatment planning strategies were used to elongate, tilt, or otherwise modify the shape of the treatment field.

The mean lesion volume was 10 ml (0.3 to 45.3 ml). Median lesion volume was 9 ml. In an effort to provide data comparable to other publications in the radiosurgical literature, the following size categories were used in this analysis: A (<1 ml), B (1 to 4 ml), C (4 to 10 ml), and D (>10 ml). The treatment volume was determined in all cases by performing a computerized dose volume histogram of the treatment isodose shell (which was constructed so as to conform to the AVM nidus).

Follow-up

Mean follow-up duration for the entire AVM group is 33 months (1 to 75 months). Follow-up consisted of clinical examination and MRI scanning every 6 months after treatment (30). If possible, follow-up was performed in Gainesville, Florida; otherwise, scan and exam results were forwarded by the patient's local physician. Clinical information is available on 184/190 patients.

Initially, all patients were asked to undergo angiography at yearly intervals, regardless of the MRI findings. After the first 50 patients were treated, it was decided to defer angiography until MRI/magnetic resonance angiography (MRA) strongly suggested complete thrombosis. Furthermore, if complete thrombosis was not identified 3 years after radiosurgery, repeat radiosurgery was undertaken in an effort to obliterate any remaining nidus.

Outcome Categories

Possible AVM outcome categories included the following:

1. Angiographically Documented Cure. This was considered to be a definitive successful endpoint for radiosurgery.

2. Angiographically Documented Failure (> 24 < 36 months after Radiosurgical Treatment.) This was not considered to be a definitive failure of radiosurgery, because several patients with small remaining nidi at 2 years post-treatment were subsequently found to have complete thrombosis at 3 years post-treatment. Recall that all patients underwent radiosurgical retreatment if angiography revealed persistent nidus 36 months after the original treatment.

3. Retreatment. This was considered to be a definitive failure endpoint for the original radiosurgical treatment.

4. MRI Suggestive of Cure. This is not definitive, as angiography sometimes reveals small amounts of persistent nidus, even when MRI or MRA does not. All patients were followed until MRI suggested complete thrombosis; then, they were scheduled for angiography. Some patients in this outcome category refused angiography or have angiography pending.

5. MRI Suggestive of Failure. When an MRI showed persistent flow at a time point less than 36 months after radiosurgery, the patient was followed-up. If an MRI suggested persistent flow at a time point greater than 36 months after treatment, the patient was scheduled for an angiogram, to be immediately followed by re-treatment (same day), if the angiogram confirmed persistent nidus. This category is not a definitive endpoint for failure—the definitive failures are re-treated (category 3).

6. Patient Refusing Follow-up. Unfortunately, in any clinical series, some patients, for a multitude of reasons, refuse suggested follow-up. Nonetheless, these patients are available for telephone interviews, and their clinical status is, therefore, known. This outcome category is not a definitive endpoint.

7. Lost to Follow-up. Again, a small number of patients are inevitably lost to follow-up. Every effort was made to contact these patients or their families to ensure that they had not suffered an untoward event related to the AVM or to radiosurgical treatment.

8. Death. A small number of patients can die from intercurrent disease or from AVM/radiosurgery-related complications. For purposes of this analysis, death related to hemorrhage was considered a definitive failure endpoint. Hemorrhage from which the patient recovered was not considered a definitive endpoint, as some of these patients went on to experience complete AVM angiographic cure later.

In summary, eight possible outcomes are presented to fully describe the entire group of patients, rather than just those undergoing angiography. Three outcome categories, including 66 patients, were considered definitive endpoints: angiographic cure, retreatment, and death due to AVM hemorrhage or radiosurgery complication. In addition, radiation-induced complications and nonfatal hemorrhages were also analyzed by size category.

Outcome Analysis

The outcome categories are tabulated *versus* AVM volume categories in Table 20.3. The detailed results in each category follow below.

TABLE 20.3
Outcome Categories versus AVM Volume Categories

	Size Category			
	A (<1 ml)	B (1–4 ml)	C (4–10 ml)	D (>10 ml)
Total No. of Patients[a]	4	40	28	45
Angiographic cure	1	25	18	12
Angiographic failure (>24<36 months)		6	1	8
Retreated (>36 months)		2	1	4
Deceased[b]		2	1	3
MRI cure (angiography pending or refused)	2	1	3	5
MRI failure (<36 months)			1	9
Refused follow-up		2	2	2
Lost to follow-up	1	2	1	2

[a]Those patients (117) followed long enough to reach one of the indicated outcome categories.

[b]Two patients died secondary to fatal hemorrhage from AVM; the others died from intercurrent disease.

1. Angiographic Cure. In general, angiography was performed when MRI and/or MRA suggested complete thrombosis or when the patient had evidence of persistent nidus at 36 months post-treatment (as part of the re-treatment procedure). Timing varied somewhat, depending on patient compliance and the logistics of long distance radiographic scheduling.

An angiographic cure required that no nidus or shunting remain on the study, as interpreted by a radiologist and the treating neurosurgeon (Fig. 20.2). A total of 56 of 71 patients who had had angiograms performed had angiographic cures (79%). These patients are considered to have achieved a definitive successful endpoint for radiosurgery. The following angiographic cure rates were seen in the various size categories: A, 100%; B, 81%; C, 95%; and D, 60%.

It is of interest that several patients with 2-year angiograms, showing small amounts of remaining nidus, had complete occlusion on 3-year follow-up angiograms.

2. Angiographic Failure (>24<36 Months after Treatment). There were a total of 15 angiograms that showed less than complete thrombosis in this category. Angiography was performed for the following reasons: routine study prior to reliance on MRI/MRA, 3; inability to detect flow on MRI/MRA, 6; prior to re-treatment, 6. Angiographic failures correlated with size as follows: B, 6; C, 1; and D, 8.

3. Re-treatment. All patients with angiographic or MRI evidence of persistent nidus 36 months after radiosurgery treatment were sched-

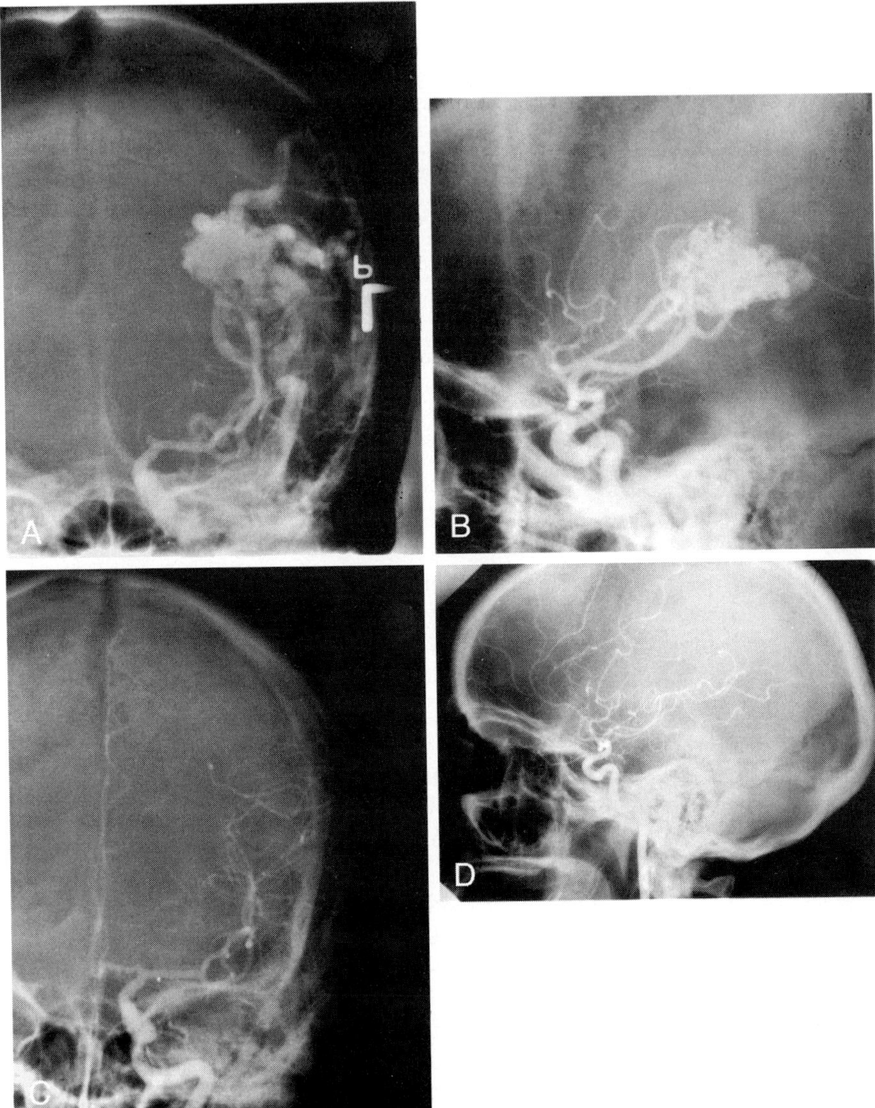

FIG. 20.2 A 36-year-old female presented with a history consistent with subarachnoid hemorrhage, as well as probable sensory seizures. Her AVM was 11.2 ml in volume and was located in the left sylvian region. (**A**) Anteroposterior angiogram. (**B**) Lateral angiogram, nidus outlined. Since it was 28 mm in diameter and had no deep venous drainage, it was only a Spetzler-Martin grade 2 lesion. Yet is was believed, because of location, that surgery had a not insignificant risk of at least temporary neurologic deficits. Angiography 24 months post-treatment revealed complete thrombosis. (**C**) Anteroposterior angiogram. (**D**) Lateral angiogram.

uled for re-treatment. If willing, all such patients have undergone re-treatment. They are considered to have reached a definitive failure endpoint for the original radiosurgical procedure (Fig. 20.3). Two patients in category B required retreatment, as did one patient in category C and three patients in category D. A single re-treated patient has reached a new definitive endpoint—angiographic cure.

4. MRI Suggestive of Cure. Ten patients are being followed-up currently with MRI evidence of AVM thrombosis, who either have angiography pending or have refused angiography. Although, these patients may reach the definitive successful endpoint (angiographic cure), we know that MRI/angiography correlation is less than perfect (see outcome category 2). In addition, two patients listed in outcome category 2 now have MRIs suggestive of cure.

5. MRI Suggestive of Failure. Ten patients are being followed currently with MRI scans suggestive of persistent AVM (one in size category C, nine in category D). These studies were performed 24 to 30 months post-treatment. All studies suggest substantial but incomplete AVM thrombosis.

These patients are not considered to have reached a definitive failure endpoint, as two patients experienced AVM thrombosis between 2 and 3 years post-treatment. When and if they reach 36 months post-treatment with evidence of persistent flow, they will be scheduled for treatment.

6. Six Patients Refusing Radiographic Follow-up (B, 2; C, 2; D, 2). Clinical information is available on all six.

7. Six Patients Lost to Follow-up (A, 1; B, 2; C, 1; D, 2). At the time of last contact, no positive or negative results referable to radiosurgery had been identified.

8. Six Patients Who Died during the Follow-up Period. In all cases, information as to the precise cause of death was obtained from the family or local physician. Four of the patients succumbed to intercurrent disease, unrelated to the AVM or to radiosurgery. Two patients died secondary to AVM hemorrhage and were considered in this study to have reached a definitive failure endpoint for radiosurgery.

Outcome Endpoint Summary

Definitive outcome endpoints included angiographic cure (category 1), re-treatment (category 3), and fatal hemorrhage (category 8). Patients currently in category 2 (angiographic failure, <36 months), category 4 (MRI suggestive of cure), and category 5 (MRI suggestive of failure) may, judged by previous experience (see above), eventually move into definitive success or failure endpoint categories. Patients in category 6 (refused follow-up) and category 7 (lost to follow-up) cannot be analyzed.

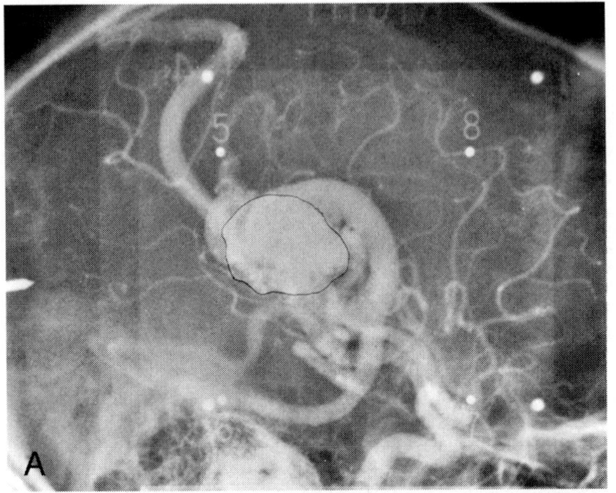

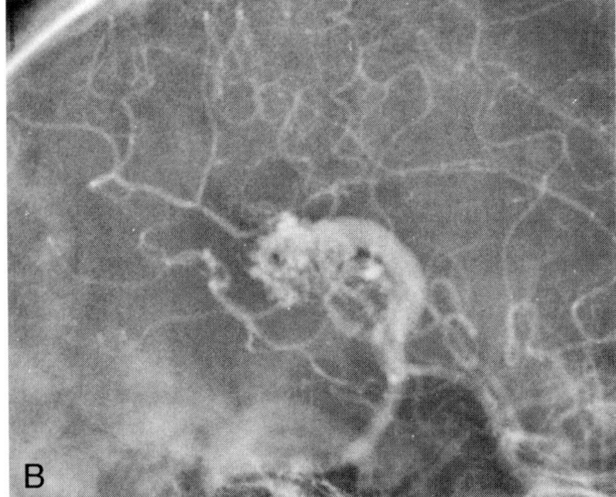

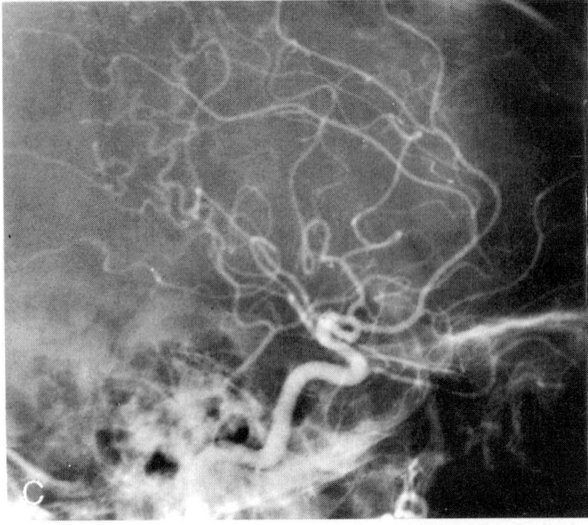

FIG. 20.3 A 37-year-old male presented with a long history of grand mal seizures. His 11.4-ml AVM was treated with a dose of 1500 cGy to the 80% isodose line of a 28-mm collimator. (**A**) Lateral angiogram, pretreatment. Three years later, a persistent but reduced (3.4-ml) nidus was re-treated with 1500 cGy to the 70% isodose line, using two 14 mm collimators. (**B**) Lateral angiogram, after one treatment. Subsequent angiography revealed complete obliteration of the AVM. (**C**) Lateral angiogram after re-treatment.

Table 20.4 summarizes endpoint outcome by size category. Successful endpoints have thus far been attained in 100% of category A patients, 93% of size category B patients, 95% of size category C patients, and 67% of size category D patients.

Complications

ACUTE MORBIDITY

Seven patients experienced seizures within 48 hours of radiosurgery. All had originally presented with a seizure disorder. Anticonvulsant levels are routinely optimized in the high normal range prior to radiosurgical therapy. Prophylactic anticonvulsants are not administered in those AVM patients with no prior seizure history. No other acute morbidity has been seen after radiosurgery.

HEMORRHAGE

Ten patients experienced intracerebral hemorrhages after radiosurgical treatment (A, 0; B, 0; C, 1; D, 9). Only one of these patients presented with a history of hemorrhage. Hemorrhages occurred 2, 3, 4, 4, 4, 5, 6, 11, 12, and 14 months after radiosurgical treatment, respectively. The hemorrhage rate for patients followed-up for 1 year is 6%. The annualized hemorrhage rate is much less (2%), because only one hemorrhage occurred later than 1 year after treatment. Four patients recovered fully; four had significant permanent neurologic deficits; and two died.

RADIATION EDEMA/NECROSIS

Six patients (3%) have experienced transient delayed complications directly attributable to radiosurgery. One of these patients experienced headache; two had mild dysphasia; two had hemiparesis; and one had bilateral fourth nerve palsies. The onset of symptoms was at 10, 10, 14, 14, 14, and 15 months post-radiosurgery, respectively. All patients had documented areas of edema around their AVMs. Four patients have fully recovered. Two are currently under treatment and are improving.

TABLE 20.4
Endpoint Outcome Summarized by Size Category

	A	B	C	D
Angiographic cure	1	25	18	12
Retreatment	0	2	1	4
Fatal hemorrhage	0	0	0	2
% Success	100%	93%	95%	67%

Two patients (1%) have experienced permanent radiation-induced complications (C, 1; D, 1). One patient has mild lower extremity weakness. The other has Parinaud's syndrome and hemibody analgesic. The onset of symptoms was 11 and 14 months after radiosurgery, respectively. Both patients had documented areas of edema, which resolved after months of steroid therapy. Both patients have subsequently been documented to have had angiographic cures.

In summary, two patients (1%) have experienced minor, but permanent, neurologic deficits due to radiation. Another three patients (3%) have experienced transient complications. Figure 20.1 shows the treatment dose and lesion size for all patients treated. The two patients with permanent complications received doses higher than the author subsequently used in other AVMs of similar volume. Conversely, the three patients with transient complications received doses that have been safely used in other patients with AVMs of similar size.

MULTIMODALITY AVM TREATMENT

Radiosurgery may be used alone in the treatment of AVMs <3.5 cm in diameter. Occasionally, larger AVMs are treated with a combination of endovascular therapy, surgery, and radiosurgery (7). Embolization and radiosurgery have been applied with increasing frequency (Fig. 20.4). Many questions remain to be answered regarding this combination of therapies. For example, what type of embolic material is best? Currently, the author treats the nidus that remains after embolization. Since radiosurgery frequently takes 2 years to produce nidus thrombosis, the possibility exists that the embolic material will "wash out" during this latent period.

It does seem reasonably clear at this point that radiosurgery combined with embolization exposes the patient to the risk of both procedures. Since embolization alone rarely produces a cure, it should be used only when the AVM is too large to be safely treated with radiosurgery alone.

CAVERNOUS MALFORMATIONS

The advent of MRI scanning as a neurologic screening test has resulted in the identification of substantial numbers of cavernous malformations. This vascular malformation differs pathologically from true AVMs. The role of radiosurgery in the treatment of angiographically occult vascular malformations (AOVMs) is not well defined. Kondziolka *et al.* reported on 24 patients treated on the gamma knife at the University of Pittsburgh (18). Radiosurgery was used conservatively; each patient had sustained two or more hemorrhages and had a magnetic res-

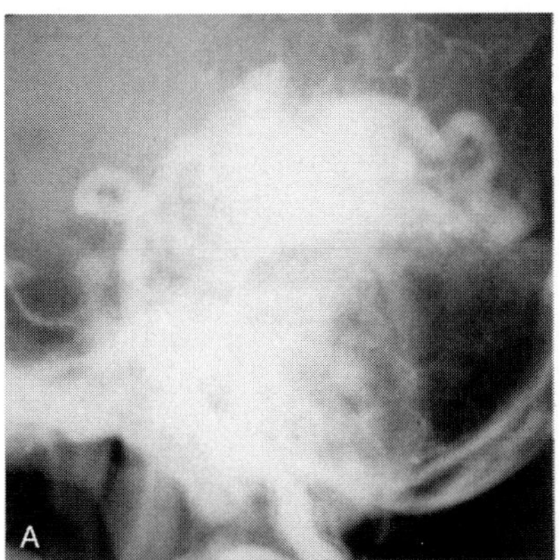

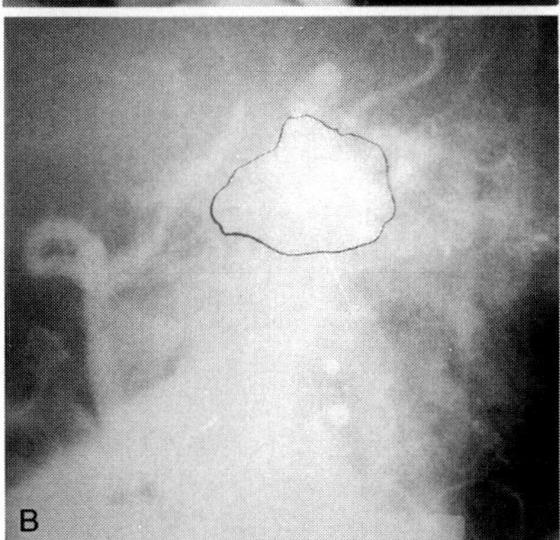

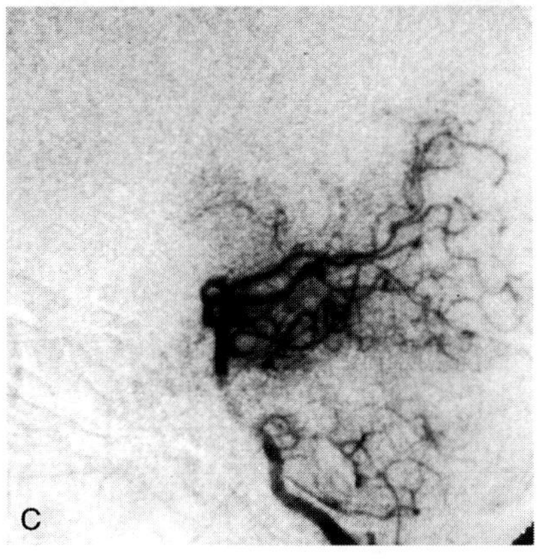

FIG. 20.4 A 40-year-old male presented with a history of headaches and seizures. He underwent multiple endovascular treatments for a large left occipitoparietal AVM (**A**, pre-embolization lateral angiography). The residual nidus (**B**, postembolization lateral angiography, with nidus outlined) was treated with radiosurgery (1500 cGy, 80% isodose line, 28 mm collimator). One-year post-treatment angiography (**C**, lateral digital angiogram) showed complete thrombosis.

onance imaging-defined AOVM located in a region of the brain where microsurgical removal was judged to pose an excessive risk. Fifteen malformations were in the medulla, pons, and/or mesencephalon, and five were located in the thalamus or basal ganglia. Follow-up ranged from 4 to 24 months. Nineteen patients either improved or remained clinically stable and did not hemorrhage again during the follow-up interval. One patient suffered another hemorrhage 7 months after radiosurgery. Five patients experienced temporary worsening of pre-existing neurologic deficits that suggested delayed radiation injury. MRI demonstrated signal changes and edema surrounding the radiosurgical target.

Steinberg *et al.* (37) reported 35 patients treated for AOVMs. The clinical outcome was excellent or good in 80% and poor in 14%. Six percent of the patients died. Six patients experienced recurrent hemorrhage. Four patients worsened from probable radiation injury.

These reports clearly indicate a significantly higher complication rate for radiosurgical treatment of cavernous malformations than for true AVMs. In addition, the fact that they are angiographically occult means that no objective criteria for "successful" treatment exist. Only by following patients with a proven propensity for hemorrhage, and demonstrating a significant decrease in hemorrhage rate, can benefit be shown. Proof of such benefit does not currently exist. At the University of Florida, aggressive surgical therapy is used on the majority of symptomatic cavernous malformations. Radiosurgery is regarded as a "last resort."

CONCLUSIONS

In summary, many reports indicate that approximately 80% of AVMs in the "radiosurgery-sized range" will be angiographically obliterated 2 years after radiosurgical treatment. Permanent neurologic complications are rare (2 to 3%). The major drawback of this treatment method is that patients are unprotected against hemorrhage during the 2-year latent period. Although radiosurgery has been used primarily as a single modality of treatment in previous studies, more recently it has been increasingly used as part of a multimodality treatment approach incorporating surgical and endovascular methods. Radiosurgery is currently of unproven value in the treatment of cavernous malformations.

REFERENCES

1. Alexander E, III, Siddon RL, Loeffler JS: The acute onset of nausea and vomiting following stereotactic radiosurgery: Correlation with total dose to area postrema. **Surg Neurol** 32:40–44, 1989.

2. Backlund EO, Johansson L, Sarby B: Studies on craniopharyngiomas. II: treatment by stereotaxis and radiosurgery. **Acta Chir Scand** 138:749–759, 1972.

3. Betti OO, Munari C, Rosler R: Stereotactic radiosurgery with the linear accelerator: Treatment of arteriovenous malformations. **Neurosurgery** 24:311–321, 1989.

4. Blatt DL, Friedman WA, Bova FJ: Modifications in radiosurgical treatment planning of arteriovenous malformations based on CT imaging. **Neurosurgery** 33: 588–596, 1993.

5. Bova FJ, Friedman WA: Stereotactic angiography: An inadequate database for radiosurgery? **Int J Radiat Oncol Biol Phys** 20:891–895, 1991.

6. Colombo F, Pozza F, Chierego G, *et al.:* Linear accelerator radiosurgery of cerebral arteriovenous malformations: An update. **Neurosurgery** 34:14–21, 1994.

7. Dawson RC, III, Tarr RW, Hecht ST, *et al.:* Treatment of arteriovenous malformations of the brain with combined embolization and stereotactic radiosurgery: Results after 1 and 2 years. **Am J Neuroradiol** 11:857–864, 1990.

8. Flickinger JC: An integrated logistic formula for prediction of complications from radiosurgery. **Int J Radiat Oncol Biol Phys** 17:879–885, 1989.

9. Flickinger JC, Schell MC, Larson DA: Estimation of complications for linear accelerator radiosurgery with the integrated logistic formula. **Int J Radiat Oncol Biol Phys** 19:143–148, 1990.

10. Friedman WA, Bova FJ: LINAC radiosurgery for arteriovenous malformations. **J Neurosurg** 77:832–841, 1992.

11. Friedman WA, Bova FJ, Mendenhall W: Linear accelerator radiosurgery for arteriovenous malformations: The relationship of size to outcome. **J Neurosurg** 82:180–189, 1995.

12. Hamilton MG, Spetzler RF: The prospective application of a grading system for arteriovenous malformations. **Neurosurgery** 34:2–7, 1994.

13. Heros RC, Korosue K, Diebold PM: Surgical excision of cerebral arteriovenous malformations: Late results. **Neurosurgery** 26:570–578, 1990.

14. Hosobuchi Y, Fabrikant JI, Lyman JT: Stereotactic heavy-particle irradiation of intracranial arteriovenous malformations. **Appl Neurophysiol** 50:248–252, 1987.

15. Kemeny AA, Dias PS, Forster DM: Results of stereotactic radiosurgery of arteriovenous malformations: An analysis of 52 cases. **J Neurol Neurosurg Psychiatry** 52:554–558, 1989.

16. Kjellberg RN, Abbe M: Stereotactic Bragg peak proton beam therapy, in Lunsford LD (ed): *Modern Stereotactic Neurosurgery.* Boston, Martinus Mijhoff, 1988, pp 463–470.

17. Kjellberg RN, Hanamura T, Davis KR, *et al.:* Bragg-peak proton-beam therapy for arteriovenous malformations of the brain. **N Engl J Med** 309:269–274, 1983.

18. Kondziolka D, Lunsford LD, Coffey RJ, *et al.:* Stereotactic radiosurgery of angiographically occult vascular malformations: Indications and preliminary experience. **Neurosurgery** 27:892–900, 1990.

19. Leksell L: The stereotaxic method and radiosurgery of the brain. **Acta Chir Scand** 102:316–319, 1951.

20. Lindquist C, Steiner L: Stereotactic radiosurgical treatment of malformations of the brain, in Lunsford LD (ed): *Modern Stereotactic Neurosurgery.* Boston, Martinus Mijhoff, 1988, pp 491–506.

21. Linskey ME, Lunsford LD, Flickinger JC: Radiosurgery for acoustic neurinomas: Early experience. **Neurosurgery** 26:736–744, 1990.

22. Loeffler JS, Alexander E, III, Siddon RL, *et al.:* Stereotactic radiosurgery for intracranial arteriovenous malformations using a standard linear accelerator. **Int J Radiat Oncol Biol Phys** 17:673–677, 1989.

23. Lunsford LD, Kondziolka D, Flickinger JC, *et al.*: Stereotactic radiosurgery for arteriovenous malformations of the brain. **J Neurosurg** 75:512–524, 1991.

24. Marks LB, Spencer DP: The influence of volume on the tolerance of the brain to radiosurgery. **J Neurosurg** 75:177–180, 1991.

25. McGinley PH, Butker EK, Crocker IR, *et al.*: A patient rotator for stereotactic radiosurgery. **Phys Med Biol** 35:649–657, 1990.

26. Nedzi LA, Kooy H, Alexander E, *et al.*: Variables associated with the development of complications from radiosurgery of intracranial tumors. **Int J Radiat Oncol Biol Phys** 21:591–599, 1991.

27. Ogilvy CS: Radiation therapy for arteriovenous malformations: A review. **Neurosurgery** 26:725–735, 1990.

28. Ondra SL, Troupp H, George ED, *et al.*: The natural history of symptomatic arteriovenous malformations of the brain: A 24-year follow-up assessment. **J Neurosurg** 73:387–391, 1991.

29. Pollock BE, Lunsford LD, Kondziolka D, *et al.*: Patient outcomes after stereotactic radiosurgery for "operable" arteriovenous malformations. **Neurosurgery** 35:1–8, 1994.

30. Quisling RG, Peters KR, Friedman WA, *et al.*: Persistent nidus blood flow in cerebral arteriovenous malformation after stereotactic radiosurgery: MR imaging assessment. **Radiology** 180:785–791, 1991.

31. Sisti MB, Kader A, Stein BM: Microsurgery for 67 intracranial arteriovenous malformations less than 3 cm in diameter. **J Neurosurg** 79:653–660, 1993.

32. Souhami L, Oliver A, Podgorsak EB, *et al.*: Radiosurgery of cerebral arteriovenous malformations with the dynamic stereotactic irradiation. **Int J Radiat Oncol Biol Phys** 19:775–782, 1990.

33. Spetzler RF, Martin NA; A proposed grading system of arteriovenous malformations. **J Neurosurg** 65:476–483, 1985.

34. Spiegelmann R, Friedman WA, Bova FJ: Liimitations of angiographic target localization in radiosurgical treatment planning. **Neurosurgery** 30:619–624, 1992.

35. Statham P, Macpherson P, Johnston R, *et al.*: Cerebral radiation necrosis complicating stereotactic radiosurgery for arteriovenous malformation. **J Neurol Neurosurg Psychiatry** 53:476–479, 1990.

36. Steinberg GK, Fabrikant JI, Marks MP, *et al.*: Stereotactic heavy-charged particle Bragg peak radiation for intracranial arteriovenous malformations. **N Engl J Med** 323:96–101, 1990.

37. Steinberg GK, Levy RP, Fabrikant JI, *et al.*: Stereotactic helium ion Bragg peak radiosurgery for angiographically occult intracranial vascular malformations. **Stereotact Funct Neurosurg** 57:64–71, 1991.

38. Steiner L: Treatment of arteriovenous malformations by radiosurgery, in Wilson CB, Stein BM (eds): *Intracranial Arteriovenous Malformations*. Baltimore, Williams & Wilkins, 1984, pp 295–313.

39. Steiner L: Radiosurgery in cerebral arteriovenous malformations, in Fein JM, Flamm ES (eds): *Cerebrovascular Surgery*. New York, Springer-Verlag, 1985, vol 4, pp 1161–1215.

40. Steiner L, Leksell L, Greitz T, *et al.*: Stereotaxic radiosurgery for cerebral arteriovenous malformations. Report of a case. **Acta Chir Scand** 138:459–464, 1972.

41. Steiner L, Lindquist C, Adler JR, *et al.*: Clinical outcome of radiosurgery for cerebral arteriovenous malformations. **J Neurosurg** 77:1–8, 1992.

42. Yamamoto M, Jimbo M, Ide M, *et al.*: Long-term follow-up of radiosurgically treated

arteriovenous malformations in children: Report of nine cases. **Surg Neurol** 38:95–100, 1992.

43. Yamamoto M, Jimbo M, Kobayashi M, *et al.:* Long-term results of radiosurgery for arteriovenous malformation: Neurodiagnostic imaging and histological studies of angiographically confirmed nidus obliteration. **Surg Neurol** 37:219–230, 1992.

21

Surgical Treatment of Intracranial Arteriovenous Malformations with an Analysis of Cost-Effectiveness

ERIC S. NUSSBAUM, M.D., ROBERTO C. HEROS, M.D.,
AND PAUL J. CAMARATA, M.D.

Several recent textbooks, chapters, and literature reports, including our own, deal exhaustively with the technical aspects of surgical procedures for cerebral arteriovenous malformation (AVM) (2, 18, 19, 32, 37, 46, 50, 53, 57, 58, 64, 65). In addition, we devoted most of our recent report in *Clinical Neurosurgery* to this topic (21). Therefore, we will limit our discussion in this chapter to the indications for surgical treatment and the results of such therapy, including an analysis of the cost-effectiveness of surgery, as compared to that of conservative management or radiosurgery.

We will not attempt to compare the results of surgery to the results of embolization because, in general, embolization is used mostly as a surgical adjunct to make surgical excision safer and easier (21). Clearly, embolization is assuming a greater role, either as lone palliative therapy or in combination with radiosurgery, for lesions that are considered inoperable (29). In addition, it is clear that embolization alone can result in complete obliteration of a minority of AVMs (9). However, there is insufficient data about the results of embolization, when used as primary therapy, to allow meaningful comparisons with surgical excision or radiosurgery.

INDICATIONS FOR SURGERY

Decision Making

There are few instances in neurosurgery where decisions as to whether to treat and how to treat are as difficult as in the case of cerebral AVMs. First of all, the surgeon must have a clear understanding of the natural history of these lesions, which will be discussed in more detail below. The surgeon must then consider a variety of factors related to the patient, to the surgeon himself, and to the specific AVM in question. We will proceed to discuss in detail some of these factors.

PATIENT'S AGE

This is one of the most critical factors in decision making. There is evidence to suggest that the likelihood of hemorrhage from an AVM decreases in later life (12, 29, 42), but there are some other studies that indicate otherwise (8, 15). Obviously, the age of the patient determines the number of years at risk for hemorrhage if left untreated. In addition, a younger patient will be able to tolerate better the type of extended surgical procedure and potentially prolonged postoperative course often associated with this type of surgery. Furthermore, a younger patient is more capable of recovering from the potential morbidity of the operation.

PATIENT'S GENERAL HEALTH AND CLINICAL CONDITION

This is another important factor. An elderly patient, with a cardiac condition that prohibits prolonged general anesthesia, would be better advised to undergo radiosurgical treatment or no therapy at all. In addition, a patient with a life-limiting condition has fewer years at risk than a healthier person of the same age.

The neurologic condition of the patient is also extremely important, because the results of surgery are going, to a large degree, to be determined by the patient's pre-operative condition. One caveat about the pre-operative neurologic condition is that considerable judgment must be exercised in treating a patient who has had a recent hemorrhage and a resulting neurologic deficit. Patients, particularly when they are young, have a great potential for neurologic recovery from a neurologic deficit secondary to an intracerebral hemorrhage from an AVM. Therefore, it is unwise to assume that a patient who is hemiplegic immediately after a hemorrhage from an AVM will remain so and, therefore, to recommend surgery of a deep ganglionic AVM that would surely make the patient unable to recover from his hemiplegia. One frequently sees examples of such surgery performed early on, with the results quoted as "good" on the basis that the patient was "unchanged" or not made worse by the operation.

Another way in which the pre-operative condition influences the decision-making process is that patients who are symptomatic from their AVM because of recent hemorrhage, because of a progressive neurologic deficit, or because of frequent seizures are much more likely to accept the risk of serious morbidity from surgical excision than patients who are asymptomatic. Yet, as will be discussed later, the risk of future hemorrhage is not so different from asymptomatic and symptomatic patients. The surgeon's decision-making expertise is most severely tested with asymptomatic patients who harbor lesions that pose significant surgical risks.

PATIENT'S OCCUPATION AND LIFESTYLE

This is another very important consideration where the patient's own judgment plays a major role. The patient must consider the risks as described by the surgeon and be aware of the effect that a potential deficit from surgery will have on his or her future occupation and ability to carry on his or her previous lifestyle. A young athlete may consider a hemiparesis as unacceptable and be willing to live with the risk of a future hemorrhage. Another patient may find the fear of a hemorrhage unacceptable and may be willing to pay the price of a significant handicap from surgery to be rid of such a risk. A mild speech deficit that would be hardly bothersome to most may be a career-ending event for a trial lawyer or a preacher.

LOCATION AND SIZE OF THE AVM

There have been many attempts in the past to grade AVMs or to identify those important characteristics of them that correlate with surgical outcome (3, 14, 24, 28, 40, 48, 51, 59). It is clear from these classifications that the larger AVMs present the greater technical challenge to the treating surgeon and that their removal is fraught with increased morbidity. Likewise, deeper lesions and those adjacent to or involving eloquent cortex are associated with increased surgical morbidity (1, 31, 51, 52). In addition, there are sites where an AVM simply cannot be excised without major resulting morbidity and, therefore, such lesions located deep in the brainstem or within the posterior limb of the internal capsule are frequently called "inoperable." The sheer size of an AVM may make it "inoperable." Although several of the classification systems used are satisfactory, we have found that the system of Spetzler and Martin is simple, easy to use, and reproducible (51). This classification is based on size, eloquence, and whether there is deep venous drainage, which is indicative of deep location or deep extension.

SURGEON'S EXPERIENCE

Although not included in any of the grading systems, and difficult to quantify, the experience that the surgeon has with surgical excision of lesions similar to the one being considered for surgery is an extremely important factor that should be dealt with honestly by the surgeon involved, by the referring physician, and by the hopefully well-informed patient.

ETHICAL CONSIDERATIONS

The neurosurgeon has the responsibility to try to determine what is best for the patient, carefully considering all of the important factors discussed above (21). When he believes that he does not have sufficient experience to reach such a judgment, he should refer the patient. However, if he reaches a distinct opinion as to what is best for the patient, the neurosurgeon must clearly convey this opinion to the patient. Only when the surgeon truly feels that there are equally satisfactory options, should he fairly present the options as valid alternatives. It is unfair to simply present a number of statistics to a patient and " wash our hands" of responsibility, placing on the patient the entire burden of the decision. Clearly, the surgeon must present alternatives but if indeed he believes that the alternatives are less satisfactory, then he should express such an opinion in a straightforward manner to the patient. Once presented with a firm recommendation, the patient may still choose what the neurosurgeon considers a less satisfactory alternative. At this stage, the surgeon must fully support the patient in whatever decision he or she makes. If the well-informed patient chooses a conservative course of action, it is unfair for the neurosurgeon to emphasize the risk of the "time bomb" in his head. The proper thing at this stage is to be reassuring and to emphasize that, in fact, the risk of hemorrhage is "only" 3 to 4% per year.

A complicated ethical dilemma may arise for the surgeon who has recommended no therapy or radiosurgery to the patient, based on the relatively high risk of surgical excision. The patient may say "I don't want any radiation to my head. I would rather have the AVM taken out and be paralyzed than live with the fear of a hemorrhage." Should the surgeon proceed with surgery under these circumstances? We feel strongly that he should not. The best course of action in this case may be to refer the patient to another surgeon for a "second opinion." The converse also applies. Should a patient be treated by radiosurgery, even when the physician feels that the best alternative is surgical excision? It is interesting that the same standard does not seem to apply in this respect and that the indication for many radiosurgical procedures for otherwise straightforward operable AVMs seems to be the "patient's choice" or, worse, the "choice of the referring physician." There is no simple answer to these difficult ethical questions (22).

NATURAL HISTORY

From these and other studies, several conclusions can be drawn (18, 19, 22, 23, 63). First, unruptured AVMs, in terms of the risk of bleeding, appear to follow a course very similar to that of AVMs that present with hemorrhage, although during the 6 months to 1 year following hemorrhage, the risk may be slightly greater (about 6%); after 1 year, the annual rate of hemorrhage is identical in ruptured and unruptured AVMs (3 to 4% per year in the largest series). Second, the risk of death associated with each hemorrhage appears to be about 10 to 15%, with an annual rate of death secondary to hemorrhage of 1% in both ruptured and unruptured AVMs. Third, there is a significant permanent neurologic morbidity associated with AVM hemorrhage that approaches 2 to 3% per year or about 30% from each episode of bleeding.

SURGICAL RESULTS AND COMPLICATIONS

It is meaningless to talk in general terms about surgical results with "AVMs." Here is where the different classifications are particularly useful in that they compare surgical results effectively. Most modern surgical series indicate that AVMs of small or moderate size, even when they are deep and/or adjacent to eloquent areas and even large AVMs in relatively silent areas of the brain, can be excised with a combined mortality and serious morbidity rate of less than 10% (3, 9, 10, 14, 20, 26, 41, 48, 51, 54, 56). In our own report of late results of surgical excision of cerebral AVMs, we encountered a serious permanent morbidity (poor result) of only about 5% when all Spetzler and Martin grade I, II, III, and IV lesions were included (20). However, as mentioned previously, there are a number of lesions that, regardless of size, cannot be excised without serious morbidity (Spetzler and Martin grade VI, or "inoperable"). In addition, the morbidity of surgical excision of large (> 6 cm) AVMs with deep extension and located in or adjacent to critical areas of the brain (Spetzler and Margin grade V) may be unacceptable; in our report the late combined morbidity and mortality rate for these lesions was 38% (20).

Table 21.1 is the recent update of our early (at the time of discharge from the hospital) surgical results in 311 patients who have undergone surgical excision of their AVMs by the senior author (RCH) since 1981. Again, the combined mortality and major morbidity (poor result) in this series was approximately 4% for Spetzler and Martin grade I to IV AVMs, when the patients are considered as a group. There was no major morbidity or mortality for AVMs in grades I or II. However, as discussed before, the serious morbidity for patients with AVMs in grade V was very high (46%). Of course, some of these patients improved with time, as was clearly shown in our analysis of late results (20); however, these data have indeed tempered our enthusiasm for operating on patients with these difficult lesions, and, in fact, since our earlier analy-

TABLE 21.1

Early [a] Surgical Results in AVM Surgery[b]

Grade (S-M)[c]	No. of Patients	Good	Fair	Poor	Dead[d]
I	41	41	0	0	0
II	74	71	3	0	0
III	84	67	11	5	1
IV	75	56	13	5	1
V	37	12	8	16	1
Totals	311	247	35	26	3

[a]Results at time of discharge from hospital.
[b]Cases of senior author (RCH) from 1981 to 1994.
[c]Grade according to the classification system of Spetzler and Martin (S-M).
[d]Two deaths were attributable to pre-operative embolization and the third to postoperative liver failure in a patient with hepatic cirrhosis.

sis of patients operated on before 1989, we have operated only on an additional 16 patients with grade V AVMs; in most of them, the reason for recommending surgery was that they already had a significant neurologic deficit or had a progressive deficit referable to the AVM.

We have analyzed our surgical complications in several recent publications (7, 19, 20, 26). In addition, there have been other recent excellent publications specifically concerning surgical complications (14, 43, 46, 48, 51, 53, 56). In our own analysis the main cause of surgical complications was faulty surgical judgment. This included problems such as midjudging the topographical extent of the lesion and undertaking surgery in lesions that extended too close to or into the primary motor and speech areas, the brainstem, or the internal capsule. This problem, of course, has been minimized since the advent of magnetic resonance imaging (MRI), and functional MRI offers even greater possibilities for determining, in a noninvasive fashion, whether an AVM involves critical areas of the brain (7). Another problem has been to undertake surgery in patients who were not in optimum medical or neurologic condition pre-operatively; one of our early patient deaths, from liver failure, is an example.

The second most important source of morbidity has been excessive intra-operative parenchymal damage, which usually results from too extensive a margin of resection around the AVM. With pre-operative embolization this problem has been minimized and, when the embolization is successful, the surgeon can develop his plane of resection right at the AVM with annoying but controllable bleeding. Occasionally, we have taken feeders too far away from the AVM, thus sacrificing perfusion to critical areas of the brain. We have also encountered problems occluding "vessels of passage," particularly with AVMs located deep in the sylvian region and in the corpus callosum. These AVMs tend to be supplied by arterial branches that pass close to, or even within, the AVM, giving only small side branches to the AVM and going on to supply normal tissue; their sacrifice at surgery can lead to significant damage. Incidentally, this is also a problem with embolization and, in our group, has frequently resulted in the decision not to embolize vessels of passage.

Intra-operative hemorrhage was another problem that we encountered more frequently before the wider use of embolization. Hemorrhage can develop because of early occlusion of important draining veins. More frequently, it develops as the result of losing control of the small fragile vessels in the deep aspect of the AVM. The recent development of "microclips" by Sundt is a very effective, but quite expensive, way of dealing with these tiny fragile vessels. Still, intra-operative hemorrhage remains one of the most important problems in AVM surgery. Patience and meticulous perseverance are necessary at a time when the surgeon is already exhausted from dealing with some of these large lesions that extend toward the ventricle. It is frequently only when the ependymal surface has been reached that bleeding can be stopped satisfactorily. Some experienced surgeons have used relatively deep hypotension successfully in dealing with this problem (Tew JM, personal communication, 1989). When this has been done, it is essential to keep the patient hypotensive and well sedated for at least 2 or 3 days after surgery. Early in our experience we had two cases of significant parenchymal and intraventricular hemorrhage from packing bleeding in the plane away from the AVM. Since then, we have avoided this practice assiduously, and we control bleeding with cottonoids and gentle retraction only against the AVM and never against the opposite plane.

Retraction damage has also been an occasional source of morbidity. This can be direct damage from retractor pressure or from damage to bridging veins, which can either tear or thrombose under excessive retraction. To minimize this problem we sometimes resect a small amount of "silent" brain, as described in a previous publication (18). Subtemporal retraction and injury to the vein of Labbé are particularly problematic. Again, a small amount of resection of the inferior aspect of the temporal lobe may alleviate this difficulty (17).

Damage to the visual radiations has been a frequently encountered but usually predictable source of morbidity in patients with temporal and occipital AVMs. It has been our experience that unless they have a complete hemianopsia, patients adjust quite well to partial visual field deficits in time. Therefore, we are quite willing to undertake surgery in some of these deep occipital or temporal AVMs, even knowing that the surgery will result in a significant visual field cut; when explained carefully to the patients, they seem to tolerate this possibility well.

Postoperative hemorrhage from retained AVM has not been a major problem in our series, and we have had only two patients who have suffered serious major morbidity from this problem. Our success in this respect may be due to our compulsiveness in checking for hemostasis after removal of the AVM. First of all, we have not generally used hypotension at all. In addition, when we believe that the AVM has been completely excised, we raise the blood pressure by approximately 15 to 20 torr and observe carefully for hemostasis. We even tend to "rub" the walls of the resection gently with a cottonoid to try to induce bleeding in any areas where a small surface clot suggests that there may be a small residual piece of AVM. To our dismay we have frequently been successful in inducing bleeding, which has resulted sometimes in hours of frustrating attempts to re-establish hemostasis after finding additional pieces of AVM, when we had previously thought we had performed a complete excision; the only consolation in this situation has been that dealing with the bleeding at the time was much better than doing so later on that first night after surgery. Over the last 3 to 4 years with increasing frequency we have used intra-operative angiography to check for complete excision, but we still depend heavily on the maneuvers described, because it is very possible that an intra-operative angiogram may miss a small piece of AVM which may nevertheless bleed profusely postoperatively.

Normal perfusion breakthrough has not been a major problem in our series, and there are only three patients in whom we can directly attribute major deficit to this complication (52). Despite the infrequency with which we have encountered this complication, we have no doubt that it exists and that it can be a very significant problem. We are convinced that the reason we have not encountered this problem more frequently is that we have routinely "staged" surgery of the large high-flow AVMs that are prone to lead to this problem. Initially, we staged these lesions surgically by occluding large feeders before the final stage. We also used intra-operative embolization frequently during our early experience. Over the last 8 to 10 years we have almost exclusively used endovascular pre-operative embolization for this purpose. As will be discussed later, we have encountered very significant complications and two deaths that we can directly attribute to pre-operative embolization; however, we have no doubt that our surgical morbidity would have been considerably higher and that we would have encountered many more cases of normal perfusion breakthrough had we not used embolization routinely for selected lesions.

Epilepsy has not been a major problem in our series. In our report of late results we encountered only a 7% incidence of postoperative epilepsy requiring chronic antiseizure medication in patients who did not have pre-operative seizures. On the other hand, of patients with pre-operative epilepsy, the frequency of seizures improved in 54%, was unchanged in 32%, and was made worse in only 12% (20, 26). Very similar results have been reported by Piepgras and colleagues (43).

Pre-operative embolization has been a serious source of morbidity in our series. Two of our patients have died, one from massive pulmonary embolization of polyvinyl alcohol that occurred during the embolization of a large AVM (grade V) that obviously had fistulous components with very rapid flow into the venous system. The second death occurred when a patient developed what initially was a "silent" carotid dissection, which was unrecognized at the time of embolization the day before surgery. The excision of his frontal AVM went very well, but the day after surgery, a thrombus from the site of dissection in the neck extended to occlude the carotid bifurcation intracranially, with a resulting massive cerebral infarct; the dissection was confirmed at autopsy to be the source of the large thrombus extending intracranially. We have also had several hemorrhages after embolization and one case of major cerebral infarction from what we interpreted as retrograde arterial thrombosis, occurring in a delayed fashion after embolization. Nevertheless, despite these very serious complications, we continue to use pre-operative embolization selectively, because we are convinced that, as indicated earlier, it has contributed positively to our overall surgical results and, in addition, it has undoubtedly made it possible for us to operate on lesions that, otherwise, we would not, or at least should not, have operated on. The point to emphasize is that pre-operative embolization is not without complications even in the best hands (9, 41, 54, 61). Therefore, exquisite judgment and restraint ought to be exercised in deciding which candidates for surgical excision should be treated by pre-operative embolization. This adjunct should not be used simply to make surgery "easier" or even "less bloody." A few extra hours in the operating room and even a few extra units of blood transfused are a small price to pay, compared to the problems that can be encountered from embolization. Only when, in the best judgment of the surgeon and the interventionist, the combined morbidity and mortality of embolization plus surgery is less than the presumed risks of surgery alone should embolization be used.

ANALYSIS OF COST-EFFECTIVENESS

Methodology

A retrospective review identified 91 patients who underwent surgical resection of a cerebral AVM by a single neurosurgeon (RCH) at the

University of Minnesota over the last 4 years. Many of these patients, mostly with medium- and large-sized AVMs, underwent one or more sessions of pre-operative endovascular embolization in an attempt to reduce flow or occlude inaccessible feeders to the AVM. The average age of these patients was 33. Discharge summaries, operative reports, and follow-up clinic notes were reviewed in all cases, and patients were then contacted by telephone. No patient was lost to follow-up. Early (immediate postoperative) and late (more than 6 months postoperative) surgical results were classified as: good (minimal or no neurologic deficit, no seizures or only well-controlled seizures, and patient able to work full time), fair (mild-to-moderate neurologic deficit and/or difficulty controlling seizures, and patient unable to work full time but fully independent), poor (moderate-to-severe neurologic deficit, patient incapacitated and dependent), or death (20). In the most recent cases, when less than 6 months of follow-up were available, the patient condition at the time of last follow-up evaluation was assumed to remain unchanged on late follow-up. AVMs were graded as small (<3 cm), medium (3 to 6 cm), or large (>6 cm). According to this standard, there were 35 small (38.5%), 43 medium (47.3%), and 13 large (14.2%) AVMs in our series. Patients with occult AVMs were excluded from the study.

OVERVIEW OF THE MODEL

We constructed a Markov decision analysis model, comparing three cohorts of 100 patients who had "operable" AVMs. "Operable" for this purpose refers to lesions chosen for operative resection, with or without pre-operative embolization, by the senior author (RCH). The size distribution of AVMs within each group was based on the results of our review; therefore, each cohort contained 39 small, 47 medium, and 14 large AVMs. In the first group, patients were treated by observation alone. In the second group, all patients underwent surgical resection of their AVMs. For the purposes of this model we made no attempt to separate patients who had or did not have pre-operative embolization; in this sense embolization was considered, for simplicity, strictly as a surgical adjunct to be used when, in the judgment of the surgeon, it enhanced overall safety. This is a valid simplification as long as the morbidity of embolization has been included in the overall surgical morbidity, as we have done. In the final group, patients with medium and large AVMs underwent surgical resection, and patients with small AVMs were treated with stereotactic radiosurgery. Surgical outcomes were based on operative results from our review. Radiosurgery results were derived from the literature; we used global results from all of the largest series of radiosurgery. This tactic may be criticized, because these series contain both "operable" and "nonoperable" AVMs; however, we could have used interchangeably the recent results reported by the Pittsburgh group for "operable" AVMs treated with the gamma knife, and the results of our analysis would have been identical (44). In a separate analysis, we compared the cost-effectiveness of treating 100 patients with small, "operable" AVMs with either conventional surgery or radiosurgery.

For convenience, we assumed that all patients were 33 years of age on initiation of therapy. Initially, all patients were "well." In each subsequent month, a patient might remain well, experience an intracerebral hemorrhage, or die of hemorrhage or another cause. Using this model, outcomes and costs were estimated on a monthly basis to age 99 years. This allowed for comparison of the life expectancy and lifetime medical care costs in each treatment group. Average life expectancy (adjusted for quality of life) was calculated by summing the probabilities of surviving each month in a given state of health (4). All dollar costs were discounted at an annual rate of 5% (62).

INTRACEREBRAL HEMORRHAGE RISK

The incidence of hemorrhage from an untreated AVM was assumed to be 3% per year (6, 8, 15, 23, 38, 45). After surviving a hemorrhage, the risk of re-hemorrhage was assumed to be 6% per year for the first year and then 3% per year thereafter (6, 8, 22). For any given year, the annual rate of hemorrhage was assumed to be distributed evenly over 12 months. Each hemorrhage was assumed to have a 30% chance of producing a major neurologic deficit (16, 23, 25, 42). After surgery, patients were assumed to be absolutely protected from future hemorrhage; an assumption supported by the literature (10, 23). After radiosurgery, patients were assumed to have no protection from hemorrhage for 24 months, an assumption which, once again, is well supported by the literature (13, 30, 44, 55). After 24 months, 80% were assumed to be protected from hemorrhage, and 20% were assumed to remain at baseline risk for future hemorrhage (13, 30, 44, 55). It could be argued that at the end of 2 or 3 years, many of the patients whose AVM was not completely obliterated by radiosurgery could either be treated again by radiosurgery or could undergo surgical excision, with a possible improvement in overall results for this cohort; however, we have no substantial data to indicate what the outcome is of such re-treated patients.

MORTALITY

Age-specific, noncerebrovascular mortality rates were estimated from life tables and Social Security Administration data (11, 35). To obtain the adjusted mortality rate after major intracerebral hemorrhage or for patients in poor condition after surgery, the age-specific population mortality rate was multiplied by a factor of 4.5; for patients in fair condition after surgery, a factor of 2.67 was used (39). For any given year, the annual mortality rate was assumed to be spread evenly over the 12 available months. Each intracerebral hemorrhage was assumed to have a 12.5% mortality rate (15, 16, 20, 29, 42). Based on the work of Ondra *et al.*, the cumulative annual mortality rate for AVM patients is approximately 1%, and the predicted mortality rates in our model matched this figure well (38). The postoperative early and late mortality rates were derived directly from our data.

COSTS OF THERAPY

The dollar costs used in our model are summarized in Table 21.2. The cost of surgical AVM resection was estimated at $24,156.34 per patient. This was based on the average allowable Medicare reimbursements for professional fees and hospital charges for DRG 001 at the University of Minnesota Hospital and Clinic (UMHC). The cost of radiosurgery was estimated to be $7416.74. Similarly this figure was based on average Medicare reimbursements for hospital and physician (neurosurgeon and radiation therapist) fees at UMHC.

For patients experiencing an intracerebral hemorrhage, we accounted for costs of the initial event, as well as ongoing costs of treatment. All patients experiencing a hemorrhage were assumed to incur costs in the acute period consisting of inpatient hospitalization and professional fees. The cost of acute hospital care was estimated to be $8906.94. This was based on a hospital charge of $8279.94, the average medicare reimbursement at UMHC for DRG 014 (cerebrovascular disease other than transient ischemic attack) and professional fees accrued during an average 11-day hospital stay. These include an initial visit by an internist at $117 (HCPCS 99223), daily follow-up visits at $31 (HCPCS 99231), discharge services at $53 (HCPCS 99238), and consultation with a neurologist at $147 (HCPCS 99255) (39).

It was further estimated that 40% of patients surviving a hemorrhage would require inpatient rehabilitation, and 80% would require

TABLE 21.2
Cost Estimates

Item	Cost
Craniotomy for AVM	$24,156.34
Radiosurgery for AVM	$ 7416.74
Acute hemorrhage	$ 8279.94
Inpatient rehabilitation	$21,233.00
Nursing home care	$ 2385.00 per month

outpatient rehabilitation services (47). After surgery, all patients in fair condition were assumed to require inpatient rehabilitation. The mean cost of inpatient rehabilitation, based on data for stroke patients, was estimated at $21,233 (33, 34). The average monthly cost of hemorrhage-related outpatient and home health care, including physician visits, other professional services, and the purchase or rental of aids and appliances, was estimated at $101 per month (39). It was further estimated that at any given time, 25% of survivors of intracerebral hemorrhage require nursing home care. Patients in poor condition after surgery were also assumed to require chronic nursing home care. The average monthly cost of nursing home care was estimated at $2385, based on a 1985 National Nursing Home Survey (36).

UTILITIES

Quality-adjustment weighting after major and minor stroke has been previously described (60). According to similar criteria, hemorrhage-free survival was assumed to have a utility weight of 1.0, survival after hemorrhage without significant deficit (70% of cases) to have a weight of 0.8, after hemorrhage with persistent major deficit (30% of cases) 0.2, and after death 0.0. In other words, for each month that a patient survives without hemorrhage (in the well state), he or she accrues 1 quality-adjusted month of life. After minor or major hemorrhage, he would accrue only 0.8 or 0.2 months, respectively. After death, no further quality-adjusted survival is accrued. After surgery, survival in good condition was given a weight of 1.0, in fair condition a weight of 0.8, and in poor condition a weight of 0.2.

Results

SURGICAL RESULTS

Among the 91 patients who underwent surgery, upon early evaluation, 73 (80%) were considered good; 9 (10%) were fair; 8 (9%) were poor; and 1 (1%) was dead (Table 21.3). On late follow-up, 81 (90%) were in good condition; 4 (4%) were fair; 2 (2%) were poor; and 4 (4%)

TABLE 21.3
AVM Surgery: Early Outcome

Result	No. of Patients (%)
Good	73 (80)
Fair	9 (10)
Poor	8 (9)
Dead	1 (1)
Total	91 (100)

TABLE 21.4
AVM Surgery: Late Outcome

Result	No. of Patients (%)
Good	81 (89)
Fair	4 (4.4)
Poor	2 (2.2)
Dead	4 (4.4)
Total	91 (100)

TABLE 21.5
Causes of Late Poor Outcomes and Death

Poor: 1. Hemiparesis and aphasia from dissection of middle cerebral artery by pre-operative embolization (grade III).
2. Postoperative hemorrhage from normal perfusion breakthrough despite embolization (grade V).

Dead: 1. Embolization of polyvinyl alcohol to lungs. Early death from pulmonary failure (grade V).
2. Poor pre-operative condition from cerebellar hemorrhage. Late death from pneumonia (grade III).
3. Poor pre-operative condition from pre-operative embolization and retrograde arterial thrombosis. Late death unrelated to AVM (grade V).
4. Patient in poor pre-operative condition from radiation necrosis after proton-beam therapy. Late death from pneumonia (grade IV).

[a]Note: The Spetzler and Martin grade (51) of the AVM is indicated in parentheses.

were dead (Table 21.4). The causes of late poor results and death are summarized in Table 21.5. There were 35 patients with small AVMs. In this subgroup, 33 were considered good and 2 were fair on early follow-up, and all were in good condition on late follow-up (Table 21.6).

LIFE EXPECTANCY

Quality-adjusted average life expectancy was estimated to be 29 years without treatment, 35 years with radiosurgery, and 41 years after surgical resection (Table 21.7).

COSTS OF TREATMENT

The average lifetime cost to society of observation of an AVM was estimated at $33,137.64 per patient. This compared to $37,484.47 for surgery, and $32,137.77 for a policy of surgery for large- and medium-sized AVMs and radiosurgery for small AVMs (Table 21.7). A policy of surgical resection of all "operable" AVMs thus costs society $4346.83 to extend the quality-adjusted life expectancy by 12 years. The cost-effectiveness of this policy is therefore $362.24 per quality-adjusted life-

TABLE 21.6
AVM Surgery: Results with Small AVMs (<3 cm)

Result	Early (%)	Late (%)
Good	33 (94)	35 (100)
Fair	2 (6)	
Poor		
Dead		
Total	35 (100)	35 (100)

TABLE 21.7
Comparison of Treatment Modalities

Treatment	Cost	Life Expectancy (yr)[a]
Observation	$33,137.64	29
Surgery[b]	$37,484.47	41
Surgery and radiosurgery[c]	$32,137.77	35

[a]Expressed as undiscounted, quality-adjusted life-years.
[b]Surgical excision performed for all "operable" AVMs regardless of size.
[c]Surgical excision performed for large- and medium-sized AVMs and radiosurgery performed for small (<3 cm) AVMs.

year gained compared to observation alone. Compared to a policy of surgical resection for large and medium size AVMs and radiosurgery for small AVMs, surgical resection of all "operable" AVMs costs $5,346.70 to extend quality-adjusted life expectancy by 6 years; this represents a cost-effectiveness of $891.12 per quality-adjusted life-year gained. These results are summarized in Table 21.7.

ANALYSIS OF TREATMENT OF SMALL AVMS

We examined the cost-effectiveness of treating cohorts of 100 patients with small AVMs with observation, surgical resection, or radiosurgery. For surgical resection, the lifetime treatment cost was $25,495.41 per patient, with an average quality-adjusted life expectancy of 44 years. For radiosurgery, the lifetime treatment cost was $18,660.82 per patient, with an average quality-adjusted life expectancy of 38 years. Compared to observation alone, surgical resection of small AVMs yields a cost savings to society of $7642.23, while extending quality-adjusted life expectancy by 15 years. Compared to radiosurgery, conventional surgery is more expensive, costing an additional $6834.59 in order to extend the quality-adjusted life expectancy by 6 years; in other words, the cost-effectiveness of surgical excision, as compared to that of radiosurgery, is $1139.09 per quality adjusted life-year gained. These results are summarized in Table 21.8.

TABLE 21.8
Comparison of Treatment Modalities for Small AVMs

Treatment	Cost	Life Expectancy (yr)[a]
Observation	$33,137.64	29
Radiosurgery	$18,660.82	38
Surgery	$25,495.41	44

[a]Expressed as undiscounted, quality-adjusted life-years.

Discussion

Laupacis *et al.*, in an attempt to establish guidelines for the comparison of available technologies, proposed a grading scale (from A to E) based on cost-effectiveness (27). In this classification, a grade A technology is both more effective and cheaper than other treatment methods, and a grade B technology costs less than $20,000 per quality-adjusted life-year gained, when compared to the cost of other treatments. Both grade A and B technologies are almost universally accepted as appropriate utilizations of limited societal and health care resources (29). Based on our model, surgical resection of "operable" AVMs qualifies as a grade B technology when compared to observation alone or to a combined surgery-radiosurgery regimen, in which large- and medium-sized AVMs are treated by surgical excision and small AVMs are treated by radiosurgery. In either case, conventional microneurosurgery is established as highly cost-effective in the treatment of AVMs.

That a combined surgery-radiosurgery regimen results in long-term cost savings is not surprising. That patients in the combined surgery radiosurgery group have such a shortened life-expectancy, compared to that of patients in the surgery group, deserves comment. This difference in survival is accounted for by the excellent results of surgical resection of small AVMs in our series—94% good early result, 100% good late result. While waiting for AVM obliteration, a certain percentage of patients treated with radiosurgery (approximately 2 of 35) suffers an intracranial hemorrhage. Two years after radiosurgery, 7 of 35 patients (20%) remain unprotected from later hemorrhage. A large portion of the lifetime "cost" of treatment with radiosurgery is therefore accrued in terms of delayed morbidity and mortality from hemorrhages that occur while the patient is waiting for AVM obliteration and in patients whose AVMs do not respond to treatment.

Analyzing the treatment of small AVMs independently, we found that surgical resection resulted in a great cost savings to society, as well as in an increased longevity over observation alone. Compared to radiosurgery, conventional surgical resection was more expensive but still extended the quality-adjusted life expectancy by a significant amount—6 years. It is worthwhile to note that 95% of the lifetime cost of resecting a small AVM is accounted for by the immediate procedural cost of the craniotomy. In contrast, the immediate procedural cost of radiosurgery accounts for only 40% of the lifetime cost of radiosurgery treatment, which is predominantly accrued in the treatment of delayed morbidity from hemorrhage. If patients undergoing radiosurgery were re-evaluated at 24 months to identify treatment failures, and then the failed cases were either retreated with radiosurgery or underwent surgical resection, the cost of treatment in this cohort would increase, but the longevity could improve as well; as indicated above, we have no substantial data to indicate what the result of such re-treatment policy could be expected to be and, therefore, we did not include in our analysis a cohort of patients in whom such re-treatment policy was used routinely. On the other hand, we did not include in our analysis the cost of morbidity from radiation necrosis since the figures for the incidence of this complication in the literature are generally small and vary widely. Inclusion of such morbidity in our analysis would have weighted against the radiosurgical approach.

It is also important to note that this series examines the cost-effectiveness of surgery in the treatment of AVMs deemed "operable" and then operated on by an experienced vascular neurosurgeon. Clearly, individual judgment in terms of which AVMs should be operated on and technical skill in terms of surgical ability will influence surgical outcomes and, therefore, alter estimates of cost-effectiveness. In this respect it is important to note that results very similar to ours were obtained by Stein and his colleagues, who experienced only 1.5% morbidity and no mortality with surgical excision of 67 consecutive AVMs of less than 3 cm in diameter (49). In contrast, Pollock *et al.* reviewed 65 patients with small (less than 3 cm) "operable" AVMs who refused microsurgery and were treated by radiosurgery; these patients experienced a hemorrhage rate of 3.7% annually and a mortality rate of 3.1% during the latency period (44); the figures coincide with the assumptions made in our analysis (44). The results of our analysis would have been very similar if we had substituted in our calculations the results for small "operable" AVMs treated by microsurgical excision or by radiosurgery, provided by Stein and colleagues and by Pollock *et al.*, respectively (44, 49).

CONCLUSIONS

Decision making with cerebral AVMs is one of the most difficult aspects of neurosurgical practice. A diversity of factors, such as the size and location of the AVM; the patient's age, medical, and neurologic condition; and his occupation, hobbies, and expectations, as well as his psychological makeup, must be considered. In addition, a thorough understanding of the natural history is necessary. There is no possible substitution for individual case-by-case analysis since every AVM and every patient is different.

Currently, we have excellent information about the natural history of cerebral AVMs. It appears that they bleed at a rate of 3 to 4% per year whether they have bled before or not. The risk of rehemorrhage after a hemorrhage is only slightly higher during the first year (6%), and after that it is the same as for AVMs that have not bled. The serious morbidity associated with each hemorrhage is about 30% and the mortality about 12.5%.

Modern surgical results indicate that all but the very large cerebral AVMs and those AVMs that involve critical deep structures, such as the internal capsule and the brainstem, can be excised with satisfactory results.

For grade I to IV AVMs (Spetzler and Martin grading system (51)) a combined morbidity and mortality rate of less than 10% can generally be expected. The surgery of grade V AVMs is accompanied by very substantial morbidity and generally should not be recommended, except for patients who have a significant pre-operative deficit or who have had multiple hemorrhages or a gradually progressing deficit.

There are many different causes of morbidity accompanying surgical excision of cerebral AVMs. Of these, probably the most important is faulty surgical judgment, although technical problems do arise frequently, even for the most experienced surgeons. Pre-operative embolization is a significant source of morbidity and mortality, and it should be used only when it is expected that the combined morbidity and mortality of embolization and surgery is less than the risk for surgery alone.

Surgical excision of "operable" cerebral AVMs, preceded by embolization in selected cases, is highly cost-effective when compared to observation alone or to a policy of surgery for large- and medium-sized lesions and radiosurgery for small (<3 cm) lesions. This conclusion assumes that an experienced team performs the surgery and embolization, as well as the selection of patients for surgery with or without embolization.

Operable small (<3 cm) AVMs should be treated by surgical excision; when compared to radiosurgery or observation alone, surgical excision is highly cost-effective and very efficacious in prolonging quality-life expectancy. This conclusion assumes that an experienced cerebrovascular surgeon makes the judgment of operability (selection for surgery) and then performs the operation.

REFERENCES

1. Amacher AL, Allock JM, Drake CG: Cerebral angiomas: The sequelae of surgical treatment. **J Neurosurg** 37:571, 1972.
2. Apuzzo MLJ: *Brain Surgery: Complication Avoidance and Management*. New York, Churchill Livingstone, 1993, vols 1 and 2.
3. Batjer HH, Devous MD, Seibert GB, *et al.:* Intracranial arteriovenous malformation: Relationship between clinical factors and surgical complications. **Neurosurgery** 24:75, 1989.
4. Beck JR, Pauker SG: The Markov process in medical prognosis. **Med Decis Making** 3:419–458, 1983.
5. Beck JR, Pauker SG, Gottlieb JE, *et al.:* A convenient approximation of life expectancy. II. Use in medical decision-making. **Am J Med** 73:889–897, 1982.
6. Brown RD, Weibers DO, Forbes G, *et al.:* The natural history of unruptured intracranial arteriovenous malformations. **J Neurosurg** 68:352–356, 1988.
7. Camarata PJ, Heros RC: Arteriovenous malformations of the brain, in Youmans JR, Smith RR (eds): *Neurological Surgery.* in press, 1994.
8. Crawford PM, West CR, Chadwick DW, *et al.:* Arteriovenous malformation of the brain: Natural history in unoperated patients. **J Neurol Neurosurg Psychiatry** 49:1–10, 1986.
9. Debrun G, Vinuela F, Fox A, *et al.:* Embolization of cerebral arteriovenous malformations with bucrylate. Experience in 46 cases. **J Neurosurg** 56:615–627, 1982.
10. Drake CG: Cerebral arteriovenous malformations: Considerations for and experience with surgical treatment in 166 cases. **Clin Neurosurg** 26:145–208, 1979.
11. Faber JF, Wade AH: *Life Tables for the United States: 1900–2050*. Washington, DC, Social Security Administration, Social Security Administration publication (SSA), 1983, pp 11515–11536.
12. Forster DMC, Steiner L, Häkanson S: Arteriovenous malformations of the brain. A long-term clinical study. **J Neurosurg** 37:562, 1972.
13. Friedman WA, Bova FJ: Linear accelerator radiosurgery for arteriovenous malformations. **J Neurosurg** 77:832–841, 1992.
14. Garretson HD: Intracranial arteriovenous malformations, in Wilkins RH, Rengachary SS (eds): *Neurosurgery.* New York, McGraw-Hill, 1985, pp 1448–1458.
15. Graf CJ, Perret GE, Torner JC: Bleeding from cerebral arteriovenous malformations as part of their natural history. **J Neurosurg** 58:331, 1983.
16. Heros RC: Arteriovenous malformations of the brain, in Ojemann RG, Heros RC, Crowell RM (eds): *Surgical Management of Cerebrovascular Disease.* Baltimore, Williams & Wilkins, 1988, ed 2, pp 347–413.
17. Heros RC: Arteriovenous malformations of the medial temporal lobe: Surgical approach and neuroradiological characterization. **J Neurosurg** 56:44–52, 1982.
18. Heros RC: Brain resection for exposure of deep extracerebral and paraventricular lesions. **Surg Neurol** 34:188–195, 1990.
19. Heros RC, Korosue K: Parenchymal cerebral arteriovenous malformations, in Apuzzo MLJ (ed): *Brain Surgery: Complication Avoidance and Management.* New York, Churchill Livingstone, 1993, pp 1175–1193.
20. Heros RC, Korosue K, Diebold PM: Surgical excision of cerebral arteriovenous malformations: Late results. **Neurosurgery** 26:570–578, 1990.
21. Heros RC, Morcos JJ, Korosue K: Arteriovenous malformations of the brain: Surgical management, in Selman W (ed): *Clinical Neurosurgery.* Baltimore, Williams & Wilkins, 1993, pp 139–173.

22. Heros RC, Tu Y-K: Unruptured arteriovenous malformations: A dilemma in surgical decision making. **Clin Neurosurg** 33:187–236, 1985.

23. Heros RC, Tu Y-K: Is surgical therapy needed for unruptured arteriovenous malformations? **Neurology** 37:279–286, 1987.

24. Höllerhage H-G, Dewenter K-M, Dietz H: Grading of supratentorial arteriovenous malformations on the basis of multivariate analysis of prognostic factors. **Acta Neurochir (Wien)** 117:129, 1992.

25. Kjellberg RN, Hanamura T, Davis KR, *et al.:* Bragg-peak proton-beam therapy for arteriovenous malformations of the brain. **N Engl J Med** 309:269–274, 1983.

26. Korosue K, Heros RC, Diebold P: Late results of complete resection of cerebral arteriovenous malformations in reference to neurologic condition, seizures and risk of bleeding, in Sugita K, Shibuya M (eds): *Intracranial Aneurysms and Arteriovenous Malformations: State of Art,* 1990, pp 399–403.

27. Laupacis A, Feeny D, Detsky AS, *et al.:* How attractive does a new technology have to be to warrant adoption and utilization? Tentative guidelines for using clinical and economic evaluations. **Can Med Assoc J** 146:473–481, 1992.

28. Luessenhop AJ, Gennarelli TA: Anatomical grading of supratentorial arteriovenous malformations for determining operability. **Neurosurgery** 1:30, 1977.

29. Luessenhop AJ, Rosa L: Cerebral arteriovenous malformations. Indications for and results of surgery, and the role of intravascular techniques. **J Neurosurg** 60:14, 1984.

30. Lunsford LD, Kondziolka D, Flickinger JC, *et al.:* Stereotactic radiosurgery for arteriovenous malformations of the brain. **J Neurosurg** 75:512–524, 1991.

31. Malik GM, McCormick PW: Surgical resection of thalamocaudate arteriovenous malformations, in Wilkins RH, Rengachary SS (eds): *Neurosurgery Update II: Vascular, Spinal, Pediatric, and Functional Neurosurgery.* New York, McGraw-Hill, 1991, pp 149–156.

32. Malik GM, Umansky F, Patel S, *et al.:* Microsurgical removal of arteriovenous malformations of the basal ganglia. **Neurosurgery** 23:209–217, 1988.

33. McGinnis GE, Osberg JS, DeJong G, *et al.:* Predicting charges for inpatient medical rehabilitation using severity, DRG, age, and function. **Am J Public Health** 77:826–829, 1987.

34. McGinnis GE, Osberg JS, Seward ML, *et al.:* Total charges for inpatient medical rehabilitation. **Health Care Finance Rev** 9:31–40, 1988.

35. National Center for Health Statistics: *Births, Marriages, and Deaths for August 1989: Monthly Vital Statistics Report.* Hyattsville, MD, National Center for Health Statistics, 1989, US Dept of Health and Human Services Publication (PHS) 89–1120.

36. National Center for Health Statistics: *The National Nursing Home Survey: 1985 Summary for the United States.* Hyattsville, MD, National Center for Health Statistics, 1989, US Dept of Public Health and Human Services Publication (PHS) 89–1758.

37. Ojemann RG, Heros RC, Crowell RM: *Surgical Management of Cerebrovascular Disease.* Baltimore, Williams & Wilkins, 1987, ed 2.

38. Ondra SL, Troupp H, George ED: The natural history of symptomatic arteriovenous malformations of the brain: A 24 year follow-up assessment. **J Neurosurg** 73:387–391, 1990.

39. Oster G, Huse DM, Lacey MJ, *et al.:* Cost-effectiveness of ticlopidine in preventing stroke in high-risk patients. **Stroke** 25:1149–1156, 1994.

40. Pasqualin A, Barone G, Cioffi F, *et al.:* The relevance of anatomic and hemodynamic factors to a classification of cerebral arteriovenous malformations. **Neurosurgery** 28:370, 1991.

41. Pasqualin A, Scienze R, Cioffi F, *et al.:* Treatment of cerebral arteriovenous malformations with a combination of preoperative embolization and surgery. **Neurosurgery** 29:358, 1991.

42. Perret G, Nishioka H: Report on Cooperative Study of Intracranial Aneurysms and Subarachnoid Hemorrhage. Section VI: Arteriovenous malformations. Analysis of 545 cases of cranio-cerebral arteriovenous malformations and fistulae reported to the Cooperative Study. **J Neurosurg** 25:467–490, 1966.

43. Piepgras DG, Sundt TM Jr, Raggowanksi AT, *et al.:* Seizure outcome in patients with surgically treated cerebral arteriovenous malformations. **J Neurosurg** 78:5, 1993.

44. Pollock BE, Lunsford LD, Kondziolka D, *et al.:* Patient outcomes after stereotactic radiosurgery for "operable" arteriovenous malformations. **Neurosurgery** 35:1–8, 1994.

45. Samson D, Batjer HH: Preoperative evaluation of the risk/benefit ratio for arteriovenous malformations of the brain, in Wilkins RH, Rengachary SS (eds): *Neurosurgery Update II: Vascular, Spinal, Pediatric and Functional Neurosurgery.* New York, McGraw-Hill, 1991, pp 129–133.

46. Samson DS, Batjer HH: Surface lesions: Lobar arteriovenous malformations, in Apuzzo MLJ (ed): *Brain Surgery: Complication Avoidance and Management.* New York, Churchill Livingstone, 1993, pp 1142–1175.

47. Scharfenberger JA, III KC: Financing of health care for elderly stroke patients. **Phys Med Rehabil: State Art Rev** 3:653–658, 1989.

48. Shi Y, Chen X: A proposed scheme for grading intracranial arteriovenous malformations. **J Neurosurg** 65:484, 1986.

49. Sisti MB, Abraham K, Stein BM: Microsurgery for 67 intracranial arteriovenous malformations less than 3 cm in diameter. **J Neurosurg** 79:653–660, 1993.

50. Solomon RA, Stein BM: Surgical resection of medial hemispheric arteriovenous malformations of the brain, in Wilkins RH, Rengachary SS (eds): *Neurosurgery Update II: Vascular, Spinal, Pediatric, and Functional Neurosurgery.* New York, McGraw-Hill, 1991, pp 140–148.

51. Spetzler RF, Martin NA: A proposed grading system of arteriovenous malformations. **J Neurosurg** 65:476–483, 1986.

52. Spetzler RF, Martin NA, Carter LP: Surgical management of large AVM's by staged embolization and operative excision. **J Neurosurg** 67:17–28, 1987.

53. Stein BM, Solomon RA: Periventricular arteriovenous malformations, in Apuzzo MLJ (ed): *Brain Surgery: Complication Avoidance and Management.* New York, Churchill Livingstone, 1993, pp 1193–1224.

54. Stein BM, Wolpert SM: Surgical and embolic treatment of cerebral arteriovenous malformations. **Surg Neurol** 7:359, 1977.

55. Steiner L, Lindquist C, Cail W, *et al.:* Microsurgery and radiosurgery in brain arteriovenous malformations. **J Neurosurg** 79:647–652, 1993.

56. Steinmeier R, Schramm J, Muller H-G, *et al.:* Evaluation of prognostic factors in cerebral arteriovenous malformations. **Neurosurgery** 24:193–200, 1989.

57. Sundt TM Jr: Operative techniques for arteriovenous malformations of the brain, in Barrow DL (ed): *Intracranial Vascular Malformations: Neurosurgical Topics,* American Association of Neurological Surgeons Publications. Park Ridge, Illinois 1990, pp 111–123.

58. Sundt TM Jr, Piepgras DG, Stevens LN: Surgery for supratentorial arteriovenous malformations. **Clin Neurosurg** 37:49–115, 1989.

59. Tamaki N, Ehara K, Lin T-K, *et al.:* Cerebral arteriovenous malformations: Factors influencing the surgical difficulty and outcome. **Neurosurgery** 29:856, 1991.

60. Torrance GW, Feeny D: Utilities and quality-adjusted life-years. **Int J Technol Assess Health Care** 5:559–575, 1989.
61. Vinuela F, Dion JE, Duckwiler G, *et al.:* Combined endovascular embolization and surgery in the management of cerebral arteriovenous malformations. Experience with 101 cases. **J Neurosurg** 75:856, 1991.
62. Weinstein MC, Stason WB: Foundations of cost-effectiveness analysis for health and medical practices. **N Engl J Med** 296:716–721, 1977.
63. Wilkins RH: Natural history of intracranial vascular malformations: A review. **Neurosurgery** 16:421–430, 1985.
64. Wilson CB, Stein BM: *Intracranial Arteriovenous Malformations.* Baltimore, Williams & Wilkins, 1984.
65. Yasargil MG: *Microneurosurgery.* New York, Thieme Medical Publishers, 1988, vol IIIB.

IV

General Scientific Session IV—Management of Low Grade Gliomas

22

Brain Tumor Gene Therapy in Mice with a Novel "Suicide" Gene: The Cyclophosphamide-activating CYP2B1 Gene

E. ANTONIO CHIOCCA, M.D., Ph.D.

The therapeutic action of numerous drugs depends on their biologic activation by enzymes. Recent technological advances have rendered feasible the transfer of almost any gene into tissues. The logical connection between these two facts is that the delivery of genes, which code for enzymes responsible for the conversion of a prodrug into its active metabolites, can be exploited for the therapy of central nervous system tumors. Over the last few years, three prodrug-susceptibility genes have been described for experimental gene therapies of solid tumors in animals: (a) the herpes simplex virus-thymidine kinase (*HSV-TK*) gene has been shown to confer chemosensitivity to ganciclovir (11, 29, 33), (b) the *Escherichia coli* cytosine deaminase gene has been shown to confer chemosensitivity to 5-fluorocytosine (25, 34), and (c) the *E. coli* guanine phosphoribosyltransferase gene has been shown to confer chemosensitivity to 6-thioxanthine (32). In these paradigms, the gene, when expressed into a tumor cell, encodes an enzyme that converts the prodrug into a nucleotide analog. this analog kills tumor cells, because it is incorporated into DNA strands during DNA replication in the course of tumor cell division. This process produces termination of nucleic acid synthesis and subsequent tumor cell death. Therefore, this type of gene therapy will be most effective for tumor cells in the S-phase of the cell cycle.

CHARACTERISTICS OF CYCLOPHOSPHAMIDE

The large majority of tumor cells in glioblastoma are in the G_0-phase of the cell cycle (36, 48) and might not provide an ideal target for the above prodrug-susceptibility genes. On the other hand, alkylating agents might constitute a useful alternative, because their tumor-killing action is not restricted to a particular phase of the cell cycle (15). Cyclophosphamide (CPA) is an inert lipophilic prodrug that requires enzymatic conversion by an hepatic cytochrome P450 2B1 gene (CYP2B1) for its anticancer effect (13). Its activated form, 4-hydroxy-cyclophosphamide (4-HCPA), is unstable and spontaneously decomposes into two metabolites, phosphoramide mustard (PM) and acrolein (Fig. 22.1). PM produces DNA alkylation, resulting in strand breaks during DNA replication. Acrolein promotes the formation of covalent links in cellular proteins, but this does not appear to contribute significantly to antitumor action *in vivo* (43). The cytotoxicity of PM is not restricted to a particular phase of the cell cycle, rendering CPA and other alkylating agents particularly suited for the treatment of solid tumors, where a large proportion of the neoplastic cells are not in S-phase. The different lipophilicities of the various agents in this pathway affects their ability to cross the blood-brain barrier and to diffuse passively into cells (2, 3, 23). The inert prodrug CPA is extremely lipophilic and readily crosses cellular membranes. 4-HCPA and acrolein are less lipophilic but can still diffuse passively across cellular membranes. PM, which is the active anticancer metabolite, is very hydrophilic and does not diffuse readily across cell membranes (Fig. 22.2). Therefore, the effectiveness of current anticancer therapy with cyclophosphamide depends on its activation into 4-HCPA by cytochrome P450 enzymes in the liver and in the diffusion of 4-HCPA into the target tumor cells before its spontaneous decomposition into acrolein and PM, the hydrophilic anticancer metabolite.

GENE THERAPY

Gene therapy refers to the transfer and expression of a gene into mammalian cells with the intent of replacing a defective function, en-

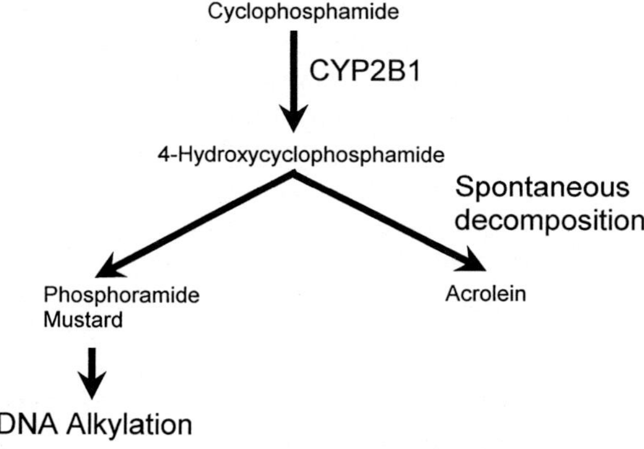

FIG. 22.1 Pathway of bioactivation of CPA.

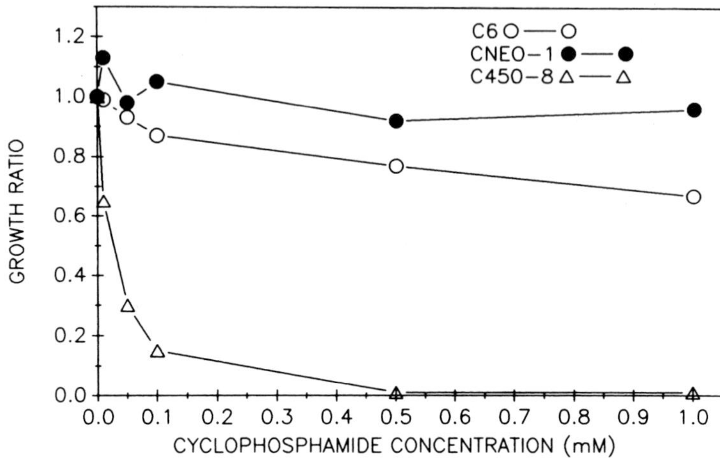

FIG. 22.2 Acquisition of CPA sensitivity after transfection of the *CYP2B1* gene into rat C6 glioma cells. The growth ratio is the number of cells that survived at a defined CPA concentration divided by the number of cells that survived without drug for each cell line. Parental *C6* and *CNEO-1* cells serve as controls. *C450-8* cells have been stably transfected with the *CYP2B1* gene. [Reproduced with permission from (47).]

hancing a beneficial phenotype, and/or decreasing/eliminating a perceived deleterious phenotype of that cell. A gene is a segment of DNA that encodes a functional protein, together with all the necessary DNA elements that serve to regulate its expression (26). Based on successful laboratory and animal experiments, several human clinical trials have been initiated to test the effectiveness of gene therapy. Some of the targeted diseases include inherited enzyme deficiencies, cystic fibrosis, hypercholesterolemia due to defective low-density lipoprotein (LDL)-receptors, and several forms of cancer (1). In cancer, there are several types of genes that might possess therapeutic effects (Table 22.1). In addition to the drug-susceptibility genes mentioned earlier, therapeutic genes include those that: (a) can enhance the immune response against tumors, such as interleukin-4 (49), the granulocyte-macrophage colony-stimulating factor (18), and insulin-like growth factor-I (46); (b) suppress the malignant phenotype, such as *p53* (21), the retinoblastoma-susceptibility gene (20), and *merlin* (45); (c) modulate programmed cell death such as *bcl-2* (24), *bax* (38), and *crmA* (22), and (d) encode highly toxic proteins, such as diphtheria toxin (31).

VECTORS USED FOR THE TRANSFER OF GENES *IN VIVO*

Viruses are used to transfer a gene into tumor cells *in vivo* efficiently. They have been genetically modified so that they can serve the func-

TABLE 22.1
Therapeutic Genes

- Prodrug-activating genes (*HSV-TK, gpt, CYP2B1, CDA*)
- Immune-response enhancer genes (*IL-4, GM-CSF*)
- Tumor suppressor genes (*p53, Rb, merlin*)
- Apoptosis genes (*bcl-2, bax, crmA*)
- Toxin genes (*DT-A*)

TABLE 22.2
Viral Vectors Used for Brain Tumor Gene Therapy[a]

- Retroviruses
- Adenovirus
- Herpes simplex virus
- Others

[a]Data compiled in 1994.

tion of the "shuttle" or "vector," with minimal toxic effect on normal tissues. Table 22.2 lists some of the most widely used vectors for gene therapy. By far, the most widely used virus vector is derived from a mouse retrovirus, named the Moloney murine leukemia virus (MoMLV). Several modifications have been engineered in the genome of this virus to allow for insertion of a foreign gene of interest (35). Briefly, the life cycle of this vector is as follows: After infecting a mammalian cell, the viral RNA (containing the foreign, therapeutic gene) is copied into double-stranded DNA, which is then integrated into the host cell's mammalian DNA. This process of integration strictly occurs only when the mammalian cell's DNA is replicating, *i.e.*, during cell division. The integrated retroviral DNA thus becomes part of the infected cell's genome, and it will be passed on to future daughter cells. In summary, some of the characteristics of retroviral vectors are: (a) they infect and transfer the foreign gene to one cell only, *i.e.*, the infecting retrovirus does not travel from cell to cell, nor does it produce progeny retroviruses in the mammalian cell. (b) Integration and expression of the foreign gene require division of the infected cell. (c) The foreign gene is passed on to the cell's progeny. These properties can be useful in brain tumor therapy, because they provide for safety (the vector will not spread infection throughout the body), tumor cell selectivity (only dividing cells will be targeted by the vector), and inheritance to numerous daughter tumor cells. In contrast, retroviral vectors possess some disadvantages, in that (a) they are relatively unstable, and direct injection of the vector into a tumor mass results in essentially little infection of tumor cells (42). (b) The safety associated with their lack of spreading may work against the delivery of the therapeutic gene to remote areas of a tumor mass. (c) Expression of the foreign therapeutic gene can be variable. (d) Only one copy of the foreign gene is found inside the tumor cell.

The first disadvantage can be circumvented by injecting the retroviral vector producer cell (RVPC) into the tumor. This consists of a murine fibroblast, derived from NIH-3T3 cells, which has been genetically engineered to produce and secrete the retrovirus vector continuously (28, 35). As shown by Short *et al.* (42), inoculation of RVPCs into rat C6 gliomas, established in the frontal lobe of athymic mice, results in the delivery and expression of a reporter gene into at least 10% of tumor cells. Using this method, other laboratories have obtained transduction efficiencies of 40 to 60% in rat 9L gliosarcoma tumors (40). This method of *in situ* retroviral gene transfer is currently used for the delivery of a therapeutic gene into patients afflicted with recurrent glioblastoma multiforme (37). Nevertheless, the other three disadvantages easily cannot be circumvented with retrovirus vectors. Therefore, other types of viral vectors have been used for the delivery of therapeutic genes into experimental brain tumors.

Vectors based on adenoviruses possess several advantages: (a) the vector can be grown to very high titers. (b) Gene expression does not require integration into host cell chromosomes. (c) Numerous copies of a gene are transferred into the cell. (d) The vector does not produce progeny virions and thus does not spread infection to normal tissues (8). There are limitations to these vectors, in that (a) 50 to 100 viral particles are needed to efficiently express a foreign gene. (b) Transferred genes are located in extrachromosomal elements and thus become diluted with each tumor cell division. (c) There is no selectivity for gene transfer into tumor cells versus endogenous neural cells. (d) Although the vector does not replicate, the injection of high doses of adenoviral proteins might have deleterious inflammatory effects on endogenous neural cells. Nevertheless, the successful delivery of a foreign gene into experimental tumors has been reported by several laboratories (5, 10, 44). Further studies that address the toxicity of adenovirus on endogenous neural cells would benefit future use of adenovirus vectors for the delivery of therapeutic genes into human brain tumors.

The third type of viral vector is based on herpes simplex virus type 1 (HSV1) (9, 12). One feature of wild-type HSV1 is that it encodes enzymes, such as thymidine kinase (TK) or ribonucleotide reductase (RR), necessary in the metabolism of its nucleic acids. An HSV that is mutated in *TK* or *RR* does not replicate in a postmitotic mammalian cell, such as a neuron (14). However, actively dividing mammalian cells, such as tumor cells, synthesize large quantities of enzymes that perform a function analogous to that of the HSV-TK and HSV-RR (17). These mammalian enzymes can thus complement the missing function in the HSV, which has been mutated in TK or RR, thus permitting it to replicate inside the cell (30). This finding provides for the selectivity of these HSV vectors for tumor cells in the brain. It also furnishes an advantage for HSV over retrovirus or adenovirus vectors, in that the former will conditionally replicate within a brain tumor, allowing for more viral spread of daughter vectors throughout the mass of the neoplasm (5). HSV vectors perform a dual function: (a) they are cytotoxic by themselves, in that their replication within a tumor cell will lead to that cell's demise. (b) They can be engineered to carry one or more therapeutic genes. The antitumor activity of an HSV vector was first shown by Martuza *et al.* (30). We have recently shown that this antitumor activity can be coupled with a drug-susceptibility function to cause long-lasting and complete regression of established intracerebral 9L gliosarcomas in approximately 50% of treated animals (6, 7). Therefore, the antitumor potential of HSV vectors appears to be relatively powerful. This enthusiasm is still tempered however, by the potent neuropathogenicity of the wild-type HSV1 (39). Efforts to further modify current HSV vectors are aimed to improve the safety of these viruses while maintaining their relative selectivity for tumor cells and their conditional spread within a tumor mass.

CYTOTOXIC MECHANISMS INVOLVED IN TUMOR CELL DEATH AFTER THE TRANSFER OF DRUG-SENSITIVITY GENES.

None of the above vectors can achieve gene transfer in all tumor cells *in vivo*. Therapeutic efficacy in gene therapy strategies that involve transfer of drug-sensitivity genes thus depends on the "bystander" effect. This effect was first described with ganciclovir/*HSV-TK* gene therapy strategy (19, 33). In this instance, ganciclovir treatment leads to the death of tumor cells expressing the *HSV-TK* gene, as well as to that of neighboring tumor cells that do not express the gene. Several mechanisms have been invoked to explain this effect, such as transfer of toxic metabolites through gap junctions (16, 27), induction of programmed cell death by transfer of apoptotic vesicles from drug-sensitive to insensitive tumor cells (19), activation of immune responses (4), and disruptions of the vascular supply to the tumor (41). It is likely that the long-term success of drug sensitivity gene therapies will involve a combination of all of the above mechanisms. This knowledge might also be used to further optimize current treatments by combining an immune-response enhancer gene or a programmed cell death gene with a drug-sensitive gene.

EXPERIMENTAL BRAIN TUMOR THERAPY WITH THE CYCLOPHOSPHAMIDE-ACTIVATING *CYP2B1* GENE

The above considerations have thus rendered feasible the use of gene therapy methodologies for the *in vivo* transfer of the cyclophosphamide-activating cytochrome P450 2B1 (*CYP2B1*) gene into experimental brain tumors. The therapeutic strategy involves the placement of the CYP2B1 gene into one of the aforementioned viral vectors, followed by inoculation of the vector (or, in the case of retrovirus, injection of RVPCs) into the tumor bed. Administration of the prodrug, cyclophosphamide, is initiated several days later to allow for gene transfer to occur. To maximize the antitumor effect and minimize toxic effects on normal cells, an intrathecal route was chosen for drug administration (47).

Before proceeding with the above strategy, we wanted to show that expression of the *CYP2B1* gene would indeed render rat C6 glioma cells susceptible to CPA. We thus inserted the rat CYP2B1 gene into the retroviral vector MFG (18) and then used the plasmid containing this vector to transfect C6 glioma cells stably. Figure 22.2 shows that rat C6 glioma cells, stably transfected with the *CYP2B1* gene (designated as C450-8), acquire chemosensitivity to CPA, whereas parental C6 glioma cells or control CNEO-1 cells (obtained by stably transfecting C6 glioma cells with a neomycin resistance gene) were not affected by the prodrug. Immunocytochemical analysis further confirmed the existence of immunoreactive *CYP2B1* in C450-8 cells but not in parental C6 cells (Fig. 22.3). Western blot analysis and enzyme activity were

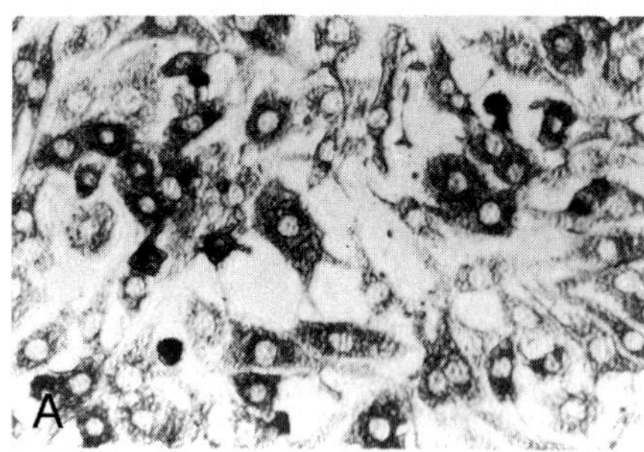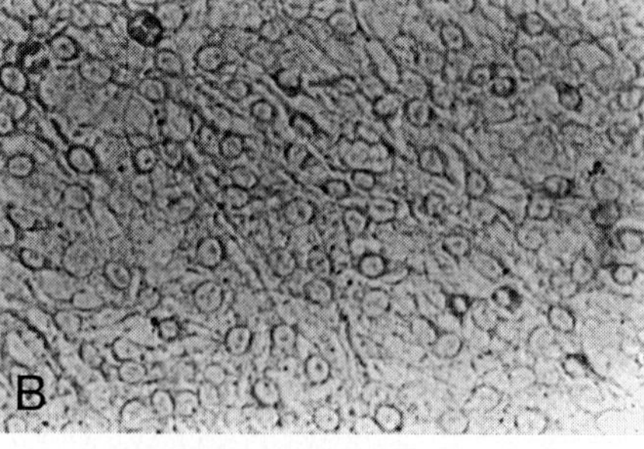

FIG. 22.3 Immunocytochemical analysis of cytochrome P450-2B1 enzyme in CPA-susceptible C450-8 and in CPA-insensitive CNEO-1. Immunoreactive protein appears as a black precipitate in a lace-like pattern in C450-8 cells (**A**), whereas no staining is present in CNEO-1 cells (**B**). [Reproduced with permission from (47).]

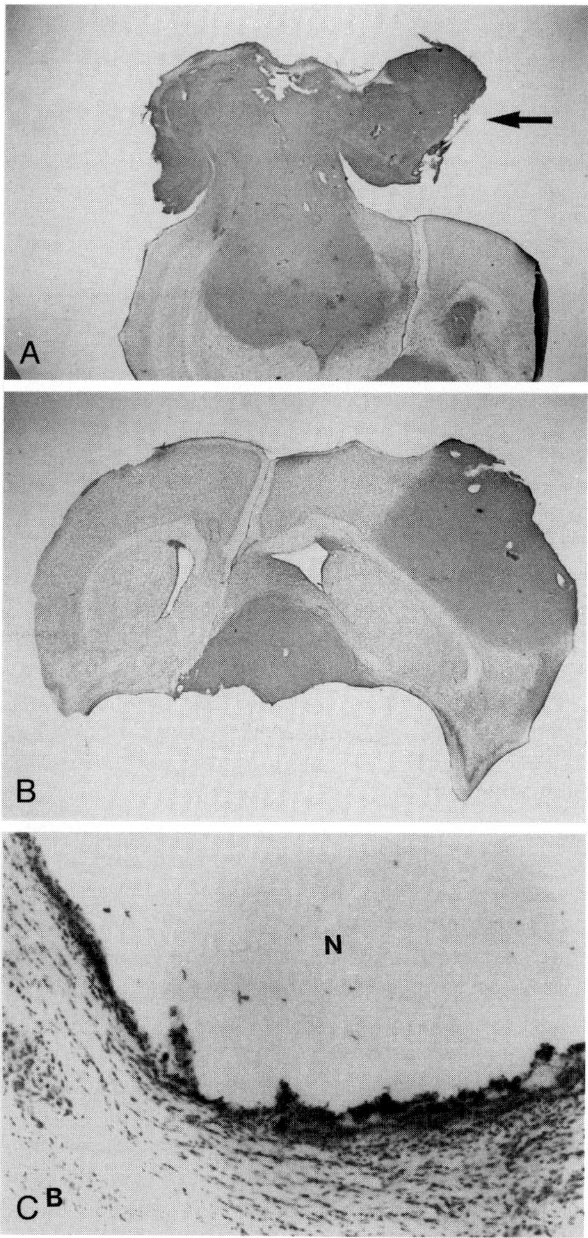

Legend for Figure 22.4 on page 378.

FIG. 22.4 Meningeal neoplasia and parenchymal tumors formed by C6 gliomas in mouse brains injected with retrovirus producer fibroblasts and CPA. Panel **A** shows a histopathologic coronal section from the brain of a control nude mouse that had been seeded with rat C6 glioma cells and then treated by stereotactic injection of *lacZ*-expressing murine cells (CRE*lacZ*) into the brain and meningeal spaces, followed by intratumoral administration of CPA. The extensive infiltration of tumor tissue into the meninges is marked by the *arrow*. Panel **B** shows a histopathologic coronal section from the brain of a nude mouse that had been seeded with rat C6 glioma cells and was then treated by stereotactic injection of cytochrome P450 2B1-expressing murine cells (R450-2) into the brain and meningeal spaces, followed by intratumoral administration of CPA. Panel **C** shows a coronal section from the brain tumor of a mouse treated with R450-2 cells and then CPA. This particular section shows the margin between normal brain on the *lower left side* of the photomicrograph *(B)* and the cavity on the *center right (N)*, which originally contained necrotic tumor tissue that could not be mounted due to its friability. Some necrotic tumor cells (exhibiting extensive nuclear fragmentation) are still visible adjacent to normal brain. No cavitary necrosis was seen in the brains of mice treated with CRE*lacZ* producer fibroblasts and CPA (results not shown). Magnification, ×100. [Reproduced with permission from (47).]

also used to determine conclusively that C450-8 cells expressed functional *CYP2B1,* whereas parental C6 or control CNEO-1 cells did not (results not shown). Taken in conjunction, these results indicate that a retrovirus vector containing the *CYP2B1* gene can render C6 tumor cells sensitive to CPA.

For practical applications to brain tumor gene therapy, we genetically engineered RVPCs that would secrete the *CYP2B1* retrovirus vector (designated as R450-2). Rat C6 glioma cells were stereotactically inoculated into the frontal lobes of athymic mice. A two-step treatment approach was then instituted: (a) 3 days after implantation of the C6 glioma cells, we stereotactically injected into the tumor the R450-2 cells or, as a control, RVPCs that produce a retrovirus vector that carries the *lacZ* reporter gene (designated as CRE*lacZ*), and (b) 7, 11, and 14 days after implantation of the C6 glioma cells, we injected the prodrug, CPA, intrathecally. Mice were then sacrificed 24 days after C6 glioma cell implantation. All mice that had received the CRE*lacZ* control fibroblasts plus CPA exhibited extensive meningeal neoplasia (8/8) (Fig. 22.4A), as well as large intraparenchymal tumors (6/6 studied). On the contrary, 7/8 mice that had received the R450-2 fibroblasts plus CPA showed no meningeal tumor (Fig. 22.4**B**). Furthermore, 3/6 mice showed extensive necrosis of the intraparenchymal tumor (Fig. 22.4**C**). Computer-assisted volumetric analysis was used to measure the volume of tumors with intraparenchymal necrosis to show that they were 1/20, 1/5, and 1/2 the volume of the other tumors (Table 22.3).

TABLE 22.3

Volumes of Parenchymal Brain Tumors after R450-2 or CRElacZ Grafts and Cyclophosphamide Administration[a]

C6 + CRE*lacZ* (mm³)	C6 + R450-2 (mm³)
47.5	3.2
51.5	14.2
54.7	28.4
62.4	87.4
72.6	105.3
85.1	171.4

[a]Reprinted with permission from (47). Tumor volumes were measured by computer-assisted contouring.

Taken in conjunction, the above experiments provide evidence that the CPA/*CYP2B1* gene therapy strategy shows promise as an adjunct in the treatment of glioblastoma. Although the therapeutic value of CPA/*CYP2B1* gene therapy has to be further studied with larger groups of animals and with other viral vectors, an experimental basis is being created for the improvement of current neuro-oncologic chemotherapy regimens through the transfer of genes that will enhance antitumor activity.

REFERENCES

1. Anderson WF: Human gene therapy. **Science** 256:808–813, 1992.
2. Arndt CAS, Balis FM, McCully CL, *et al.:* Cerebrospinal fluid penetration of active metabolites of cyclophosphamide and ifosfamide in rhesus monkeys. **Cancer Res** 48:2113–2115, 1988.
3. Arndt CAS, Colvin OM, Balis FM, *et al.:* Intrathecal administration of 4-hydroperoxycyclophosphate in rhesus monkeys. **Cancer Res** 47:5932–5934, 1987.
4. Barba D, Hardin J, Sadelain M, *et al.:* Development of anti-tumor immunity following thymidine kinase-mediated killing of experimental brain tumors. **Proc Natl Acad Sci USA** 91:4348–4352, 1994.
5. Boviatsis EJ, Chase M, Wei MX, *et al.:* Gene transfer into experimental brain tumors mediated by adenovirus, herpes simplex virus (HSV), and retrovirus vectors. **Hum Gene Ther** 5:183–191, 1994.
6. Boviatsis EJ, Park JS, Sena-Esteves M, *et al.:* Long-term survival of rats harboring brain tumors treated with ganciclovir and a herpes simplex virus vector that maintains an intact thymidine kinase gene. **Cancer Res,** 54:5745–5751, 1994.
7. Boviatsis EJ, Scharf JM, Chase M, *et al.:* Antitumor activity and reporter gene transfer into rat brain neoplasms inoculated with herpes simplex virus vectors defective in thymidine kinase or ribonucleotide reductase. **Gene Ther** 1:323–331, 1994.
8. Breakefield XO: Gene delivery into the brain using virus vectors. **Nature Genet** 3:187–189, 1993.

9. Breakefield XO, DeLuca NA: Herpes simplex virus for gene delivery to neurons. **New Biol** 3:203–218, 1991.
10. Chen SH, Shine HD, Goodman JC, *et al.:* Gene therapy for brain tumors: Regression of experimental gliomas by using adenovirus-mediated gene transfer *in vivo.* **Proc Natl Acad Sci USA** 91:3054–3057, 1994.
11. Chiocca EA, Andersen JK, Takamiya Y, *et al.:* Virus-mediated genetic treatment of rodent gliomas, in Wolff JA (ed): *Gene Therapeutics.* Boston, Birkhauser Publishers, 1994, pp 245–262.
12. Chiocca EA, Choi BB, Cai W, *et al.:* Transfer and expression of the lacZ gene in rat brain neurons mediated by herpes simplex virus insertion mutants. **New Biol** 2:739–746, 1990.
13. Clarke L, Waxman DJ: Oxidative metabolism of cyclophosphamide: Identification of the hepatic monooxygenase catalysts of drug activation. **Cancer Res** 49:2344–2350, 1989.
14. Coen DM, Kosz-Vnenchak M, Jacobson JG, *et al.:* Thymidine kinase-negative herpes simplex virus mutants established latency in mouse trigeminal ganglia but do not reactivate. **Proc Natl Acad Sci USA** 86:4736–4740, 1989.
15. Colvin OM: Alkylating agents and platinum compounds, in Holland JF, *et al.* (eds): *Cancer Medicine.* Philadelphia, Lea & Febiger, 1993, pp 733–734.
16. Culver KW, Ram Z, Wallbridge S, *et al.: In vivo* gene transfer with retroviral vector-producer cells for treatment of experimental brain tumors. **Science** 256:1550–1552, 1992.
17. Dou Q-P, Markell PJ, Pardee AB: Thymidine kinase transcription is regulated at G_1/S phase by a complex that contains retinoblastoma-like protein and a *cdc2* kinase. **Proc Natl Acad Sci USA** 89:3256–3260, 1992.
18. Dranoff G, Jaffee E, Lazenby A, *et al.:* Vaccination with irradiated tumor cells engineered to secrete murine granulocyte-macrophage colony-stimulating factor stimulates potent, specific, and long-lasting anti-tumor immunity. **Proc Natl Acad Sci USA** 90:3539–3543, 1993.
19. Freeman SM, Abboud CN, Whartenby KA, *et al.:* The "bystander effect": Tumor regression when a fraction of the tumor mass is genetically modified. **Cancer Res** 53:5274–5283, 1993.
20. Friedmann T: Gene therapy of cancer through restoration of tumor-suppressor functions? **Cancer** 70:1810–1817, 1992.
21. Fujiwara T, Grimm EA, Mukhopadhyay T, *et al.:* Induction of chemosensitivity in human lung cancer cells *in vivo* by adenovirus-mediated transfer of the wild-type *p53* gene. **Cancer Res** 54:2287–2291, 1994.
22. Gagliardini V, Fernandez PA, Lee RK, *et al.:* Prevention of vertebrate neuronal death by the *CrmA* gene. **Science** 263:826–828, 1994.
23. Genka S, Deutsch J, Stahle PL, *et al.:* Brain and plasma pharmacokinetics and anticancer activities of cyclophosphamide and phosphoramide mustard in the rat. **Cancer Chemother Pharmacol** 27:1–7, 1990.
24. Hockenbery DM, Oltvai ZN, Yin XM, *et al.: Bcl-2* functions in an antioxidant pathway to prevent apoptosis. **Cell** 75:241–251, 1993.
25. Huber BE, Austin EA, Good SS, *et al.: In vivo* antitumor activity of 5-fluorocytosine on human colorectal carcinoma cells genetically modified to express cytosine deaminase. **Cancer Res** 53:4619–4626, 1993.
26. Lewin B: DNA as a store of information, in Lewin B (ed): *Genes IV.* Cambridge, MA, Cell Press, pp 41–109, 1990.
27. Li Bi W, Parysek LM, Warnick R, *et al.: In vitro* evidence that metabolic cooperation

is responsible for the bystander effect observed with *HSVtk* retroviral gene therapy. **Hum Gene Ther** 4:725–731, 1993.

28. Mann R, Mulligan RC, Baltimore D: Construction of a retrovirus packaging mutant and its use to produce helper-free defective retrovirus. **Cell** 33:153–159, 1983.

29. Martuza RL: Viral vectors for experimental brain tumor therapy, in Levine AJ, Schmidek HH (eds): *Molecular Genetics of Nervous System Tumors.* New York, Wiley-Liss, 1993, pp 381–386.

30. Martuza RL, Malick A, Markert JM, *et al.:* Experimental therapy of human glioma by means of a genetically engineered virus mutant. **Science** 252:854–856, 1991.

31. Maxwell IH, Maxwell F, Globe LM: Regulated expression of diphteria toxin A-chain gene transfected into human cells: A possible strategy for inducing cancer cell suicide. **Cancer Res** 46:4660–4664, 1986.

32. Mroz PJ, Moolten FL: Retrovirally transduced *E.coli gpt* genes combine selectability with chemosensitivity capable of mediating tumor eradication. **Hum Gene Ther** 4:589–595, 1993.

33. Moolten FL: Tumor chemosensitivity conferred by inserted thymidine kinase genes: Paradigm for a prospective cancer control strategy. **Cancer Res** 46:5276-5281, 1986.

34. Mullen CA, Kilstrup M, Blaese RM: Transfer of the bacterial gene for cytosine deaminase to mammalian cells confers lethal sensitivity to 5-fluorocytosine: A negative selection system. **Proc Natl Acad Sci USA** 89:33–37, 1992.

35. Mulligan RC: The basic science of gene therapy. **Science** 260:926–932, 1993.

36. Nagashima T, Hoshino T: Rapid detection of S-phase cells by anti-bromodeoxyuridine monoclonal antibody in 9L brain tumor cells *in vitro* and *in situ.* **Acta Neuropathol (Berl)** 66:12–17, 1985.

37. Oldfield EH, Ram Z, Culver KW, *et al.:* Gene therapy for the treatment of brain tumors using intra-tumoral transduction with the thymidine kinase gene and intravenous ganciclovir. **Hum Gene Ther** 4:39–69, 1993.

38. Oltvai ZN, Milliman CL, and Korsmeyer SJ: Bcl-2 heterodimerizes with a conserved homolog, Bax, that accelerates programmed cell death. **Cell** 74:609–619, 1993.

39. Pakzaban P, Chiocca EA: Nerve growth factor protects against herpes simplex virus type 1 neurotoxicity in the rat striatum. **Neuroreport** 5:993–996, 1994.

40. Ram Z, Culver KW, Wallbridge S, *et al.: In situ* retroviral-mediated gene transfer for the treatment of brain tumors in rats. **Cancer Res** 53:83–88, 1993.

41. Ram Z, Walbridge S, Shawker T, *et al.:* The effect of thymidine kinase transduction and ganciclovir therapy on tumor vasculature and growth of 9L gliomas in rats. **J Neurosurg** 81:256–260, 1994.

42. Short MP, Choi BC, Lee JK, *et al.:* Gene delivery to glioma cells in rat brain by grafting of a retrovirus packaging cell line. **J Neurosci Res** 27:427–433, 1990.

43. Sladek NE: Oxazaphosphorines, in Powis G, Prough RA (eds): *Metabolism and Action of Anti-Cancer Drugs.* New York, Taylor and Francis, 1987, pp 48–90.

44. Smythe WR, Hwang HC, Amin KM, *et al.:* Use of recombinant adenovirus to transfer the herpes simplex virus thymidine kinase (HSV-TK) gene to thoracic neoplasms: An effective *in vitro* drug sensitization system. **Cancer Res** 54:2055–2059, 1994.

45. Trofatter JA, MacCollin M, Rutter JL, *et al.:* A novel moesin-, ezrin-, radixin-like gene is a candidate for the neurofibromatosis 2 tumor suppressor. **Cell** 72:791–800, 1993.

46. Trojan J, Johnson TR, Rudin SD, *et al.:* Treatment and prevention of rat glioblastoma by immunogenic C6 cells expressing antisense insulin-like growth factor I RNA. **Science** 259:94–97, 1993.

47. Wei MX, Tamiya T, Chase M, *et al.:* Experimental tumor therapy in mice using the cyclophosphamide-activating cytochrome P4502B1 gene. **Hum Gene Ther** 5:969–978, 1994.
48. Yoshii Y, Maki Y, Tsuboi K, *et al.:* Estimation of growth fraction with bromodeoxyuridine in human central nervous system tumors. **J Neurosurg** 65:659–663, 1986.
49. Yu JS, Wei MX, Chiocca EA, *et al.:* Treatment of glioma by engineered interleukin 4-secreting cells. **Cancer Res** 53:3125–3128, 1993.

23

Surgery for Low-Grade Glioma: Rationale for Early Intervention

CHARLES B. WILSON, M.D., AND MICHAEL D. PRADOS, M.D.

Low-grade glioma is a pathologic term that includes a number of different histologic types of intracranial tumors. In general, adult patients with these tumors are relatively young, often presenting with clinical signs and symptoms of a space-occupying lesion. In many cases magnetic resonance imaging (MRI) reveals a tumor that diffusely infiltrates one or more lobes of the brain with increased signal on T2-weighted images and hypodensity on T1 images. More often than not, these tumors do not exhibit contrast enhancement. Management of these tumors can vary from physician to physician and may include symptomatic treatment based on the clinical and radiographic exam without surgical intervention; surgical treatment that may include either biopsy, partial resection, or an attempt at total removal; and either radiotherapy or chemotherapy. The dose of radiotherapy and/or the type of chemotherapy that may be used is also subject to physician preference, rather than being based on prospective clinical trail data. Physician bias is often the major reason that one or several of the these options is chose. Unfortunately, few if any well-conducted clinical research trials have been undertaken that help to define the natural history or treatment outcome of these patients with low-grade gliomas, which means there are no data that would allow physicians and patients to make rational decisions about specific treatments or to decide to go through follow-up without therapy until further tumor growth has been documented either clinically or radiographically.

The timing for surgical intervention is an important aspect of this clinical problem. Patients are frequently referred to a neurosurgeon with a nonenhancing lesion seen on MRI and a clinical history suggestive of a tumor. Often, the first question that arises is when and how to intervene surgically. A tumor that is producing mass effect and acute neurologic deterioration is an indication for surgical treatment. A lesion that is not producing mass effect and is diffusely infiltrative in a patient who is neurologically intact is more problematic. Should such a patient be watched expectantly, or should some surgical approach be undertaken? Specific surgical techniques are not the focus of this review, and we have excluded discussions about pediatric low-grade gliomas. The goal of this article is to define our reasons for suggesting early surgical intervention in adult patients with presumed low-grade glial neoplasms. We believe that clinical and radiographic assessment alone is often inaccurate for determination of neuropathology and that surgical intervention is indicated to establish a specific histologic diagnosis. Surgery also allows the physician an opportunity to sample tumor tissue for the assessment of proliferative potential, a biologic predictor of individual patient outcome. Finally, newly published data suggest that more extensive surgery may favorably influence disease-specific progression-free survival and decrease the incidence of malignant transformation. It is for all of these reasons that we recommend early surgical intervention.

RADIOGRAPHIC DIAGNOSIS

Pathologic diagnosis based entirely on MRI is often inaccurate. Although many patients will present with a noncontrast-enhancing lesion on MRI, some low-grade gliomas will enhance and, conversely, many higher-grade anaplastic tumors will not exhibit contrast enhancement. Earlier studies based on computerized tomography (CT) and recent experience with MRI show convincingly that MRI alone is not reliable in predicting the pathologic grade of tumors. McDermott *et al.* reviewed the results of contrast enhancement on CT in a series of patients who had undergone surgical resection at the University of California, San Francisco (9). Patients in this series were also studied with bromodeoxyuridine (BUdR) *in vivo,* and a labeling index (BUdR-LI) was determined. The goal of the review was to correlate CT contrast enhancement with results of histopathologic diagnosis and the proliferative potential of the surgically resected tumors. A total of 71 cases were analyzed who had surgical confirmation of either an anaplastic astrocytoma (35 patients) or a low-grade astrocytoma (36 patients). For the anaplastic astrocytoma group, 28.6% of cases did not show enhancement on CT imaging. In the low-grade astrocytoma group 36.1% did show enhancement. Thus, if contrast enhancement with CT was to be the sole determining factor in assigning a pathologic diagnosis, the radiographic error rate was significant for both low-grade and high-grade glioma. In addition, for those nonenhancing cases that were pathologically shown to be low-grade astrocytomas, the BUdR-LI was found to be high (>1%) in 39% of cases. We feel this last fact is biologically significant, as patients with low-grade astrocytomas with a high BUdR-LI tend to progress earlier and die sooner than similar patients with a lower BUdR-LI(5, 6, 10). Tissue sampling helps to identify those patients with lower-grade lesions who may benefit form more aggressive therapy. Even if a BUdR-LI were not done, a radiographic diagnosis alone would have resulted in some high-grade glioma patients being treated very differently from those treated with our standard approach used for these tumors, which is to use higher doses of radiotherapy and adjuvant chemotherapy, as compared to radiotherapy alone in low-grade tumors.

Similar errors will be made if MRI is used to try to predict grade of tumor. Kondziolka *et al.* recently reviewed their experience with 20 consecutive adult patients, who were suspected of having a low-grade astrocytoma based on clinical history and MRI (7). None of the lesions showed contrast enhancement. All patients underwent biopsy, and a surgical diagnosis was made in every case. Only 10 patients were documented as having a low-grade astrocytoma; 9 were shown to have an anaplastic astrocytoma; and 1 had a diagnosis of encephalitis. Thus, at least 50% of patients were incorrectly diagnosed with clinical and radiographic criteria. It is possible that more extensive surgical resection with more tissue sampling could have additionally "upgraded" some of the low-grade astrocytomas that underwent biopsy only. Thus, even in a recent series of patients imaged with MRI, there is significant variation in the pathologic diagnoses seen.

Because of the uncertainty of the pathologic nature of the lesion seen on MRI or CT imaging, early surgical intervention is warranted for histologic confirmation of disease. We believe that at least a biopsy is indicated to document disease. If a high-grade glioma is diagnosed, immediate therapy is indicated, which may include the decision to perform a more extensive resection before radiotherapy and chemotherapy is delivered. The general term "low-grade glioma" represents a heterogeneous group of biologically different diseases. Thus, once the surgical diagnosis is confirmed, specific therapies can be prescribed. For instance, patients with dysembryoplastic neuroepithelial tumor (DNET) are often treated with surgery alone and have a favorable clinical course, even if tumor tissue remains on postoperative imaging (3). Knowing that a particular patient will have a favorable outcome without further therapy will spare that patient potentially harmful side effects of treatment. Other tumor types, surgically confirmed, may be treated in a more "disease-specific" manner as well. Recent reports of successful therapy, using chemotherapy as primary treatment for anaplastic oligodendroglioma, may suggest a role for chemotherapy in patients with low-grade oligodendroglioma or mixed low-grade oligoastrocytoma as well (2, 4). As we learn more about chemotherapy for low-grade glioma in young children, which is documented to produce high objective response rates with durable disease control for many years, similar strategies for young adults will probably emerge (11). A biologic assessment of the tumor may help to stratify those patients who should be treated more aggressively as well, as will be discussed below.

PROLIFERATIVE POTENTIAL

Even in those cases of young adults with surgically confirmed low-grade astrocytomas or mixed oligodendroglioma, biologic diversity exists. With similar surgery and radiotherapy, some patients have a worse outcome than other patients and should be considered for additional treatment to attempt to improve disease-free survival. We and others have studied the proliferative potential of low-grade tumors, in an attempt to identify individual patients who may be considered as having a higher-risk tumor (5, 10). The technique of studying the BUdR-LI has been published many times, but in general, patients receive an intravenous infusion of BUdR just prior to surgical removal of tumor. The tumor specimen is fixed in ethanol, embedded in paraffin, and sectioned. The specimens are incubated in hydrogen peroxide to block endogenous peroxidase activity, denatured in hydrochloric acid and immersed in anti-BUdR monoclonal antibody. The sections are then incubated with a dilution of peroxidase-conjugated antimouse immunoglobulin and then counterstained with Gill hematoxylin. The BUdR-LI is calculated as the average percentage of BUdR-labeled cells seen in a representative field of tumor. At least 3000 cells in three high-powered fields are counted for each specimen. A BUdR-LI of greater than 1% is felt to represent a high proliferative potential in patients with low-grade astrocytomas. Recently, Ito *et al.* reviewed a series of surgically confirmed cases of low-grade gliomas treated at the University of California at San Francisco, who were studied with a BUdR-LI (6). A total of 87 patients were included, with a mean age of 28 years. Of these, 69 patients were studied at the time of first surgical diagnosis and 18 at the time of tumor recurrence. Patients with juvenile pilocytic astrocytoma were excluded. A Cox proportional-hazards model was used to assess the relative effects of patient variables on the duration of survival and time to tumor progression. Survival was estimated by Kaplan-Meier analysis, and survival curves were compared with a log-rank test. A summary of these results is shown in Tables 23.1 to 23.4. The range of the BUdR-LI was from <1% to as high as 9.3%, with a mean of 1.3%. The BUdR-LI was not associated with age, sex, tumor location, or whether the tumor was primary or recurrent. The extent of surgery and the BUdR-LI were both predictive for survival and progression-free survival in all patients, and the BUdR-LI

TABLE 23.1
Proliferative Potential: Effect of the BUdRLI on Survival

BUdRLI	Survival at 1 yr (%)	Survival at 2 yr (%)
LI < 1%	92	89
LI > 1%	82	64
	$P = 0.007^a$	

[a]The survival rate was estimated by Kaplan-Meier analysis, and the curves were compared, using a log-rank test (log-rank test, BUdRLI <1% *versus* >1%).

TABLE 23.2
Proliferative Potential: Effect of the BUdRLI on Progression-free Survival

BUdRLI (%)	PFS at 1 yr (%)	PFS at 2 yr (%)
<1	85	83
>1	60	32
	$P = < .001^a$	

[a]Progression-free survival (PFS) was estimated with Kaplan-Meier analysis, and the curves were compared, using a log-rank test (log-rank test, BUdRLI <1% *versus* >1%).

TABLE 23.3
Proliferative Potential: Patient and Outcome Variables Used in the Cox Proportional-Hazards Stepwise Regression Analysis in Patients with Low-Grade Gliomas

Patient variables
    Primary *versus* recurrent tumor
    BUdRLI
    Age
    Sex
    Extent of surgery (biopsy, STR, GTR)
    Tumor location
Outcome variables
    Survival[a]
    Progression-free survival

[a]Survival and progression-free survival, estimated using Kaplan-Meier analysis. STR = subtotal resection; GTR = gross total resection.

TABLE 23.4.
Proliferative Potential: Cox Proportional-Hazards Analysis for All 87 Patients with Low-Grade Glioma

Survival[a]	BUdRLI ($P = .0142$)
	Surgery ($P = .0011$)
PFS[a]	BUdRLI ($P = .0006$)
	Surgery ($P = .0149$)

[a]Survival and PFS were negatively influenced by a higher BUdR LI and a lesser extent of surgery. PFS, progression-free survival.

alone was predictive of progression-free survival for patients with recurrent tumors.

The assessment of proliferative potential in a given patient may be very helpful for physician and patient in discussing treatment strategies. There are several methods available for determining the proliferative potential of individual tumors, including BUdR-LI, and the measurement of Ki[67] DNA polymerase alpha, as well as other techniques. The higher the proliferative potential, the greater the possibility of early treatment failure. Tumor tissue is necessary to obtain this information at this time and, again, establishes a role for surgery for presumed low-grade tumors. Although not a subject of this review, there are many other important biologic questions that remain unanswered about these diseases, and the ability to study human tumor tissue at the molecular level will hopefully prove to be one of the most important reasons for surgical intervention.

EXTENT OF SURGICAL RESECTION

The rationale for surgical intervention is to establish an accurate diagnosis and to allow biologic studies to be performed. These two reasons for surgery only require single or multiple biopsies to obtain the required amount of tissue. An important, unanswered question still remains about the role that extensive surgical intervention plays in improving clinical outcome. This question was recently studied by investigators at the University of Washington, who retrospectively reviewed 53 patients with a surgical diagnosis of low-grade glioma (1). Pre- and postoperative tumor volumes were measured, using the prior CT or MRIs available from the patient's surgical records. The authors used these volume measurements to analyze the extent of resection and its impact on progression-free survival and the rate of later higher-grade relapses. All patients who underwent a total resection were recurrence-free in their review, and there were no recurrences in patients who initially presented with a lesion volume <10 cm^3. For the remainder of these patients, a statistically significant difference was noted in progression-free survival when comparing patients who had less than or greater than 10-cm^3 tumor volumes postoperatively. Patients with a tumor volume <10 cm^3 had a 14.8% relapse rate, and a median time-to-tumor progression of 50 months, whereas those who had a larger tumor volume postoperatively had a 46% relapse rate and a median time to tumor progression of 30 months ($P = .002$). Patients with a postoperative tumor volume >10 cm^3 had a 46% incidence of "high-grade" relapse, defined as the histologic appearance of a more anaplastic lesion, as compared to the original tumor sample.

Although retrospective, and uncontrolled, these and other reports suggest a role for surgery in patients with low-grade astrocytoma that favors a more extensive resection (1, 8). Prospective trials will be needed to further clarify the role of extensive surgical resection with specific tumor types and in carefully defined clinical situations. The ultimate goal of these trials would be to define disease-specific therapies that include extent of resection recommendations, as well as recommendations for chemotherapy and/or radiotherapy.

CONCLUSIONS

We feel that early surgical intervention is appropriate in the patient who presents with a clinical picture suggesting a low-grade glioma. Neuroimaging is not adequate to make an accurate diagnosis of the underlying pathology. Tumor tissue sampling allows a more specific diagnosis and testing for biologic factors such as the proliferative potential of the lesion. Surgical diagnosis allows a disease-specific therapy to be more appropriately prescribed to the patient, including the option for no further treatment, radiotherapy, and/or chemotherapy. There is compelling early data that suggest that the extent of surgery and the postoperative tumor volume will be predictive of outcome in at least some tumor types. We encourage participation of physician and patients in well-designed clinical trails that will ultimately answer the many questions that remain about these unique diseases.

ACKNOWLEDGEMENTS

This work was supported in part by NCI CA 13525.

REFERENCES

1. Berger MS, Deliganis AV, Dobbins J, *et al:* The effect of extent of resection on recurrence in patients with low grade cerebral hemisphere gliomas. **Cancer** 74:1784–1791, 1994.
2. Cairncross JG, Macdonald DR, Ramsay DA: Aggressive oligodendroglioma: A chemosensitive tumor. **Neurosurgery** 31:78–82, 1992.
3. Daumas-Duport C, Scheithauer BW, Chodkiewicz J-P, *et al.:* Dysembryoplastic neuroepithelial tumor: A surgically curable tumor of young patients with intractable partial seizures. Report of thirty-nine cases. **Neurosurgery** 23:545–556, 1988.
4. Glass J, Hochberg FH, Gruber ML, *et al.:* The treatment of oligodendrogliomas and mixed oligodendroglioma-astrocytoma with PCV chemotherapy. **J Neurosurg** 76:741–745, 1992.
5. Hoshino T, Prados M, Wilson CB, *et al.:* Prognostic implications of the bromodeoxyuridine labeling index of human gliomas. **J Neurosurg** 71:335–341, 1989.
6. Ito S, Chandler KL, Prados MD, *et al.:* Proliferative potential and prognostic evaluation of low-grade astrocytoma. **J Neurooncol** 19:1–9, 1994.

7. Kondziolka D, Lunsford LD, Martinez AJ: Unreliability of contemporary neurodiagnostic imaging in evaluating suspected adult supratentorial (low grade) astrocytoma. **J Neurosurg** 79:533–536, 1993.
8. Laws ER, Taylor WF, Clifton MB, *et al.:* Neurosurgical management of low-grade astrocytoma of the cerebral hemispheres. **J Neurosurg** 61:665–673, 1984.
9. McDermott MW, Krouwer HGJ, Asai A, *et al.:* Comparison of CT contrast enhancement and BUDR labeling indices in moderately and highly anaplastic astrocytomas of the cerebral hemispheres. **Can J Neurol Sci** 19:34–39, 1992.
10. Nishizaki T, Orita T, Kajiwara K, *et al.:* Correlation of in vitro bromodeoxyuridine labeled index and DNA aneuploidy with survival or recurrence in brain tumor patients. **J Neurosurg** 73:396–400, 1990.
11. Packer RJ, Lange B, Ater J, *et al.:* Carboplatin and vincristine for recurrent and newly diagnosed low-grade gliomas of childhood. **J Clin Oncol** 11:850–856, 1993.

24

Low-Grade Glioma:
The Case for Delayed Surgery

J. GREGORY CAIRNCROSS, M.D.

Some researchers have argued that the natural history of nonpilocytic low-grade glioma of the cerebral hemispheres is sufficiently variable and therapies for this condition sufficiently imperfect, that early aggressive multimodality treatment is not necessary in every instance. Some researchers believe that early aggressive treatment, including biopsy or surgical resection, can be delayed for many patients and that a conservative "wait-and-see" approach to management of these low-grade gliomas is not only reasonable (2, 3,) but also safe and effective (13).

This chapter focuses on the issue of early surgical intervention *versus* delayed surgical intervention for patients with a computerized tomography (CT) or magnetic resonance imaging (MRI) abnormality compatible with a low-grade glioma of the cerebral hemispheres. Based on recent data and, to a lesser degree, on the author's personal experience, this chapter identifies two groups of patients, those for whom early surgery is likely to be of particular benefit and those for whom the wait-and-see management approach is likely to be an acceptable course of action.

PILOCYTIC ASTROCYTOMAS AND SPECIAL GLIOMA VARIANTS

Many low-grade gliomas in children and a minority in adults are well circumscribed, indolent neoplasms, often curable by surgical resection. Tumors with these characteristics include pilocytic astrocytomas of the cerebral hemispheres, thalamus, rostral brainstem and cerebellum (usual location); gangliogliomas of the temporal lobe (and other locations); and the rare pleomorphic xanthoastrocytoma. These tumors frequently appear on CT or MRI as discrete cystic masses with an intensely enhancing mural nodule; usually become symptomatic during childhood, adolescence, or early adult life; and eventually cause disabling symptoms, such as headaches, ataxia, focal weakness, and intractable seizures. Whenever possible, they should be removed without delay. Early surgical intervention is also recommended for low-grade gliomas growing in the midline and causing ventricular obstruction, such as subependymal giant cell astrocytomas at the foramen of Monro in patients with tuberous sclerosis and low-grade ependymomas arising from the floor of the fourth ventricle. Based on clinical and radiologic features, pilocytic astrocytomas and special glioma variants are often suspected prior to surgery, and in clinical practice, there is rarely if ever disagreement about the timing of surgical intervention. To this author's knowledge no one advocates delayed surgery for these types of low-grade glioma.

Whereas few would question the wisdom of early curative surgery for a pilocytic astrocytoma of the cerebellum, causing headaches, vomiting, and gait unsteadiness in a young child, the merits of urgent partial removal of a diffuse glioma of the cerebral hemispheres, causing but a single seizure in a young adult, are far from clear-cut, at least in the minds of some surgeons and physicians.

DIFFUSE GLIOMAS OF THE CEREBRAL HEMISPHERES

Tumors in this category include fibrillary astrocytomas (called ordinary astrocytomas by some researchers) (14), oligodendrogliomas, and mixed gliomas. They frequently present with seizures, less often headaches; appear on CT or MRI as diffuse nonenhancing space-occupying lesions; and vary considerably in location and size. In this era of modern brain imaging, low-grade gliomas of the cerebral hemispheres are recognized at a much earlier stage in their natural history than was the case 3 decades ago, and it is now unusual for patients to have papilledema or focal neurologic deficits at diagnosis (9, 18). In the absence of any new treatment, lead-time bias introduced by earlier diagnosis has resulted in significantly longer patient survival rates in retrospective studies of patients diagnosed since the advent of CT. The debate over the timing of potentially toxic aggressive treatment, including surgical treatment, for hemispheric low-grade glioma is now more important, not less, and conclusions gleaned from older retrospective studies of low-grade glioma are now less relevant not more (18).

Although the timing of surgery is unlikely to be the subject of a randomized clinical trial, a century of experience in neurosurgery of brain tumor and common sense would suggest that early surgery is appropriate for some patients with low-grade glioma of the cerebral hemispheres. Patients with raised intracranial pressure and threatened transtentorial herniation due to large tumors or cystic masses and those with progressive neurologic deficits are candidates for early surgery. Patients with tumors containing enhancing regions likely to be undergoing malignant transformation or those with tumors, which by virtue of their smaller size and polar location can be "completely" resected, are also candidates for early surgical intervention. Other factors that should lead to one to consider earlier surgery, as opposed to later intervention, are older age at radiologic diagnosis, because tumors in older patients are more likely to behave aggressively or have anaplastic pathology (17); patient preference; and patient inaccessibility to follow-up clinical evaluation or neuro-imaging.

At radiologic diagnosis, many patients with diffuse hemispheric low-grade glioma are young (*i.e.,* < age 40), present with a single seizure, do not have papilledema or other evidence of raised intracranial pressure, have a normal neurologic examination, have small nonenhancing unresectable tumors with little mass effect and, in America, have ready access to follow-up state-of-the-art brain imaging. It is open to question whether these patients should be exposed to the risks of stereotactic biopsy or tumor resection simply for diagnosis at a time when they are "perfectly well," especially for an "incurable" illness with a relatively long and largely unpredictable natural history. Frequent reassessment with MRI scans, delaying aggressive multi-modality treatment to a later date when the tumor-controlling benefits of treatment clearly outweigh its toxic effects, is an alternative management strategy worth considering for these patients. The author's personal views on the indications for early surgery and delayed surgery are summarized in Table 24.1.

DELAYED SURGERY—BENEFITS AND RISKS

Delayed surgery is unlikely to yield a more favorable overall clinical outcome than early surgery for patients with diffuse hemispheric low-grade glioma, but it may yield the equivalent. Postponing the possibility of surgical misadventure, that is, surgical mortality and morbidity,

TABLE 24.1
Indications for Early Surgery and Delayed Surgery

Early Surgery	Delayed Surgery
Raised intracranial pressure	Single seizure
Neurologic deficit	Normal neurologic examination
Large tumor mass	Small tumor mass
Contrast enhancing lesion	Nonenhancing lesion
Possible complete resection	Eloquent area—not completely resectable
Older age at diagnosis	Younger age at diagnosis
Patient unavailable for follow-up	Patient available for follow-up
Patient preference	Patient preference

is the major benefit of delayed surgery. This statement begs the following question: What is the risk of death or neurologic injury following stereotactic biopsy or tumor resection for supratentorial low-grade glioma in neurosurgery's modern era? Based on three recent studies summarized in Table 24.2, the 30-day mortality is 1%, and the risk of significant neurologic morbidity is 4% (1, 9, 18). These are low rates or, at least they would be for glioblastoma multiforme, for which the natural history is such that serious disability, if not already present, is likely to occur within 6 months, death within a year, but are these considered low rates of surgical mortality and morbidity for an illness with a highly favorable short-term natural history? For low-grade glioma of the cerebral hemispheres, death and serious neurologic disability (with the possible exception of intractable seizures) are unlikely to occur spontaneously for several years at least.

Misdiagnosis and poorer outcome are the arguments put forward by advocates of early surgery for all patients. As such, misdiagnosis and poorer outcome must be considered the risks of delayed operative intervention; both warrant discussion. Misdiagnosis can take two forms, first underestimating the degree of malignancy by assuming the tumor to be low-grade when, in fact, it is anaplastic and, second, assuming the lesion is a neoplasm when, in fact, it is some other pathologic process altogether. Similarly, inferior outcome as a result of delayed surgery can take two forms, either poorer neurologic function or shorter survival. Advocates of delayed surgery must be prepared to address these issues.

How often is a CT or MRI abnormality typical of a diffuse hemispheric low-grade glioma, not a low-grade glioma? Three recent studies summarized in Table 24.3 have addressed this issue, with strikingly different findings and conclusions (1, 7, 13). Two studies from surgical neuro-oncology units put the error rate at 20 to 50%, the com-

TABLE 24.2

Surgical Complications: Supratentorial Low-Grade Glioma

Case Series	No. of Cases	Stereotactic Biopsy	Mortality (30-day)	CNS Morbidity
Vertosick *et al.* (18)	25	16	0	0
McCormack *et al.* (9)	53	9	1[a]	3[b]
Bernstein and Guha (1)	48	48	0	2[c]
Totals	126	73	1 (1%)	5 (4%)

[a]Myocardial infarction.
[b]Recovery over several months.
[c]Hemorrhages.

TABLE 24.3
Misdiagnosis: Delayed Surgical Intervention

Case Series	No. of Cases	Low-Grade Glioma	Anaplastic Glioma	Other	Error Rate (%)
Kondziolka *et al.* (7)	20	10	9	1	50
Bernstein and Guha (1)	48	39	6	3	19
Recht *et al.* (13)	20	19	0	1	5

mon error being underestimation of the degree of malignancy, whereas one study drawing on consecutive cases at a medical neuro-oncology unit found only a 5% rate of misdiagnosis, and the single error involved an inflammatory lesion for which there was no specific therapy. The explanation for these differences may lie in the complex process of selecting patients for surgery; patients with atypical clinical presentations are more likely to be referred to surgeons, are more likely to have a surgical procedure,and are more likely to have an unexpected pathologic diagnosis. Admittedly, failure to obtain a biopsy inevitably leads to some rate of diagnostic error, but one must consider other issues as well: Does it really matter whether the diagnosis of an anaplastic glioma is somewhat delayed? How often is there a specific therapy for the occasional non-neoplastic pathology? Finally, on this issue of erroneous diagnosis, it must be acknowledged by the advocates of early surgery that biopsy procedures (less so, tumor resections) have a false-negative/false-positive rate while always exposing the patient to some degree of surgical risk.

Does delaying surgery compromise the quality of life or length of life for patients with diffuse hemispheric low-grade glioma? This is a critical issue; it would be foolish to advocate delayed surgery if delay would compromise quality of or length of life for the patient. There is no information in the literature that pertains specifically to quality and length of life in relation to the timing of surgical intervention. However, several often-cited retrospective studies of the treatment of low-grade glioma, recently reviewed by Vecht *et al.* and summarized in Table 24.4, suggest that the extent of surgical resection is a significant independent predictor of patient survival (5, 8, 11, 14, 15). Patients with completely resected tumors tend to live longer than those with partially removed tumors, who in turn tend to live longer than those with tumors that underwent biopsy. These studies have guided our thinking on the management of low-grade glioma for many years and constitute the strongest evidence in support of early aggressive surgery (and radiotherapy). Conclusions drawn from retrospective studies run a higher risk of being incorrect than those based on the results of randomized clinical trials, but nevertheless they give the practicing clinician some path to follow when treating individual patients. Not all studies have found a statistically significant correlation between extent of surgical removal and length of life, but certainly none have found that minimal surgery enhances survival (10, 12).

This was the state of affairs until Recht and colleagues, at the University of Massachusetts, published the results of an ingenious "cohort-style" study (13). Two comparable, concurrently "treated," contemporary groups of patients were identified: one group had early surgery and radiotherapy for biopsy-proven low-grade glioma and the other, patients with suspected low-grade glioma, was followed clinically and radiologically, delaying surgery and radiotherapy until a later date when and if deterioration occurred. The quality of life, length of life, and rate of malignant conversion were identical in the two groups. This, too, was a retrospective study, but patients were ascertained in an entirely different way, and a radically different conclusion ensued. The important outcomes were identical, whether one intervened immediately or later. Those who think that a probable diagnosis of diffuse hemispheric low-grade glioma based on CT or MRI demands early surgery (and radiotherapy) are challenged by this new data to reconsider the matter.

Clearly, those who recommend a wait-and-see approach for their patients must remain vigilant, because sooner or later, as the study by Recht *et al.* also demonstrated, most patients with a diffuse low-grade glioma of the cerebral hemispheres will require stereotactic biopsy or

TABLE 24.4
Independent Prognostic Factors in Low-Grade Glioma[a, b]

Study	No. of Patients Studied	Grade of Tumor	Age	Performance Status	Extent of Surgical Resection	Radio-therapy
Laws *et al.* (8)	461	S[c]	S	S	S	S
Garcia *et al.* (5)	86	S	NS	ND	S	S
Piepmeier (12)	60	ND	S	ND	NS	NS
Medbery *et al.* (10)	50	NS	S	ND	NS	S[d]
Shaw *et al.* (14)	126	S	S	ND	S	S
Sofietti *et al.* (15)	85	ND	NS	S	S	NS
North *et al.* (11)	77	NS	S	S	S	NS

[a]Reproduced with permission from (17).
[b]All studies were evaluated by multivariate analysis, except for the report by Garcia *et al.,* which was evaluated by univariate analysis.
[c]S, statistically significant; NS, not significant; *ND*, no data.
[d]According to dose of radiation (P = 0.07).

TABLE 24.5
When to Reconsider Delaying Surgery

Increasing symptoms (including seizures)
Emerging neurologic deficit
Increasing tumor size
Appearance of enhancing regions
Patient preference

tumor resection and radiotherapy, which is best done before irreversible neurologic deficits develop (13). Guidelines for reconsidering the wait-and-see approach are listed in Table 24.5. Perhaps in the near future, patients needing early aggressive treatment will be unambiguously identified by studies of proliferation or molecular markers (6, 16), but until then, this author strongly suggests that neurosurgeons consider making their treatment decisions on an individual basis.

REFERENCES

1. Bernstein M, Guha A: Biopsy of low-grade astrocytomas. **J Neurosurg** 80:776–777, 1994.
2. Cairncross JG, Laperriere NJ. Low-grade glioma. To treat or not to treat? **Arch Neurol** 46:1238–1239, 1989.
3. Cairncross JG, Laperriere NJ: Low-grade gliomas: To treat or not to treat? A reply. **Arch Neurol** 47:1139–1140, 1990.
4. Chandrasoma PT, Smith MM, Apuzzo MLJ: Stereotactic biopsy in the diagnosis of brain masses: Comparison of results of biopsy and resected surgical specimens. **Neurosurgery** 24:160–165, 1989.
5. Garcia DM, Fulling KH, Marks JE: The value of radiation therapy in addition to surgery for astrocytomas of the adult cerebrum. **Cancer** 55:919–927, 1985.
6. Hoshino T, Ahn D, Prados MD, *et al.:* Prognostic significance of the proliferative potential of intracranial gliomas measured by bromodeoxyuridine labeling. **Int J Cancer** 53:550–555, 1993.
7. Kondziolka D, Lunsford LD, Martinez AJ: Unreliability of contemporary neurodiagnostic imaging in evaluating suspected adult supratentorial (low-grade) astrocytoma. **J Neurosurg** 79:533–536, 1993.
8. Laws ER, Taylor WF, Clifton MB, *et al.:* Neurosurgical management of low-grade astrocytoma of the cerebral hemispheres. **J Neurosurg** 61:665–673, 1984.
9. McCormack BM, Miller DC, Budzilovich GN, *et al.:* Treatment and survival of low-grade astrocytoma in adults: 1977–1988. **Neurosurgery** 31:636–642, 1992.
10. Medbery CA, Straus KL, Steinberg SM, *et al.:* Low-grade astrocytomas: Treatment results and prognostic variables. **Int J Radiat Oncol Biol Phys** 15:837–841, 1988.
11. North CA, North RB, Epstein JA, *et al.:* Low-grade cerebral astrocytomas. Survival and quality of life after radiation therapy. **Cancer** 66:6–14, 1990.
12. Piepmeier JM: Observations on the current treatment of low-grade astrocytic tumors of the cerebral hemispheres. **J Neurosurg** 67:177–181, 1987.

13. Recht LD, Lew R, Smith TW: Suspected low-grade glioma: Is deferring treatment safe? **Ann Neurol** 31:431–436, 1992.
14. Shaw EG, Daumas-Duport C, Scheithauer BW, *et al:* Radiation therapy in the management of low-grade supratentorial astrocytomas. **J Neurosurg** 70:853–861, 1989.
15. Soffietti R, Chio A, Giordana MT, *et al.:* Prognostic factors in well-differentiated cerebral astrocytomas in the adult. **Neurosurgery** 24:686–692, 1989.
16. Van Meyel DJ, Ramsay DA, Casson AG, *et al:* p53 mutation, expression and DNA ploidy in evolving astrocytic gliomas: Evidence for two pathways of progression. **J Natl Cancer Inst** 86:1011–1017, 1994.
17. Vecht CJ: Effect of age on treatment decisions of low-grade glioma. **J Neurol Neurosurg Psychiatry** 56:1359–1364, 1993.
18. Vertosick FT, Selker RG, Arena VC: Survival of patients with well-differentiated astrocytomas diagnosed in the era of computed tomography. **Neurosurgery** 28:496–501, 1991.

25

Surgical Issues in the Management of Supratentorial Low-Grade Gliomas

PATRICK J. KELLY, M.D., F.A.C.S.

Low-grade supratentorial gliomas present special problems to a surgeon attempting to resect them. First, many low-grade gliomas in adult patients comprise intact parenchyma infiltrated by isolated tumor cells (5, 17,18). Resecting the tumor is, in fact, resecting intact brain tissue as well. Low-grade gliomas in children, on the other hand, tend to be histologically circumscribed, and many displace, rather than infiltrate, brain tissue (13, 19, 20). However, many of these tumors are deep-seated: in the thalamus, hypothalamus, basal ganglia, and bainstem deep in the subcortical white matter.

Since a surgeon's 3-dimensional orientation decreases as surgical exposure descends below the cortical surface, the surgeon can get "lost" in attempts to find the tumor. In addition, low-grade glial tumors are not infrequently irregular in shape, and maintaining surgical orientation within the various extensions of the tumor is difficult. Finally, the histologic distinction between tumor and surrounding normal brain tissue may not always be clear to a surgeon at an open operation. Not wishing to inflict neurologic deficit on the patient, most surgeons tend to be conservative with low-grade gliomas, with the inevitable result that much of the tumor remains following surgical attempts to "resect" it.

For these reasons methods of computerized tomography (CT)- and magnetic resonance imaging (MRI)-based stereotactic data acquisition, mapping, surgical planning, and volumetric resection have been developed (12–15, 20). These are all methods for achieving the maximum possible cytoreduction that should, in a low-grade glioma, represent a beneficial, and cytokinetically significant, reduction of tumor burden in infiltrating as well as histologically circumscribed lesions. However, in low-grade glial neoplasms, selection of appropriate surgical candidates is very important.

The risk:benefit ratio for surgical resection of a low-grade glioma is directly related not only to the anatomic location of the lesion but also to its individual biology and growth pattern. Significant neurologic complications can follow attempted resections of low-grade gliomas in eloquent brain regions. A need for a better understanding of these tumors prompted investigations into the growth patterns of low-grade glial tumors, their 3-dimensional spatial structure, the histologic nature of the glial tumor/brain interface, and the reliability with which glioma margins were detected on stereotactic CT and MRI examinations.

High-grade gliomas are more straightforward in their surgical microanatomy than low-grade gliomas. In high-grade gliomas contrast enhancement on CT and gadolinium-diethylenetriamine-penta-acetic acid enhancement on MRI correlates with the volume of solid tumor tissue that can be safely resected (17, 18, 20). In contrast, tumor tissue in some low-grade gliomas may not appear any different on imaging from infiltrated parenchyma and may be only a small part of the global lesional volume. Other low-grade lesions may comprise a mass of solid tumor tissue only, which will demonstrate intense enhancement on imaging studies (2, 17, 20, 24).

In high-grade gliomas the abnormality defined by hypodensity on CT corresponds to perilesional edema which, in turn, is frequently, but not always, related to the presence of isolated tumor cells that infiltrate the edematous parenchyma. CT hypodensity usually resembles the T2 signal prolongation on MRI, even though the T2 abnormality may be more extensive due to the fact that MRI is much more sensitive to unbound water than CT is. In low-grade gliomas, hypodensity can be infiltrated parenchyma, solid resectable tumor, or just plain edema without tumor. In low-grade as well as in high-grade glial tumors, isolated tumor cells can be found well outside the CT- and MRI-defined limits in most fibrillary astrocytomas, oligo-astrocytomas, and oligodendrogliomas (17, 18).

Previously reported correlation studies of CT- and MRI-defined abnormalities with histologic limits defined by imaging-based stereotactic serial biopsy were expanded to focus on the biology and growth patterns of low-grade lesions (16–18). These, in turn, resulted in the formulation of a management plan for the proper selection of surgical patients harboring low-grade glial tumors.

STEREOTACTIC SERIAL BIOPSY STUDIES IN LOW-GRADE GLIOMAS

The stereotactic serial biopsy procedure developed at Hôpital Sainte-Ann (Paris, France) was adapted to the CT- and MRI-based stereotactic instrumentation and biopsy methods used at our institution (17, 18). Prospective and retrospective correlation studies of specimen histology and imaging characteristics use computer-assisted multimodality-image cross registration, in which the location of each biopsy specimen is displayed on stereotactic slice images (Fig. 25.1). Stereotactic angiography is used to select safe avascular trajectories for the biopsy sampling. In the usual surgical procedure one or several biopsy trajectories sample normal, hypodense CT-defined abnormal, and contrast-enhancing regions. Since stereotactic MRI is not always included, in the pre-operative database in a biopsy procedure for a glial neoplasm, CT correlations only are considered in this chapter.

Stereotactic serial biopsy procedures are typically performed under general anesthesia. This is especially important when sampling low-grade gliomas in patients presenting with seizures. The biopsy probe is inserted through a twist drill hole 3mm in diameter, with the drill guided by the stereotactic arc-quadrant frame. Biopsy specimens obtained with a Sedan-type biopsy instrument are typically 1 cm in length and 1.5 mm in diameter. The position of each biopsy is cross correlated to its location on CT and documented by AP and lateral teleradiographs.

Specimens are studied by means of hematoxylin and eosin (H&E)-stained smear preparations and standard paraffin-embedded sections. Specimens are examined for the presence or absence of tumor tissue, necrosis, or isolated tumor cells within infiltrated parenchyma (4, 6). The smear preparations, which separate the tissue into its individual cellular elements, are useful in distinguishing isolated tumor cells from reactive gliosis. Tumors are graded, using the classification scheme developed by Daumas-Duport and colleagues (3, 4).

This study concerns serial stereotactic biopsy examinations in 178 consecutive low-grade glioma patients operated on between August 1984 and June 1989 (see Table 25.1). Some of this material has been published elsewhere. These patients, as a group, had 100 astrocytomas (grade 2, 76 patients; grade 1, 24 patients), 18 pilocytic astrocytomas,

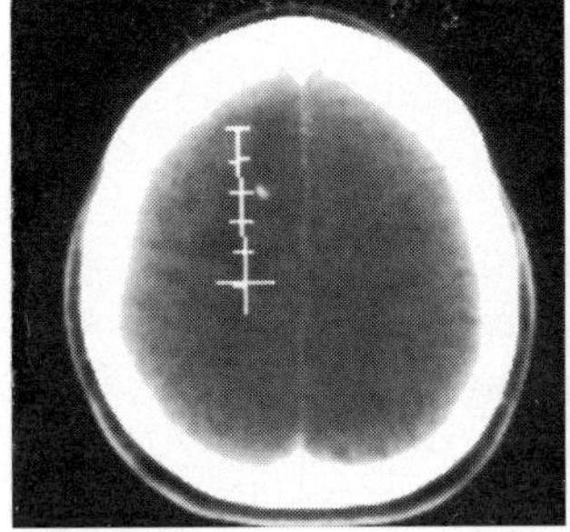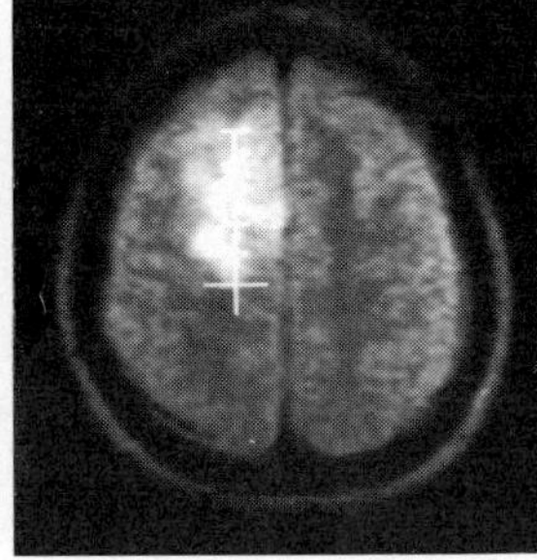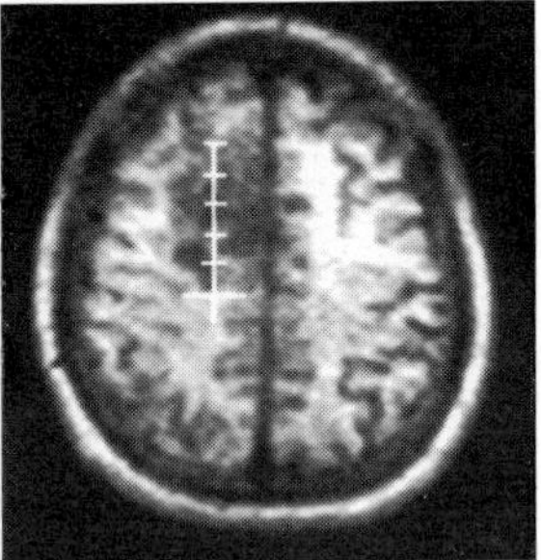

FIG. 25.1 Stereotactic serial biopsy registered on CT, T2, and T1 MRI slices. The *vertical line* represents the biopsy tract. The biopsy specimen locations will be located between the *"hash marks."* For this low-grade glioma, six biopsy specimens were obtained.

TABLE 25.1

Histology and CT in Grade I and II Lesions

	Hypodense	Isodense	Contrast Enhancement
Normal tissue	25	21	
Tumor tissue	31	4	28[a]
Isolated tumor cells	377	99	
Necrosis	1		
	434	124	28

[a]Twenty specimens were obtained from pilocytic astrocytomas.

and 35 oligodendrogliomas (grade 3, 6 patients; grade 2, 25 patients; grade 1, 10 patients). An additional 25 patients had mixed gliomas (oligo-astrocytomas), comprising the following grades: grade 2, 23 patients; grade 1, 2 patients.

RESULTS

A total of 586 specimens were obtained: 434 specimens from hypodense areas, 28 specimens from contrast-enhancing areas, and the remaining 124 specimens from isodense areas on CT scanning (Table 25.1). Histologic review of this material confirmed the following two growth patterns in glial neoplasms.

Tumor Tissue

Neoplastic cells of the tumor tissue component are packed together tightly. Neovascularization and necrosis are noted with high-grade tumor tissue masses. Cells within tumor tissue masses tend to have cytoplasm; some have short and numerous glial processes. Mitotic figures can be noted within these regions. *There is no intervening parenchyma in tumor tissue.* Bodian or myelin stains performed on this tissue reveal no myelinated fibers. As shown in Table 25.1 tends to enhance with contrast in high-grade gliomas, whereas enhancement patterns for tumor tissue are inconsistent or absent in low-grade lesions.

Infiltrated Parenchyma

Isolated tumor cells infiltrate intact and usually functional parenchyma. Mapping studies at the author's institution have clearly shown that this infiltrated parenchyma is functioning brain tissue. Frequently, the involved parenchyma exhibits edema. Occasionally, small patches of tumor tissue can exist within larger zones of isolated tumor cell-infiltrated parenchyma. Isolated tumor cells have little or no discernible cytoplasm when identified on smear preparations; nuclei are frequently large with prominent nucleoli. These features provide a means of distinguishing isolated tumor cells from reactive gliosis on smear preparations: reactive astrocytes have small nuclei in comparison to those found in tumor cells. In addition, reactive astrocytes feature long glial processes; when isolated tumor cells demonstrate cytoplasm and glial processes, the latter are short and too numerous to be confused with those seen in reactive astrocytes.

As shown in Table 25.1, parenchyma infiltrated by isolated tumor cells tends to be hypodense on CT in high-grade and low-grade lesions. In general, many low-grade glial neoplasms have both tumor tissue and isolated tumor cells infiltrating surrounding parenchyma. However, in contrast to many high-grade gliomas, biopsies obtained from low-grade gliomas (with the exception of pilocytic astrocytomas) demonstrate infiltrated parenchyma more often than tumor tissue does.

CT/HISTOLOGIC CORRELATIONS

Low-grade glial tumors of astrocytic, oligodendroglial, or mixed glioma types usually manifest an area of hypodensity on CT or prolonged T1 or T2 on MRI. There is little or no contrast enhancement. As shown in Table 25.1, the majority of the 586 specimens were obtained from hypodense areas on CT. Most of those specimens in that majority demonstrated isolated tumor cells infiltrating intact parenchyma. However, 99 of the 124 specimens obtained from isodense ("normal") areas on CT scanning also demonstrated isolated tumor cells.

Tumor tissue can be found in low-grade glial tumors. In fact, tumor tissue was found in 63 of 586 specimens: 31 of these specimens were obtained from CT hypodense areas; 4 were obtained from isodense areas; and 28 specimens were obtained from areas that demonstrated contrast enhancement. However, and notably, 20 of the 28 tumor tissue specimens obtained from areas that demonstrated contrast enhancement on CT were retrieved from patients with pilocytic astrocytomas. In fact, most pilocytic astrocytomas consist of tumor tissue only, which typically exhibits contrast enhancement. As in high-grade gliomas, contrast enhancement is directly related to the presence of neovascularization within the tumor tissue.

Forty-six specimens demonstrated no evidence of tumor tissue or isolated tumor cells. Twenty-five of these specimens had been obtained from CT hypodense areas, but the other 21 had been obtained from isodense areas on CT scanning.

Therefore, in nonpilocytic low-grade gliomas, isolated tumor cells are usually found in areas that manifest hypodensity on CT scanning. However, tumor cells can be found in areas far afield of the CT-, or for that matter, MRI-defined abnormality.

GLIAL TUMOR SPATIAL TYPES IN LOW-GRADE GLIOMAS

As Daumas-Duport demonstrated, low-grade glial neoplasms can be classified into three types based on the growth patterns and presence or absence of tumor tissue with or without surrounding tumor cell-infiltrated parenchyma.

Type I: Tumor Tissue Only without Surrounding Parenchymal Tumor Cell Infiltration. In general, type I tumors include gangliogliomas, most pilocytic astrocytomas, many xantho-astrocytomas, rare protoplasmic astrocytomas, and some oligodendrogliomas in young patients. Complete surgical resection can, in theory, cure these patients. Some, but not all, type I tumors present as contrast-enhancing mass lesions that can be resected without fear of a neurologic deficit, as shown in Figure 25.2. Other type I tumors show only a hypodense but apparently circumscribed mass in which the CT hypodensity comprises the same volume as the T1 and T2 signal abnormalities. These tumors can also be resected with good postoperative results.

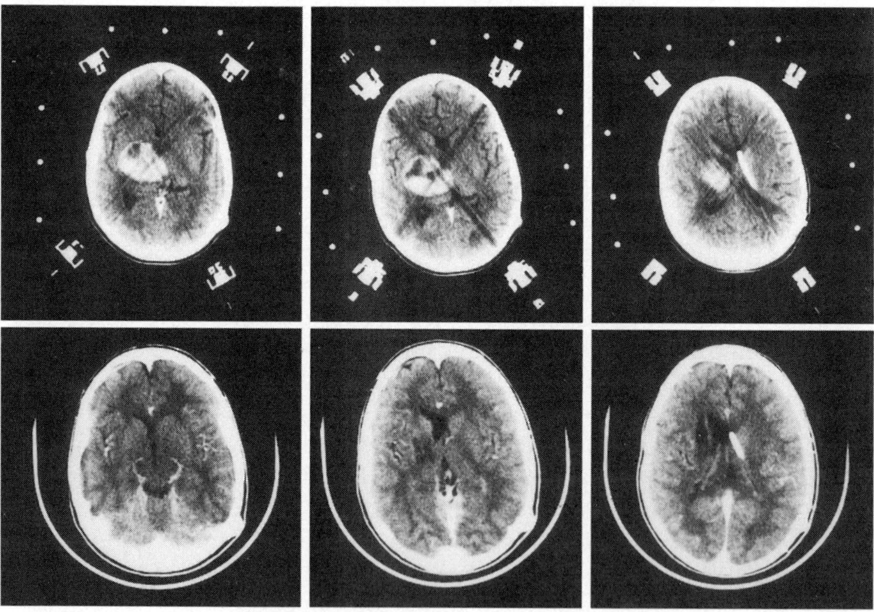

FIG. 25.2 Pilocytic astrocytoma of right thalamus, internal capsule, and basal ganglia in a young girl with mild left hemiparesis. The tumor was completely removed, utilizing an anterior approach through the anterior limb of the internal capsule. Her postoperative gadolinium-enhanced MRI is shown at the **bottom**. Here hemiparesis was improved postoperatively.

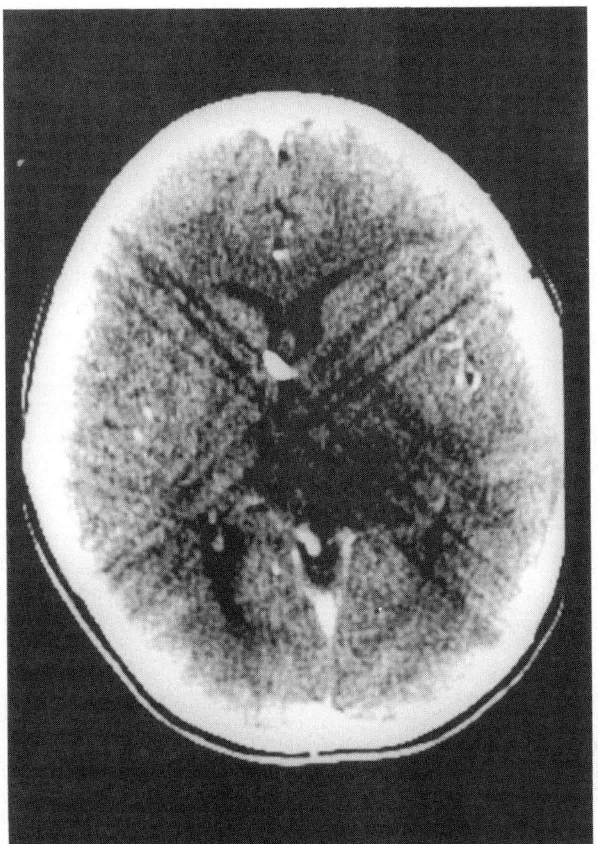

FIG. 25.3 Type II oligodendroglioma. Stereotactic serial biopsy demonstrated that the majority of the tumor is composed of isolated tumor cells within intact parenchyma. However, small patches of solid tumor tissue were noted in the posterior aspect of the thalamus. This is not a resectable tumor.

Type II: Tumor Tissue Parenchyma Surrounded by Isolated Infiltrated Tumor Cells. Low-grade tumors can have a mass of tumor tissue that is frequently hypodense on CT within a field of infiltrated parenchyma that is also hypodense (Fig. 25.3). Surgical resection of the tumor tissue mass will benefit the patient in direct relationship to the proportion of the lesional volume that tumor tissue proper comprises. Resection of a small mass of tumor tissue within a large field of infiltrated parenchyma is of questionable benefit. In "silent" brain regions, however, the infiltrated parenchyma, as well as the solid tumor tissue mass, can be resected *en bloc* as a stereotactically defined volume in space.

Type III: Parenchyma Infiltrated with Isolated Tumor Cells and No Tumor Tissue. This pattern is most frequently noted in low- and intermediate-grade gliomas in adult patients (Fig. 25.4). In nonessential brain areas, the volume of the lesion defined by hypodensity on CT scanning or T2 prolongation on MRI can be resected by a computer-assisted volumetric stereotactic technique. In essential brain regions, however, resection of these lesions is, in essence, resection of viable, albeit infiltrated, brain tissue and will be associated with a postoperative neurologic deficit.

SURGICAL PLANNING AND CASE SELECTION

Resective surgery is not appropriate for all glial neoplasms; some lesions are best suited for stereotactic biopsy alone, followed by external beam radiation therapy. As stated above, patient selection for low-grade glial neoplasms, as in all surgeries, is based on a risk:benefit ratio, which can be anticipated using the following guidelines. Figure 25.5 presents an algorithm, developed over the years, for surgical selection and planning in the management of low-grade glial tumors.

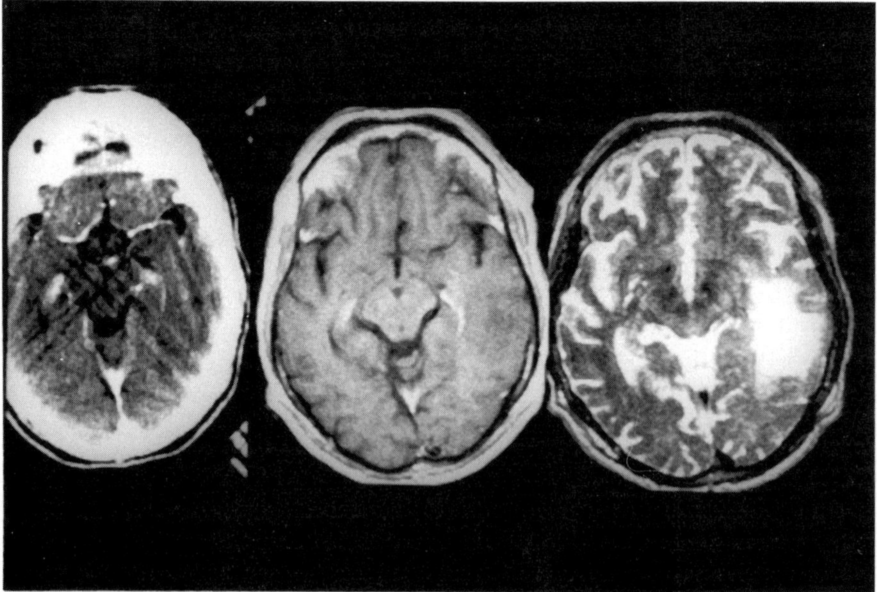

FIG. 25.4 Type III glioma in the left midtemporal lobe in an elderly woman. A stereotactic biopsy demonstrated edematous parenchyma infiltrated by isolated tumor cells.

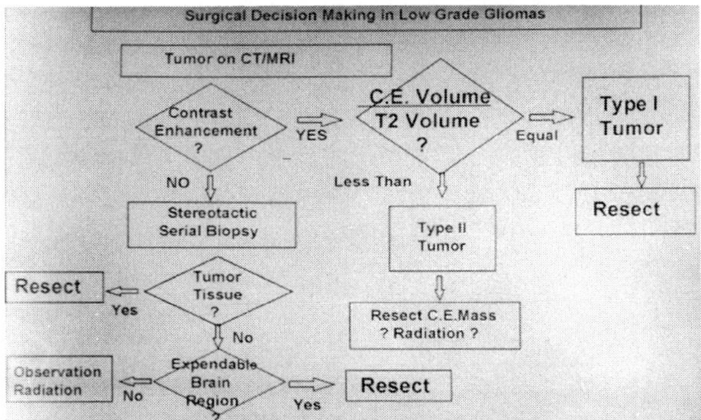

FIG. 25.5 Surgical decision making in patient selection in treatment of low-grade glial tumors.

Removal of cytokinetically significant portions of low-grade glial neoplasms is dependent on: (a) the ability to recognize tumor boundaries on imaging studies, (b) the ability to transfer this information to the surgical field, (c) the knowledge of whether or not the tumor is comprised of solid tumor tissue that can be resected or parenchyma infiltrated by isolated tumor cells and (d) the determination of the functionality of infiltrated brain areas that are intended for resection. Infiltrated parenchyma must not be resected in eloquent brain areas. Resecting infiltrated brain regions in a low-grade glioma is resecting functioning, albeit "sick," brain tissue—a neurologic deficit will usually result.

If the tumor volume defined by contrast enhancement on CT scanning (or by gadolinium enhancement on MRI) is roughly equal to the volume defined by the T2-weighted image of the MRI (or the volume of perilesional hypodensity on CT), the lesion is frequently a type I tumor. Pilocytic astrocytomas are a good example of this type. In most instances, they can (and should) be resected. The postoperative results will be good and the morbidity low (Fig. 25.6).

An important exception can be noted in type I lesions in patients with seizures: the perilesional hypodensity or surrounding regions of T2 prolongation in these cases may represent edema and not infiltrated parenchyma. A stereotactic serial biopsy can be performed to exclude the presence of infiltrating tumor cells prior to consideration for definitive surgery.

In type II lesions located in nonessential brain regions, volumetric stereotactic resection of the entire volume of tumor tissue as well as infiltrated brain tissue can provide very significant cytoreduction, and

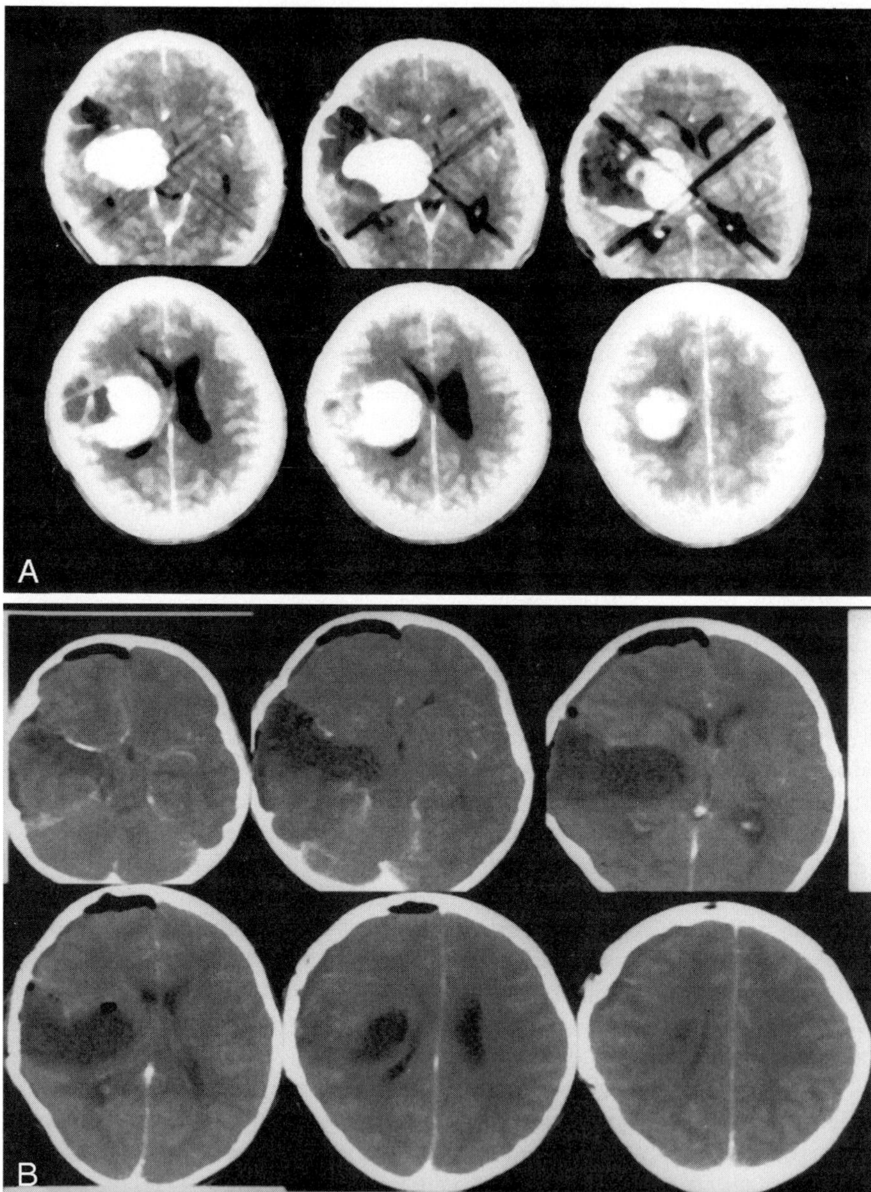

FIG. 25.6 Pre-operative (**A**) and postoperative (**B**) contrast-enhanced CT scans in a 3-year-old girl with a large pilocytic astrocytoma located in the thalamus and basal ganglia. A previous attempt had been made at resection at another institution. The tumor was totally resected, as confirmed on the postoperative scan. The patient had a mild hemiparesis pre-operatively, which did not significantly worsen after surgery. Since discharge from the hospital, progressive improvement in neurologic function has been noted.

should theoretically prolong survival in low-grade glial tumors. However, no imaging method can prospectively differentiate nonenhancing solid tumor tissue from parenchyma infiltrated by isolated tumor cells in tumors that do not exhibit contrast enhancement on CT or MRI. In most adult low-grade gliomas, the absence of contrast enhancement usually indicates that the lesion comprises isolated tumor cells within parenchyma only. Resection of the imaging-defined lesional volume is, in fact, resection of intact and usually functional brain parenchyma and, when done in important brain areas, neurologic deficit can result.

However, in some low-grade glial tumors, tumor tissue is present and is hypodense. This situation is not infrequently encountered in children presenting with seizures (Fig. 25.7). If in doubt, a serial stereotactic biopsy procedure can establish whether the lesion comprises tumor tissue, infiltrated parenchyma, or both. CT hypodense nonenhancing tumor tissue lesions can be resected from essential brain regions with low morbidity.

In particular, very low-grade oligodendrogliomas, dysembryoplastic neuroepitheliomas (DNEs), and some gangliogliomas in young patients frequently manifest a solid tumor tissue mass that is hypodense

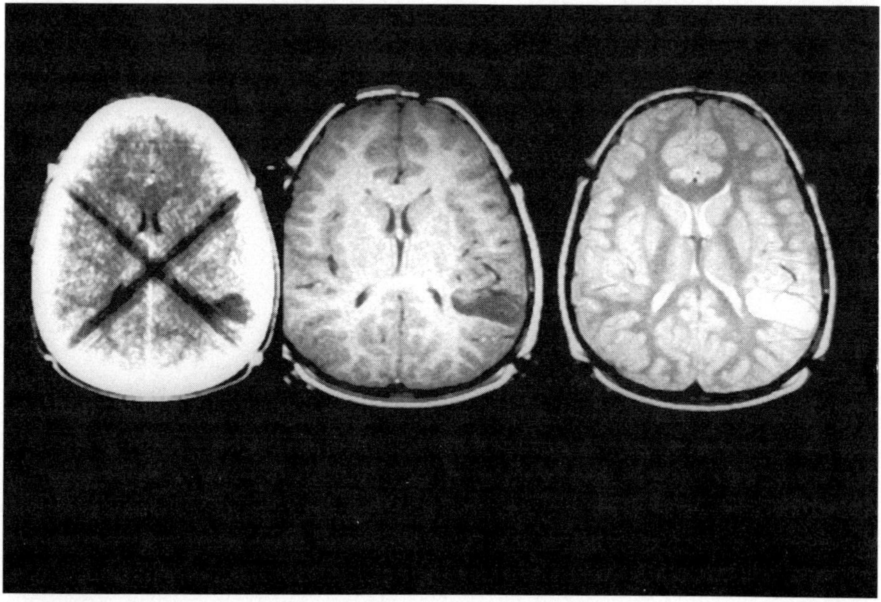

FIG. 25.7 Type I nonenhancing tumor in an 11-year-old boy presenting with seizures. Note that the configuration and size of the lesion on CT, T1, and T2 are virtually identical. This tumor was resected and found to be a ganglioglioma. The patient was neurologically intact pre- and postoperatively.

and nonenhancing on CT scanning. Serial biopsies in these lesions will show only tumor tissue, with minimal or no surrounding infiltrated parenchyma (type 1 tumor).

Tumors located in eloquent brain, which on biopsy are found to comprise isolated tumor cells within parenchyma with or without tumor tissue (types II or III, respectively), should not be resected unless careful cortical mapping techniques establish that the involved parenchyma is "silent."

Hypodense type II or III tumors located in nonessential brain tissue can be resected in their entirety. Low-grade oligodendrogliomas, mixed gliomas, and astrocytomas located in frontal, anterior, or medial temporal lobes or superior parietal lobule can be selectively resected by imaging-based volumetric stereotactic methods with rewarding postoperative results (Fig. 25.8).

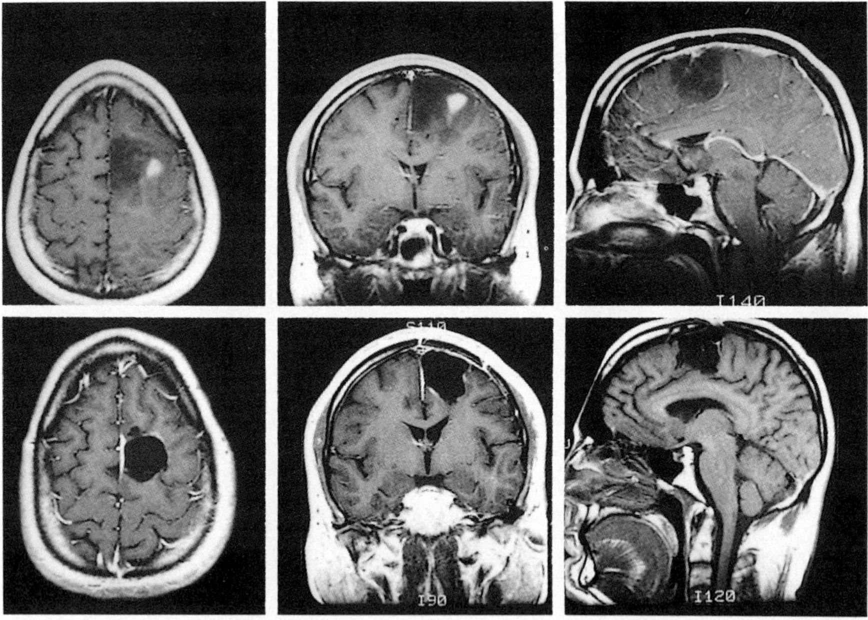

FIG. 25.8 Type II tumor located in the posterior portion of the left superior frontal convolution. The lesion extends from the inner hemispheric face to the superior frontal sulcas, inferiorly into the cingulate sulcus and posteriorly to the precentral sulcus. Gross total en bloc resection of the lesion was achieved, as documented in the postoperative gadolinium-enhanced MRI. Histologic examination of the tissue revealed a grade II oligoastrocytoma. Examination of the contrast-enhancing nodule demonstrated tumor tissue with neovascularization. The remainder of the tumor consisted of tumor cell-infiltrated edematous parenchyma.

The resectability of low-grade gliomas depends on the degree of *histologic circumscription*. In adults, low-grade astrocytomas, mixed gliomas, and oligodendrogliomas most often manifest an area of low density on CT scanning and prolongation of signal on MRI. Stereotactic serial biopsy studies of these lesions reveals that the "tumor" is comprised almost entirely of infiltrated but intact parenchyma. There is little tumor tissue proper. Therefore, resection of the tumor is, in fact, resection of intact but infiltrated parenchyma, which is defined by hypodense areas on CT scanning and signal prolongation on MRI. The volumetric resection technique, which will be discussed below, can be used to achieve this end. In the author's opinion, resection of a low-grade infiltrating glioma involves an en bloc resection of the entire CT- and MRI-defined volume. The concept of "internal decompression" applies to high-grade gliomas with significant mass effect and is not valid for most low-grade infiltrating gliomas.

However, in important brain regions, resection can result in a postoperative neurologic deficit. Resection, if contemplated, should be attempted only after careful mapping procedures have established that the infiltrated brain tissue is silent neurophysiologically. Mapping techniques comprise various methods of noninvasive mapping including magnetoencephalotomography, positron emission tomography (PET) scanning, transcranial magnetic field motor stimulation, and functional MRI. Invasive mapping can also be performed with chronically implanted epidural electrodes or subdural grids. Direct cortical simulation can be performed in an awake patient at craniotomy prior to tumor resection. Finally, direct cortical stimulation can be used to map out the motor strip. In some cases, the lesion is confined to expendable brain tissue, such as the posterior portion of the superior frontal convolution.

Pilocytic astrocytomas are very different from the tumors described above in biology, prognosis, and growth patterns. Most occur in children and young adults. They are histologically circumscribed and grow by volume expansion, with displacement of surrounding brain tissue— few are associated with isolated tumor cell infiltration into surrounding brain tissue. Despite the fact that many are located in the thalamus and other important subcortical locations, most can be completely resected with excellent postoperative results. These lesions exhibit prominent enhancement on CT or on MRI with gadolinium and the histologic borders are defined accurately by the contrast enhancement.

SURGICAL PROCEDURES FOR LOW-GRADE GLIOMAS

Conventional classical craniotomy techniques have been used in the surgical management of low-grade gliomas for many years. They continue to be appropriate in the management of lesions located at frontal, temporal, and occipital poles, where a lobectomy can provide significant cytoreduction and relief of mass effect. However, stereotactic techniques have particular advantages over nonstereotactic classical surgical techniques in the management of nonpolar low-grade cerebral gliomas. CT- and MRI-based point-in-space stereotactic biopsy procedures for the diagnosis of intracranial tumors are now commonplace. Adult low-grade gliomas, which comprise isolated tumor cells within intact functioning eloquent parenchyma, require a tissue diagnosis by means of stereotactic biopsy. No further surgery should be attempted in these lesions. Treatment with radiation and/or chemotherapy is controversial in low-grade gliomas but is usually administered in fibrillary astrocytomas or, when signs of anaplasia are apparent on histologic review of the surgical specimens.

Many surgically resectable low-grade gliomas, usually noted in the pediatric age group, are deep-seated and not infrequently are located in the thalamus, hypothalamus, and basal ganglia. With nonstereotactic craniotomy, these lesions may be difficult to find, and it may also be difficult to ascertain where tumor stops and normal brain begins. Nonetheless, most pilocytic and nonpilocytic low-grade gliomas are clearly visible on CT and MRI. CT and MRI provide precise 3-dimensional databases, which can easily be incorporated into a stereotactic coordinate system. Volumetric stereotaxis provides a means of locating, staying oriented within, and identifying the imaging-defined histologic planes at open surgical resection procedures.

Imaging-based stereotactic volumetric resections are useful for the resection of superficial as well as deep-seated lesions. In volumetric stereotaxis, a CT- and MRI-defined tumor volume is represented in stereotactic space. This information is reformatted and displayed to the surgeon. Technical innovations have increased the facility and accuracy with which these operations are performed. In particular an operating-room computer system and appropriate software are used for the transposition of volumetric information derived from axial stereotactic CT scans and MRIs into 3-dimensional space and to display the position of stereotactically directed instruments in relation to computer-generated reconstructions of the tumor volume.

COMPUTER-ASSISTED STEREOTACTIC VOLUMETRIC RESECTION

Volumetric stereotaxis is a method for gathering, storing, and reformatting imaging-derived 3-dimensional volumetric information, defining an intracranial lesion with respect to the surgical field (13–16, 19, 20). With this technique a surgeon can plan and simulate the surgical procedure beforehand to reach deep-seated or centrally located brain tumors, using the safest and least invasive route possible.

Most importantly, this computer-generated information is displayed to the surgeon intra-operatively on computer monitors in the operating room and into a "heads-up display unit" (similar to that used in jet fighter aircraft), mounted on the operating microscope. These images, which provide a CT- and MRI-defined map of the surgical field, are scaled to the actual size and location. This map guides the surgeon in finding and defining the boundaries of brain tumors for more complete and safer removal of the lesions. The computer-generated images are indexed (registered) to the surgical field by means of robotics-controlled stereotactic frame, which positions the patient's tumor within a defined targeting area.

Volumetric stereotaxis allows the smallest possible skin incision, craniotomy openings, and brain incisions, which minimizes injury to normal brain tissue. A more complete tumor removal can be accomplished with much less risk to surrounding brain tissue, because the surgeon knows exactly where tumor ends and normal brain begins. In our experience the postoperative neurologic results are better than those associated with conventional (nonstereotactic, nonvolumetric) surgical techniques for similar lesions. The method has been well described elsewhere (13, 20) and will be outlined briefly below.

METHODS

Database Acquisition

A CT/MRI-compatible stereotactic headframe, applied under local anesthesia, is attached to the patient's skull by means of four-flanged carbon fiber pins inserted through drill holes made in the outer table of the skull. A detachable micrometer registration system allows removal of the head holder following data acquisition and accurate replacement for surgery. A pre-operative database comprising stereotactic CT, MRI, and digital angiography (DA) is acquired. These studies use imaging localization systems that have been reported on previously.

CT, MRI, and DA data are transferred by data link from the imaging host computers to the operating-room computer system (COM-PASS, Admiral Series; Stereotactic Medical Systems, Inc., Rochester, MN). The surgeon traces around the contours of the tumor detected on serial CT slices and MRIs. These slices are suspended within a 3-dimensional computer image matrix that corresponds directly to the coordinate system of the stereotactic frame. An interpolation program creates intermediate slices between the digitized slices and then fills these slices in with cubic voxels, thus creating a volume in abstract stereotactic space.

Surgical Planning

Slices through the CT- and MRI-defined lesional volume scaled to the proper image size can also be displayed in the correct location within the stereoscopic angiogram or upon a map of the brain sulci and fissures derived from the stereoscopic angiogram so that a surgical viewline, defined in arc and collar stereotactic arc-quadrant settings, is then selected on the display screen. In general the viewline defines the surgical approach from the surface of the brain to the tumor in a direction that is parallel to major white matter fibers and that spares important brain tissue and vascular structures.

This volume can be sliced perpendicular to the intended surgical viewline to present to the surgeon the appearance of the lesion as it will be encountered at surgery. All of this data can be displayed within a shaded graphics rendition of the patient's skull that has been extracted from the stereotactic CT scan. Such displays are used in surgical simulations for planning the stereotactic trajectory to an intracranial lesion so as to approach and extract a tumor in the safest possible manner.

Surgical Procedures

These procedures use a COMPASS stereotactic frame, a heads-up video display terminal that is attached to the operating microscope, a carbon dioxide laser system, and various custom microsurgical instruments that have been designed specifically for these surgical procedures. The COMPASS stereotactic frame is basically a Cartesian robotics system in which the patient's head, fixed in the stereotactic head holder, is moved in X, Y, and Z space by a stepper motor-controlled 3-dimensional slide system to position the intracranial target volume in the isocenter of a fixed arc-quadrant. Surgical trajectories are expressed in terms of settings on the arc-quadrant: collar (angle from the horizontal plane) and arc (angle from the vertical plane) angles.

Computer-generated images of the imaging-defined tumor volume sliced perpendicularly to the surgical approach trajectory are projected into a heads-up display unit mounted on the operating microscope. These images are scaled to the exact size of the surgical field viewed through the operating microscope and are superimposed upon it. Thus, during these procedures, the surgeon views not only the surgical field itself but also a computer-generated rendition of what that surgical field should look like based on the CT, MRI, and DA data bases.

The carbon dioxide surgical laser is useful in vaporizing tissue from a deep cavity into which there is limited access. This is very appropriate in the stereotactic approach to and resection of deep-seated neoplasms, which are removed through stereotactically directed retractors 140-cm long but no more than 2 cm in diameter.

Computer-assisted stereotactic resections can be performed in superficial and deep-seated lesions. In superficial lesions a circular trephine is turned on a stereotactically placed cranial pilot hole centered over the lesion. The trephine must be slightly larger than the largest cross sectional diameter of the CT/MRI-defined tumor slice. The trephine defect, having a known configuration and size, serves as a reference structure for indexing of the scaled image within the heads-up display of the operating microscope. The computer-generated image of the trephine with respect to the CT/MRI-defined tumor volume is superimposed over the actual trephine in the surgical field viewed through the operating microscope (Fig. 25.9). Thus the computer-generated tumor slice images serve as a template which guides the dis-

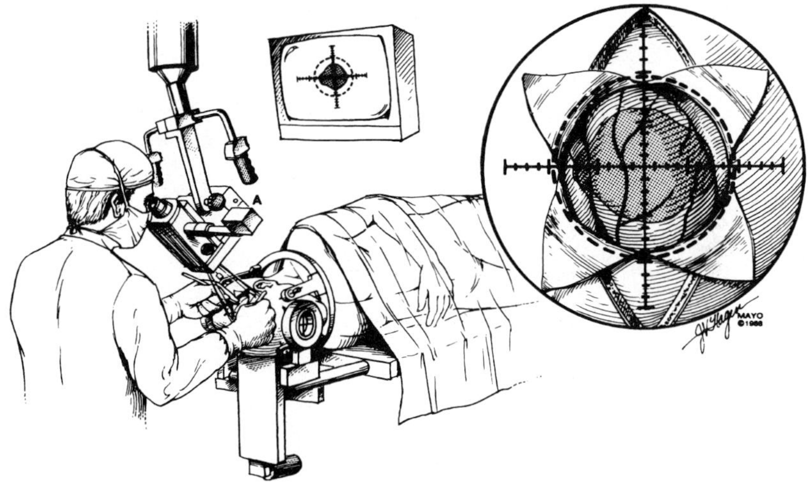

FIG. 25.9 Method for the stereotactic resection of a superficial tumor. A trephine opening of the skull is performed, centered on a pilot hole drilled by means of the stereotactic frame. The computer displays the position of a tumor slice in proper position with respect to the location of the trephine at a specified distance along the viewline on the display monitor and into the "heads-up" display unit of the operating microscope (A). The image is scaled in the heads-up display and the microscope moved until the configuration of the trephine in the image display is exactly the same size as the actual trephine in the surgical field and aligns to the trephine. The surgeon then uses the tumor slice image as a template, which will aid in identification of the surgical plane between CT/MRI-defined tumor and surrounding brain tissue. This facilitates isolation of the tumor from surrounding brain tissue [Reproduced with permission from (13).]

section around subcortical tumors and facilitates identification of the plane between the lesion and the surrounding brain parenchyma.

Deep-seated lesions are resected by means of a stereotactically directed cylindrical retractor, which is inserted through a dilated cortical and subcortical white matter incision (Fig. 25.10). The incision is made, using the carbon dioxide laser and is dilated by means of the retractor-dilator system. The configuration of the deep end of the retractor is represented in the computer-generated slice images so that this may be superimposed over the actual surgical field by means of the heads-up display unit on the operating microscope. In practice a plane is developed between tumor and surrounding brain tissue before the lesion is vaporized with a high-powered defocused carbon dioxide laser. Lesions which are much larger than the retractor can be removed by multiple image translations on the display screen which result in the calculation of new stereotactic coordinates. These, once executed on the stereotactic slide system, position a new part of the tumor under the stereotactic retractor. A plane can then be developed between tumor

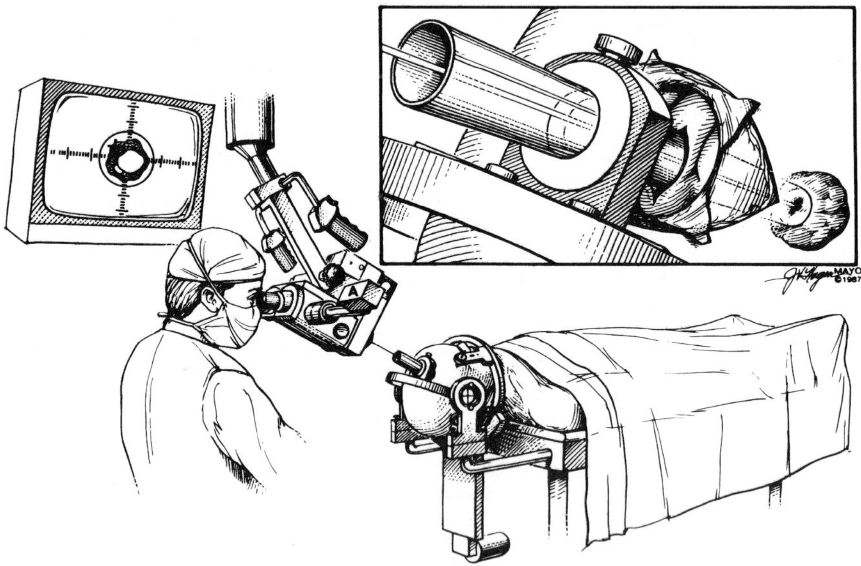

FIG. 25.10 The stereotactic cylindrical retractor is used during the resection of deep-seated lesions. The computer displays the configuration of a cross section of the retractor (*inset*) with respect to a selected slice through the tumor volume cut perpendicularly to the surgical viewline. This information is displayed on a computer monitor in the operating room as well as in the "heads-up" display unit of the operating microscope (*A*). [Reproduced with permission from (13).]

and brain for some distance beyond the retractor using the computer-generated slice images depicting the CT/MRI-defined limits and the image of the retractor as a guide. Once the lesion has been isolated from surrounding brain tissue, it can be removed piecemeal with biopsy forceps, defocused carbon dioxide laser, or suction.

Technical Aspects in the Resection of Low-Grade Gliomas

To prevent the shifting of intracranial structures following dural opening and approaches to stereotactically defined intracranial lesions, the following precautions are necessary. In the absence of hydrocephalus and cystic tumors, dural relaxation can usually be achieved by elevating the head of the operating table (reverse Trendelenburg table position) and hyperventilation in order to keep the arterial pCO_2 about 25 mm Hg. Spinal drainage and hyperosmotic agents should never be used in stereotactic tumor resections. In more than 1100 stereotactic tumor resection procedures, the author has never found it necessary to use either mannitol or spinal drainage to achieve satisfactory brain relaxation.

The trephine craniotomy should also be put in the least dependent position of the surgical field. This is accomplished by rotating the patient's head in the stereotactic head holder so that the arc angle approximates zero, with a target and entry point trajectory calculation yielding a zero arc angle, and recalculating and setting the target coordinates to account for that rotation. The collar angle can be compensated by reverse Trendelenburg table position, which will raise the patients head. The trephine craniotomy will then be at the least dependent position within the surgical field. This is similar to the opening of a jar of liquid that is held upright: the contents of the jar stay in place after the lid of the jar has been removed. So, too, will the contents of the cranial vault remain in place unless the ventricle or tumor cyst is entered and fluid lost.

In cystic tumors, intraventricular tumors, or those near the ventricular system, the monitoring of possible movements of the tumor during the procedure may be necessary. This is accomplished by using a series of 0.5-mm stainless steel reference balls, which are deposited at 5-mm intervals along the surgical viewline in the tumor by a stereotactically directed biopsy cannula inserted through a ⅛-inch drill hole in the skull. Anteroposterior and lateral radiographs are obtained (Fig. 25.11). The position of these steel balls on subsequent radiographs after exposure of the lesion may indicate shifts in the position of the tumor that can be adjusted in the computer software for updated accurate tumor slice images.

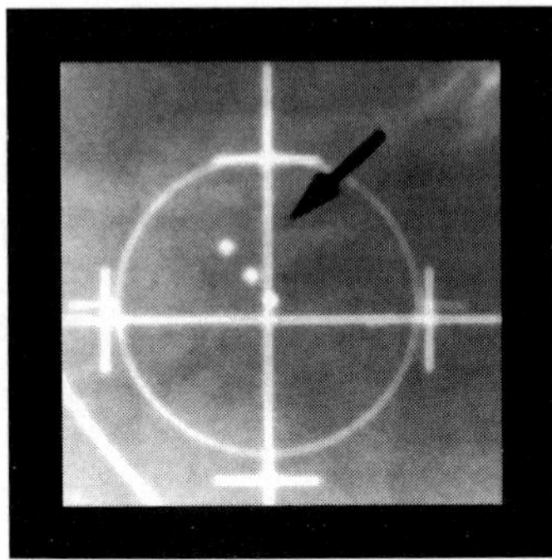

FIG. 25.11 In cystic tumors, radiographically opaque marker balls are placed by stereotactic probe prior to craniotomy and approach to the tumor. Movements of the stainless steel reference balls documented by subsequent stereotactic x-ray pictures can be measured, and the CT/MRI-defined tumor volume can be shifted in the computer matrix accordingly for updated slice images, which account for possible movements of the tumor volume within the cranial cavity.

In contrast to standard intra-axial tumor resection techniques, in which an internal decompression is done before trying to dissect the edges free from surrounding brain, in stereotactic resection the tumor edges are separated from brain tissue before the central mass of the tumor is entered. If the tumor is too large for complete isolation from surrounding brain tissue (usually encountered in the resection of large deep tumors through a stereotactically directed cylindrical retractor), the superficial aspects of the lesion are dissected free of surrounding brain, then removed layer by layer, progressing from the most superficial to the deepest (Fig. 25.12). The purpose of the volumetric stereotactic technique is to facilitate identification of a plane between tumor and surrounding brain tissue. However, the tumor must remain intact for as long as possible; otherwise, the brain around it can fill into the cavity produced by internal decompression.

RESULTS

A series of 1165 patients underwent computer-assisted volumetric stereotactic resection procedures performed at the Mayo Clinic and New York University Medical Center in the 10-year period between August 1984 and December 1994 (Mayo 8/84 to 7/93; NYU 9/93 to 12/94) Of these, 268 volumetric stereotactic resections were performed on 264 patients harboring low-grade gliomas. Histologic subtypes and pre-operative and postoperative neurologic examination results with morbidity and mortality rates are provided in Table 25.2.

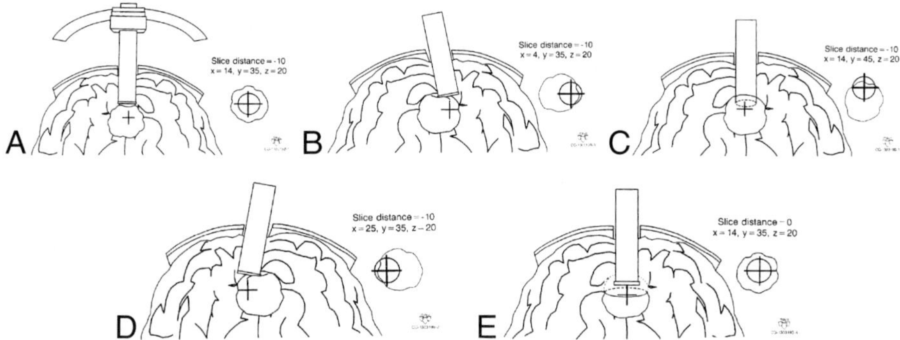

FIG. 25.12 **(A)** Method of stereotactic removal of a larger, deep-seated tumor, through a stereotactically directed retractor 2 cm in diameter. A computer image demonstrates the limits of the lesion defined by CT and MRI. The configuration of the retractor is shown on the computer-generated tumor outline. **(B)** The image is translated on the computer screen to place the edge of the tumor under the edge of the retractor. New stereotactic coordinates are calculated. The surgeon then develops a plane between tumor and surrounding brain tissue, using the sequential slice images as a guide. In this example, the plane of dissection can be created around the right side of the tumor. **(C)** After developing a plane between the tumor and surrounding brain on the right side of the tumor to a level of 10 to 15 mm beyond the end of the stereotactic retractor, the retractor is withdrawn to the superficial aspect of the tumor, and the lesion image is translated on the computer screen. New stereotactic co-ordinates are calculated on the computer and executed on the stereotactic frame. Then the surgeon creates a plane of dissection between tumor and brain on the posterior aspect of the tumor. **(D)** The position of the tumor relative to the retractor has been changed again in order to develop a plane of dissection between the left side of the tumor and surrounding brain tissue. **(E)** After circumscribing the superficial aspects of the tumor for distance for about 10 to 15 mm beyond the end of the retractor, the superficial aspects of the tumor are vaporized slice by slice by a CO_2 laser progressing from the most superficial slices to the deepest. The retractor is then advanced to this level, and the remainder of the tumor is separated from surrounding brain tissue by means of the translation procedure listed above.

Two deaths occurred within 1 month of surgery: one from massive brainstem edema after removal of a ventral thalamic mixed pilocytic/fibrillary astrocytoma in a 30-year-old man, the other a 28-year-old woman who underwent a herniation syndrome and died because of a subdural hygroma, which had developed 2½ weeks after resection of a large intraventricular neurocytoma. There was one infection: an abscess in the resection bed, which occurred in a 15-year-old boy following removal of a partially cystic pleomorphic xanthoastrocytoma, in which a cyst catheter to an Ommaya reservoir drainage system had been placed at another institution. This patient responded to drainage, debridement, and appropriate antibiotics. He was neurologically intact pre- and postoperatively and has had no long-term sequela from his infection.

TABLE 25.2

Histologies, Pre- and Postoperative Neurologic Examination, Mortality, and Morbidity following 268 Stereotactic Volumetric Resections for Low-Grade Gliomas

	Pre-operative		Postoperative					
Lesion	Resections	Normal (Seizures)	Deficit	Improved	Unchanged	Worse (Dead)	Morbidity (%)	Mortality (%)
Astrocytoma								
Grade II	27	17 (1)	10	9	12	6	22	
Grade I	6	6(4)		1	5			
Pilocytic	97	36 (6)	61	44	46	7(1)	7.2	1.1
Oligodendroglioma	47	43 (23)	4	2	43	2	4.25	
Oligo-astrocytoma	33	23 (17)	10	14	17	2	6.1	
Subependymoma	12	9	3	4	8			
Ependymoma	12	9(2)	3	1	11			
Neurocytoma	4	2	2	1	2	1 (1)		25
Ganglioglioma	19	14 (5)	5	4	14	1		
Xanthoastrocytoma	2	2 (1)		1	1			
Tuberous sclerosis	9	8 (8)	1	8	1			
Totals	268	169 (67)	99	89	160	19 (2)	7.08%	0.75%

Of the 268 patients, 169 were neurologically normal on pre-operative examination (67 of these had medically intractable seizures); 99 additional patients had a documented neurologic deficit. Postoperatively, 160 patients were neurologically unchanged when examined prior to hospital discharge. Neurologic improvement, in comparison to the pre-operative level, was documented in the 3-month follow-up exam in 78 of the 99 patients in whom a pre-operative neurologic deficit had been noted.

Nineteen additional patients were neurologically worse when examined at the time of hospital discharge or at 2 weeks following the procedure (morbidity, 7.08%). At the 3-month postoperative exam 6 had returned to their neurologic pre-operative baseline; 4 of these had neurologic deficits that initially were worse following surgery but had improved to a level better than that their pre-operative examination had documented. Included in these 19 patients were 7 patients who experienced a contralateral superior quadrantanopsia, which followed a transcortical approach to mesial posterior temporal (5 patients) or ventral posterior thalamic (2 patients) lesions. The remaining four patients had a hemiparesis following surgery, from which they recovered to a functional level (all were able to walk) but not to their pre-operative neurologic examination level.

Specific Tumor Types

PILOCYTIC ASTROCYTOMAS

Ninety-seven procedures were performed on 93 patients harboring pilocytic astrocytomas. The mean age of the patients was 19 years (range, 2 to 47 years). Four procedures were repeated for residual tumor in two patients, recurrent tumor in another, and a new tumor in a fourth patient. Tumor locations were as follows: thalamus in 35 patients (right, 18; left, 17), midbrain in 12 patients, basal ganglia in 9 patients (right, 3; left, 6), Lateral ventricle in 4 patients (right, 1, left, 3), septum pellucidum in 2 patients, third ventricle in 2 patients, hypothalamus in 2 patients, posterior hippocampus in 7 patients (right, 2; left, 5), deep cerebellum, including middle cerebellar peduncle, in 12 patients, and various other subcortical locations, including mesial parieto-occipital in 6 patients (right, 2; left, 4) and posterior frontal-central in 6 patients (right, 2; left, 4).

Postoperative contrast-enhanced imaging studies confirmed a complete or gross total tumor resection in 86 patients (Fig. 25.13) with a less than 10% residual in 8 others and a 25% or greater residual in the remaining 3 patients. The pre-operative examination revealed that 36 patients were neurologically normal, whereas 61 patients had a neurologic deficit (see Table 25.2). Postoperatively, 46 patients were neu-

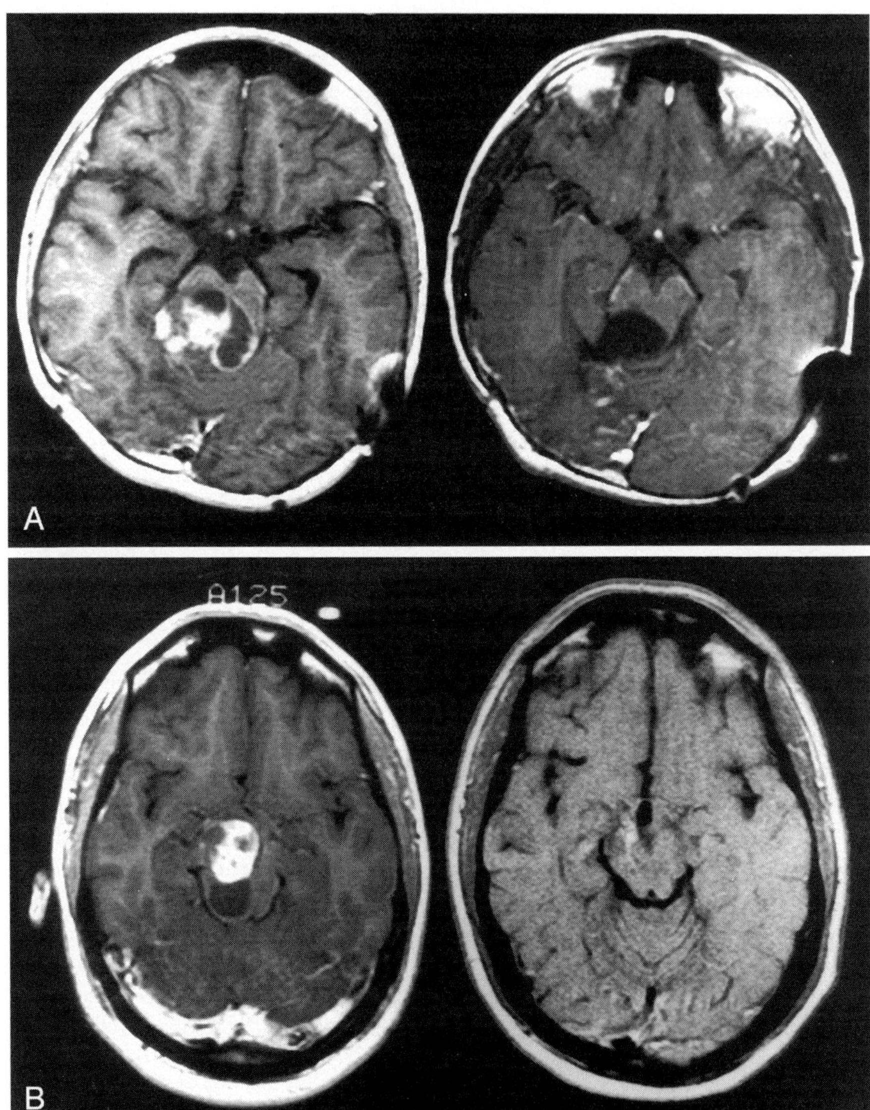

FIG. 25.13   Pre-operative (*left*) and 3 months postoperative (*right*). Gadolinium-enhanced MRI scans. (**A**) Pilocytic astrocytoma of the dorsal midbrain in a 12-year-old boy. (**B**) Pilocytic astrocytoma with cyst in the anterior midbrain/ventral right thalamus in a 20-year-old man. Neither of these patients had neurologic deficits following surgery. Both patients are now neurologically normal 3 years (**A**) and 3 years and 3 months (**B**) postoperatively.

rologically unchanged; 44 were neurologically improved; and 7 were worse at time of hospital discharge or 2 weeks following surgery. Two of these sustained a contralateral superior quadrantanopsia following a posterior temporal transcortical approach to ventral thalamic lesions. Four others had worsening of a pre-operatively noted hemiparesis due to lesions that extended to or invaded the internal capsule. One patient with a very mild hemiparesis pre-operatively, with a cystic lesion in the left ventral thalamus and midbrain, sustained a moderately severe right hemiparesis postoperatively. She ultimately made a satisfactory recovery and walks almost normally but notes distal weakness in the right hand. There was one death in the postoperative period, a man with a mixed pilocytic/fibrillary astrocytoma, which is discussed in more detail above.

Thirty four additional patients underwent stereotactic biopsies of what was found to be a pilocytic astrocytoma. Aspiration of a cyst was accomplished concurrent with the biopsy in six patients, and a third ventriculostomy was performed to treat hydrocephalus in two others. One additional patient underwent a ventriculoperitoneal shunt. Seventeen of these patients subsequently underwent stereotactic volumetric resection and are included in the above statistics. Two had their cyst treated with intracavitary radionuclide above statistics. Two had their cyst treated with intracavitary radionuclide (colloidal $_{32}$P). An additional three patients unwilling to accept the risk of volumetric resection underwent external beam irradiation therapy at other institutions.

MISCELLANEOUS WELL-CIRCUMSCRIBED LESIONS

This group of 58 patients had the following 12 subependymomas, 12 low-grade ependymomas, 4 neurocytomas, 19 gangliogliomas, 2 xanthoastrocytomas, and 9 superficial lesions associated with seizures and the clinical syndrome of tuberosclerosis. This group is lumped together, because the lesions were histologically well circumscribed, biologically indolent, and could be resected without much difficulty, using the volumetric stereotactic technique. The subependymoma patients fell within two age bands: mean age 11 years with a range 5 to 16 years ($n = 7$) and 52 years with a range of 47 to 68 years ($n = 5$). All of the younger patients had tuberosclerosis (TS); there was no sign of TS in the older patients. All of the lesions were at the foramen of Monro (right, 8; left, 4) and were either obstructing the foramen, or obstruction appeared imminent. The adult patients had much larger lesions than the younger patients (Fig. 25.14). All of these lesions were removed without any neurologic morbidity.

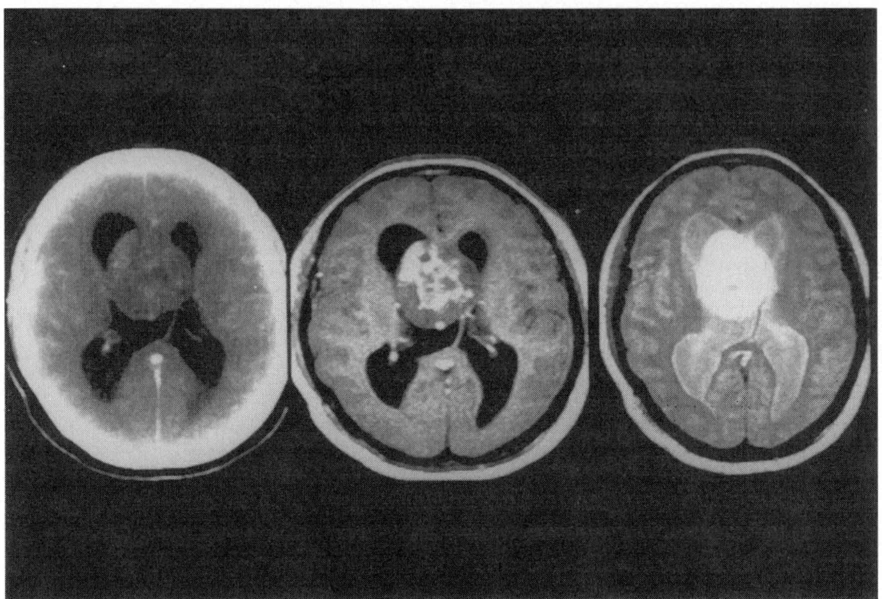

FIG. 25.14 Giant subependymoma in a 47-year-old Chinese-American female, causing obstruction of the foramen of Monro. This lesion was easily resected, and the patient recovered with no postoperative neurologic deficit.

Low-grade ependymomas were also resected without much difficultly, with good postoperative results and no morbidity. There were two age ranges; 4 to 20 years (7 patients, mean 13 years) and 32 to 47 years (5 patients, mean 37 years). Lesions were located in the left frontal lobe in three patients, the posterior third ventricle in two patients, and one each in left basal frontal, left thalamus, right occipital, right subinsular, left lateral ventricle, left central, and laterally in the cerebellar hemisphere. All of these lesions were completely resected without postoperative morbidity.

There were four neurocytomas resected, three from the right and one from the left lateral ventricle. All patients were neurologically intact following the procedure. However, one patient, a 28-year-old-woman with an extensive lesion involving the frontal horn and body of the right lateral ventricle and third ventricle with obstructive hydrocephalus, underwent two procedures: the first for the lateral ventricular component; the second for a more aggressive resection of the third ventricular component several weeks after when her hydrocephalus persisted. A small subdural hygroma was noted on CT when she was discharged within a week following the second procedure. She was

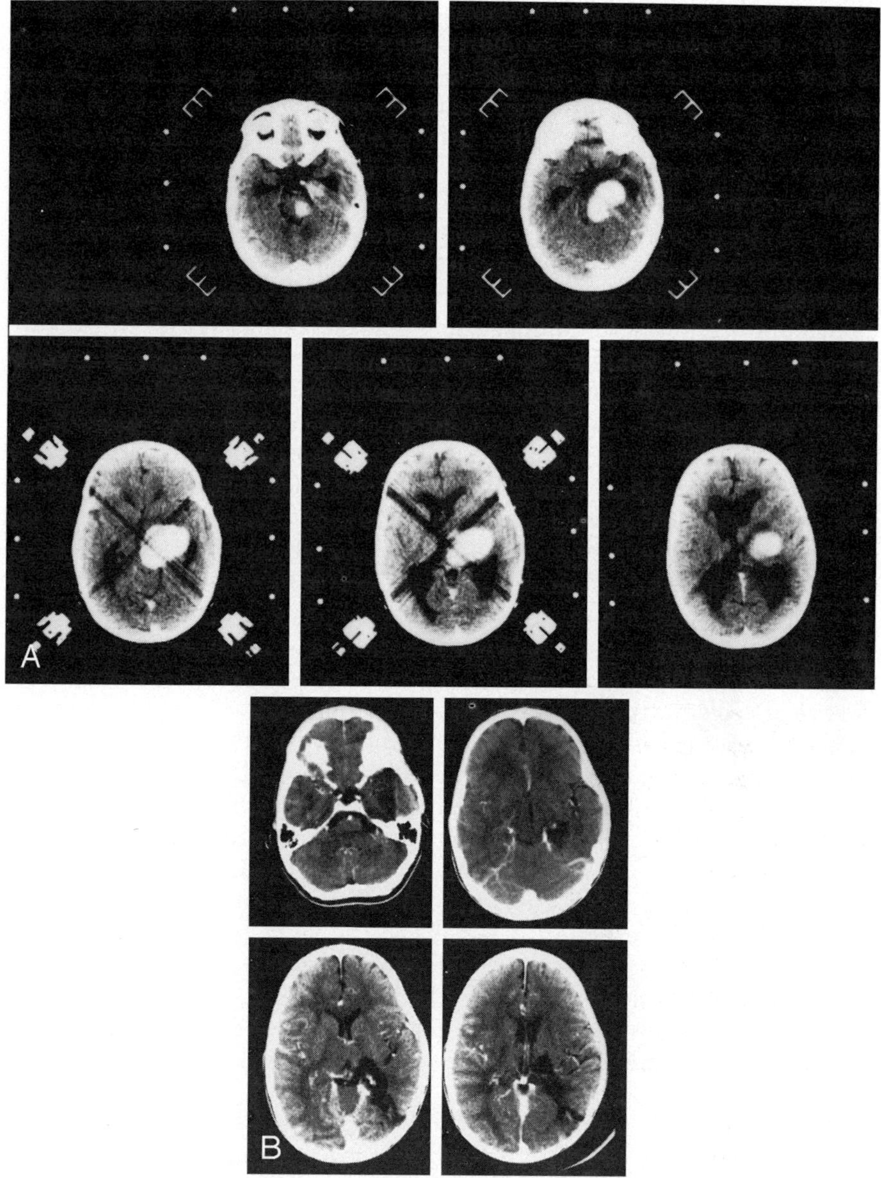

FIG. 25.15 A 32-year-old man presenting with seizures and increasing right hemiparesis with a giant ganglioglioma involving the posterior thalamus and lateral basal ganglia, as well as an exophytic component that extended out the choriodal fissure and into the posterior fossa. (**B**) Postoperative contrast-enhanced CT scan, demonstrating complete resection of the lesion.

taken to a local hospital 2 weeks later in a coma; the subdural hygroma had enlarged and caused her to herneate during the night. She died shortly thereafter.

Of the 19 patients harboring ganglioglioma, 5 of the 7 patients with gangliogliomas in the mesial temporal lobe (right, 3; left, 4) presented with medically intractable seizures. All had excellent seizure control (on medication) following stereotactic resection at 1-year follow-up. Some of these lesions were very large but could be completely removed (Fig. 25.15). Other patients presented with mass effect, including four lesions in the posterior frontal area, two in the left basal ganglia, two in the pons, and one in the thalamus. There was one lesion in the left caudate head, causing mild unilateral hydrocephalus. There were two other large lesions in the cerebral hemispheres, causing midline shift. The results of surgery in this group were excellent. One patient, however, a 32-year-old woman from Germany, had undergone multiple operations, radiation therapy, and interstitial irradiation for an "anaplastic astrocytoma" in the left basal ganglia. She presented with progressive right hemiparesis, an enlarging cyst, and a contrast-enhancing lesion 5 cm in diameter. The lesion was completely resected. The patient had a dense right hemiparesis post-operatively but went on to make an impressive recovery over the next several months and is now at a better neurologic level than she was pre-operatively, with imaging studies showing no evidence of residual tumor.

Nine patients with tuberosclerosis underwent resection of subcortical tubers, causing medically intractable seizures in eight patients and mass effect in another. These lesions were well delineated by MRI, were immediately subcortical, and removal was straightforward without postoperative morbidity. Similarly, two young patients (ages 15 and 19 years) with xanthoastrocytomas underwent gross total stereotactic volumetric resection of lesions in the right temporal/basal ganglia area and right superior parietal lobule, respectively. There were no postoperative neurologic sequellae. However, the 15-year-old patient developed an abscess in the resection and cyst bed, as described above, that responded to drainage and appropriate antibiotics.

INFILTRATING GLIOMAS (TYPES II AND III)

The information provided below presents the author's experience in the resection of gliomas composed mostly of isolated tumor cells within intact parenchyma. The number of patients undergoing stereotactic biopsy procedures for each histologic type is also presented. Note that the percentage of patients suitable for resection is relatively small in comparison to the percentage of patients who undergo stereotactic biopsy in each group. This should indicate that not all patients are good candidates for resection, even with stereotactic volumetric technology, and that the patients undergoing resection are well selected, utilizing the guidelines described above.

NONPILOCYTIC ASTROCYTOMAS

One-hundred fifty-seven patients with low-grade astrocytomas underwent stereotactic procedures between August 1984 and December 1994. Most of these were stereotactic biopsies only. There were few volumetric excisions. In fact, only 33 patients with low-grade astrocytomas underwent volumetric excision for lesions: in the posterior frontal lobe in 10 patients (right, 4; left, 6), the parietal lobe in 2 patients (right, 1; left, 1), the left temporoparietal area in 1 patient, the right occipital lobe in 1 patient, the posterior medial temporal lobe in 11 patients (left, 7; right, 4), the thalamus in 3 patients (left, 2; right, 1), the cerebellum in 2 patients, and the pons in 1 patient. Patients who underwent volumetric excision of lesions in the thalamus had undergone a previous stereotactic serial biopsy that revealed an unusual tumor comprised mostly of solid tumor tissue.

The pontine lesion was in a 4-year-old girl who had undergone empirical irradiation for a glioma. She presented with an enlarging contrast-enhancing mass which, when examined following resection, proved to be a grade II astrocytoma with radiation changes. She ultimately died 8 months later of either progressive tumor or radiation necrosis.

Five pre-operatively neurologically intact patients had some neurologic deficit postoperatively: four of them had superior temporal quadrantanopsia contralateral to a transcortical approach to posterior medial temporal lesions (the author has since adopted a subtemporo-occipital approach to these lesions). Two others (one normal pre-operatively, the other with a hemiparesis) had a contralateral hemiparesis or worsening of a hemiparesis following resection of precentral lesions.

OLIGOASTROCYTOMAS

Of 106 patients harboring low-grade oligoastrocytomas undergoing stereotactic tumor procedures, only 33 underwent volumetric resection; the remainder had stereotactic biopsy only. Nineteen patients had posterior frontal lesions (right, 12; left, 7); four had posterior medial temporal lesions (right, 3; left, 1); six had posterior lateral temporal lesions (right, 2; left, 4); two had basal ganglia lesions (right, 1; left, 1) that were partially resected; and two had right central cingulate lesions. As shown in Table 25.2, two of these patients were worse following surgery—one had a worsened hemiparesis following partial resection of a basal ganglia lesion; the other had a new hemiparesis following resection of a posterior frontal precentral lesion. Histologically, all of these lesions were type I or type II in character, and their resection involved resection of intact but infiltrated brain parenchyma.

OLIGODENDROGLIOMAS

Forty-seven of 142 patients with low-grade oligodendrogliomas underwent stereotactic resection. Stereotactic biopsies were performed in the remainder. Resected lesions were in the posterior frontal area in 27 patients (right, 12; left, 15), the superior parietal lobule in 6 (right, 3; left, 3), under the central sulcus in three (right, 1; left, 2), deep to the cingulate gyrus in four (right, 2; left, 2); one in the septum pellucidum (see Fig. 25.11), one in the left thalamus and one in the middle cerebellar peduncle, and four in other locations (left temporoparietal, deep left occipital, posterolateral right temporal lobe, and left hippocampus). Two patients were neurologically worse: a 22-year-old man with a right inferior quadrantanopsia following removal of a left supracalcarine lesion and a 36-year-old man with a slightly worsened, pre-operatively noted right hemiparesis following removal of a partially cystic, partially calcified tumor in the left thalamus. This lesion had been noted to progressively enlarge over a 4-year period despite empirical radiation therapy delivered at another institution. Only four of these resected tumors were composed of solid tumor tissue only; the rest had small nests of tumor tissue residing within a field of tumor cell-infiltrated parenchyma.

DISCUSSION

The selection of low-grade glioma patients for surgical procedures requires an understanding of the growth patterns of each individual lesion. Not all low-grade gliomas are resectable: a lesion comprised almost entirely of isolated tumor cells within intact parenchyma located in an eloquent brain area is not a resectable lesion. Although any CT/MRI-defined tumor volume is theoretically removable with computer-assisted stereotactic technologies, the risk of deficit in these lesions far exceeds the supposed benefit. In addition a low-grade glioma of type II (solid tumor tissue surrounded by infiltrated parenchyma) located in eloquent brain is also a nonresectable lesion: the solid tumor tissue will be indistinguishable from the infiltrated parenchyma on CT, MRI, and probably at surgery as well. Type I tumors (solid tumor tissue only) in most cortical and subcortical locations and type II and type III tumors located in nonessential brain tissue are usually resectable with low morbidity.

The benefit of resection in low-grade gliomas depends on cell type, age of the patient (which may relate, in part, to the cell type), location of the lesion, and neurologic condition of the patient (3, 7, 21, 22, 25, 28). Within defined tumor cell types, differences in benefit can be noted: resection of a basal ganglionic pilocytic astrocytoma with increasing size on serial imaging studies and progressive neurologic deficit will be great; the benefit for resection of a similar lesion in an asymptomatic patient that does not enlarge on serial imaging studies is questionable. The major problem in many of these decisions is our inability to predict which lesions will grow and/or undergo malignant transformation. There are only three ways to predict course of illness: histology, labeling indices, and clinical behavior over time.

Histologic studies with retrospective correlations to survival have been of some value: astrocytomas seem more aggressive than mixed gliomas, which have a greater likelihood of malignant transformation than pure oligodendrogliomas (31, 32, 36). Pilocytic and microcystic astrocytomas are reported to have a better prognosis than any of the above (2, 3, 20, 24, 31, 36). Ganglioneuromas and subependymomas are thought to be relatively indolent (26). Xanthoastrocytomas are also very slow-growing and a high percentage can be cured surgically (37). An entire class of cortically based indolent lesions referred to as dysembryoplastic neuroepithelial tumors can be confused with oligodendrogliomas, mixed gliomas, and anaplastic astrocytomas (4).

Unlike high-grade gliomas, which rarely cause a problem in histologic interpretation, there seems to be no uniformity among pathologists in calling cell type and grade in low-grade gliomas. Patients and families not infrequently request "second opinions" on most physician judgment calls—including the histologic interpretation of the surgical specimen. Low-grade gliomas open a Pandora's box, with wide variation in interpretations between pathologists. It has been the author's not altogether uncommon, but nevertheless unsettling, experience to have a low-grade glioma interpreted as a grade II astrocytoma by one neuropathologist, as an anaplastic astrocytoma by another, as a "low-grade oligoastrocytoma" by a third, as a "low-grade oligodendroglioma with reactive astrogliosis" by a fourth, as a ganglioglioneurocytoma by a fifth, and as a DNE by a sixth neuropathologist.

Grading systems between institutions are nonuniform. Some neuropathologists prefer a simple three-tiered classification scheme: low-grade, anaplastic, and glioblastoma; others prefer a numerical grading system, usually a variation of that proposed by Kernohan. In the three-tiered schemes one mitotic figure (not unusual in very slow-growing, indolent tumors, such as pilocytic astrocytomas, DNEs, or even astrogliosis) will prompt some pathologists to call what ordinarily would be a low-grade astrocytoma an anaplastic astrocytoma. Thus, it is not unusual to have some institutions quote a 10-year mean survival rate for low-grade astrocytoma while others report a mean survival of less than 5 years (7, 25, 31, 35, 36). A uniform grading system for low-grade gliomas is clearly needed so that the natural history, as well as the effects of therapy, can be studied multi-institutionally. The grading system proposed by Daumas-Duport *et al.* (5) in which the cumulative score was derived from defined criteria, such as nuclear abnormalities, mitotic figures, neovascularization, and necrosis, is used to define a grade. This method seems to have the highest degree of concordance among pathologists but applies only to astrocytomas (3).

Labeling indices (by [3H] thymidine (11), bromodeoxyuridine (BUdR) (8, 9, 30), proliferating cell nuclear antigen (PCNA) (23) and 67Ki (39) provide a numerical quantitative value for a tumor that may have prognostic significance in high-grade as well as in low-grade gliomas. Hoshino (10) studied cell kinetics in gliomas by means of a [3H]thymidine-labeled pulse and found that the labeling index in low-grade gliomas was less than 1% in comparison to that of anaplastic astrocytomas, in which the LI was 4.0% (+/−0.8%), and glioblastomas, in which the LI was 9% (+/−1.0%). Autopsy studies showed that low-grade gliomas harbored labeled cells for 2 1/2 to 7 years. He concluded that the higher the LI, the faster the tumor grows.

BUdR labels cells in S-phase and was more dramatic in indication of the level of biologic malignancy (5 to 20% for glioblastomas, as opposed to less than 1% for low-grade and anaplastic gliomas) (9). Hoshino *et al.* (8), in a study of BUdR labeling in 47 patients, found that low-grade gliomas fell within two groups: those with low BUdR LIs and those with high BUdR LIs. Those with high LIs recurred and were associated with shorter survival.

PCNA accumulates in the nucleus during the S-phase of the cell cycle. Immunohistochemical labeling indices for this 36-kilodalton DNA polymerase delta auxiliary protein increase as the grade (Daumas-Duport) of the glioma increases (23). Louis *et al.* found that low-grade gliomas had a PCNA labeling index of less then or equal to 1%.

Similarly, Ki67 recognizes a nuclear antigen expressed by proliferating cells. In low-grade gliomas the LI with Ki67 is significantly less than in anaplastic astrocytomas or glioblastoma (27, 34, 39). However, considerable variability in LI is noted within individual specimens obtained along a biopsy tract within the same tumor (0.0 to 12%) (27). Interestingly, pilocytic astrocytomas were found to have a high Ki67 labeling index (5.6%) in comparison to nonpilocytic low-grade astrocytomas (Ki67 LI less than 1) (27, 37).

Unfortunately, there are two major problems with labeling indices in low-grade gliomas. First, most adult low-grade gliomas are infiltrating tumors, isolated tumor cells that permeate intact brain parenchyma. The number of labelled cells must be divided by the total number of tumor cells in a microscopic field. The identification and counting of isolated tumor cells within a field of reactive astrocytes in a paraffin section is difficult, if not impossible. Smear preparations, though not routinely done, facilitate the identification of isolated tumor cells in distinction to background elements and gliosis (6). Nonetheless, it should be noted that low-grade and anaplastic fibrillary astrocytomas (where the denominator may have included a significant number of normal and astrogliotic cells) had lower BUdR and Ki67 labelling indices in comparison to pilocytic astrocytomas (composed of tumor tissue only) despite the fact that pilocytic astrocytoma is a much more slowly growing neoplasm (9, 34). In addition, labeling indices do not account for cells that undergo apoptosis and balance off the number of cells undergoing mitosis, so that the net result is tumor stability-no growth. This is probably the case with dysembryoplastic neuroepithelial tumors wherein labeling indices can be as high as in malignant glial neoplasms, yet the lesions are totally benign and do not enlarge when followed over time (4).

The Benefit of Treatment

With the advent of CT and MRI, low-grade gliomas are now detected much more commonly than ever before. In addition, they are also being detected earlier. Piepmeier (28) reported that patients presenting for treatment in the past 10 years survive longer following "diagnosis" than those presenting for treatment in pre-CT era. He noted that a higher percentage of his study population of 60 patients had a normal neurologic examination and total resection of their lesions. Medbery *et al.* (25) noted better survival in post-CT era patients but also noted that less radiation was given in the pre-CT era and concluded that the improved survival was due to the increased dose of radiation. Shaw *et al.* (31, 32) also lumped pre- and post-CT era patients together to arrive at similar conclusions regarding the efficacy of higher radiation dosages in low-grade gliomas. However, studies comprising a large group of patients, gathered over a time during which a significant advance in technology (such as CT scanning, microsurgery, or tumor stereotaxis) has occurred, should be interpreted with caution.

Each low-grade glioma cell type may be associated with fixed-length survival. Lesions diagnosed earlier in their clinical course by means of modern imaging techniques will be associated with longer survival times than those diagnosed later in their clinical course, as occurred in the pre-CT era. In the pre-CT era, the diagnosis and histologic limits of the tumor had to be inferred from mass effect detected on angiography and pneumoencephalography. No radiologic diagnosis was possible until the tumor exhibited some mass effect, produced elevated intracranial pressure, neurologic deficit, or underwent malignant degeneration, leading to neovascularization, blood-brain barrier breakdown, and uptake on radionuclide scintigrams.

With stereotactic biopsy being so available and relatively safe, few patients now go without a "tissue diagnosis" and referral to radiation or neuro-oncologist. Many undergo radiation therapy and chemotherapy, in some cases inappropriately. Retrospective studies lump together heterogeneous groups of patients gathered form pre- and post-CT eras and consisting of lesions having very different prognoses in attempts to show the efficacy of various forms of treatment on survival (21, 22, 31, 32). However, confounded by "treatment," information on the natural history of low-grade glioma, from which we can determine the benefit of any treatment modality over the natural history of the disease, is lacking.

Surgery

There is little question that resection in pilocytic astrocytomas that are growing and/or producing symptoms should be removed. In addition, xanthoastrocytomas, subependymomas threatening to cause obstructive hydrocephalus, or gangliogliomas and DNEs causing intractable epilepsy can be removed with a significant degree of benefit to the patient. The benefit of resective surgery is raised for low-grade nonpilocytic fibrillary astrocytoma, mixed oligoastrocytoma, and oligodendroglioma.

On a cytokinetic basis, the concept of surgical reduction of tumor burden seems more valid in low-grade gliomas than in high-grade lesions (8, 11). A significant reduction of tumor burden in tumors having only a small percentage of mitotically active and mitotically capable cells should theoretically slow the tumor's growth significantly and reduce the chances of malignant transformation. Unfortunately, a prospective randomized study on survival following resective surgery *versus* biopsy is unlikely: there are probably less than 5000 low-grade gliomas in the United Sates annually with 4200 neurosurgeons willing to operate on them. Accrual in all but the busiest academic centers will be painfully slow, considering that many of these patients have good long-term prognosis a long time before the survival results reach any significant level before interpretation. Nonetheless, the benefit of surgery in low-grade gliomas is difficult to prove, using retrospective data.

Phillippon *et al.* (29), in a retrospective study of 179 adult patients with supratentorial low-grade astrocytomas, found that 80% of patients in whom complete removal of the tumor had been achieved at surgery were alive at 5 years following surgery, as compared to 52% of patients alive 5 years following partial resection and 42% 5 years following biopsy. Berger *et al.* (1) noted that low-grade glioma patients with tumor volumes greater than 10 cm^3 did significantly better following aggressive resection in terms of recurrence and recurrent tumor phenotype than patients who underwent a partial resection or biopsy. Furthermore, patients with a residual tumor volume greater than 10 cm^3 had a higher incidence of recurrence at a higher grade and a shorter time to recurrence than patients with a lesser tumor burden (1). Winger *et al.* (38) noted that survival in high-grade gliomas was better in patients with a past history of a known low-grade tumor than in an anaplastic glioma starting *de novo.*

Certainly, seizure control, when a problem can be improved by resection of a low-grade glioma—the more histologically circumscribed, the better for seizure control (26). Others have noted a positive benefit on length of survival in patients who underwent radical or subtotal removal of low-grade gliomas (21, 22, 31, 32). Vecht (35), based on a review of the literature on surgery and radiation therapy in low-grade gliomas, concluded that surgery and radiation therapy are beneficial only in the group of patients over 35 years of age. However, many of these studies have lumped together a heterogeneous group of patients those with pilocytic and nonpilocytic astrocytomas, xanthoastrocytomas, and DNEs, as well as those presenting with seizures and those presenting with neurologic deficits. Smith *et al.* (33) noted that resective surgery and postoperative radiation therapy provided a survival advantage in patients presenting with neurologic deficit but no benefit in those neurologically normal patients presenting with seizures.

In the author's experience low-grade fibrillary astrocytomas, oligoastrocytomas, and oligodendrogliomas most commonly present with epilepsy. These lesions can be resected only in nonessential brain regions in neurologically intact patients. The appearance of a neurologic deficit in these individuals is frequently associated with malignant transformation of the lesion, the formation of tumor tissue with destruction of the underlying parenchyma, and neovascularization with patches of contrast enhancement on CT and MRI. These lesions can no longer be considered "low-grade."

Radiation Therapy

The role of radiation therapy in the management of low-grade gliomas remains controversial. There are major proponents of radiation therapy in all low-grade fibrillary astrocytomas and mixed oligoastrocytomas (31, 32). Meybery *et al.* (25) in a study of 50 patients noted a significant correlation between postoperative radiation therapy and the dose of radiation therapy on survival. Whitton *et al.* (36), in a review of 88 adult patients with low-grade gliomas, were able to establish a benefit for surgery but not for postoperative radiation therapy.

In their opinion the role of radiation therapy, the proper dose, and the timing of radiation therapy remained unclear. Phillippon *et al.* (29) were unable to demonstrate benefit of radiation therapy following surgery: 65% of surviving patients had received postoperative radiation therapy, and 55% had received no radiation therapy. Benefit of radiation therapy was noted only in patients over the age of 40 with partially resected tumors. Others claim no measurable benefit from postoperative radiation therapy (1).

Volumetric Stereotactic Resection

Volumetric stereotaxis provides the following major advantages to the surgeon in the management of low-grade gliomas. First, it allows the surgeon to find the lesion. Second, the technique imparts a concept of the 3-dimensional shape of the lesion to be removed. It allows pre-operative surgical simulation with surgical trajectory planning for selection of the safest and most effective surgical approach to the lesion, which takes into account surrounding normal brain and vascular anatomy delineated by pre-operative imaging.

This method maintains surgical orientation as the procedure extends below the cortical surface, and the approach is preplanned to disrupt as little important brain tissue as possible. Finally, the volumetric stereotactic technique indicates, by means of a scaled real-time intra-operative display, where the CT- and MRI-defined tumor ends and normal brain begins. This information augments the gross appearance of a tumor at surgery and its apparent margins on visual inspection in circumscribed lesions such as pilocytic astrocytomas, circumscribed oligodendrogliomas, dysembryoplastic, neuroepithelial tumors, xanthoastrocytomas, gangliogliomas, subependymomas and infiltrating fibrillary astrocytomas, oligoastrocytomas, and oligodendrogliomas in nonessential brain tissue.

The volumetric stereotactic method allows us to resect as much of a CT/MRI-defined lesion as we choose to remove. However, infiltrating lesions in important brain regions are beyond the resection capabilities of any responsible surgeon using any surgical technique or "gimmick" microsurgery, frame-based or frameless stereotaxis, laser technology, ultrasonic aspiration, and radiosurgery. Further research must be done to better understand the biology of the isolated tumor cell and the ecological environment in which it seems to thrive.

As in high-grade gliomas, future therapies directed at cell surface or nuclear membrane receptors, the metabolism, mitotic potential, or motility of isolated tumor cells must be developed. These therapeutic agents must be delivered selectively to each of these cells residing within the cellular elements of the normal brain parenchyma that must be preserved if we are ever to cure infiltrating lesions without inflicting a neurologic deficit on our patients.

REFERENCES

1. Berger MS, Deliganis AV, Dobbins J, et al.: The effect of extent of resection on recurrence in patients with low grade cerebral hemisphere gliomas. **Cancer** 74(6): 1784–1791, 1994.
2. Clark GB, Henry JM, McKeever PE: Cerebral pilocytic astrocytoma. **Cancer** 56(5):1128–1133, 1985.
3. Daumas-Duport C, Scheithauer B, O'Fallon J, et al.: Grading of astrocytomas. A simple and reproducible method. **Cancer** 62(10):2152–2165, Nov 15, 1988.
4. Daumas-Duport C, Monsaingeon V, Szenthe L, et al.: Serial stereotactic biopsies: A double histological code of gliomas according to malignancy and 3-D configuration, as an aid to therapeutic decision and assessment of results. **Appl Neurophysiol** 45:431–437, 1982.
5. Daumas-Duport C, Scheithauer BW, Kelly PJ: A histologic and cytologic method for the spatial definition of gliomas. **Mayo Clin Proc** 62:435–449, 1987.
6. Daumas-Duport: Dysembryoplastic neuroepithelial tumours. **Brain Pathol** 3:283–295, 1993.
7. Eyre HJ, Crowley JJ, Townsend JJ, et al.: A randomized trial of radiotherapy versus radiotherapy plus CCNU for incompletely resected low-grade gliomas: A Southwest Oncology Group study. **J Neurosurg** 78(6):909–914, 1993.
8. Hoshino T, Rodriguez LA, Cho KG, et al.: Prognostic implications of the proliferative potential of low-grade astrocytomas. **J Neurosurg** 69(6):839–842, 1988.
9. Hoshino T, Nagashima T, Murovic JA, et al.: In situ cell kinetics studies on human neuroectodermal tumors with bromodeoxyuridine labeling. **Neurosurg** 64(3): 453–459, 1986.
10. Hoshino T: A commentary on the biology and growth kinetics of low-grade and high-grade gliomas. **J Neurosurg** 61(5):895–900, 1984.
11. Hoshino T, Barker M, Wilson CB, et al.: Cell kinetics of human gliomas. **Neurosurgery** 37:15–26, 1972.
12. Kelly PJ: Stereotactic imaging, surgical planning and computer assisted volumetric resection of intracranial lesions: Methods and results, in Symon L (ed). *Advances and Technical Standards in Neurosurgery.* New York, Springer-Verlag, 1990, vol 17, pp 77–118.
13. Kelly PJ: Volumetric stereotactic surgical resection of intra-axial brain mass lesions. **Mayo Clin Proc** 63:1186–1198, 1988.
14. Kelly PJ, Alker GJ Jr: A stereotactic approach to deep seated CNS neoplasms using the carbon dioxide laser. **Surg Neurol** 15:331–334, 1980.
15. Kelly PJ, Alker GJ Jr, Goerss S: Computer assisted stereotactic laser microsurgery for the treatment of intracranial neoplasms. **Neurosurgery** 10:324–331, 1982.
16. Kelly PJ: Computer tomography and histologic limits in glial neoplasms: Tumor types and selection for volumetric resection. **Surg Neurol** 39:458–465, 1993.
17. Kelly PJ, Daumas-Duport C, Kispert DB , et al.: Imaging-based stereotactic serial biopsies in untreated intracranial glial neoplasms. **J Neurosurg** 66:865–874, 1987.
18. Kelly PJ, Daumas-Duport C, Scheithauer BW, et al.: Stereotactic histologic correlations of computed tomography and magnetic resonance imaging defined abnormalities in patients with glial neoplasms. **Mayo Clin Proc** 62:450–459, 1987.

19. Kelly PJ, Kall B, Goerss S, et al.: Computer-assisted stereotaxic resection of intra-axial brain neoplasms. **J Neurosurg** 64:427–439, 1986.
20. Kelly PJ: *Tumor Stereotaxis.* Philadelphia, W.B. Saunders, 1991, 400 p.
21. Laws ER Jr, Taylor WF, Bergstrahl EJ, et al.: The neurosurgical management of low-grade astrocytoma. **Clin Neurosurg** 33:575–588, 1986.
22. Laws ER Jr, Taylor WF, Clifton MB, et al.: Neurosurgical management of low-grade astrocytoma of the cerebral hemispheres. **J Neurosurg** 61(4):665–673, 1984.
23. Louis DN, Edgerton S, Thor AD, et al.: Proliferating cell nuclear antigen and Ki-67 immunohistochemistry in brain tumors: A comparative study. **Acta Neuropathol** 81(6):675–679, 1991.
24. McGirr SJ, Kelly PJ, Scheithauer BW: Stereotactic resection of juvenile pilocytic astrocytomas of the thalamus and basal ganglia. **Neurosurgery** 20:447–452, 1987.
25. Medbery CA 3d, Straus KL, Steinberg SM, et al.: Low-grade astrocytomas: Treatment results and prognostic variables. **Int J Radiat Oncol Biol Phys** 15(4): 837–841, 1988.
26. Packer RJ, Sutton LN, Patel KM, et al.: Seizure control following tumor surgery for childhood cortical low-grade gliomas. **J Neurosurg** 80(6):998–1003, 1994.
27. Parkins CS, Darling JL, Gill SS, et al.: Cell proliferation in serial biopsies through human malignant brain tumours: Measurement using Ki67 antibody labelling. **Br J Neurosurg** 5(3):289–298, 1991.
28. Piepmeier JM: Observations on the current treatment of low-grade astrocytic tumors of the cerebral hemispheres. **Neurosurg** 67(2):177–181, 1987.
29. Phillippon JH, Clemenceau SH, Fauchon FH, et al.: Supratentorial low grade astrocytomas in adults. **Neurosurgery** 32(4):554–559, 1993.
30. Prados MD, Krouwer HG, Edwards MS et al.: Proliferative potential and outcome in pediatric astrocytic tumors. **J Neurooncol** 13(3):277–282, 1992.
31. Shaw EG, Daumas-Duport C, Scheithauer BW, et al.: Radiation therapy in the management of low-grade supratentorial astrocytomas. **J Neurosurg** 70(6):853–861, 1989.
32. Shaw EG, Scheithauer BW, Gilbertson DT, et al.: Postoperative radiotherapy of supratentorial low-grade gliomas. **Int J Radiat Oncol Biol Phys** 16(3):663–668, 1989.
33. Smith DF, Hutton JL, Sandemann D, et al.: The prognosis of primary intracerebral tumours presenting with epilepsy: The outcome of medical and surgical management. **Neurol Neurosurg Psychiatry** 54(10):915–920, 1991.
34. Tsanaclis AM, Robert F, Michaud J, et al.: The cycling pool of cells within human brain tumors: In situ cytokinetics using the monclonal antibody Ki-67. **Can J Neurol Sci** 18(1):12–17, 1991.
35. Vecht CJ: Effect of age on treatment decisions in low-grade glioma. **J Neurol Neurosurg Psychiatry** 56(12):1259–1264, 1993.
36. Whitton AC, Bloom HJ: Low grade glioma of the cerebral hemispheres in adults: A retrospective analysis of 88 cases. **Int J Radiat Oncol Biol Phys** 18(4):783–786, 1990.
37. Whittle IR, Gordon A, Misra BK, et al.: Pleomorphic xanthoastrocytoma. Report of four cases. **J Neurosurg** 70(3):463–468, 1989.
38. Winger MJ, Macdonald DR, Cairncross JG: Supratentorial anaplastic gliomas in adults: The prognostic importance of extent of resection and prior low-grade glioma. **J Neurosurg** 71(4):487–493, 1989.
39. Zuber P, Hamou MF, de Tribolet N: Identification of proliferating cells in human gliomas using the monoclonal antibody Ki-67. **Neurosurgery** 22(2):364–368, 1988.

26

Functional Mapping-guided Resection of Low-Grade Gliomas

MITCHEL S. BERGER, M.D., F.A.C.S.

The surgical approach to management of low-grade cerebral hemisphere tumors in children and adults remains controversial and is influenced by current data based on the natural history of these lesions, which is somewhat sparse. There has never been a prospective study to analyze the effects of extent of resection, although several retrospective analyses are available that are based on the surgeon's impression of tumor removal or qualitative assessment of postoperative imaging studies (26, 28, 31, 36). Therefore, when a patient presents with a diagnosis based on computerized tomography (CT) or magnetic resonance imaging (MRI), the critical therapeutic issue is whether to follow the lesion conservatively with serial imaging studies or to operate, *e.g.,* to perform a biopsy or resect, and perhaps follow either of those options with focal radiotherapy. The natural history of a low-grade glial lesion is quite difficult to predict, although recent evidence seems to indicate that most of these tumors will progress within 24 to 40 months of diagnosis (38). The argument against conservative management is based on the assumption that the lesion will eventually increase in size, possibly converting an operable lesion into a diffuse tumor not readily resectable, and malignant transformation is almost certainly influenced by the duration of the tumor's existence. The likelihood of change toward a malignant phenotype varies between 30 and 70% in most series (1, 30, 41), and it is difficult to predict what influences this phenomenon, although tumor volume is clearly an important parameter (2, 40).

The vast majority of low-grade astrocytic tumors are difficult to grossly distinguish from the surrounding gliotic white matter because of their firm consistency and whitish color. This factor, combined with the infiltrative nature of these tumors adjacent to or within functional areas, has discouraged neurosurgeons from radically resecting most low-grade gliomas. However, localization techniques, such as intraoperative ultrasound (27), computerized volumetric resection, using

CT or MRI (24), and frameless surgical navigation systems (14), will allow for more precise and extensive resections in regions that are microscopically infiltrated, yet grossly normal appearing. In addition, neurophysiologic methods are now available and may be used routinely to stimulate functional pathways and record epileptogenic foci. The latter technique is especially critical for influencing the seizure outcome in patients with medically refractory epilepsy and a low-grade tumor.

EXTENT OF TUMOR RESECTION INFLUENCING OUTCOME

Several recent studies have confirmed the role of radical tumor resection in prolonging survival for patients with low-grade gliomas (17, 31, 41), especially early after the diagnosis is made (25, 29, 43). We have followed a similar approach and recently analyzed the influence tumor volume, prior to and following resection, had on recurrence patterns in these lesions (2). For example, when the pre-operative tumor volume was less than 10 cm^3, no recurrences were noted *versus* those in the groups with tumors measuring 10 to 30 cm^3 and greater than 30 cm^3, where the incidence of recurrence was 13.6% and 41.2%, respectively. As expected, the time to tumor progression was shorter for the bigger tumors, and all recurrences were malignant when the tumor measured more than 30 cm^3 at the onset (Table 26.1). When a complete T2 weighted MRI resection was performed, no recurrences were documented at a 54-month postoperative interval. Yet, patients with more

TABLE 26.1

The Effect of Pre-operative Tumor Volumes on Recurrence, Recurrence at a Higher-Grade Histology, and Time-to-Tumor Progression[a]

Pre-operative Tumor Volume	<10 cm^3	10–30 cm^3	>30 cm^3
Patients (no.)	14	22	17
Age (yr)	35.9 (7–64)	39.6 (19–70)	36.3 (6–74)
Follow-up (months) (range)	41.7 (24–121)	51.4 (26–150)	50.4 (24–172)
Postoperative tumor volume (cm^3) (range)	0.46 (0–3.84)	5.38 (0–24.89)	19.93 (0–83.18)
Pathology (%)			
Astrocytoma	71	23	24
Oligodendroglioma	21	45	29
Mixed glioma	8	32	47
Radiotherapy (% received)	43	86	88
Recurrence (%), patients (no.)	0	13.6, $n = 3$	41.2, $n = 7$
Recurrence at higher-grade histology (%), patients (no.)	0	0	41.2, $n = 7$
Time-to-tumor progression (months) (range)	N/A	58 (12–91)	30 (13–45)

[a]Age, follow-up, postoperative tumor volume, and time to tumor progression are expressed as a mean value, and ranges are shown in parentheses. N/A, not applicable.

TABLE 26.2
The Effect of Postoperative Tumor Volumes on Recurrence, Recurrence at a Higher Grade Histology, and Time-to-Tumor Progression[a]

Postoperative Tumor Volume	$0\ cm^3$	$<10\ cm^3$	$>10\ cm^3$
Patients (no.)	13	27	13
Age (yr), (range)	29.8 (6–59)	39.6 (7–74)	41.2 (31–55)
Follow-up (months), (range)	54.4 (24–172)	47.9 (24–150)	44 (24–60)
Preoperative tumor volume (cm^3) (range)	14.16 (1.9–48.95)	21.72 (1.04–53.06)	49.07 (18.95–115.86)
Percent of resection (range)	100	83.1 (24.5–98.3)	38.8 (10.7–67.2)
Pathology (%)			
Astrocytoma	77	18	31
Oligodendroglioma	0	56	23
Mixed glioma	23	26	46
Radiotherapy (% received)	46	85	85
Recurrence (%), patients (no.)	0	14.8, $n = 4$	46.2, $n = 6$
Recurrence at higher-grade histology (%), patients (no.)	0	3.7, $n = 1$	46.2, $n = 6$
Time-to-tumor progression(months), (range)	N/A	50 (12–91)	30 (13–45)

[a]Age, follow-up, pre-operative tumor volume, percent of resection and time-to-tumor progression are expressed as a mean value, and ranges are shown in parentheses. N/A, not applicable.

than 10 cm^3 remaining after resection had 46.2% incidence of recurrence within 30 months of surgery. Nearly half of these patients developed a malignant tumor at the time of recurrence. This was significantly more likely than those patients with a residual tumor volume of less than 10 cm^3 (Table 26.2). Thus, our data support the concept that the risk of recurrence is lessened with a more aggressive initial operation that leaves the least amount of residual tumor. The volume of residual disease was more important than the actual percent of tumor resection in determining recurrence at a higher-grade histology. Thus, delaying surgical intervention may not be in the best interest of the patient, contrary to what some investigators have reported (8, 38). The goal of early surgery is to maximize the chances of achieving a radical resection that will hopefully diminish the likelihood of malignant transformation. The remainder of this chapter will describe intraoperative methods that may be used to perform radical tumor resections around and within critical functional regions. In addition, the role of electrocorticography in helping to control seizure activity in those low-grade glioma patients who are considered intractable will be discussed.

STIMULATION MAPPING OF FUNCTIONAL AREAS

The primary regions of interest for functional mapping encompass the dominant hemisphere temporal, posterior frontal, and anterior parietal lobes, where the concentration of language related cortex is greatest. The motor pathways are comprised of the cortical sites of origin, *i.e.*, Rolandic cortex, and corona radiata, internal capsule, cerebral peduncles, and corticospinal tracts. The same may be said for the primary somatosensory cortex and its subcortical pathways. Any lesion located adjacent to these areas, *e.g.*, supplementary motor area, insula, thalamus, *etc.*, are excellent targets for the mapping procedure. These techniques have been found to be very safe and accurate (7), with studies in human and monkey cortex showing only a 2- to 3-mm spread of current as detected with optical imaging (20, 21). Particularly relevant during the removal of low-grade gliomas is the capability of resecting infiltrating tumor and adjacent white matter with the aid of subcortical stimulation. This can detect both motor and sensory descending pathways with similar or slightly higher currents than those used for cortical mapping.

If any doubt exists regarding the localization of language functions to the left hemisphere, considering handedness and perhaps a history of speech deficits during or subsequent to a seizure, a WADA test (intracarotid sodium amytal) should be performed (42). Although mesial temporal lobe tumors on the left side may be removed while the patient is asleep, consideration should be given to operating while awake when the tumor extends posteriorly toward the region of the tectal plate. In this setting, lateral cortex may need to be removed to facilitate exposure of the mesial tumor, thus necessitating knowledge of essential temporal lobe language sites. Another important area to consider approaching while the patient is awake is the paramedian posterior frontal or anterior parietal region, when the lesion extends beyond 4 to 5 cm from the midline. Not infrequently, high suprasylvian language sites may be present, thus making radical tumor resection dangerous unless these sites are mapped.

Prior to surgery, the pre-operative MRI study should be evaluated to determine where the sensory and motor cortex is located by identifying the central sulcus on rostral T1- or T2-weighted axial images. A characteristic mirror-image sulcal pattern will be identified that localizes the Rolandic cortex. Regardless of mass effect, this landmark will be readily found and should be carefully looked for. A sagittal view will show the sensorimotor cortex as the collective bundle of tissue directly in front of the termination of the cingulate sulcus, *i.e.,* marginal sulcus. Using the far parasagittal image, drawing a perpendicular line from the back of the insular triangle will bisect the Rolandic cortex. Thus, with any of these three imaging planes, the relationship of the tumor to these functional regions will be easily identified (11). Currently, similar landmarks to identify Broca's area responsible for fluent speech output, or posterior essential naming and reading sites, do not exist although work is in progress to elucidate this. Functional MRI is in its infancy yet may soon be capable of pre-operatively localizing functional cortex in relation to the tumor nidus.

Several caveats exist that must be considered prior to performing these intra-operative mapping techniques. For example, if the patient is under 5 years old, direct stimulation mapping of the motor cortex may not yield localizing information because of the relatively unexcitable nature of the "young" motor cortex (5). Therefore, should this information be essential, it will be necessary to have somatosensory evoked potentials available during surgery to identify the central sulcus based on the phenomenon of phase reversals (16, 44). Alternatively, a subdural electrode array may be placed prior to the definitive tumor resection, so that the motor and sensory cortex may be stimulated with the patient awake on the hospital ward.

Another critical issue that influences the success of the mapping procedure is the extent of neurologic deficit seen prior to the operation. No matter how high the current is, if an extremity is densely paretic or plegic, stimulation either awake or asleep will be unable to evoke motor responses; thus, mapping will not provide the necessary information. In a similar fashion, deficits in reading, object naming, and speaking fluently will limit the effectiveness of stimulation mapping. Therefore, it is essential to test the patient prior to surgery by having him or her count from 1 to 10 (Broca's area), read short phrases (posterior temporal sites), and name common objects (temporal, parietal, and posterior frontal lobes). When deficits are present, it may be helpful to start a short trial of dexamethasone to determine whether these problems are related to swelling. On occasion we have attempted to use "conversation mapping" in mildly dysphasic patients, *i.e.,* talking while stimulation takes place, although the results of this have been disappointing and unreliable.

Stimulation Parameters for Sensory and Motor Mapping

A bipolar electrode with 5-mm spacing is used to stimulate the cortex. A constant current generator is used to produce a train of biphasic square-wave pulses, which have a frequency of 60 Hz and a single peak duration of 1.25 msec. Thus the peak to peak duration is 2.5 milliseconds. When the patient is asleep, a starting current of 4 mA should be used and increased in 2-mA increments up to 16 mA. At first, a train of four twitches should be present to ensure that the patient is not paralyzed. Secondly, the muscle adjacent to the craniotomy should be depolarized with the bipolar stimulator to again make certain that the electrical system is functional. If motor movements cannot be evoked with a current as high as 16 mA, functional tissue is not present at the stimulation site; higher currents will not produce motor responses in this setting. The bipolar stimulator is best oriented parallel to the sulcus, as opposed to perpendicular to the main axis of the gyral segment that is stimulated. Sometimes, the bone and dural flap are just at the margin near the Rolandic cortex. In this situation, a strip electrode may be inserted subdurally and stimulation delivered *via* the contacts spaced 1 cm apart to evoke a motor response. Likewise, the leg motor cortex is typically hidden under the midline dura and then descends in a parallel fashion along the falx. To find the leg motor cortex, a strip electrode may be inserted between the falx and the cortex and subsequently stimulated. When using strip electrodes, it is critical to remember that the contact points are separated by a distance of 1 cm. Therefore, if the first two contacts evoke a motor response, it is necessary to stimulate through the second and third contact points to determine whether the key contact is the first or second electrode. If the second and third contacts do not elicit a motor response when stimulated, then it is the first contact that is overlying functional tissue.

At times, stimulation will evoke a focal motor seizure. This is usually not a problem if it is brief and does not spread. However, when using smaller currents, *i.e.,* 2 to 4 mA, in awake patients, the seizure may last longer and may spread. At that point in time, it will be necessary to administer a short-acting barbiturate such as Ativan (0.5 to 1.0 mg). Sensory mapping can only be done in the awake patient, and as such, small currents should be used. In general, the somatosensory cortex is more readily depolarized, and it may take a slightly higher current to elicit motor responses. Resection of nonfunctional cortex should be carried out until the resection cavity is directly adjacent to the functional sensory or motor portions of the gyrus. At this point, the somatosensory cortex may be resected if involved with tumor (Fig. 26.1). In the early postoperative period, the patient may complain of hypesthesia in the involved extremity without loss of pain or temperature sensation. Although proprioceptive difficulties usually resolve over the ensuing months, a very mild hypesthesia will persist without being disabling.

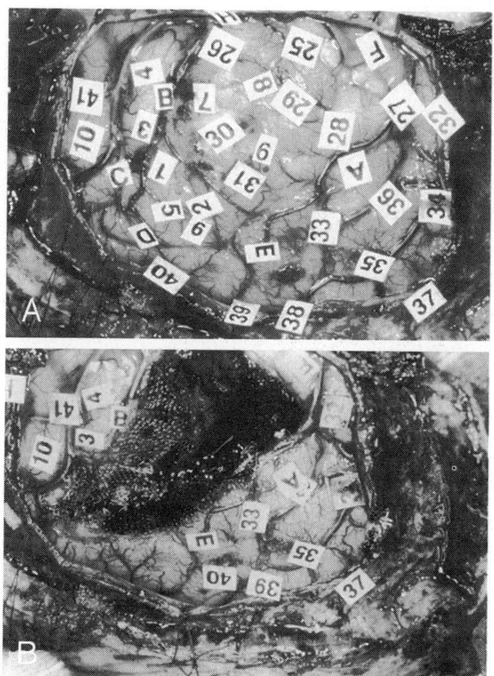

FIG. 26.1 Prior to resecting the tumor, awake cortical mapping revealed localization of the lesion within the somatosensory cortex (**A**, *1–9*). This functional area is removed and the resection cavity lined with Surgicel (**B**).

Notwithstanding, this may bother the patient whose dominant hand is affected; thus, that individual must be counseled about the deficit prior to surgery. At the end of the tumor resection, the motor cortex should be restimulated before paralyzing the patient for the closure. If the motor pathways are still stimulatable, whatever temporary deficits are present in the postoperative period will resolve after several days to weeks.

One particular pattern of postoperative motor deficits that routinely occurs following removal of tumors within the supplementary motor cortex (Fig. 26.2) (39) is a reversible recovery of motor function in a stepwise fashion after an immediate hemiplegia. Within a week, the arm, and then the leg, motor function will return and achieve its pre-operative level of strength within weeks to a few months. If the dominant hemisphere supplementary motor area is resected, this afore-mentioned deficit is accompanied by muteness, which slowly resolves,

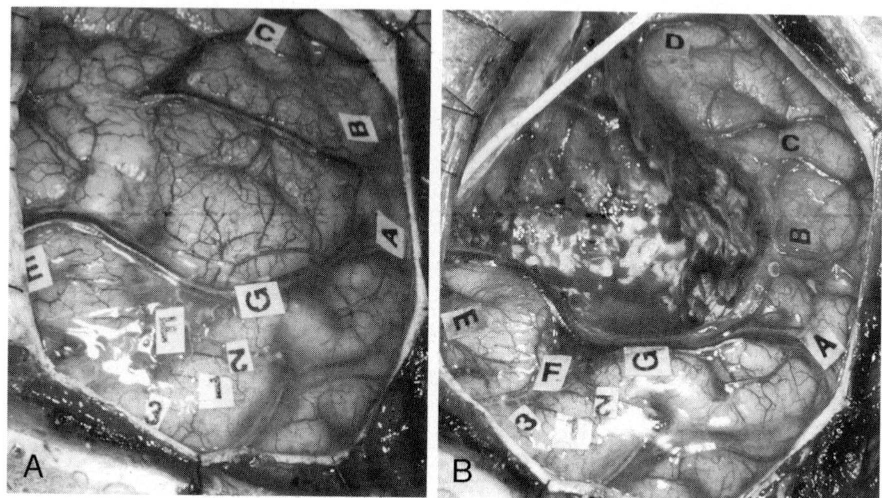

FIG. 26.2 The supplementary motor cortex is infiltrated with tumor (*A–F*) and is located just in front of the motor cortex (**A**, *1–3*). Resection is carried out to the premotor sulcus (**B**).

starting within the week following surgery and regaining nearly complete return of function within a month. This syndrome is particularly pronounced when the cingulate gyrus is part of the tumor removal. Although it does not have motor pathways within its boundaries, the cingulate gyrus is part of the motor initiation circuit that is synonymous with the supplementary motor area.

While removing infiltrative low-grade gliomas, subcortical motor and sensory pathways must be identified and preserved. This is accomplished by stimulating deep within the region adjacent to overlying functional cortex until stimulation-induced movements or sensations occur. As previously mentioned, current spread is minimal, thus allowing the surgeon to stop removing tumor, without incurring deficits, before damaging the descending motor tracts (6) (Fig. 26.3). In doing this, subcortical motor and sensory pathways may be identified throughout the region of the corona radiata and internal capsule. This is quite helpful during resection of large mesial temporal lobe tumors that are contiguous with the cerebral peduncles, as well as while removing thalamic tumors. In the latter circumstance, the resection proceeds in a piecemeal fashion until the posterior limb of the internal capsule is identified. In the location of the spinal cord, motor responses may be evoked with currents ranging from 0.5 to 2.0 mA. This occurs *via* depolarization of anterior horn cells or stimulation of corticospinal

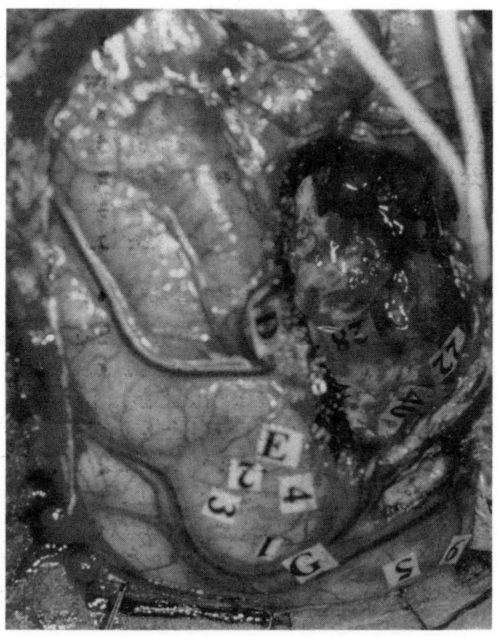

FIG. 26.3 Descending subcortical motor fiber are stimulated and identified following removal of the cortex (*22, 28, 40*). The motor strip is just behind the resection cavity (*1–6*).

tracts. Thus, this is a very effective way to maximize extent of resection for spinal cord tumors without causing motor deficits.

Stimulation Parameters for Language Mapping

Perhaps the most complicated form of intra-operative mapping during removal of low-grade gliomas is that which involves awake language localization. The patient is briefly anesthetized with the sedative hypnotic agent, propofol (Diprivan), while the scalp is injected with a regional lidocaine-marcaine field block, and the bone is removed. Following this procedure, the patient is awakened prior to the opening of the dura just in case coughing occurs so as not to cause herniation of a swollen brain infiltrated with tumor. When the dura is tender upon incising it, the local anesthetic mixture can be infiltrated along the middle meningeal artery with a 30-gauge needle. It is important to create a generous bone flap in order to allow for a large cortical area to be mapped. A skull clamp is fixed to the cut edge of the craniotomy bone margin to allow for fixation of the electrodes. Following localization of the face motor and sensory region, and hand area, if far enough above the sylvian fissure, Broca's area is located by having the patient count from 1 to 50 while the surgeon stimulates multiple cortical sites contiguous with the inferior aspect of the Rolandic cortex (Fig. 26.4). The same current used to stimulate the face motor cortex should be applied to localize Broca's area. During stimulation, counting should cease without any movement of the mouth or pharynx. Should motor movements occur, speech arrest may be secondary to these motor responses and may not truly represent Broca's area. All functional sites should be labeled with small, sterile numbered "tickets" for photographic and record keeping purposes.

At this point the electrodes are mounted on the horseshoe head holder, which is fixed to the skull clamp. With the surgeon starting at 2 mA and working upward to 1-mA increments, the cortical site directly under the electrode should be stimulated to try and evoke an after discharge potential, which can be readily seen on the intraoperative electrocorticogram. When an afterdischarge potential(s) is seen, the current is too high for language mapping and should be reduced by 1 mA. This will avoid an unnecessarily high current, which could provoke seizure activity in the awake patient. Once the proper current for language mapping has been determined, multiple numbered tickets are placed on the surface with 8 to 10 mm spacing throughout the exposed cortex. Common object naming is the most accurate way to assess language function, as originally determined by Penfield (33, 35). Naming is used because deficits in this task are commonly seen in all aphasias. Although object naming most clearly defines essential language sites when deficits are present during stimulation, posterior temporal lobe cortex may be additionally tested with sentence reading (34).

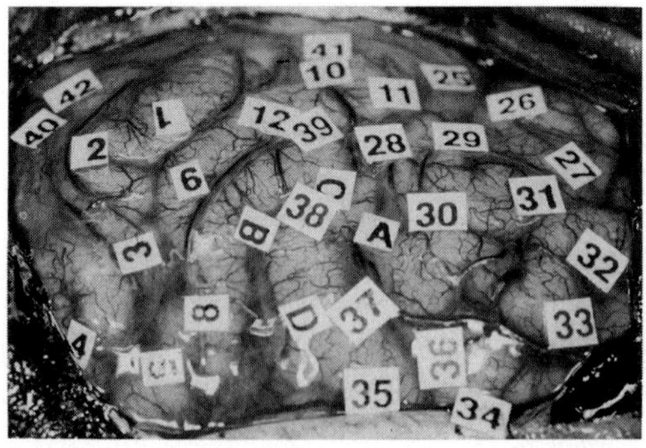

FIG. 26.4 Speech arrest (Broca's area, *11, 12*) is located in front of the face motor cortex (*1, 2, 3, 6*).

Thus, the two most important aspects of mapping language during removal of low-grade gliomas is to determine the adequate stimulating current that does not provoke seizure activity during testing and to select a battery of objects to be named, *i.e., via* a slide presentation, in which the baseline error rate in naming those objects is 20% or less.

Multiple cortical sites should be tested to find out not only where language is located but also where it is not found (Fig. 26.5). A completely negative stimulation is somewhat worrisome in terms of confidently removing a wide margin around the tumor. Thus, time should be taken to test at least 20 cortical sites during the stimulation mapping. Every 4 seconds the patient is presented with a slide of the common object preceded by a short leader phrase, *e.g.,* "This is a . . . CAT (object)." After one site is tested, a slide is allowed to pass without stimulating the cortex to ensure that the baseline error rate in naming has not increased. No site in particular is stimulated twice in a row without an intervening slide to be named without stimulation. A site(s) found to demonstrate repetitive, *i.e.,* 2 out of 3, errors, is essential for language and should not be violated. The error made should be a clear anomia; hesitation or a minor dysnomia is not acceptable as a criterion to delineate that site as essential. Errors in reading are evidenced by a slow, almost staccato sound to the sentence, often with errors in syntax (32).

Previous experience from a functional mapping database (34) has shown that the location of essential language sites in the perisylvian region is variable in every individual tested. Most sites are small, *i.e.,* having a 2-cm^2 surface area, and there appears to be a very sharp distinction in the brain directly adjacent to the language site in that none or few errors are made in this so-called "penumbra." Language sites may be found within 3 to 4 cm of the temporal lobe tip or in the inferior

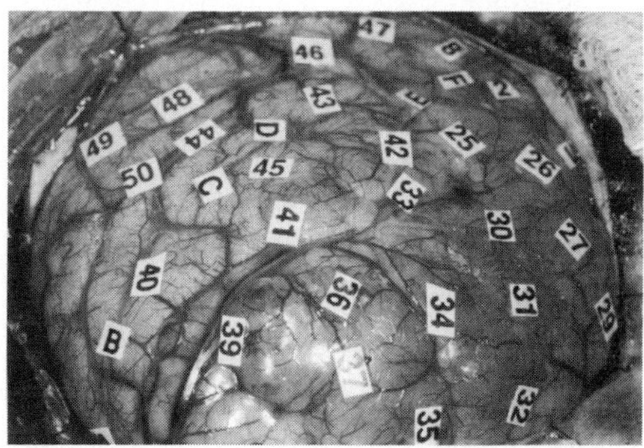

FIG. 26.5 Suprasylvian essential language size (*D*) is identified inferior to the tumor nidus (*36, 37*).

frontal lobe just behind the sphenoid wing. In addition, 16% of the 117 patients tested in this study failed to show any language localization in the temporal lobe. In a follow-up study (19) assessing language in patients with temporal lobe gliomas, most of whom had low-grade glial tumors, researchers found a similar percentage of patients without temporal lobe language and up to 16% of patients with language located within 4 cm of the temporal lobe tip. No language sites were found in the inferior temporal gyrus, and female glioma patients were more likely to have essential language sites in the posterior portion of the middle and superior temporal gyrus than were their male counterparts. Postoperative deficits in naming were also critically assessed as a function of how close the resection came to an essential site (Fig. 26.6). When the resection came within 7 mm of a language site, permanent naming errors were documented in 40% of cases. However, when the tumor removal stayed at least 1 cm away from the naming site, no permanent deficits were seen. This again emphasizes the role of a "supplementary" penumbra, located directly adjacent to cortex, that produces naming errors when stimulated, which must be preserved. This is certainly not the case with the motor or sensory cortex, where the resection margin may come into contact with, but not violate, functional cortex.

MANAGEMENT OF INTRACTABLE EPILEPSY ASSOCIATED WITH LOW-GRADE GLIOMAS

The most common presentation of a patient harboring a low-grade glioma is seizure activity, which reflects the slow-growing nature of

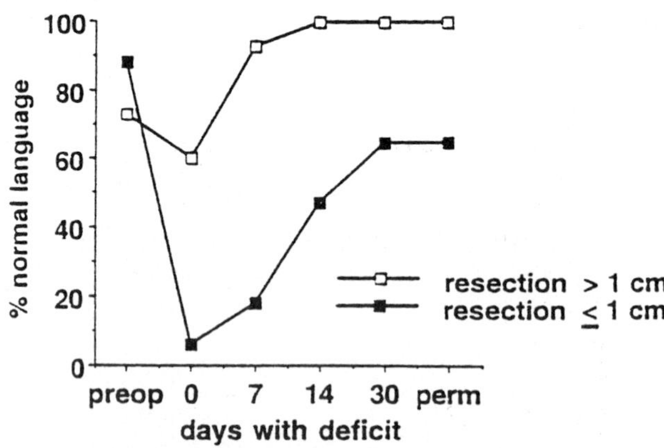

FIG. 26.6 Graph illustrates the time course of postoperative language outcome, based on the patient's pre-operative status and the tumor resection margin distance from a language site.

these lesions. Chronic compression of the surrounding brain by the tumor leads to morphologic changes and alterations of neurotransmitter levels (18, 22). Because of this pathophysiologic alteration in the brain contiguous with the mass lesion, consideration must be given as to whether or not this factor should be included in the resection strategy. Control of infrequent seizure activity is typically obtained when the tumor is removed without the adjacent surrounding brain (9, 13, 15). Yet, when intractable epilepsy accompanies the diagnosis of a low-grade glioma, removal of the tumor and epileptogenic foci, determined with the use of intra-operative electrocorticography, appear to offer superior results in terms of seizure control, more so than lesion removal alone (12, 37). In the author's experience, 88% of adults with low-grade gliomas were seizure free, with nearly half of these patients off antiepileptic drugs (4). In pediatric patients, slightly more than 90% of patients were seizure-free and not taking antiepileptic drugs (3). This emphasizes the need to address the seizure problem early in the patient's history in the hope of gaining the best degree of control of the epilepsy associated with the indolent low-grade glioma. Removing the tumor without using electrocorticography to identify and resect seizure foci will often reduce the incidence and frequency of intractable epilepsy, yet will seldom allow the patient to discontinue his or her anticonvulsant medications (10, 15, 23). Interestingly enough, several of the patients who were better controlled postoperatively often had a wide resection performed around the lesion, which almost certainly encompasses the surrounding epileptogenic foci. Several of our patients were also documented as having multiple seizure foci, which was commensurate with a longer duration of seizures. This again supports the use of electrocorticography and post-tumor resection recordings to ensure that all epileptogenic foci are identified and removed in this select group of patients with intractable seizures (Fig. 26.7).

CONCLUSION

In summary, evidence exists with quantitative volumetric resection of low-grade gliomas in adults and children that a greater extent of tumor resection affects the time to tumor recurrence and the recurrent tumor phenotype. Radical resections of infiltrating low-grade glial tumors may be enhanced with the aid of intra-operative mapping methods to identify sensory, motor, and language cortex. Subcortical, descending functional pathways within white matter may also be localized using these techniques. For patients with intractable epilepsy associated with a low-grade glioma, optimal control of seizure activity, without anti-epileptic medication, is often made possible with the use

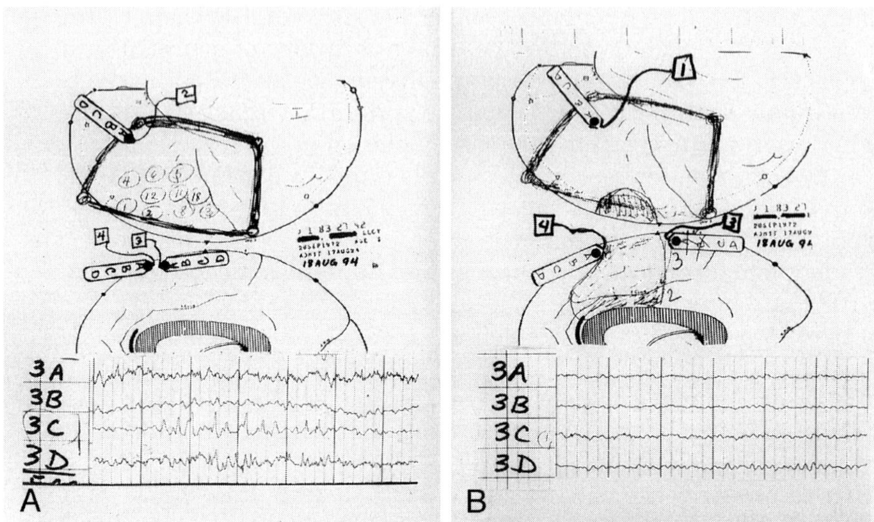

FIG. 26.7 Preresection electrocorticography *via* strip electrode in the interhemispheric fissure identifies epileptogenic areas in *3C* and *3D* (**A**). Postresection electrocorticography, demonstrating no further seizure activity from the region of *3C* and *3D* (**B**).

of electrocorticography before and following the tumor resection, as opposed to lesion resection alone.

ACKNOWLEDGMENTS

This work was supported by the American Cancer Society Professor of Clinical Oncology Grant 071, NIH-NINCDS T32 NS07289, American Cancer Society Grant #EDT-53, and American Cancer Society's Rex and Arlene Garrison Summer Fellowship Training Grant.

REFERENCES

1. Afra D, Muller W, Benoist G, *et al.*: Supratentorial recurrences of gliomas: Results of operations on astrocytomas and oligodendrogliomas. **Acta Neurochir** 43:217–227, 1978.
2. Berger MS, Deliganis AV, Dobbins J, *et al.*: The effect of extent of resection on recurrence in patients with low grade cerebral hemisphere gliomas. **Cancer** 74:1784–1791, 1994.
3. Berger MS, Ghatan S, Geyer JR, *et al.*: Seizure outcome in children with hemispheric tumors and associated intractable epilepsy: The role of tumor removal combined with seizure foci resection. **Pediatr Neurosurg** 17:185–191, 1992.
4. Berger MS, Ghatan S, Haglund MM, *et al.*: Low-grade gliomas associated with intractable epilepsy: Seizure outcome utilizing electrocorticography during tumor resection. **J Neurosurg** 79:62–69, 1993.
5. Berger MS, Kincaid J, Ojemann GA, *et al.*: Brain mapping techniques to maximize

resection, safety, and seizure control in children with brain tumors. **Neurosurgery** 25:786–792, 1989.

6. Berger MS. Ojemann GA: Intraoperative brain mapping techniques in neuro-oncology. **Stereotact Funct Neurosurg** 58:153–161, 1992.

7. Berger MS, Ojemann GA, Lettich E: Neurophysiological monitoring during astrocytoma surgery. **Neurosurg Clin North Am** 1:65–80, 1990.

8. Cairncross JG, Laperriere NJ: Low-grade glioma: To treat or not to treat? **Arch Neurol** 46:1238–1239, 1989.

9. Cascino GD: Epilepsy and brain tumors: Implications for treatment. **Epilepsia** 31 (Suppl 3):37–44, 1990.

10. Cascino GD, Kelly PJ, Hirschorn KA, *et al.:* Stereotactic resection of intra-axial cerebral lesions in partial epilepsy. **Mayo Clin Proc** 65:1053–1060, 1990.

11. deLanerole NC, Kim JH, Robbins RJ, *et al.:* Hippocampal interneuron loss and plasticity in human temporal lobe epilepsy. **Brain Res** 49:387–395, 1989.

12. Drake J, Hoffman HJ, Kobayashi J, *et al.:* Surgical management of children with temporal lobe epilepsy and mass lesions. **Neurosurgery** 21:792–797, 1987.

13. Falconer MA, Driver MV, Serafetinides EA: Temporal lobe epilepsy due to distant lesions: Two cases relieved by operation. **Brain** 85:521–534, 1962.

14. Galloway RL Jr, Berger MS, Bass WA: Registered intraoperative information: Electrophysiology, ultrasound and endoscopy, in Maciunas RJ (ed): *Interactive Image-Guided Neurosurgery*. AANS Publications Committee, Publishers, 1993, pp 247–258.

15. Goldring S, Rich KM, Picker S: Experience with gliomas in patients presenting with a chronic seizure disorder. **Clin Neurosurg** 33:15–42, 1986.

16. Gregori EM, Goldring S: Localization of function in the excision of lesions from the sensorimotor region. **J Neurosurg** 60:457–466, 1984.

17. Guthrie BL, Laws ER: Supratentorial low-grade gliomas. **Neurosurg Clin North Am** 1:37–48, 1990.

18. Haglund MM, Berger MS, Kunkel DD, *et al.:* Changes in gamma-aminobutyric acid and somatostatin in epileptic cortex associated with low-grade gliomas. **J Neurosurg** 7:209–216, 1992.

19. Haglund MM, Berger MS, Shamseldin M, *et al.:* Cortical localization of temporal lobe language sites in patients with gliomas. **Neurosurgery** 34(4):567–576, 1994.

20. Haglund MM, Ojemann GA, Blasdel GG: Video imaging of bipolar cortical stimulation. **Epilepsia** 32 (Suppl 3):22, 1991.

21. Haglund MM, Ojemann GA, Blasdel GG: Video imaging of neuronal activity, in Stamford JA (ed): *Monitoring Neuronal Activity: A Practical Approach*. New York, Oxford University Press, 1992, pp 85–114.

22. Hanna GR: Morphological changes in primary and secondary epileptic foci, in Mayersdorf A, Schmidt RP (eds): *Secondary Epileptogenesis*. New York, Raven Press, 1982, pp 115–130.

23. Hirsch JF, Sainte Rose C, Pierre-Khan A, *et al.:* Benign astrocytic and oligodendrocytic tumors of the cerebral hemispheres in children. **J Neurosurg** 70:568–572, 1989.

24. Kelly PJ: Image-directed tumor resection. **Neurosurg Clin North Am** 1:81–95, 1990.

25. Laws ER, Taylor WF, Bergstralh EJ, *et al.:* The neurosurgical management of low-grade astrocytoma. **Clin Neurosurg** 33:575–588, 1985.

26. Laws ER, Taylor WF, Clifton MB, *et al.:* Neurosurgical management of low-grade astrocytoma of the cerebral hemispheres. **J Neurosurg** 61:665–673, 1984.

27. LeRoux PD, Winter TC, Berger MS, *et al.:* A comparison between preoperative mag-

netic resonance scans and intraoperative ultrasound tumor volumes and margins. **J Clin Ultrasound** 22:29–36, 1994.

28. Medbery CA, Straus KL, Steinberg SM, *et al.:* Low-grade astrocytomas: Treatment results and prognostic variables. **Int J Radiat Oncol Biol Phys** 15:837–841, 1988.

29. Morantz RA: Radiation therapy in the treatment of cerebral astrocytoma. **Neurosurgery** 20:975–982, 1987.

30. Muller W, Afra D, Schroder R: Supratentorial recurrences of gliomas: Morphological studies in relation to time intervals with astrocytomas. **Acta Neurochir** 37:75–91, 1977.

31. North CA, North RB, Epstein JA, *et al.:* Low-grade cerebral astrocytomas: Survival and quality of life after radiation therapy. **Cancer** 66:6–14, 1990.

32. Ojemann GA: Brain organization for language from the perspective of electrical stimulation mapping. **Behav Brain Sci** 6:189–206, 1983.

33. Ojemann GA: Some brain mechanisms for reading, in Vol Euler C, Lundberg I, Lennerstrand G (eds): *Brain and Reading.* New York, Macmillan, 1989, pp 47–59.

34. Ojemann GA, Ojemann J, Lettich E, *et al.:* Cortical language localization in left, dominant hemisphere. An electrical stimulation mapping investigation in 117 patients. **J Neurosurg** 71:316–326, 1989.

35. Penfield W, Roberts L: *Speech and Brain Mechanisms.* Princeton, NJ, Princeton University Press, 1959.

36. Piepmeier JM: Observations on the current treatment of low-grade astrocytic tumors of the cerebral hemispheres. **J Neurosurg** 67:177–181, 1987.

37. Rasmussen TB: Surgery of epilepsy associated with brain tumors. **Adv Neurol** 8:227–239, 1975.

38. Recht LD, Lew R, Smith TW: Suspected low-grade glioma: Is deferring treatment safe? **Ann Neurol** 46:1238–1239, 1989.

39. Rostomily RC, Berger MS, Ojemann GA, *et al.:* Postoperative deficits and functional recovery following removal of tumors involving the dominant hemisphere supplementary motor area. **J Neurosurg** 75:62–68, 1991.

40. Shibamoto Y, Kitakabu Y, Takahashi M, *et al.:* Supratentorial low-grade astrocytoma: Correlation of computed tomography findings with effect of radiation therapy and prognostic variables. **Cancer** 7:190–195, 1993.

41. Soffietti R, Chio A, Giordana MT, *et al.:* Prognostic factors in well-differentiated cerebral astrocytomas in the adult. **Neurosurgery** 24:686–692, 1989.

42. Wada J, Rasmussen T: Intracarotid injections of sodium amytal for the lateralization of cerebral speech dominance. **J Neurosurg** 17:266–282, 1960.

43. Weingart J, Olivi A, Brem H: Supratentorial low-grade astrocytomas in adults. **Neurosurg Q** 1:141–159, 1991.

44. Woolsey CN, Cividosan TC, Gibson WE: Localization in somatosensory and motor areas of human cerebral cortex as determined by direct recording of evoked potentials and electrical stimulation. **J Neurosurg** 51:476–506, 1979.

27

Management of Low-Grade Gliomas: Results of Resections without Electrocorticography

ITZHAK FRIED, M.D., PH.D.

SURGICALLY REMEDIABLE SYNDROMES OF EPILEPSY

In the past, epilepsy surgery posed a unique challenge to the neurosurgeon since in most of these procedures no apparent structural abnormality was evident. Epilepsy surgery pioneers, such as Penfield, often gazed upon cortical surfaces with no gross abnormality and had to rely on intra-operative electrocorticography (ECoG) to define "epileptogenic" regions that subsequently became targets for resection. The definition of these zones was based largely on sharp waves or spikes, identified by the electro-encephalographer, during surgery (31).

Over the last decade a number of surgically remediable syndromes of epilepsy have been identified and studied. Rather than looking on seizure disorders as a continuum of interictal abnormalities and irritative zones, these new developments emphasize discrete syndromes, based on structural abnormalities that can often be identified by advanced magnetic resonance imaging (MRI) techniques. These structural, rather than physiologic, abnormalities then have become the focus of the surgical effort.

Surgically remediable syndromes fall into three major categories: (*a*) epilepsy related to mesial temporal sclerosis; (*b*) epilepsy related to mass lesions such as tumors and vascular malformations; and (*c*) epilepsy related to developmental disorders, including neuronal migration disorders.

Low-grade gliomas are lesions that fall into the second of these general syndrome categories. These lesions are unique in that they present the neurosurgeon with the challenge of achieving control of both tumor and seizures, subject to anatomic and functional considerations, related mostly to limbic and perilimbic circuitry.

GLIOMAS ASSOCIATED WITH INTRACTABLE SEIZURES: A DISTINCT CLINICOPATHOLOGIC GROUP

Although seizures are often the presenting symptom of low-grade gliomas, not all gliomas are associated with chronic intractable seizures.

There is increasing evidence that tumors associated with seizures constitute a distinct clinicopathologic type (16). Most patients with these tumors experience seizure onset in the 2nd decade of life. The seizures almost invariably are intractable to pharmacologic agents. Modern neuro-imaging techniques have allowed the identification of space-occupying lesions not formerly apparent. It is common for patients with these tumors to experience years of intractable seizures without deterioration in their neurologic examination, which is almost invariably normal. In a recent series of 65 patients with chronic seizures and gliomas, 82% of the patients were found to have tumors involving the gray matter of the cortex (Fig. 27.1) (16). Most of the these tumors were in limbic locations or in neocortex close to the limbic system (Fig. 27.2). On the basis of these clinical findings the author postulated that gliomas associated with intractable seizures constitute a distinct clinicopathologic groups of tumors that involve gray matter, arise in a young host, and have a stable course over many years (16). The gray matter location of these low-grade gliomas probably explains their epileptogenicity.

These lesions can be contrasted with low-grade astrocytomas, which present in adult patients, usually during the 4th or 5th decades of life, and which are limited to the white matter. The latter lesions probably

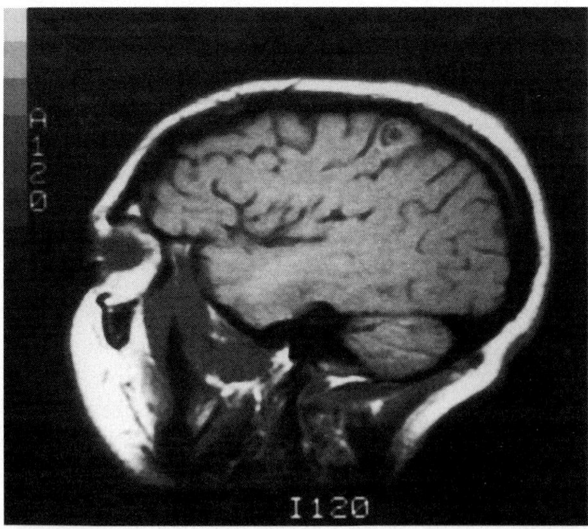

FIG. 27.1 Low-grade astrocytoma with oligodendrocytic differentiation in the left parietal lobe in a 24-year-old woman with chronic seizures since the age of 6. Note gray matter involvement of this small lesion. Resection of the lesion alone was carried out to tumor-free margins, resulting in a seizure-free outcome at 3 years postoperative follow-up.

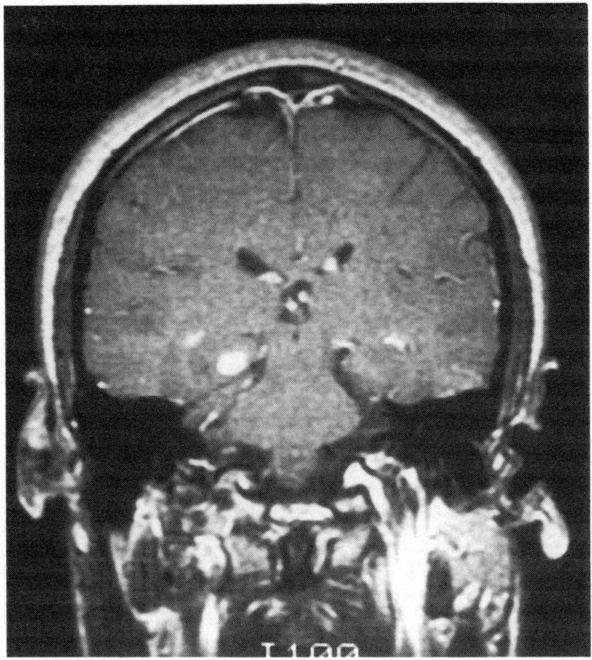

FIG. 27.2 Low-grade astrocytoma, which enhances with gadolinium in a 20-year-old man with intractable seizures since age 15. Note involvement of the right hippocampus and parahippocampal gyrus. In this case anteromedial temporal resection, including the lesion, was carried out.

disrupt white matter connections and usually do not give rise to chronic seizures. Recent data suggest that low-grade astrocytomas associated with a long history of seizures may arise from a different astrocytic lineage than low-grade astrocytomas, which are limited to the white matter and associated with a short history of symptoms (18, 33).

The unique nature of glial tumors associated with chronic seizures was suggested by early observations of Cavanagh (6), who described eight such lesions in the temporal lobe. From his description of these tumors it is apparent that they involved gray matter. Cavanagh regarded these lesions as hamartomatous in nature and suggested that they be considered potential points for further development of gliomas. Intracortical location was a salient feature of a group of tumors associated with chronic seizures described by Daumas-Duport and associates (7). They suggested that these are benign, surgically curable tumors, and offered the term "dysembrioplastic neuroepithelial tumors" (DNETs) for these lesions.

Although most of the glial tumors associated with chronic seizures are low-grade, nearly 20% are anaplastic by histology. Even these tumors have clinical features suggesting an indolent biological behavior (9, 16).

EXTENT OF RESECTION

When a lesion suspected of being a low-grade glioma is identified in a patient without seizures or with seizures that are well under control, there is no reason to contemplate a resection that exceeds the boundaries of the lesion. Resection in this case should be limited to the lesion and its margins and should follow the principles of tumor surgery. However, in patients with intractable seizures, the consideration of seizure control is added to the need to treat the tumor. Should additional resection be carried out in these cases, and what should be the basis for such additional resection? The concern in these cases is that, in addition to the structural lesion apparent on neuro-imaging studies, there might be other abnormalities either adjacent to the lesion or distant from it. These abnormalities are sometimes referred to in a physiologic sense as additional "epileptogenic foci" or "epileptogenic zones" (15). The literature is replete with reports of various resections undertaken to treat patients with gliomas and intractable seizures, but many of these reports also include other lesions associated with chronic seizures, such as vascular malformations and hamartomas.

The most direct and focused approach to extirpation of a low-grade glioma is "stereotactic lesionectomy." This is the approach reported in a series from the Mayo Clinic, using volumetric stereotactic computer-assisted resection (4). The resection is based entirely on definition of the lesion by MRI or computerized tomography (CT) abnormality. The initial experience in the application of this approach to a series of patients with structural lesions associated with chronic seizures showed 26 out of 30 patients with favorable outcome. However, in a long-term follow-up of 23 patients, only 57% were seizure-free. Interestingly, there was a clear association of lesion location with seizure outcome. Only 22% of patients with temporal lobe lesions were rendered seizure-free, while 64% of the patients with extratemporal lesions had a seizure-free outcome (5). These results indicate that removal of the lesion itself, as it appears on the radiologic study, may not be sufficient, and that lesions in the temporal lobe pose a particularly difficult challenge for seizure control, requiring additional resection beyond the lesion boundaries.

There are several other reports in the literature concerning resection of gliomas in patients with intractable seizures without the use of ECoG. Falconer and associates (12) reported two cases of low-grade gliomas in posterior temporal cortex in patients with chronic seizures. Removal of the lesion alone was carried out in each case, with eventual (although not immediate) seizure-free outcome. Goldring and colleagues (19) reported 82% seizure-free outcome following surgery on 40 patients with gliomas. Resections were done by open craniotomy and were focused on the lesion; however, seven patients had anterior temporal lobectomies, and ECoG was used in three additional patients. Goldring and associates concluded that in patients with chronic seizures and gliomas, simple excision of the tumor is usually all that is necessary for seizure control.

Fried and associates (16) reported that the most important factor in achieving seizure control in these patients is complete removal of the lesion. Their surgical approach was based on extirpation of the gliomas to tumor-free margins by frozen-section histology. (Fig. 27.1) However, when tumors were close to or infiltrated the mesial temporal lobe structures—amygdala, uncus, hippocampus, or parahippocampus gyrus— these were removed as well (Fig. 27.2). Seizure-free outcome was 82%, with better results when complete removal was accomplished (85%) and poor results (50%) when only partial resection was achieved. The importance of complete tumor removal as a prerequisite to good seizure outcome is corroborated by other investigators (1, 13). In a series limited to tumors of the pediatric age group in patients with chronic seizures, Blume and colleagues (3) reported 87% seizure-free outcome with "complete" removal of the tumor, but only 33% seizure-free outcome following partial resection. The results of other series with low-grade gliomas are sometimes difficult to interpret, because data for patients with chronic seizures are combined with data for patients without intractable seizures (*e.g.,* ref. 21). Many of the larger series of low-grade gliomas have been concerned with survival rates, rather than with seizure outcome and, although they usually included some patients with chronic seizures, this group was not analyzed separately (26, 32, 39).

There are several reports that substantiate the use of "temporal lobectomy" to treat glial tumors that are located in the temporal lobe. Lindsay and colleagues (28) reported good seizure outcome in two children with low-grade gliomas treated with radical temporal lobectomy. Kirkpatrick and associates (24) reported 81% seizure-free and 10% "almost seizure-free" outcome following en bloc temporal lobectomy for low-grade gliomas. Summarizing the UCLA experience with an anterior temporal lobectomy for lesions associated with chronic seizures, Eliashiv and associates (9) reported a 78% seizure-free outcome in patients with long-term follow-up (mean, 6 years; range, 1–20 years).

LOW-GRADE GLIOMAS: LOCAL AND REMOTE EPILEPTOGENESIS

One of the difficulties in establishing criteria for optimal resection of low-grade gliomas associated with chronic seizures is our poor understanding of the relationship between the tumor and seizures. The eminent neurologist Hughlings Jackson pointed out that seizures do not originate from the tumor itself and suggested that they arise from instability of the surrounding gray matter (22). Zulch (41) pointed to slow growth rate of tumors and their proximity to the cortex as important factors in enhancing epileptogenicity. Several animal models of experimental cortical lesions based on application of aluminum cream (25), cobalt (20), or ferric compounds (40) to the cortex have been developed to investigate local changes giving rise to chronic seizures. These changes include local neuronal injury, glial proliferation, vascular changes, and neurotransmitter changes in surrounding cortex. However, there is no animal tumor model that includes chronic seizures.

It is likely that most open resections of low-grade gliomas result in removal of surrounding brain parenchyma affected by the presence of the tumor. Indeed removal of the lesion to tumor-free margins is often sufficient to obtain excellent seizure outcome. A more difficult problem is the potential presence of remote epileptic foci, which might suggest the need for extensive resection in areas that are not contiguous with the tumor. These remote foci are sometimes attributed to the mechanism of secondary epileptogenesis (30). According to this model, irreversible lesions develop in patients as a result of frequent seizures experienced over a long period of time. This process may well result in independent, secondary foci, which are often bilateral. In these patients resection of the primary lesion, *e.g.*, tumor, may not be sufficient to control seizures. It has been suggested that the earlier the age of onset of seizures, the more rapid the development of the secondary focus (34).

Another model used to explain the presence of epileptogenic regions distant from the "primary" lesion, is that of dual pathology (27). In this model a second area of *structural* pathology is postulated to contribute to the chronic seizures. The existence of dual or additional pathology may depend on several variables, including seizure history and the type of lesion. This is perhaps the reason why chronic seizures associated with certain types of lesions, such as ganglioglioma, are more difficult to control with simple excision of the lesion (8, 23, 38).

The model of dual pathology has been invoked to explain involvement of the hippocampus in cases of lesions outside the hippocampus (17, 27). There is evidence that the degree of cell loss in hippocampus in these patients depends on several variables. These variables include the type of lesion (27), the distance of the lesion from the hippocampus

(17, 29), the age at seizure onset (17), and the presence of prolonged first seizures (29). Patients with gliomas, patients with lesions distant from the hippocampus, and patients with late age of seizure onset are usually less likely to have hippocampal cell loss.

The presence of dual pathology may sometimes be demonstrated by MRI techniques. Specifically, structural measures of the hippocampus, as seen on MRI, may correlate with hippocampal pathology in patients with ipsilateral temporal lobe tumors. Indirect inference of hippocampal integrity or pathology may be based on neuropsychologic tests, as well as on the results of intracarotid Amytal procedure (Wada test). For instance, patients with selective memory deficits or patients who fail the memory part of the Wada test following injection in the carotid contralateral to the tumor, are more likely to have hippocampal damage (35–37).

The determination of the need for resection beyond the immediate margins of the tumor needs to be based on evidence of extralesional or dual pathology. Furthermore, the surgeon contemplating resections beyond and remote from the tumor should weigh the evidence for such pathology against the probability of inflicting neuropsychologic deficits as a result of wide resection. For instance, in a patient with chronic seizures of adult onset who has good verbal memory and is found to harbor a glioma in the dominant middle temporal gyrus, there may be little reason to believe that the hippocampus is affected. In this patient a large resection in the form of a "standard" temporal lobectomy or ECoG-based resection may result in significant decline in verbal memory.

IS ECoG NECESSARY?

While pathology extraneous to the tumor may be present, there has been no clear evidence that it can be identified by ECoG, nor has it been substantiated that basing the resection on ECoG offers a significant advantage.

Although the interictal spike is considered by many to be a diagnostic criterion in clinical epilepsy and is believed to indicate epileptogenicity, the relationship between surgical outcome with respect to seizures and the presence or absence of interictal spikes is puzzling. There is conflicting evidence about the relationship between improvement of scalp EEG and surgical outcome. Engel and colleagues (11) reported no correlation of outcome following temporal lobectomy with postoperative scalp-recorded interictal spikes. Thirty-eight patients who underwent temporal lobectomy were analyzed. Sixty percent of the patients who had persistent seizures had interictal spikes, but 75% of patients who were rendered seizure-free also had interictal spikes. There is evidence that some types of interictal spiking activity actually correlate with decreased seizure potential in epileptic patients (11). In amygdaloid-kindled rats interictal EEG spikes are correlated with decreased, rather than increased, epileptogenicity (10).

There is also no evidence that preresection or postresection ECoG has any bearing on outcome with respect to seizure control. Falconer and associates (12) reported two cases in which resection of posterior temporal low-grade gliomas did not result in improvement in the ECoG, yet the patients became seizure-free. In a series reported by Kirkpatrick and colleagues (24), relief of seizures following en bloc temporal lobectomy for low-grade gliomas could not be predicted by pre- or postresection intra-operative ECoG. Similar findings were observed by Tran and associates (personal communication). In this study ECoG was recorded intraoperatively before and after glioma resection, which was not based on the ECoG information. There was no difference in spike data between patients who had good seizure outcome and patients who had poor outcome. Awad and colleagues (1) found that, when complete resection of a structural lesion was accomplished, the extent of "focus" resection based on ictal and interictal recordings did not affect seizure outcome.

Undeniably, resection of low-grade gliomas based on ECoG yields excellent seizure outcome (see Berger *et al.* (2) for results and review). However, the hazard of relying on ECoG to determine the extent of resection is that it may give license to larger resections than are needed. For instance, in a report by Berger and associates (2) on 15 patients with lateral temporal lobe focus, 13 had a concomitant mesial temporal focus. ECoG in such cases may lead to extensive mesial temporal resection, including the hippocampus, for lesions involving lateral neocortex. ECoG-based license to perform large resections is often taken in regions of association cortex that are dismissed as "noneloquent," probably because their removal does not produce a deficit that can be detected in a cursory bedside examination (14). Clearly, larger resections carry a higher probability of success with respect to seizure outcome than do smaller resections. However, the role of surgery is to remove the minimal amount of brain parenchyma necessary to achieve the therapeutic goal. Such removal should be taken after rational consideration of the variables that might contribute to secondary or other pathology, in addition to the lesion. This pertains particularly to removal of the mesial temporal structures for a low-grade glioma in the temporal lobe. One should always keep in mind the option of performing a two-stage procedure, *i.e.,* removal of the tumor and, if seizures persist, removal of the hippocampus at a later stage.

Clearly, before ECoG can be used as an aid to the resection of low-grade gliomas in patients with chronic seizures, the pathophysiology of interictal spikes should be better understood. Furthermore, the advantage of this method should be demonstrated by prospective comparison with more conservative resections that are not based on ECoG. This comparison should include not only seizure outcome but also outcome with respect to neuropsychologic function.

SUMMARY

Low-grade gliomas associated with chronic seizures constitute a distinct clinicopathologic group of tumors that arise in young hosts, are based in gray matter of limbic or adjacent cortex, and usually have an indolent course. The most important factor in achieving long-term seizure control in these patients is complete removal of the lesion, to tumor-free margins.

For low-grade gliomas in the temporal lobe, additional mesial temporal resection may be required, but there is no evidence that it need be based on ECoG. Using this procedure to define the epileptogenic zone for surgery may result in resections that are larger than necessary. The decision on extralesional hippocampal resection should be based on evaluation of the structural and functional status of the hippocampus by considering several variables, including seizure history, proximity of the tumor to the hippocampus, and the neuropsychologic profile of the patient, especially with regard to memory function.

ACKNOWLEDGMENT

The author would like to thank Irene M. Wainwright, Ph.D., for editorial assistance.

REFERENCES

1. Awad I, Rosenfeld J, Ahl J, *et al.*: Intractable epilepsy and structural lesions of the brain: Mapping, resection strategies, and seizure outcome. **Epilepsia** 32:179–186, 1991.
2. Berger M, Ghatan S, Haglund M, *et al.*: Low-grade gliomas associated with intractable epilepsy: Seizure outcome utilizing electrocorticography during tumor resection. **J Neurosurg** 79:62–69, 1993.
3. Blume W, Girvin J, Kaufmann J: Childhood brain tumors presenting as chronic uncontrolled focal seizure disorders. **Ann Neurol** 12:538–541, 1982.
4. Cascino G, Kelly P, Marsh W, *et al.*: Stereotactic resection of intra-axial cerebral lesions in partial epilepsy. **Mayo Clin Proc** 65:1053–1060, 1990.
5. Cascino G, Kelly P, Sharbrough R, *et al.*: Long-term follow-up of stereotactic lesionectomy in partial epilepsy. **Epilepsia** 33:639–644, 1992.
6. Cavanagh J: On certain small tumors encountered in the temporal lobe. **Brain** 81:389–405, 1951.
7. Daumas-Duport C, Scheithauer B, Chodkiewicz J, *et al.*: Dysembryoplastic neuroepithelial tumor: A surgically curable tumor of young patients with intractable partial seizures. **Neurosurgery** 23:545–556, 1988.

8. Demierre B, Stichnoth FA, Hori A. *et al.:* Intracerebral ganglioglioma. **J Neurosurg** 65:177–182, 1986.
9. Eliashiv S, Dewar S, Engel J Jr, *et al.:* Chronic seizures associated with temporal lobe lesions: Seizure outcome following uniform anterior temporal lobectomy. **Epilepsia** 35(Suppl 8):100, 1994 (abstr).
10. Engel J Jr, Ackermann RF: Interictal EEG spikes correlate with decreased, rather than increased, epileptogenicity in amygdaloid kindled rats. **Brain Res** 190:543–548, 1980.
11. Engel J Jr, Ackermann RF, Caldecott-Hazard S, *et al.:* Epileptic activation of antagonistic systems may explain paradoxical features of experimental and human epilepsy: A review and hypothesis, in Wada JA (ed): *Kindling 2.* New York, Raven Press, 1981, pp. 193–217.
12. Falconer M, Driver M, Serafetinides E: Temporal lobe epilepsy due to distant lesions: Two cases relieved by operation. **Brain** 85:521–534, 1962.
13. Fish D, Andermann F, Olivier A: Complex partial seizures and small posterior temporal or extratemporal structural lesions: Surgical management. **Neurology** 41:1781–1784, 1991.
14. Fried I: The myth of eloquent cortex, or what is non-eloquent cortex? **J Neurosurg** 78:1009–1010, 1993.
15. Fried I, Cascino G: Lesional surgery, in Engel J Jr (ed): *Surgical Treatment of the Epilepsies 2.* New York, Raven Press, 1993, pp. 501–509.
16. Fried I, Kim J, Spencer D: Limbic and neocortical gliomas associated with intractable seizures: A distinct clinicopathological group. **J Neurosurg** 34:815–823, 1994.
17. Fried I, Kim JH, Spencer DD: Hippocampal pathology in patients with intractable seizures and temporal lobe masses. **J Neurosurg** 76:735–740, 1992.
18. Fried I, Piepmeier JM, Makuch R: Low-grade astrocytomas associated with chronic seizures may arise from type I astrocyte lineage. **Epilepsia** 34(Suppl 6):126, 1993. (abstr).
19. Goldring S, Rich K, Picker S: Experience with gliomas in patients presenting with a chronic seizure disorder. **Clin Neurosurg** 33:15–42, 1986.
20. Hartman E, Colasanti B, Craig C: Epileptogenic properties of cobalt and related metals applied directly to cerebral cortex of rat. **Epilepsia** 15:121–129, 1974.
21. Hirsch, J-F, Sainte Rose C, Pierre-Khan A, *et al.:* Benign astrocytic and oligodendrocytic tumors of the cerebral hemispheres in children. **J Neurosurg** 70:568–572, 1989.
22. Jackson JH: Case of tumor of the right temporo-sphenoidal lobe, bearing on the localization of the sense of smell and the interpretation of a particular variety of epilepsy, in Taylor J (ed): *Selected Writings of J. Hughlings Jackson.* New York, Basic Books, 1958, pp 406–411.
23. Kalyan-Raman UP, Olivero WC: Ganglioglioma: A correlative clinicopathological and radiological study of ten surgically treated cases with follow-up. **Neurosurgery** 20:428–433, 1987.
24. Kirkpatrick P, Honavar M, Janota I, *et al.:* Control of temporal lobe epilepsy following en bloc resection of low-grade tumors. **J Neurosurg** 78:19–25, 1993.
25. Kopeloff L, Barrera S, Kopeloff N: Recurrent convulsive seizures in animals produced by immunological and chemical means. **Am J Psychiatry** 98:881–902, 1942.
26. Laws ER, Taylor WF, Clifton MB, *et al.:* Neurosurgical management of low grade astrocytoma of the cerebral hemisphere. **J Neurosurg** 61:665–673, 1984.

27. Levesque M, Nakasato N, Vinters H, *et al.:* Surgical treatment of limbic epilepsy associated with extrahippocampal lesions: The problem of dual pathology. **J Neurosurg** 75:364–370, 1991.
28. Lindsay J, Ounsted C, Richards P: Long-term outcome in children with temporal lobe seizures. V: Indications and contra-indications for neurosurgery. **Dev Med Child Neurol** 26:25–32, 1984.
29. Mathern G, Babb T, Pretorius J, *et al.:* Pathogenic clinical mechanisms in temporal seizures. **Epilepsia** 35(Suppl 7):2, 1994 (abstr).
30. Morrell F: Secondary epileptogenesis in man. **Arch Neurol** 42:318–335, 1985.
31. Penfield W, Jasper H: *Epilepsy and the Functional Anatomy of the Human Brain.* Boston, Little Brown, 1954.
32. Piepmeier JM: Observations on the current treatment of low-grade astrocytic tumors of the cerebral hemispheres. **J Neurosurg** 67:177–181, 1987.
33. Piepmeier J, Fried I, Makuch R: Low-grade astrocytomas may arise from two different astrocyte lineages. **Neurosurgery** 33:632–637, 1993.
34. Rasmussen T: Surgical treatment of complex partial seizures: Results, lessons, and problems. **Epilepsia** 24(Suppl 1):S65–S76, 1983.
35. Rausch R, Babb TL: Hippocampal neuron loss and memory scores before and after temporal lobe surgery for epilepsy. **Arch Neurol** 50:812–817, 1993.
36. Sass KJ, Lencz T, Westerveld M, *et al.:* The neural substrate of memory impairment demonstrated by the intracarotid amobarbital procedure. **Arch Neurol** 48:48–52, 1991.
37. Sass KJ, Spencer DD, Kim JH, *et al.:* Verbal memory impairment correlates with hippocampal pyramidal cell density. **Neurology** 40:1694–1697, 1990.
38. Sutton LN, Packer RJ, Rorke LB, *et al.:* Cerebral gangliomas during childhood. **Neurosurgery** 13:124–128, 1983.
39. Vertosick FT, Selker RG, Arena VC: Survival of patients with well-differentiated astrocytoma diagnosed in the era of computed tomography. **Neurosurgery** 28:496–501, 1991.
40. Willmore M, MacDonald D, Cairncross J: Recurrent seizures induced by cortical iron injection. **Ann Neurol** 4:329–334, 1978.
41. Zulch K: Röntgendiagnostik beim cerebralen Anfall. Verh Dtsch Ges Inn Med 56:24, 1951.

28

Brain Astrocytomas: Biopsy, Then Irradiation

L. DADE LUNSFORD, M.D., F.A.C.S., SALVADOR SOMAZA, M.D.,
DOUGLAS KONDZIOLKA, M.D., M.Sc., F.R.C.S.(C.),
AND JOHN C. FLICKINGER, M.D.

DEFINITION OF THE PROBLEM

Astrocytomas represent approximately 15% of brain tumors diagnosed by means of surgery (33). They usually develop in young adults and have a peak incidence in the third decade of life (20), when the patients are just entering their peak earning capacity. Physicians find it difficult to recommend a definitive approach to their patients with astrocytomas because neurosurgeons have reached no consensus regarding the need for and timing of diagnosis, the optimal initial management strategy, or the long-term risk that such tumors present.

Any discussion of the management of astrocytomas must first define the entity in question: the nonanaplastic, nonpilocystic glial neoplasm. Because survival is longer than with histologically malignant tumors, they are often considered "benign." This term belies the insidious progression of these tumors and the unfortunate outcomes with which they are associated in the vast majority of patients (16). Although their growth rate is slower than that of anaplastic astrocytomas or glioblastomas (that is, their initial histopathologic features do not meet the criteria for malignancy), almost all astrocytomas eventually lead to death. Median survival of 5 years or less is common, even in more recent series (28, 39, 40). Only 20 to 30% of patients live 10 years or more after the onset of symptoms (28).

With no consensus regarding the effectiveness of initial cytoreductive surgery or radiation therapy (30), the recommendations for initial management at various centers include simple observation, biopsy and irradiation, or radical resection with or without postoperative radiation therapy. These diverse approaches underscore the confusion that reigns concerning current management.

In 1982, the senior author (LDL) initiated a prospective phase I-II study to determine the outcome of early stereotactic biopsy followed by external-beam fractionated coned-down radiation therapy. In this report, we will analyze the results for 35 consecutive patients and compare these to some of the data available from the brain tumor literature.

ASTROCYTOMAS ARE NOT BENIGN

Analyses of survival after the diagnosis of a cerebral astrocytoma emphasize the significant problem that this tumor presents. Soffietti *et al.* reported 5-year survival rates of 51, 23.5, and 0%, respectively, for patients who underwent total, subtotal, and partial tumor removal (40). North *et al.* reported overall actuarial survival rates of 55 and 43% at 5 and 10 years, respectively (31), and McCormack *et al.* noted a 5-year survival rate of 64% (27). More recently, Vertosick *et al.* reported a median survival of 8.2 years for 25 patients with astrocytomas (43).

A re-examination by Shaw *et al.* (38), of a large series at the Mayo Clinic indicates the importance of stratification variables in determining and reporting outcomes related to astrocytoma management. This study of a series originally analyzed by Laws *et al.* (21), found the 5- and 10-year survival rates to be 51 and 23%, respectively. The original report included a large group of patients with pilocystic astrocytomas, all of whom had significantly better survival than the patients with nonpilocystic tumors (21); for example, those who underwent total or radical subtotal removal of the tumor alone had a 10-year survival rate of 100%. Moreover, for patients with a nonpilocystic astrocytoma, the re-analysis was unable to show that the extent of surgical removal significantly improved survival when radiation therapy was also administered (38). Other series are similarly flawed in failing to stratify variables that influence survival, namely, tumor location, tumor volume, patient age, and completion of an adequate tumor dose of fractionated external-beam radiation therapy (approximately 50 Gy).

Most patients with astrocytomas die because the original nonanaplastic tumor progresses to a more malignant lesion (21, 27, 28, 30, 32, 33, 39). In our series of 35 patients, such delayed transformation to a malignant glial neoplasm was evident in six patients (17%). In two of these patients, craniotomy and resection confirmed progression of the tumor to an anaplastic form, and stereotactic biopsy verified this finding in a third patient. For the remaining three patients, delayed but distinct imaging signs of tumor progression and new marginal or intratumoral contrast enhancement of central necrosis combined with a deteriorating clinical condition were considered indicative that the tumor had become malignant.

CYTOREDUCTIVE SURGERY: NECESSARY FOR SOME PATIENTS

Even today, some astrocytomas are not diagnosed until the patient has a large intracranial mass associated with a significant neurologic deficit. When such tumors are located in polar or subcortical lobar locations and are large enough to cause a significant mass effect (often larger than 40 to 50 mm in average diameter), cytoreductive surgery is often the only measure that will allow the patient to complete subsequent adjuvant therapy.

The modern cytoreductive surgery has been enhanced by modern technological achievements, including stereotactically guided craniotomy, computer-assisted laser vaporization, intraoperative monitoring, electrocorticography, and high-resolution frameless stereotactic imaging (8, 17, 23). Thus, the debatable issue is not whether such surgical adjuncts improve the surgeon's ability to resect the tumor safely, but whether such resection actually improves outcomes and long-term survival. The concept of gross total or even radical resection of astrocytomas is tenuous at best. Since astrocytomas often contain 3 to 6 $\times$ 10^{10} tumor cells at presentation, a 99% surgical resection still leaves as many as 10^8 tumor cells remaining (37). We believe that cytoreductive surgery *alone* *never* cures nonpilocytic glial neoplasms. Thus, although we have performed cytoreductive surgery as the initial procedure on more than half of the patients with an astrocytoma who have presented to our service since 1981, all of them had significant mass effect and/or significant neurologic deficits. The 35 patients who did not have these findings underwent stereotactic biopsy and fractionated radiation therapy. The completeness of a cytoreductive resection is impossible to ascertain because the tumor extends beyond the area of hypodensity on the computerized tomography (CT) scan or the abnormality on T2-heightened magnetic resonance imaging (MRI) (29, 30). This feature contributes to the lack of consensus about the value of "radical" surgery inasmuch as few surgeons even agree on the terminology used (6, 17–19).

Cytoreductive surgery is often recommended as the initial procedure for all patients with glial neoplasms, based on the theory that this will reduce the number of cells that can differentiate into a more malignant neoplasm (27). However, it is also possible that initial fractionated radiation therapy reduces the same cell population, even without causing cell death, by rendering these cells incapable of mitosis. Unfortunately, no surgical procedure can completely remove an astrocytoma, and therefore the validity of the cytoreductive hypothesis has proven difficult to test. To date, there is no substantive evidence to support this intriguing concept.

RADIATION THERAPY CONTROVERSY

The controversy concerning subsequent management of an astrocytoma is surprising given the overwhelming evidence that radiation therapy significantly improves survival (3, 4, 12–14, 22, 29, 33, 39, 40). In their initial report on Mayo Clinic series, Laws *et al.* concluded that radiation therapy did not strongly improve survival rates, although patients who received doses above 40 Gy survived longer than those who received smaller doses (21). The re-analysis by Shaw *et al.* showed that radiation therapy had statistically favorable benefits (38). Survival curves differed depending on the dose administered: patients who received high-dose irradiation (>53 Gy) had a 5-year survival of 68%, compared with 47% for those who had low-dose irradiation and 32% for those who underwent surgery alone. Medbery *et al.* reported that doses above 50 Gy were associated with better outcomes than were lower doses (28).

Before high-resolution neurodiagnostic imaging became readily available, radiation therapists advocated whole-brain irradiation because the tumor volume was difficult to define (35, 43). We concur with current radiation oncology regimens wherein external-beam radiation therapy, to a total dose of 50 to 60 Gy, is administered in fractions of 1.8 Gy over approximately 7 weeks. The target volume should be the imaging-defined tumor mass plus a 2- to 3-cm margin (31).

NOT ALL ASTROCYTOMAS REQUIRE SURGICAL DEBULKING

To clarify the role of various management strategies, we have analyzed in detail our experience using stereotactic biopsy plus fractionated external-beam radiation therapy on 35 patients who had histologically verified nonanaplastic nonpilocystic astrocytomas. The biopsies were performed within 6 months of onset of symptoms in 27 (77%) of these patients. We were able to obtain long-term follow-up evaluations for all 35 patients (median, 62 months; range, 11 to 128 months). We calculated their survival from both the time of biopsy and the onset of tumor-related neurologic symptoms. The endpoint of the analysis was death or latest available follow-up evaluation. Survival curves were constructed using the life table method (2).

Neurodiagnostic Technique

Table 28.1 shows the clinical features of our patients. More than two-thirds of them were between the ages of 21 and 40 when first examined, and symptoms included seizures in more than 60%. All patients underwent neurodiagnostic imaging initially with CT (Table 28.2). Since 1987, we have also performed MRI on most patients. A low-attenuation area on a CT and a high T2 signal lesion on MRI, often associated with relatively little mass effect, suggested the possibility of an astrocytoma. Their tumors were lobar or deep lesions without contrast enhancement (Table 28.2). Patients who entered this prospective

TABLE 28.1
Clinical Features in 35 University of Pittsburgh Patients[a] with an Astrocytoma

	No. of Patients (%)
Sex	
Male	22 (63)
Female	13 (37)
Age (y)	
<20	6 (17)
21–40	24 (69)
41–60	5 (14)
Symptoms	
Seizures	22 (63)
Headaches	14 (40)
Decreased vision	2 (6)
Signs	
Sensory loss	4 (11)
Motor weakness	10 (29)
Speech disorder	3 (9)
Cranial neuropathy	4 (11)
Personality changes	2 (6)

[a]Data gathered from 1981 to 1983.

TABLE 28.2
CT-Defined Characteristics of Astrocytomas (n = 35)[a]

	No. of patients (%)
Lobar location	22 (63)
Deep location[b]	13 (37)
Low attenuation	30 (86)
Local mass effect	2 (6)
Cystic	2 (6)
Calcification	1 (3)
Contrast enhancement	5 (14)
Mean diameter:	
≤3 cm	15 (43)
>3 cm	18 (51)
unspecified	2 (6)

[a]Reprinted with permission from (23).
[b]Basal ganglia or brainstem.

study did not have significant mass effect or signs of increased intracranial pressure, and patients with anaplastic astrocytomas or other histologic diagnoses were excluded from this trial.

All of our patients underwent biopsies using the Leksell stereotactic system. A dedicated intra-operative CT system has been used since 1981 and since 1987 has been supplemented by MRI. MRI proved to be a superior method for target selection owing to its accuracy and multiplanar imaging. All stereotactic procedures were performed with the patient under local anesthesia, and all lesions were sampled at multiple points along a single trajectory. In this series, the average tumor diameter was 35 mm (range, 15 to 55 mm).

Histologic touch preparations (25) were performed intraoperatively, and then the specimens were fixed with paraffin for analysis. Using the dedicated CT scanner in our operating suite, we were able to assess target accuracy and detect possible complications immediately after biopsy. Neuropathologic analysis revealed a nonpilocystic astrocytoma in all patients included in this series. No tumor had features of anaplasia (marked hypercellularity, nuclear pleomorphism, necrosis, or endothelial proliferation). We used the astrocytoma grading system of Burger, a three-tiered system that classifies tumors as an astrocytoma, an anaplastic astrocytoma, or a glioblastoma (5, 7). Histopathologic analysis of the tumors in this study showed mild hypercellularity, the fairly uniform morphologic characteristics of mature astrocytic tumor cells, and an absence of oligodendroglia. Occasional nuclear atypism or pleomorphism was noted. In more recent years, immunocytochemistry stains have also been used, but they have not been particularly valuable.

All patients underwent conventional fractionated external-beam radiation therapy as outpatients. We selected coned-down fractionated radiation therapy, basing the tumor volume targeted for irradiation on the neurodiagnostic imaging studies. The average radiation dose was 56 Gy (range, 45 to 60 Gy) for an average dose per fraction of 1.8 Gy. The median number of fractions was 31 (range, 22 to 36), delivered over a median of 5.5 weeks. For two patients whose tumors subsequently became neoplastic, we administered delayed intracavitary irradiation using colloidal radioactive phosphorus (^{32}P). In both cases, we calculated the cyst volume using standard stereotactic software and stereotactically injected the ^{32}P to provide a dose of 200 to 250 Gy to the cyst wall over five lives of the isotope. Four other patients received delayed intravenous chemotherapy after documentation that their tumors had taken a more malignant form.

Clinical Response

We were able to control seizures in 20 of the 22 patients who had seizures initially. For many of these patients, seizure control was obtained with anticonvulsant medications and paralleled the reduction in local tumor mass effect noted on serial imaging studies after radiation therapy (Fig. 28.1). No patient had a biopsy-related complication, and 91% of the patients who had a good or excellent neurologic condition before biopsy had the same afterward (Table 28.3). Two patients

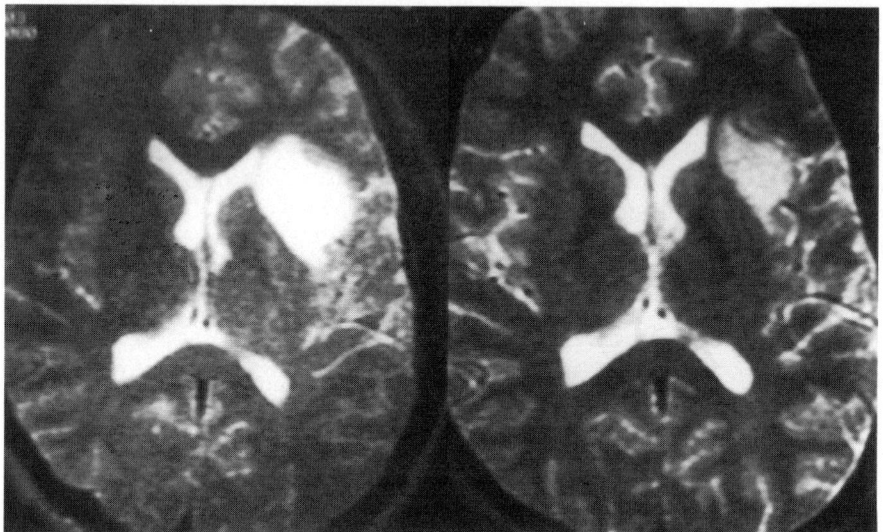

FIG. 28.1 Pre- **(left)** and postbiopsy **(right)** MRI scan on a 21-year-old male who presented with a single seizure. The astrocytoma regressed 10 months after completely fractionated radiation therapy.

TABLE 28.3
Karnofsky Performance Rating Associated with Stereotactic Biopsy and Irradiation of Astrocytomas

Karnofsky Performance Rating	No. of Patients		
	Before Biopsy	Immediately after Biopsy	At Last Available Follow-up[a]
100	27	29	15
90	5	3	6
80	3	3	5
70			5
60			3
50			1

[a]Median, 62 months. Six patients subsequently died of tumor progression.

actually improved, perhaps related to the usage of oral corticosteroids. According to the Brain Tumor Study Group, the Karnofsky Performance Scale (KPS) rating is significantly related to the survival rate when each KPS component is treated as an independent variable (15, 30). Low preoperative KPS scores are significantly associated with higher death rates (15, 30). At last follow-up (median, 62 months) 60% of the surviving patients had KPS ratings of 90 or 100, and four patients had a rating of less than 70. Delayed hydrocephalus developed in four patients (all with deep-seated tumors), and they required ventriculoperitoneal shunts. After a median follow-up of 57 months, almost 70% of patients maintained their full working capacity.

Imaging-Defined Response

Serial neurodiagnostic imaging studies for all patients were performed every 6 months for the first 3 postoperative years and then yearly thereafter. The response of the tumor volume to radiation therapy was judged by monitoring the low-attenuation area on CT images and, for patients who had MRI, the T2-weighted increased-signal area. As it was for target selection, MRI was clearly the superior imaging tool for assessing the response to treatment (Fig. 28.2). The serial imaging studies showed tumor regression in 16 of the 35 patients (46%), with tumor shrinkage occurring gradually. Most tumors regressed within 2 years after radiation therapy (Fig. 28.3).

During the follow-up interval, significant tumor growth and increased mass effect associated with new symptoms occurred in only three patients, and they underwent craniotomy and delayed cytoreductive surgery (Fig. 28.4). One of these patients had a residual astrocytoma (56 months after biopsy); the second patient had an anaplastic astrocytoma (96 months after biopsy); and the third patient had a glioblastoma (14 months after biopsy).

Survival curves were stratified according to several clinical variables. We identified no differences in this rather small study sample

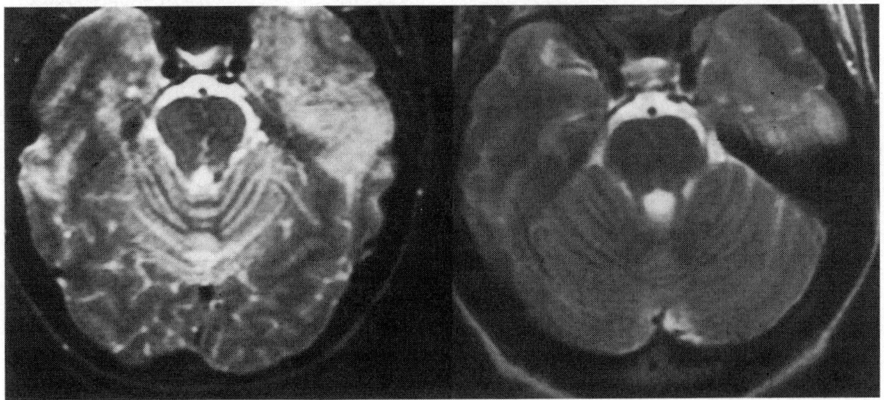

FIG. 28.2 Pre- (left) and 18 months postbiopsy (right) T2-weighted MRI of a 27-year-old woman who presented with partial complex seizures. The biopsy revealed an astrocytoma (left). The tumor regressed 16 months after fractionated radiation therapy (right).

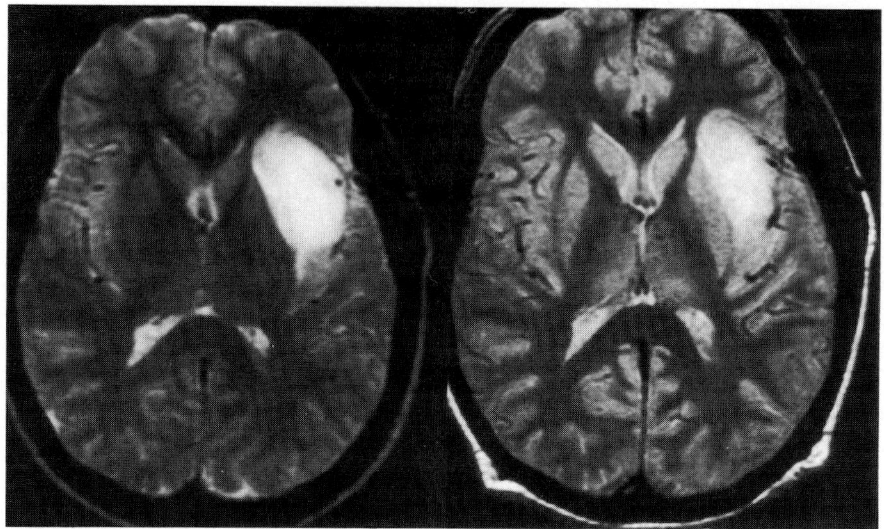

FIG. 28.3 Pre- (**left**) and postbiopsy (**right**) T2-weighted MRI on a 22-year-old male with an astrocytoma. Tumor regression was noted 18 months after completion of fractionated radiation therapy.

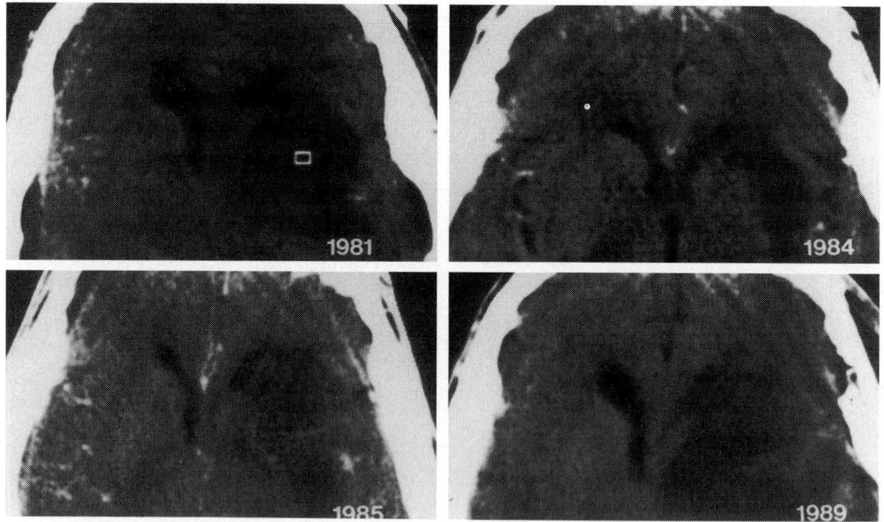

FIG. 28.4 Serial imaging studies of a 46-year-old man who presented with a 7-month history of seizures. Stereotactic biopsy in *1981* showed an astrocytoma. He had fractionated radiation therapy and remained asymptomatic until *1989*. A craniotomy and cytoreductive surgery were performed. Pathology analysis again reported an astrocytoma (without anaplastic change).

when survival rates were stratified by the following variables: tumor diameter (≤30 mm *versus* >30 mm; *P* = .34), tumor location (brainstem *versus* lobar, *P* = .47), total fractionated radiation therapy dose (≤56 Gy *versus* >56 Gy, *P* = .99), and patient age (*P* = .84) all failed to influence survival. By the time this study was completed, nine patients had died: six from tumor progression and three from other illnesses. The latter three patients were excluded from survival analysis because they were stable neurologically before they died. Figure 28.5 shows the survival curves constructed using the life table method. The median survival after stereotactic biopsy was 118 months and after symptom onset, 148 months (Table 28.4). Median survival did not seem to be significantly influenced by the interval between symptom onset and diagnostic biopsy, which was much less than 6 months for most patients. Table 28.5 compares 5- and 10-year survival data from the literature, and Table 28.6 compares median length of survival among representative series during the last 4 decades.

BIOPSY *VERSUS* RESECTION

Even more controversial than the benefit of radical surgical resection for patients with astrocytomas is the role of stereotactic biopsy in initial management. Patients who have subcortical or polar lesions generally undergo craniotomy and resection, while stereotactic biopsy is often reserved for patients with deep-seated lesions (who are thought

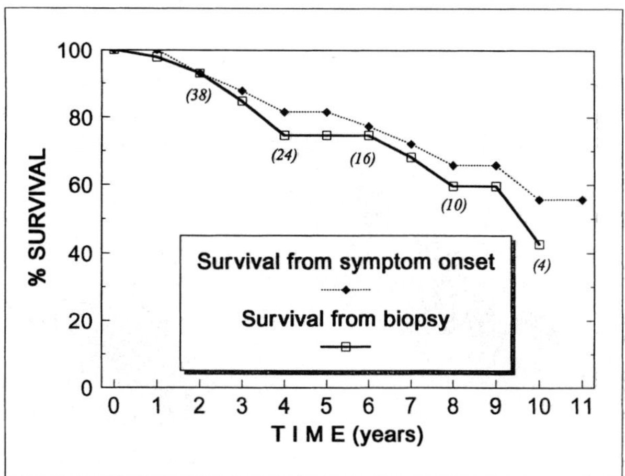

FIG. 28.5 Survival curves in a series of 35 patients with nonanaplastic, nonpilocystic astrocytomas. All patients had stereotactic biopsy at the University of Pittsburgh followed by fractionated external-beam radiation therapy.

TABLE 28.4
Stereotactic Biopsy and Radiation of Astrocytomas: Survival Statistics[a]

	Survival Rates (Median ± SD)			
	Beginning of Survival Calculation	5 yr (%)	10 yr (%)	Median Survival Rate (mo)
Disease-specific survival[b]	Date of biopsy	88.4 ± 6.5	47.2 ± 20.9	118
Overall[b] survival	Date of biopsy	81.6 ± 7.5	36.3 ± 17.3	118
Disease-specific survival	Symptom onset	88.4 ± 6.5	64.3 ± 16.3	148
Overall survival	Symptom onset	81.4 ± 7.6	51.8 ± 15.2	148

[a]Reprinted with permission from (23).
[b]Disease specific indicates survival until death related to the brain tumor; overall includes death from any cause.

TABLE 28.5
Survival Rates in Series of Patients with Cerebral Astrocytomas

			Survival Rates	
Investigators	Study Interval	No. of Patients (by Treatment Type)	5-yr (%)	10-yr (%)
Uihlein *et al.* (42) (*n* = 83)	1955–1959	33 (S)[a]	65	
		50 (S+R)	54	
Stage and Stein (41) (*n* = 45)	1956–1970	17 (S)	20	
		28 (S+R)	40	
Marsa *et al.* (24) (*n* = 40)	1957–1973	40 (S+R)	41	22
Leibel *et al.* (22) (*n* = 147)		76 (S)	19	11
	1942–1967	71 (S+R)	46	35
Laws *et al.* (21) (*n* = 241)		167 (S)	34	~10
	1915–1975	74 (S+R)	49	~15
Fazekas (12) (*n* = 68)		23 (S)	32	26
	1958–1974	45 (S+R)	54	32
Medbery *et al.* (28) (*n* = 50)	1960–1986	50 (S+R)	45	32
McCormack *et al.* (27) (*n* = 48)	1977–1988	48 (S+R)	64	
North *et al.* (31) (*n* = 66)	1975–1984	66 (S+R)	55	43
Philippon *et al.* (32) (*n* = 134)[b]	1978–1987	32 (S)	35	
		102 (S+R)	50	
Lunsford *et al.* (23) (*n* = 35)	1982–1992	35 (S+R)	81	51

[a]S, surgery only (biopsy, subtotal, or total resection); S+R, surgery plus fractionated radiation therapy.
[b]Subtotal removal and biopsy

to be poor candidates for surgical resection) or for those who are ill, in poor health, or elderly (21, 27, 31, 36). This practice alone is probably sufficient to account for the rather poor outcomes associated with biopsy. For example, in the Mayo Clinic series, Laws *et al.* noted that resection tended to be performed on tumors that were relatively small and superficial. Therefore, it is not surprising that in their initial report on this series, the 5-year survival rates were linked to whether the patient underwent biopsy only (32%), subtotal resection (44%), or radical removal (61%) (21). The re-analysis by Shaw *et al.* eliminated the pilocytic tumors and failed to disclose any significant benefit of surgical resection (38).

When the appropriate stratification variables (age, tumor volume, radiation technique, and tumor location) are considered, the reputed benefits of cytoreductive surgery are less convincing. McCormack *et al.* stated that radical extirpation is indicated, although they provided little compelling data to support this philosophy (27). They reserved biopsy for patients with tumors that were deep-seated or located in critical brain regions; such patients often had a median survival of less than 2 years.

Some surgeons do not perform stereotactic biopsy because they believe it has a high risk of morbidity and mortality, even though modern and neurodiagnostic imaging studies show a less than 1% risk of either. In contrast, the combined medical and neurologic morbidity after cytoreductive surgery may exceed 32% (11). The main objectives of cytoreductive surgery are to provide an adequate tissue sample to obtain a definitive diagnosis and to reduce intracranial pressure when it is elevated. In the past, some surgeons emphasized that craniotomy and tumor resection provide a larger sample of tissue for pathologic evaluation than needle biopsy does (10, 34, 41). Contemporary neuroimaging techniques coupled with advanced biopsy tools have modified that concept substantially (1, 8, 17, 18, 43). In 1988, Fadul *et al.* reported that, of 104 patients who underwent surgery for supratentorial gliomas, 2% had significant postoperative neurologic deterioration (11). Moreover, new postoperative neurologic deficits developed in 13%

TABLE 28.6

Median Survival of Patients with Astrocytoma in the Last Four Decades

Series	No. of Patients Treated	Study Interval	Median Survival (yr)
Soffietti *et al.* (40)	85	1950–1982	3.2
Fazekas (12)	68	1958–1974	~5
Shaw *et al.* (38)	24	1976–1983	4.5
Piepmeier *et al.* (33)	50	1975–1985	7.5[a]
Medbery *et al.* (28)	50	1960–1986	4
Vertosick *et al.* (43)	25	1978–1988	8.2
Philippon *et al.* (32)	179	1978–1987	9
McCormack *et al.* (27)	53	1977–1988	7.25
Lunsford *et al.* (23)	35	1982–1992	9.8

[a]Mean value.

TABLE 28.7

Surgical Mortality Rates for Cerebral Astrocytomas

Series	No. of Patients	Study Interval	Surgical Mortality Rates (%)
Piepmeier *et al.* (33)	60	1975–1985	3.3
Philippon *et al.* (32)	179	1978–1987	5
McCormack *et al.* (27)	53	1977–1988	11.3[a]
Laws *et al.* (21)	499	1915–1975	7.6
Fadul *et al.* (11)	109	1985–1987	3.3
North *et al.* (31)	77	1975–1984	6.5
Vertosick *et al.* (43)	25	1978–1988	0
Lunsford *et al.* (23)	35	1982–1992	0

[a]Five patients died during an extended hospital stay (beyond 30 days).

of patients who were normal pre-operatively. The authors concluded that the risks for developing a significant new neurologic deficit after unsuccessful total resection was approximately 20%. McCormack *et al.* found that 5.6% of 53 patients (who were neurologically normal before surgery) had postoperative deficits. Three recent studies (1987, 1990, 1993) found mortality rates of 3.3 to 6.5% after the resection of low-grade astrocytomas (31–33). (Table 28.7).

The morbidity and mortality of tumor biopsy were high in the years before modern neurodiagnostic imaging became available (9, 26). The likelihood of an inaccurate stereotactic biopsy is rare because sampling of the length of the lesion volume in a single trajectory provides multiple specimens for the neuropathologist to analyze (8, 25). Some surgeons still offer patients only cytoreductive surgery as the initial management procedure because they are unfamiliar with stereotactic biopsy techniques. Others may have a rather high complication rate if they use technology that requires sampling of the target volume laterally in a plane parallel to the base of the stereotactic frame. Such lateral-entry trajectories run the risk of penetrating a branch of the middle cerebral artery, especially in the region of the sylvian fissure. The approach selected for a stereotactic biopsy should have an entry point that minimizes the risk of traversing a pial artery. MRI is very helpful in identifying these vessels. We have found absolutely no value in using intra-operative stereotactic angiography to reduce the risk of morbidity. Table 28.7 shows various surgical mortality rates reported in the literature.

CONCLUSIONS

We believe that every patient who has clinical symptoms and neurodiagnostic imaging signs suggesting a low-grade glial neoplasm should undergo early diagnosis and treatment. Observation is not warranted for a tumor that has a median survival of 5 years. The value of cytoreductive surgery for many patients has yet to be proven. It is incumbent on neurosurgeons who advocate this approach to show that this more aggressive treatment strategy is preferable to minimally invasive techniques, such as stereotactic biopsy followed by radiation therapy. Clearly, some patients who have a glial tumor require early cytoreductive surgery: those with mass effect and significant neurologic deficits. Otherwise, they will not be able to tolerate fractionated radiation therapy. Because the long-term survival rate is very poor, observation is not warranted in patients with suspected glial neoplasm. Early stereotactic biopsy immediately identifies those patients who, in fact, have more anaplastic tumors and a much worse prognosis. Such patients may benefit from early, aggressive treatments such as cytoreductive surgery, chemotherapy, and radiation. Applying this philosophy, we have achieved a median survival of more than 10 years in patients with astrocytomas. Most patients maintain a high KPS rating, and most do not require delayed cytoreductive surgery. Although we believe that the outcomes of future patients with astrocytomas will improve, we must establish whether such improvement is related to better therapeutic options, earlier recognition enabled by advanced neuroimaging, or the availability of corticosteroids (28, 30).

We also believe that neurosurgeons and neuro-oncologists should stop arguing over whether cytoreductive surgery is warranted. For some patients it is, and for others it is not. This prolonged controversy indicates the basic impotence with which neurosurgeons approach glial tumors. Our energy and efforts should be devoted toward more concrete and positive goals in terms of glial tumor management. These goals include prolonged and higher-quality survival, reduced surgical and postoperative morbidity, and the development of new surgical, chemotherapeutic, and molecular tools that will allow us to improve clinical outcomes. Needless and senseless arguing over cytoreductive surgery *versus* biopsy, radiation *versus* no radiation, or any of these procedures *versus* observation alone trivialize the issues that face us and our patients: astrocytomas of the brain are neither indolent nor benign. The vast majority of our patients with astrocytomas are dead within 5 years, and almost all within 10. Our papers, our meetings, our approach should encourage us to pursue new basic science and clinical strategies to fight glial neoplasms. Surgery alone cures no patient with a glioma. Radiation therapy cures relatively few, and chemotherapy cures none. New ideas and new approaches are needed to improve the plight of our patients.

REFERENCES

1. Apuzzo MLJ, Chandrasoma PT, Cohen D, *et al.:* Computed imaging stereotaxy: Experience and perspective related to 500 procedures applied to brain masses. **Neurosurgery** 20:930–937, 1987.
2. Berkson J, Gage RP: Calculation of survival rates for cancer. **Proc Staff Meet Mayo Clin** 25:270–286, 1950.
3. Bloom HJG: Intracranial tumors: Response and resistance to therapeutic endeavors, 1970–1980. **Int J Radiat Oncol Biol Phys** 8:1083–1113, 1982.
4. Boyages J, Tiver KW: Cerebral hemisphere astrocytoma: Treatment results. **Radiother Oncol**: 8:209–216, 1987.
5. Burger PC: Gliomas: pathology, in Wilkins RH, Rengachary SS (eds): *Neurosurgery.* New York, McGraw-Hill, 1985, vol 1, pp 553–563.
6. Burger PC, Heinz ER, Shibata T, *et al.:* Topographic anatomy and CT correlations in the untreated glioblastoma multiforme. **J Neurosurg** 68:698–704, 1988.
7. Burger PC, Vogel FS, Green SB, *et al.:* Glioblastoma multiforme and anaplastic astrocytoma. Pathologic criteria and prognostic implications. **Cancer** 56:1106–1111, 1985.
8. Colbassani HJ, Nishio S, Sweeney KM, *et al.:* CT-assisted stereotactic brain biopsy: Value of intraoperative frozen section diagnosis. **J Neurol Neurosurg Psychiatry** 51:332–341, 1988.
9. Cushing H: *Intracerebral Tumors: Notes upon a Series of Two Thousand Verified Cases with Surgical-Mortality Percentages Pertaining Thereto.* Springfield, IL, Charles C Thomas, 1932.
10. Davis L, Martin J, Goldstein SL, *et al.:* A study of 211 patients with verified glioblastoma multiforme. **J Neurosurg** 6:33–34, 1949.
11. Fadul C, Wood J, Thaler H, *et al.:* Morbidity and mortality of craniotomy for excision of supratentorial gliomas. **Neurology** 38:1374–1379, 1988.
12. Fazekas JT: Treatment of grades I and II brain astrocytomas: The role of radiotherapy. **Int J Radiat Oncol Biol Phys** 2:661–666, 1977.
13. Garcia DM, Fulling KH, Marks JE: The value of radiation therapy in addition to surgery for astrocytomas of the adult cerebrum. **Cancer** 55:919–927, 1985.
14. Gol A: The relatively benign astrocytomas of the cerebrum: A clinical study of 194 verified cases. **J Neurosurg** 18:501–506, 1961.
15. Grieco A, Long CJ: Investigation of the Karnofsky Performance Status as a measure of quality of life. **Health Psychol** 3:129–142, 1984.
16. Hoshino T, Rodriguez LA, Cho KG, *et al.:* Prognostic implications of the proliferative potential of low-grade astrocytomas. **J Neurosurg** 69:839–842, 1988.
17. Kelly PJ: Stereotactic technology in tumor surgery. **Clin Neurosurg** 35:215–253, 1987.
18. Kelly PJ, Daumas-Duport C, Kispert DB, *et al.:* Imaging-based stereotaxic serial biopsies in untreated intracranial glial neoplasm. **J Neurosurg** 66:865–874, 1987.
19. Kelly PJ, Daumas-Duport C, Scherthauer BW, *et al.:* Stereotactic histologic correlations of computed tomography and magnetic imaging-defined abnormalities in patients with glial neoplasms. **Mayo Clin Proc** 62:450–459, 1987.
20. Koivukangas J, Koivukangas P: Treatment of the low-grade cerebral astrocytoma: New methods and evaluation of results. **Ann Clin Res** 18(Suppl):115–124, 1986.
21. Laws E, Taylor W, Clifton M, *et al.:* Neurosurgical management of low grade astrocytoma of the cerebral hemispheres. **J Neurosurg** 61:665–673, 1984.
22. Leibel S, Sheline G, Wara W, *et al.:* The role of radiation therapy in the treatment of astrocytomas. **Cancer** 35:1551–1557, 1975.

23. Lunsford LD, Somaza S, Kondziolka D, *et al.*: Survival after stereotactic biopsy and irradiation of cerebral (non-anaplastic, non-pilocystic) astrocytoma. **J Neurosurg** 82:530–535, 1995.

24. Marsa GW, Goffinet DR, Rubenstein LJ, *et al.*: Megavoltage irradiation in the treatment of gliomas of the brain and spinal cord. **Cancer** 36:1681–1689, 1975.

25. Martinez AJ, Pollack I, Hall W, *et al.*: Touch preparations in the rapid intraoperative diagnosis of central nervous system lesions. **Mod Pathol** 1:387–384, 1988.

26. McCarty CS: Surgical treatment of gliomas of the brain. **J Int Coll Surg** 23:290–297, 1955.

27. McCormack B, Miller D. Budzilovich G, *et al.*: Treatment and survival of low-grade astrocytoma in adults 1977–1988. **Neurosurgery** 31:636–642, 1992.

28. Medbery CA III, Strauss KL, Steinberg SM, *et al.*: Low-grade astrocytomas: Treatment results and prognostic variables. **Int J Radiat Oncol Biol Phys** 15: 837–841, 1988.

29. Morantz R: Radiation therapy in the treatment of cerebral astrocytoma. **Neurosurgery** 20:950–982, 1987.

30. Nazzaro J, Neuwelt E: The role of surgery in the management of supratentorial intermediate and high-grade astrocytomas in adults. **J Neurosurg** 73:331–344, 1990.

31. North C, North R, Epstein J, *et al.*: Low-grade cerebral astrocytomas: Survival and quality of life after radiation therapy. **Cancer** 66:6–14, 1990.

32. Philippon J, Clemenceau S, Fauchon F, *et al.*: Supratentorial low-grade astrocytomas in adults. **Neurosurgery** 32:554–559, 1993.

33. Piepmeier JM: Observations on the current treatment of low-grade astrocytic tumors of the cerebral hemispheres. **J Neurosurg** 67:177–181, 1987.

34. Pool JB, Kamrin RP: The treatment of intracranial gliomas by surgery and radiation. **Prog Neurol Surg** 1:258–299, 1966.

35. Salazar OM, Rubin P, McDonald JV, *et al.*: Patterns of failure in intracranial astrocytomas after irradiation analysis of dose and field factors. **Am J Roentgenol** 126:279–292, 1976.

36. Salcman M: Radical surgery for low-grade glioma. **Clin Neurosurg** 36:353–366, 1990.

37. Shapiro WR: Multimodality therapy of malignant gliomas. **BNI Q** 3:48–52, 1985.

38. Shaw E, Daumas-Duport C, Scheithauer B, *et al.*: Radiation therapy in the management of the low-grade supratentorial astrocytomas. **J Neurosurg** 70:853–861, 1989.

39. Shaw E, Earle J, Scheithauer B, *et al.*: Postoperative radiation for supratentorial low-grade gliomas. **Int J Radiat Oncol Biol Phys** 13(Suppl 1):148, 1987 (abstr).

40. Soffietti R, Chio A, Giordana M, *et al.*: Prognostic factors in well-differentiated cerebral astrocytomas in the adult. **Neurosurgery** 24:686–692, 1989.

41. Stage WS, Stein JJ: Treatment of malignant astrocytomas. **Am J Roentgenol** 120:7–18, 1974.

42. Uihlein A, Colby MY, Layton DD, *et al.*: Comparison of surgery and surgery plus irradiation in the treatment of supratentorial gliomas. **Acta Radiol** 5:67–68, 1966.

43. Vertosick F, Selker R, Arena V: Survival of patients with well-differentiated astrocytomas diagnosed in the era of computed tomography. **Neurosurgery** 28:496–501, 1991.

29

Radical Resection for the Treatment of Glioma

EDWARD R. LAWS, JR., M.D., F.A.C.S.

Gliomas comprise 30 to 50% of primary intracranial brain tumors, and their prevalence is on the order of 7 to 10 per 100,000 people per year. One of the reasons for the relatively imprecise statistical data lies in the poor definition of the term, "glioma." This category of brain tumor includes very common lesions, such as the glioblastoma multiforme and the astrocytoma, and it also includes very unusual and uncommon lesions, such as the ganglioglioma and the xanthoastrocytoma. Some classifications of gliomas also include tumors, such as colloid cysts and ependymomas. For the purpose of this discussion, the term glioma will be meant to focus on astrocytomas, oligodendrogliomas, and their derivatives as neoplasms.

Epidemiologic studies of gliomas of the brain have provided a number of insights as to their biology and natural history. There seems to be an age-specific increase in incidence, which is particularly true for malignant astrocytomas and glioblastomas. In most analyses, age has become one of the strongest predictors of outcome management, but this feature is clouded by the fact that certain very benign astrocytomas occur in the younger age groups (7). The incidence of gliomas appears to be increasing somewhat, but it is uncertain at this time whether this is an actual biologic phenomenon, or whether it is simply a reflection of increased detection with modern imaging techniques.

Despite numerous advances in diagnosis, surgical methodologies, adjunctive therapies, and basic scientific knowledge about the molecular biology of these tumors, the outcome for patients has changed very little over the past 25 years. Management philosophies have continued to depend on surgical resection, followed by radiation and/or chemotherapy, and attempts at innovative treatment with immunotherapy, hyperthermia, photodynamic therapy, and other methods have generally been unimpressive.

Basic concepts in oncology do apply to the management of gliomas of the brain. These include attempts to reduce the overall tumor burden, taking advantage of the peculiarities of the regional blood supply and metabolism of these tumors, and utilizing adjunctive therapies designed to prevent tumor cell replication and spread.

Radical surgical resection remains one of the pillars of the basic oncologic approach to gliomas of the brain and will be the focus of this discussion.

PRE-OPERATIVE DIAGNOSIS

The clinical diagnosis of glioma of the brain is usually made by the development of signs of increased intracranial pressure, progressive neurologic deficit, or seizures. Seizures, in general, tend to be a favorable clinical feature, as it is usually the lower-grade gliomas that present with chronic irritation of the brain, manifested in the form of seizures. Rapidly growing tumors, such as glioblastomas, frequently evolve so quickly that a seizure disorder does not develop.

Once clinical features lead to the suggestion of the presence of an intracranial tumor, imaging diagnosis is critical in making an accurate anatomic and, sometimes, pathologic diagnosis. Magnetic resonance imaging (MRI) has become the standard for evaluation of patients with gliomas, and the MRI scan can show a number of important features of the tumor. These include the degree of circumscription or invasiveness, the presence or absence of cystic components, the presence of necrosis, alterations in the blood-brain barrier, and secondary effects on the surrounding brain, such as edema, shift, and herniation. Contrast-enhancing characteristics of gliomas can also help in ensuring precision of pre-operative diagnosis. Many of the more benign pilocytic astrocytomas show dramatic homogeneous contrast enhancement, and many of the more malignant infiltrative astrocytomas show heterogeneous enhancement patterns.

Functional imaging techniques are evolving rapidly. Positron emission tomography scanning can monitor glucose utilization and protein turnover in gliomas. Single-photon emission computerized tomography scanning can show regional blood flow and, potentially, can image receptors. Functional MRI and MR spectroscopy are on the horizon as useful techniques in the diagnosis of gliomas.

Assessment of the clinical features and the imaging characteristics of an individual glioma can give the managing physicians significant information with regard to the anatomic aspects of the tumor and, secondarily, can influence the type of management recommended. Clearly, well-circumscribed homogeneous low-grade tumors in accessible locations represent the most favorable situations, and infiltrative high-grade tumors in dangerous locations within the brain represent much more difficult challenges to management and may require a number of different strategies.

The concept of radical surgical resection must be at least considered for all types of gliomas, and its relative utility will depend on the nature and location of the individual tumor.

ARGUMENTS FOR RADICAL RESECTION

Perhaps the most compelling argument in favor of radical resection of gliomas is the fact that there are certain types of gliomas that can be permanently cured by radical resection (Table 29.1). These tumors include cystic cerebellar astrocytomas in children, unilateral optic nerve gliomas, various juvenile pilocytic astrocytomas, and some microcystic low-grade gliomas. In addition, related tumors, such as gangliogliomas and dysembryoplastic neuroepithelial tumors, also carry a very favorable prognosis and can be cured by complete resection. The fact that at least some gliomas can be cured with surgical methods alone strengthens the concept that radical removal should lead to favorable outcomes.

From a theoretical standpoint, if one considers the current multistep theory of progression of malignancy in various types of tumors, including brain tumors, then radical resection also makes sense for gliomas of the brain. If malignancy is the result of a multistep process

TABLE 29.1

Arguments for Radical Resection

A. "Cytoreduction" is good; it
  1. reduces tumor burden
  2. relieves elevated intraspinal pressure
  3. reverses neurologic deficits
  4. may reduce or eliminate seizures
B. Some gliomas can be cured by radical removal
  1. Ganglioglioma
  2. Juvenile pilocytic astrocytoma
  3. Microscopic astrocytoma
  4. Cystic cerebellar astrocytoma
  5. Unilateral optic nerve glioma
C. The multistep theory of malignant progression
  1. the fewer cells at risk, the less likely a malignant progression
  2. other "statistical" factors
D. The immune surveillance theory
  1. given a small enough tumor burden, immunologic defenses may be adequate to control the tumor
E. A definitive pathologic diagnosis can be made
  1. "sampling error" is reduced

over a relatively long period of time, with a large number of cells at risk, then clearly the fewer cells that are available to undergo this process, the less likely is a malignant transformation to occur.

The multistep theory leads to a basic statistical concept with regard to the pathogenesis of gliomas. Scherer showed many years ago that the frequency of distribution of gliomas is related to the basic numbers of glial cells in the various lobes of the brain; therefore, one can make an argument that the more glial cells at risk, the more likely is a tumor to occur. Logically, the fewer tumor cells that exist at risk in any area of the brain, the less likely the tumor is to progress or to spread.

The concept of cytoreduction is central to the idea of immune surveillance, namely, the method by which the body deals with neoplastic transformation on a regular basis. The theory here is that with a very small number of tumor cells, the body's own defenses can prevent the development of a large malignancy, assuming that the immune system is capable of dealing with the occasional cell that undergoes a malignant change. This system is effective only when the tumor burden is small, and radical resection is the most effective means of providing a reduction in the number of tumor cells to be dealt with by the immune system.

Additional arguments in favor of radical resection include the elimination of mass effect and the potential for reversal of neurologic deficit. In patients who present with seizure disorders, removing the tumor and eliminating the mass and the irritative effects associated with it may improve or eliminate a seizure disorder.

ARGUMENTS AGAINST RADICAL RESECTION

Perhaps the most compelling argument against radical resection for most astrocytomas of the brain is that the majority of these tumors are inherently invasive lesions (3) (Table 29.2). They are poorly circumscribed, infiltrative of the surrounding tissue, and experimental studies have demonstrated the capacity of individual tumor cells to migrate long distances, thus giving rise to multifocal lesions as the tumor progresses over time. Such infiltrative tumors and multifocal tumors clearly cannot be cured by radical resection.

Previous studies have shown that even hemispherectomy is inadequate to prevent the ultimate spread of a malignant glioma, leading some researchers to suggest that the tumorigenesis is related to a "field effect." This kind of tumor clearly would not be amenable to resective therapy.

It is clear that radical resection carries with it the risk of complications of surgery and the potential for a new neurologic deficit to develop or for aggravation of a previously existing neurologic deficit.

TABLE 29.2
Arguments against Radical Resection

A. Inherent invasiveness of most gliomas
B. Multifocal gliomas
C. Difficulty of "total" resection of infiltrative tumors
D. "Field effect" in glial tumorigenesis
E. Potential for new neurologic deficit and surgical complications

METHODS OF RADICAL RESECTION

Technological advances have improved both the concept and the methods for radical resection of gliomas of the brain. As mentioned previously, modern imaging with MRI gives the surgeon an excellent anatomic, and in some cases pathologic, assessment of the tumor and its affect on surrounding structures. Image-based stereotactic volume resection, pioneered by Patrick Kelly, has allowed the surgeon to perform highly accurate and consistently complete resections of certain gliomas that are well circumscribed and approachable, using stereotactic concepts (5, 6). This allows the surgical removal even of deep-seated lesions and is aided by modern approaches, such as the trans-sulcal approach to lesions in the deep white matter. Other technical advances have improved the capability of the surgeon to detect and to remove gliomas of the brain. These include diagnostic ultrasound, which can accurately delineate subcortical lesions at the time of surgery; methods of resection, such as the laser and the ultrasonic aspirator, which help to ensure radical removal of neoplastic tissue; and microsurgical techniques that preserve the normal function of the surrounding brain. For lesions associated with "eloquent" areas of brain, electrophysiologic mapping can be combined with surgical resection to preserve important function. This can be accomplished by the operative insertion of grid or strip electrodes and subsequent stimulation mapping or, alternatively, electrophysiologic recording can be performed at the time of surgery with the patient awake or, in some cases, with more limited goals, with the patient asleep, to answer vital questions about the relation of the tumor to functioning areas of the adjacent brain.

RESULTS OF RADICAL RESECTION

Virtually every retrospective study of the management of gliomas of the brain has shown that the most favorable results occur in those patients who undergo radical resection of the tumor (1, 4, 7, 8). This finding is consistent with the theories of cytoreduction and decrease of tumor burden which, until recently, have generally been accepted. The problem with most of these retrospective studies is that a significant selection bias exists, and it is clear that those patients with the most favorable lesions, that is, the most benign tumor types and the most favorable anatomic locations, are those who are most likely to receive a radical resection. Infiltrative tumors in dangerous areas of the brain are much more likely to be treated by less radical techniques; these tumors clearly progress more rapidly, and therefore, the outcome for the patients is poorer. It is essential that prospective studies be done in order to answer the question as to the actual role of radical resection in the management of various types of gliomas. What is required is careful definition of the tumor types and a carefully conducted prospective randomized trial that adequately considers matching patients with regard to age, tumor type, tumor location, and method of management. Until adequate studies appear, the current published data strongly indicate that the best patient outcomes occur when radical resection is accomplished.

ALTERNATIVES TO RADICAL RESECTION

In discussing the management of the glioma with the patient and his or her family, the treating physicians must consider all of the available alternatives. The least invasive alternative, and one that may be appropriate for a number of low-grade gliomas, is simply to observe the patient and to treat symptomatically the seizure disorder or headache that may have led to the diagnosis of the tumor.

For many patients, to give an accurate prognosis and to design therapy, it will be necessary to perform a biopsy of the tumor. At present, most tumor biopsy procedures are image directed and usually use stereotactic techniques. Open biopsies still are occasionally recommended.The major disadvantage of stereotactic biopsy in low-grade gliomas is the small sample size and the occasional difficulty in confirming whether the biopsy actually includes tumor or just represents reactive brain tissue (2). This problem of sampling error is a considerable one in the diagnosis of gliomas of the brain, as many tumors contain areas of differing degrees of malignancy, and a small biopsy may not actually be representative of the majority of the tumor. Sampling error can lead to suboptimal treatment recommendations and can also confound the outcome of prospective or retrospective studies wherein the diagnosis of the tumor was based on a stereotactic biopsy.

Radiation therapy can be recommended for gliomas, either on the basis of imaging studies alone, on the basis of a biopsy sample, or as adjunctive therapy after major resection (9–11). Although the efficacy of standard-dose conventional radiation therapy for malignant astrocytomas and glioblastomas has been more or less proven, considerable controversy remains as to whether radiation therapy is effective for low-grade gliomas. The definitive answer awaits the results of one of the prospective trials that are currently underway or under analysis. Preliminary information suggests that for infiltrative hemispheric low-grade gliomas in adults there is some benefit derived from conventional radiation therapy. Radiation therapy in the form of implants or brachytherapy has been applied to gliomas of the brain, and more recently stereotactic radiosurgery, using the Gamma Knife or a stereotactic linear accelerator, has also been utilized for the management of some gliomas. Reports thus far are so contaminated by selection bias that it is impossible to know the actual value of these more focal forms of radiation therapy for gliomas of the brain. Under certain circumstances there does appear to be definite benefit for some patients, usually for those with fairly well-circumscribed supratentorial hemispheral lesions, in adults, in noneloquent areas of brain.

Other forms of adjunctive management, including chemotherapy, immunotherapy, hyperthermia, and photodynamic therapy, have been used for the treatment of malignant gliomas and, to a much lesser extent, for low-grade gliomas. At the present time, none of these modalities confers a significant survival advantage for patients with typical gliomas of the brain.

CONCLUSION

The surgical management of gliomas of the brain continues to be an area for investigation and of some controversy. Many of the questions can be answered by careful clinical investigation, using modern techniques of epidemiology and carefully controlled prospective studies. Until these studies are available, a strong case can be made for the treatment of many gliomas of the brain with radical surgical resection. In some cases this strategy can provide cures or long-term remissions, and in others it can provide disease control when combined with adjunctive measures, such as radiation therapy.

ACKNOWLEDGMENT

The author is grateful to Ms. Pamela Leake for her expert assistance in the preparation of this chapter.

REFERENCES

1. Berger MS, Keles GE, Ojemann GA, *et al.:* Extent of resection affects recurrence patterns in patients with low grade gliomas. **Cancer** 74:1784–1791, 1994.
2. Bernstein M, Parrent AG: Complications of CT-guided stereotactic biopsy of intraaxial brain lesions. **J Neurosurgery** 81:165–168, 1994.

3. Ito S, Chandler KL, Prados MD, *et al.:* Proliferative potential and prognostic evaluation of low grade astrocytomas. **J Neurooncol** 19:1–9, 1994.
4. Janny P, Cur H, Mohr M, *et al.:* Low grade supratentorial astrocytomas. Management and prognostic factors. **Cancer** 73:1937–1945, 1994.
5. Kelly PJ, Alker GJ, Goerss S: Computer assisted stereotactic laser microsurgery for the treatment of intracranial neoplasms. **Neurosurgery** 10:324–331, 1982.
6. Kelly PJ, Kall BA, Goerss SJ, *et al.:* Computer assisted stereotaxic resection of intra-axial brain neoplasms. **J Neurosurg** 64:427–439, 1986.
7. Laws ER, Taylor WF, Clifton MB, *et al.:* Neurosurgical management of low-grade astrocytoma of the cerebral hemispheres. **J Neurosurg** 61:665–673, 1984.
8. McCormack BM, Miller DC, Budzilovich GN, *et al.:* Treatment and survival of low grade astrocytomas in adults, 1977–1988. **Neurosurgery** 31:636–642, 1992.
9. North CA, North RP, Epstein JA, *et al.:* Low-grade cerebral astrocytomas. Survival and quality of life after radiation therapy. **Cancer** 66:6–14, 1990.
10. Shaw EG, Daumas-Duport C, Scheithauer BW, *et al.:* Radiation therapy in the management of low-grade supratentorial astrocytomas. **J Neurosurg** 70:853–861, 1989.
11. Shaw EG, Scheithauer BW, O'Fallon JR: Management of supratentorial low-grade gliomas. **Oncology** 7:97–107, 1993.

30

The Low-Grade Glioma Debate: Evidence Defending the Position of Early Radiation Therapy

EDWARD G. SHAW, M.D.

The question of whether adult patients with histologically verified supratentorial low-grade gliomas (LGGs) should routinely receive postoperative radiation therapy (RT) has recently received a great deal of attention. In 1994 alone, it was the topic of debates at three major national or international forums, including the 6th Canadiation Neuro-Oncology Meeting, the 36th Annual Meeting of the American Society for Therapeutic Radiology and Oncology, and the Annual Meeting of the Congress of Neurological Surgeons.

The arguments against the use of postoperative RT are essentially twofold (1, 4): first, that the natural history of the disease is "benign" or "favorable"; second, that the risks of RT outweigh the potential benefits. In this article, evidence will be presented that refutes both of these arguments, at least in the setting of an adult with a histologically verified supratentorial LGG. This evidence by necessity will include information on the pathology and natural history of LGGs as well as the efficacy and toxicity of RT. From this information, a logical set of conclusions will then be drawn supporting the position of early RT.

SUPPORTING EVIDENCE

Pathology and Natural History of LGGs

Supratentorial LGGs are an uncommon but diverse group of central nervous system (CNS) neoplasms. Of the 1,250 cases diagnosed annually in the United States, 47% are diffuse fibrillary astrocytomas, 21% pilocytic astrocytomas, 19% mixed oligo-astrocytomas, and 13% oligodendrogliomas (8).

The median age at diagnosis and 5- and 10-year survival rates are shown in Table 30.1. As seen, median age at diagnosis for supratentorial pilocytic astrocytomas is 14 years, compared to the mid-30s for the other histologic subtypes. Survival is very much a function of histology

TABLE 30.1[a]

Histologic Subtype	Median Age	Survival		
		Median (yr)	5-yr (%)	10-yr (%)
Pilocytic astrocytoma	14		85	79
Diffuse fibrillary astrocytoma	34	4.7	46	17
Mixed oligo-astrocytoma	36.5	7.0	63	33
Oligodendroglioma	36	9.8	73	49

[a]Adapted from (9).

and is best for pilocytic astrocytomas. Among the nonpilocytic supratentorial LGGs, it is best for oligodendrogliomas, intermediate for mixed oligo-astrocytomas, and poorest for diffuse fibrillary astrocytomas (9). Figure 30.1**A** through **D** shows the survival curves for the four major histologic subtypes of supratentorial LGGs compared to an age- and sex-matched control population (Shaw EG, Suman VJ, unpublished data, 1994). In each case, even for pilocytic astrocytomas, the observed survival is statistically significantly worse than the control group, which has an expected 10-year survival rate of approximately 95%. Further information about the natural history of supratentorial LGG can be derived from the series by Recht *et al.*, in which 26 patients who presented with a seizure from the series by Recht *et al.*, in which 26 patients who presented with a seizure disorder and an imaging diagnosis of supratentorial nonpilocytic LGG were followed until the therapeutic interventions of surgery and postoperative RT were required. With follow-up of 4 months to 10 years, 58% of patients developed either tumor growth, malignant transformation, or uncontrolled seizures (4).

Efficacy of Radiation Therapy

In order to accurately assess the potential benefits of postoperative RT in patients with supratentorial nonpilocytic LGG, series must be selected in which histologic subtyping was done and patients received "modern" or megavoltage radiation. Several series meet these criteria. In the Mayo Clinic experience, of 121 patients, 10 underwent surgery alone, whereas 102 received postoperative RT, 67 of whom were treated with low doses (<5,300 cGy) and 35 with high doses (>5,300 cGy). The 5-and 10-year survival rates were 23 and 11% for the surgery-alone patients, 47 and 21% for the low-dose RT patients, and 68 and 39% for those receiving high-dose RT, respectively ($P = .04$) (Fig. 30.2). These data were even more striking in adults greater than the median age of 34 years. Comparable survival figures were 37 and 5% for the 45 patients who underwent surgery alone or low-dose RT *ver-*

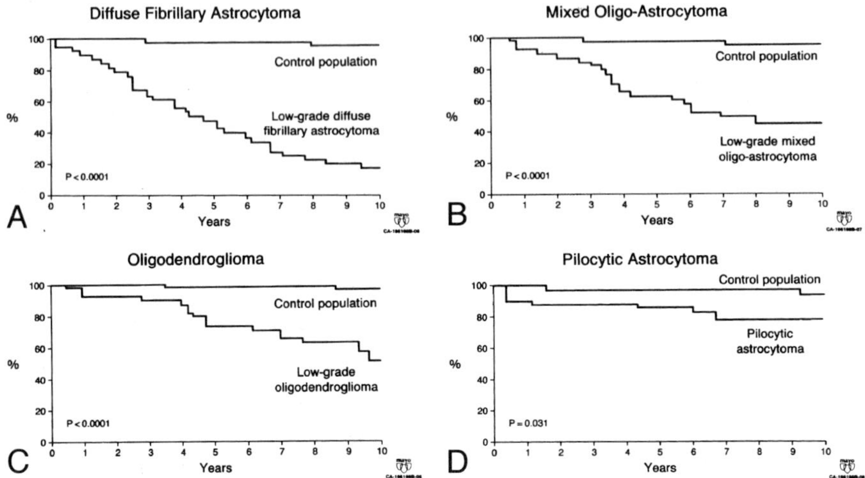

FIG. 30.1 Survival curves for supratentorial low-grade diffuse fibrillary astrocytoma (**A**) mixed oligo-astrocytoma (**B**), oligodendroglioma (**C**) and pilocytic astrocytoma (**D**), compared to an age- and sex-matched control population.

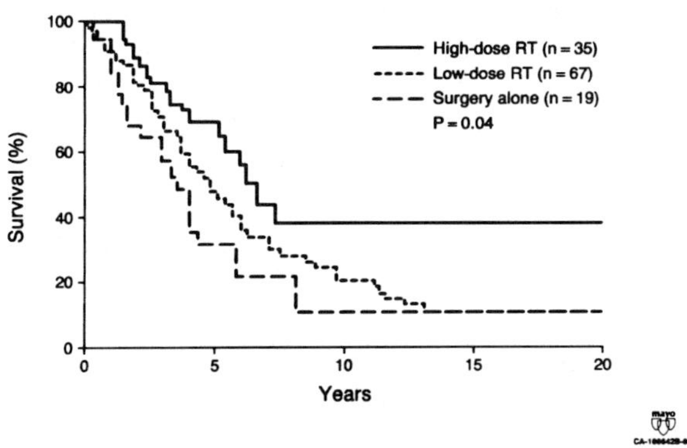

FIG. 30.2 Survival curves for 121 patients with supratentorial diffuse fibrillary astrocytoma and mixed oligo-astrocytoma according to treatment received: high-dose RT (≥5,300 cGy), low-dose RT (<5,300 cGy), or surgery alone.

sus 67 and 45% in those receiving high-dose RT, respectively ($P = .008$) (Fig. 30.3) (6). Garcia *et al.* made similar observations. The 5-year survival rate was increased from 21 to 50% with the addition of postoperative RT. In the subset of patients ≥30 years old, the apparent benefit in median survival from RT was threefold, increasing from 2 years with surgery alone to 6 years with the addition of postoperative RT (2). Importantly, in both of these series, there appeared to be a "flattening" of the survival cures by 10 years, implying that RT may be curative for at least a subset of patients with supratentorial nonpilocytic LGGs. Two key issues regarding the efficacy of RT are being or have been addressed by ongoing or recently completed phase III prospective randomized clinical trials, two by the European Organization for the Research and Treatment of Cancer (EORTC), and one of the North Central Cancer Treatment Group (NCCTG). The EORTC "nonbelievers" trial is ongoing, and randomizes patients with resected supratentorial LGGs to either delayed RT (*i.e.,* RT at the time of progression) or immediate RT, 5,400 cGy, to localized treatment fields. To date, 230 of a planned 250 patients have been accrued (Karim ABMF, personal communication, October 1994). The EORTC "believers" trial, which completed patient accrual in 1991, randomized 379 patients with incompletely resected pilocytic and incompletely or completely resected nonpilocytic LGGs to either low-dose (4,500 cGy) or high-dose localized RT (5,940 cGy). A recent preliminary data analysis failed to demonstrate a difference in survival between the two groups. The 5-year survival rate was 58% for all patients (Karim ABMF, personal communication, October 1994). The NCCTG dose-response trial, comparing 5,040 to 6,480 cGy in a similar patient population, just completed patient accrual of 200 patients in October 1994.

Toxicity of Radiation Therapy

In order to assess the toxicity of RT, it is necessary to understand the "morbidity" of the disease itself, *i.e.,* what neurologic and cognitive dysfunction results from an adult having a supratentorial nonpilocytic

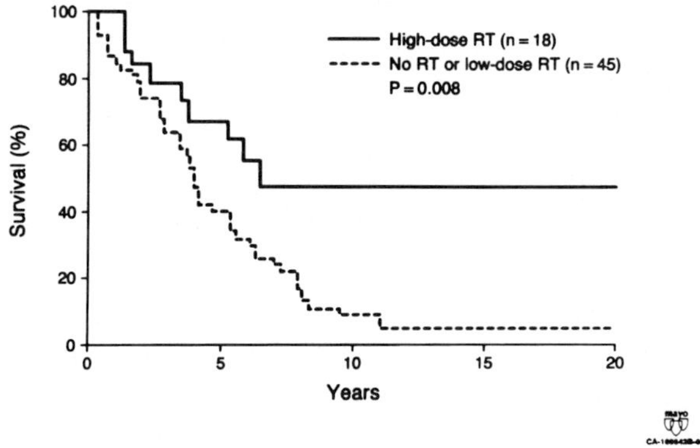

FIG. 30.3 Survival curves for 63 adult patients ≥35 years old with supratentorial diffuse fibrillary astrocytoma and mixed oligo-astrocytoma according to treatment received: high-dose RT (≥5,300 cGy), low-dose RT (<5,300 cGy), or no RT (*i.e.,* surgery alone).

LGG, and how does radiation affect this? In a unique and recently published series from the Netherlands, Taphoorn *et al.* reported on three groups of prospectively evaluated patients. Approximately 20 patients were in each group. Group 1 (RT−) had histologically verified supratentorial LGG but did not receive postoperative RT. Group 2 (RT+) did receive postoperative RT (4,500 to 6,300 cGy using multiple shaped localized treatment fields). Group 3 (control) consisted of patients with hematologic malignancies in the absence of CNS involvement. Assessment tools included neurologic examination, Karnofsky Performance Status (KPS), neuropsychological tests of attention, memory, language, visuospatial, and frontal function, a quality of life (QOL) questionnaire, and a profile of mood states. With mean follow-up of 3.5 years following surgery +/− RT, 93% of the RT−/RT+ patients had normal neurologic exams with a KPS of 85 to 90, compared to 100% with normal neurologic exams and a KPS of 95 for the control group. Neuropsychological test scores were similar for the RT−/RT+ patients and were significantly worse than the control group, implying that the disease, and not the RT, was the underlying cause of cognitive dysfunction. Furthermore, patients with left hemispheric tumors in the RT+ group scored significantly better on two of the tests (Wechsler Intelligence Scale for Children and the Stroop Color-Word Test) than similar patients in the RT− group. The QOL questionnaire and profile of mood states also resulted in similar outcomes for RT− group and RT+ patients, revealing findings such as more fatigue, memory, concentration, speech difficulties, depression, tension, and impediment of activities of daily living than those in the control group. The authors concluded that ". . . radiotherapy had no negative impact on neurological, functional, cognitive, and affective status . . ." (10). In another interesting and recent publication, Kleinberg *et al.* measured QOL in 30 adult patients with supratentorial gliomas (23 of whom had low- to intermediate grade tumors) who were recurrence-free ≥1 year after surgery and postoperative RT. KPS, employment history, and memory function were compared at 1 year and at last follow-up to baseline as a function of the radiation treatment field, using localized or whole brain radiation. The KPS declined in 0/14 patients treated with localized fields *versus* 3/16 (19%) receiving whole brain radiation. About two-thirds of patients were employed at baseline; however, 80% of those treated with localized fields were employed at 1-year or last follow-up compared to 46% at 1-year and 38% at last follow-up for those receiving whole brain radiation. Moderate to severe memory deficits occurred in 43% of patients receiving whole brain radiation as opposed to 6% in the localized RT group (3). Failure pattern studies following RT for supratentorial LGG also support the use of localized treatment fields. Tumor recurrence almost universally occurs within the treatment field at the site of the original tumor (7). Lastly, the benefit of RT on seizure control was recently reported in a small series from the Cleveland Clinic. Of five adults with supratentorial LGGs and intractable epilepsy refractory to standard drugs, one became seizure-free, two had a >90% reduction in seizure frequency, and one had a >75% but <90% reduction (5).

CONCLUSIONS

From the preceding supporting evidence, the following conclusions can be drawn:

- Supratentorial LGGs are a pathologically diverse group of CNS neoplasms whose natural history is primarily dependent upon histologic subtypes.
- The observed survival of all histologic subtypes of supratentorial LGGs are statistically significantly worse than that of an age- and sex-matched control population.
- Moderate-dose postoperative RT appears to improve survival in, and may cure, a subset of patients with supratentorial nonpilocytic LGG, particularly in those in their 30s and older.
- Multiple shaped localized treatment fields should be utilized because whole brain radiation is both unnecessary and associated with greater toxicity.
- Patients with supratentorial LGGs are usually neurologically "intact" but do exhibit cognitive impairment.
- Neurologic, functional, cognitive, and affective status do not appear to be negatively impacted by modern postoperative RT in adults with supratentorial LGG.

Therefore, all adult patients with histologically verified supratentorial low-grade nonpilocystic astrocytomas (diffuse fibrillary astrocytoma, mixed oligo-astrocytoma, or oligodendroglioma) should routinely receive postoperative RT. Localized treatment fields should be employed. The optimum dose of radiation within the range of 4,500 to 6,480 cGy has yet to be determined.

REFERENCES

1. Cairncross JG, Laperriere NJ: Low-grade glioma—to treat or not to treat? **Arch Neurol** 46:1238, 1990.
2. Garcia DM, Fulling KH, Marks JE: The value of radiation therapy in addition to surgery for astrocytomas of the adult cerebrum. **Cancer** 55:919–927, 1985.

3. Kleinberg L, Wallner K, Malkin MG: Good performance status of long-term disease-free survivors of intracranial gliomas. **Int J Radiat Oncol Biol Phys** 26:129–133, 1993.
4. Recht LD, Lew R, Smith TW: Suspected low-grade glioma: Is deferring treatment safe? **Ann Neurol** 31:431–436, 1992.
5. Rogers LR, Morris HH, Lupica K: Effect of cranial irradiation on seizure frequency in adults with low-grade astrocytoma and medically intractable epilepsy. **Neurology** 43:1599–1601, 1993.
6. Shaw EG, Daumas-Duport C, Scheithauer BW, *et al.:* Radiation therapy in the management of low-grade supratentorial astrocytomas. **J Neurosurg** 70:853–861, 1989.
7. Shaw EG, Scheithauer BW, Gilbertson DT, *et al.:* Postoperative radiotherapy of supratentorial low-grade gliomas. **Int J Radiat Oncol Biol Phys** 16:663–668, 1989.
8. Shaw EG, Scheithauer BW, O'Fallon JR: Management of supratentorial low-grade gliomas. **Oncology** 7:97–107, 1993.
9. Shaw EG, Scheithauer BW, O'Fallon JR: Supratentorial gliomas: A comparative study by grade and histologic type. **J Neurooncol,** in press, 1995.
10. Taphoorn MJB, Klein-Schiphorst A, Snoek FJ, *et al.:* Cognitive functions and quality of life in patients with low-grade gliomas: The impact of radiotherapy. **Ann Neurol** 36:48–54, 1994.

31

Management of Low-Grade Gliomas: Radiation Therapy at Time of Recurrence

JOSEPH M. PIEPMEIER, M.D., F.A.C.S., AND MURAT GUNEL, M.D.

Lesions that are traditionally classified as low-grade gliomas include a broad range of tumors, including pilocytic astrocytomas, fibrillary astrocytomas, protoplasmic astrocytomas, oligodendrogliomas, mixed oligoastrocytomas, gangliogliomas, and a few rare special variants, such as pleomorphic xanthoastrocytomas (2, 17, 37). Although the classification of low-grade gliomas can encompass a variety of pathologies, these lesions share basic clinical, histologic and radiologic characteristics that contrast them with high-grade tumors (23, 38, 43, 51). For example, low-grade gliomas tend to occur in children and young adults and commonly cause seizures, which can precede the surgical diagnosis of a tumor for many years. Many of these patients have minimal-to-no neurologic deficits at the time they reach medical attention. Imaging studies must often reveal a diffuse hypodense mass lesion on computerized tomography (CT) or a high-intensity mass on T2-weighted magnetic resonance imaging (MRI), and the majority of these tumors (with the exception of midline lesions in children) do not enhance with contrast material. Calcification and/or cysts frequently are present. On routine histopathologic examination these tumors are notable for their lack of anaplasia, the rarity of mitoses, and the absence of vascular hyperplasia and necrosis.

The general characteristics that separate low-grade neoplasms from high-grade anaplastic tumors and glioblastomas correlate with genotypic profiles that segregate primary brain tumors. While genomic instability is the hallmark of glioblastoma, the opposite appears to be true in low-grade lesions (5, 13, 31). Aneuploidy, deletions, translocations, and amplifications commonly found in poorly differentiated neuroepithelial tumors are notably less frequent in low-grade tumors (1, 5, 16, 19, 36). These basic observations have stimulated intensive investigation in an attempt to identify the genetic mutations that mark the evolution from a low-grade to a high-grade lesion. Since most patients with a low-grade glioma die from a high-grade glioma, a discussion regarding the relative usefulness of a particular form of therapy in the management of these patients is tangential to the fundamental issues that underlie the genesis, growth, invasiveness, and malignant evolution of a primary malignant brain tumor. Ultimately, the identification of the genetic alterations (inheritable and spontaneous) and environmental stimuli (external as well as intracellular) that result in a primary malignant brain tumor will provide the basis for rational and effective therapy. In the absence of this information, the physician must try to make treatment decisions based on currently available data.

FACTORS THAT RELATE TO PROGNOSIS FOR LOW-GRADE GLIOMAS

A number of retrospective clinical series have reported several factors that influence prognosis in patients with low-grade gliomas (6, 7, 10, 15, 21, 23, 24, 26, 27, 29, 32, 34, 35, 38–41, 43, 47, 51, 52). Table 31.1 illustrates those parameters that have been most commonly reported to be associated with prognosis and survival. For the purposes of this report, they are divided into clinical, biologic, and therapeutic categories. This subjective classification should be interpreted with the understanding that each category is not mutually exclusive, inasmuch as clinical indices may be surrogates for biologic issues and that both clinical and biologic factors strongly influence the results of therapeutic intervention. What is most notable about the literature on low-grade gliomas is that while most studies demonstrate similar findings, they often present very different conclusions regarding the interpretation of data and optimal therapy. Another common finding derived from clinical reports is that multivariate analyses typically show that it is the clinical and biologic factors that impact prognosis much more than any specific therapy. Therefore, understanding the relevance of clinical and biologic parameters is critical in determining the best treatment and the optimal timing for intervention.

TABLE 31.1

Clinical, Biologic and Therapeutic Factors That Have Been Reported to Influence Survival in Patients with Low-Grade Gliomas

Clinical	Biologic	Therapeutic
Age	Histology	Surgical resection
Seizures	Labeling index	Radiation therapy
Length of symptoms	Astrocyte ontogeny	Chemotherapy?
Performance status	Genetic mutations	
Imaging		
Location		

Clinical Factors

The current method of tumor classification identifies a heterogeneous group of low-grade tumors with different histologies and variable natural histories within the same category. It is generally accepted that pilocytic astrocytomas have a more favorable prognosis and that gross total resections of these tumors are associated with prolonged disease-free survival or cures, with 5- and 10-year survivals more than 75 to 90% (15, 40, 51). However, pilocytic astrocytomas generally occur in childhood and represent less than 10% of tumors classified as low-grade gliomas. Many clinical studies combine fibrillary and protoplasmic astrocytomas into a group defined as "ordinary astrocytomas" (15, 23, 26, 27, 29, 32, 34, 39, 40, 47, 52). This classification is reasonable, because these lesions tend to have similar natural histories and are often treated in the same manner. In most studies, ordinary astrocytomas comprise over 70 to 90% of the patients. Median survival for patients with ordinary astrocytomas ranges from 5 to 8 years. Oligodendrogliomas and mixed oligoastrocytomas are often reported as a distinct pathologic entity (21, 39–40). The incidence of these tumors is variable, but they can represent up to 15 to 20% of low-grade gliomas, with median survivals ranging from 3 to 6 years.

Within the spectrum of patients with low-grade gliomas, selected clinical markers have been identified that correlate with prognosis. A younger patient (<40 years old) with a long pre-operative history (usually seizures) and an unimpaired neurologic examination found to have a lesion that does not enhance with contrast will have a better prognosis than an older patient with rapidly evolving neurologic deficit caused by a tumor mass from an enhancing lesion (23, 26, 27, 29, 32, 34, 43, 47, 51, 52). Of all these indices, age less than 40 years is the most commonly cited and most powerful variable associated with better prognosis (23, 26, 32). It is not uncommon for a patient to have seizures for many years prior to the identification of his or her tumor, indicating that some of these lesions have been present for an extended period of time and have very slow growth (23, 32, 47). Performance status, tumor location, and imaging characteristics are closely related. Deep lesions and brainstem tumors are more likely to produce neurologic deficits than polar tumors, and there have been two reports that indicate that contrast enhancement in a low-grade hemispheric glioma correlates with a more aggressive tumor (26, 32, 43). Although patients often have a mixture of both favorable and unfavorable findings, the natural history of low-grade gliomas suggests that one group of tumors has very indolent growth while others transform to high-grade tumors within 1 to 2 years (32, 34). Malignant transformation is the most common cause of mortality in low-grade glioma patients, and the rate of transition to a higher grade increases over time. Based on published reports, the risk of recurrence with a malignant glioma ranges from 20% within 2 years to 70% over the 1st decade (23, 26, 29, 32).

Biologic Factors

All tumors, including gliomas, arise as a result of disruption of normal control mechanisms that regulate cellular proliferation (12). At a cellular level, development of a tumor starts with a genetic mutation that imparts a specific growth advantage, resulting in clonal expansion (30). Subsequent to this, cells within this initial clone undergo further mutations, which result in more aggressive subclones and thus progression of the lesion. Recent studies on gliomas have revealed interesting associations between the histologically defined tumor grade and the genetic alteration(s) associated with that grade (1, 4, 5, 12, 13, 16, 19, 36, 46). Both oncogenes and tumor suppressor genes have been implicated in this development and progression (1, 3–5, 8, 9, 12–14, 16, 18, 19, 22, 25, 28, 30, 36, 42, 45, 46, 48, 50). For example, clonal expansion of cells containing a mutation in the tumor suppressor gene *p53* has been observed during transition from a low-grade astrocytoma to a glioblastoma (42).Thus, evolution from a low-grade to a high-grade glioma is associated with progressive mutations at the genomic level, resulting in uncontrolled cell proliferation (1, 3–5, 8, 9, 12–14, 16, 18, 19, 22, 25, 28, 30, 36, 42, 45, 46, 48, 50). If characterization of specific genetic mutations can be achieved, then the treatment of low-grade tumors could be based on whether they have the elements that will result in their progression. Further identification of these factors will not only establish the molecular basis of gliomas but also will help to direct treatment.

Since there are variations in the natural history of tumors with similar histologic features, a better (nonmorphologic) classification based on the genetic and biologic abnormalities observed within these tumors may be more informative. For example, one way to quantify the proliferative capacity of a tumor is to determine the proportion of cells actively dividing by calculating the labeling index (LI). A recent study has shown a significant difference in time to progression and survival between low-grade tumors with a LI <1% *versus* those with a LI >1% (11). Similarly, decreased time to progression and survival in patients with mixed gliomas have been correlated with a LI >5% (49). Clearly, prognosis can be correlated with the proliferative capacity of each low-grade tumor.

Our patient population reflects the variability of low-grade astrocytomas (34). The authors recently compared a group of patients with long pre-operative histories of epilepsy (mean, 12.9 years) commonly caused by a cortically based tumor with a group of patients with relatively short histories of seizures (<1 year), headache, and cognitive impairment associated with white matter-based lesions (34). Through an immunohistochemical analysis we found that cortical tumors expressed antigens consistent with astrocytes derived from the type 1 lineage while the white matter tumors had a phenotype consistent with the type 2 astrocyte lineage (34). This analysis suggests that the biologic behavior of selected low-grade gliomas also may be related to their histogenesis and that variations in the natural histories may be correlated with the ontogeny of astrocytes. These findings suggest that variations in biologic activity of low-grade astrocytomas may relate to inherent differences associated with the development history of astrocytes.

Therapeutic Factors

The controversy regarding the optimal management of low-grade gliomas is the result of conflicting recommendations derived from retrospective clinical series. Part of the divergence in treatment recommendations is related to the variability in low-grade tumors noted above. That is to say that because patients were selected according to histologic parameters, prior clinical studies cannot segregate indolent low-grade gliomas from more aggressive tumors. Within these limitations, several reports have noted that aggressive surgical resection of localized and accessible tumors results in longer relapse-free time periods (7, 15, 23, 38, 41, 43, 52). Gross total resection is accomplished in 10 to 40% of patients. Many of these patients received no further tumor therapy, and adjuvant irradiation in this selected population has minimal influence on survival (7, 23, 24, 27, 43, 51). It should be remembered that the ability to resect a low-grade glioma is dependent on the invasive nature of the tumor. Localized, polar, and well-demarcated lesions are much more likely to be resectable than diffuse lesions that invade more than one lobe of the brain (43). Consequently, improved survival following aggressive surgical resection may be related to differences in the growth potential and invasiveness of diffuse *versus* discrete tumors.

For the majority of patients, a gross total resection of the tumor is not possible. The number of reports that demonstrate improved survival following adjuvant radiotherapy in this group (7, 23, 24, 39, 41) is matched by an equal number of studies that show no benefit (15, 21, 35, 43, 51). Some reports recommend radiotherapy, even after it has shown no significant benefit, or recommend radiotherapy only for a selected population of older patients with poor prognostic signs (23, 27, 38). A similar divergence of opinion exists regarding the effectiveness of adjuvant radiotherapy for treatment of oligodendrogliomas (21, 41). No chemotherapeutic regimen has been identified that significantly improves survival for low-grade astrocytomas (6). Mixed oligoastrocytomas have been shown to respond to combination therapy with procarbazine, lomustine, and vincristine (10).

RADIATION THERAPY: ADJUVANT *VERSUS* TIME OF RECURRENCE

Although there are a number of publications that examine the outcome of irradiated and nonirradiated patients, there is very little information that can be used to compare survival of low-grade glioma patients who receive adjuvant radiotherapy with those who are treated at the time of recurrence. Recht *et al.* (35) reported a retrospective analysis of 26 patients with presumed low-grade gliomas in whom diagnosis and therapy were withheld until it was deemed necessary (*e.g.,* until there were evidence of tumor growth, increased seizures, malignant transformation). This patient population was compared with 20 matched patients who received immediate treatment for their tumors. No differences in the length of survival and quality of life or in the time to malignant transformation were detected in the two groups. However, a higher incidence of anaplastic tumors was found at the time of intervention in the patients who were initially observed following radiologic diagnosis, indicating potential false identification of low-grade gliomas by radiologic criteria and/or malignant transformation by the time of biopsy. It is presumed that at least some of the assumed low-grade tumors (those that recurred as anaplastic tumors within a few months) may have been reclassified as anaplastic gliomas, had a biopsy been performed at the time of discovery. This is suggested by the fact that identifying low-grade gliomas by means of radiologic criteria can result in the incorrect diagnosis in as much as 50% of patients (20). Consequently, Recht's data actually may be artificially biased in favor of immediate treatment.

Müller *et al.* (29) reported the histologic features of recurrent tumors in 72 patients with low-grade gliomas, and although they did not analyze their findings with reference to the timing of radiotherapy, they provided sufficient data for this to be done (Fig. 31.1). They used a grading system for the low-grade lesions that is a modification of the Ringertz system. In this series the strongest variable that determines overall survival and time to recurrence for patients with low-grade gliomas is the histology of the tumor at recurrence. The recurrence of a low-grade glioma occurs at a mean of over 5 years from the time of diagnosis, whereas when a low-grade glioma recurs as an anaplastic tumor, it recurs at a mean of 3 years. This change in histology has a profound effect on survival. Patients whose tumors continue to remain low-grade survive for more than 7 years while the survival of patients whose recurrent tumor has progressed to anaplasia survive for less than 4 years.

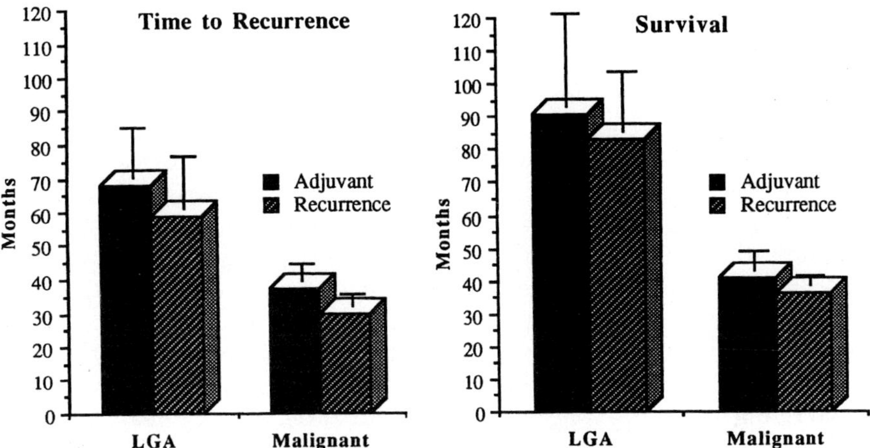

FIG. 31.1 Mean time to recurrence and total survival calculated from data published by Muller *et al.* (29). Patients are divided according to histology at recurrence and according to whether they received adjuvant radiotherapy or radiotherapy at recurrence. *LGA*, low-grade astrocytoma; *Malignant*, anaplastic tumors and glioblastomas.

There were no significant differences in time to recurrence or length of survival among patients who received adjuvant radiotherapy at the time of diagnosis of a low-grade glioma, as compared to patients who received radiotherapy at the time of recurrence. Müller's data suggest that adjuvant radiotherapy does not prolong the time to recurrence or prevent malignant degeneration and that it is the histology of the tumor at recurrence that determines survival more than any other factor. No histologic features that could be used to select tumors likely to recur as anaplastic gliomas were found.

We have adopted a strategy that radiotherapy for low-grade gliomas is best utilized when there is clinical and/or radiographic evidence that the tumor is actively growing. This treatment strategy is based on several hypotheses.

1. Most patients with low-grade gliomas die from high-grade gliomas.
2. Most low-grade glioma patients will, at some point in the course of their disease, require radiotherapy.
3. Radiotherapy is most effective when administered to a patient with an actively growing tumor.
4. Changes in the tumor's proliferative potential can be determined by close clinical and radiologic monitoring.

5. Adjuvant radiotherapy does not delay or prevent transformation to a high-grade tumor.

Since 1984 we have conducted a prospective treatment protocol based on the strategy that low-grade gliomas may be best managed by irradiation at the time they show clinical or radiographic evidence of proliferation. Between 1984 and 1994, 109 patients with low-grade gliomas (excluding pilocytic or gemistocytic astrocytomas and cerebellar and brainstem lesions), including 75 patients with ordinary astrocytomas and 34 patients with oligodendrogliomas or mixed oligoastrocytomas (mean follow-up of 5.8 years), have been treated. When this population is examined for survival according to the use of adjuvant radiotherapy (16 patients) *versus* radiotherapy at the time of recurrence (15 patients) or no radiotherapy (78 patients) there is no difference in mean survival (6.8 years *versus* 7.7 years *versus* 4.6 years, respectively).

Recurrences have occurred in 23 of these 109 patients (7 oligodendrogliomas and 16 astrocytomas) at a mean of 4.6 years following diagnosis. Neither survival nor time to recurrence differed between patients with astrocytoma or oligodendroglioma, nor were they affected by the timing of radiotherapy (adjuvant in 8 patients or at recurrence in 15 patients). The mean survival for 16 patients in whom the recurrent tumors were anaplastic gliomas or glioblastomas was 6.7 years, with a 75% mortality rate. The mean survival of the 7 patients whose recurrent tumor had not changed to a more malignant histology is 8.6 years with a 16% mortality (Fig. 31.2).

Of the remaining 87 patients who have not had a tumor recurrence, 65 received a gross total resection of their tumors, and all are alive at a mean of 5.3 years from diagnosis; 22 patients who received a subtotal resection or biopsy have a mean survival of 3.3 years (21 remain alive with 1 death from a second malignancy). Survival in the 10 patients without recurrence who received adjuvant radiotherapy (mean 6 years) is no different than that of the 77 without radiotherapy (mean 5 years). Based on the results of the studies mentioned above, radiation therapy at the time of recurrence appears to be equally effective (or ineffective) as adjuvant irradiation in the treatment of low-grade gliomas.

The Strategy for Delayed Radiation Therapy

There exists a biologic basis for proposing that radiation therapy may be more effective when delivered to an actively proliferating cell population. For nearly 3 decades it has been recognized not only that proliferating cells are more sensitive to the cytotoxic effects of ionizing radiation than resting (nonproliferating) cells, but that cells in the M-phase of the cell cycle are the most susceptible to loss of clonogenic ca-

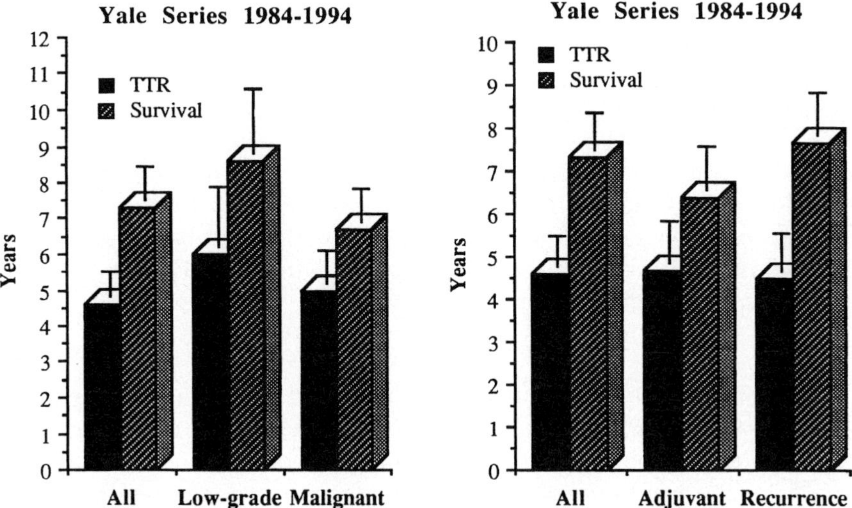

FIG. 31.2 Median time to recurrence (*TTR*) and survival in patients with recurrent tumors in a prospective trial at Yale. Patients are divided according to histology at recurrence and timing of radiation therapy (adjuvant *versus* at recurrence).

pacity (44). Synchronization of glioma cells also has been shown to sensitize them to irradiation (53). Since the proliferating population of cells in a low-grade glioma is very low (around 1%), it is anticipated that these lesions would be relatively radioresistant.

In determining the frequency of follow-up monitoring and imaging, one must consider the clinical and biologic parameters that are associated with prognosis. At the present time it is not possible to stratify these parameters with regard to the relative significance of each. That is to say, it is not known whether age is more important than the LI or length of symptoms is more significant than contrast enhancement in identifying aggressive tumors.

To address this question, the authors have started to examine each of these parameters in a consecutive series of patients with low-grade gliomas to determine the relative significance of each in determining outcome and response to therapy (33). It is anticipated that the use of a grading system that is not based on histology alone will improve our ability to classify these tumors. In addition, the authors are using positron emission tomography (PET) in the pre-operative evaluation and during follow-up of presumed low-grade gliomas to determine whether changes in glucose utilization, as identified by PET, will be useful for directing biopsies and for predicting tumor transformation.

Hypometabolic regions identified by PET corresponding to the area of tumor identified on MRI have been found in 11 of 12 patients with low-grade gliomas. A focal region of hypermetabolism corresponding to a region of contrast enhancement was detected in the remaining patient with an oligodendroglioma. One of these patients has had a recurrence. Follow-up imaging in this patient with a history of oligodendroglioma revealed a hypometabolic mass lesion consistent with the operative findings of a recurrent low-grade lesion. Further analysis and follow-up imaging will be required to determine whether PET is useful for monitoring patients with low-grade tumors.

DISCUSSION

While it is often difficult to predict the natural history for a patient with a low-grade glioma, once the tumor has transformed into a high-grade lesion, the patient's prognosis becomes very predictable. In other words, for most patients with low-grade gliomas, it is the seminal event of malignant evolution of their tumor that will determine the patient's length of survival. The literature demonstrates that, over time, the majority of subtotally resected low-grade gliomas and even some presumed totally resected lesions will regrow and change into more malignant lesions. However, the ability of adjuvant radiotherapy to prevent or at least delay this event remains in question. At the present, preliminary data have indicated several possible strategies for characterizing the biologic basis for the change in growth potential and clinical variability of low-grade tumors (33). To better represent the potential aggressive behavior of each tumor, future pathologic analyses may include not only a morphologic description of the histologic features of the tumor but also an evaluation of astrocyte lineage, LI, *p53* status, glucose utilization, and possibly other genetic markers (Table 31.2). This type of analysis is within the capability of most neuro-oncology centers and not only may

TABLE 31.2

Hypothetical Data Sheet for Analysis of Patient with an Indolent/Low-Grade Glioma

Clinical Profile	Morphologic Description	PET
Age <40 years, Symptoms >1 year	Demarcated tumor boundary p53 status	Hypometabolic lesion Astrocyte lineage
Karnovsky Performance Scale >90	Negative	Type 1
No contrast enhancement	Labeling index	Genetic analysis
Polar location	<1%	LOH 10, 17 negative
Gross total resection		Diploid

contribute to a better understanding of the risks for malignant transformation but also may generate data important to understanding the origins of gliomas and the progression from a low-grade to a more malignant tumor. Designing a radiotherapy treatment strategy based on an accurate assessment of each tumor will help us demonstrate which patients to irradiate and when.

REFERENCES

1. Brandt R, Zveibil D: Clinical significance of DNA content in neuroepithelial tumors. Proceedings of the American Association of Neurological Surgeons, 1993 Annual Meeting, p. 471.
2. Burger P, Scheithauer B, Vogel S: *Surgical Pathology of the Nervous System and Its Coverings.* New York, Churchill Livingstone, 1991, pp 193–209.
3. Chozick B, Finch P, Finkelstein S, *et al.:* Pattern of p53 in human gliomas suggests that malignant tumors can develop from different genetic pathways. Proceedings of the American Association of Neurological Surgeons, 1993 Annual Meeting, p 479.
4. Collins V, James C: Gene and chromosomal alterations associated with the development of human gliomas. **FASEB J** 7:926–930, 1993.
5. Coons S, Davis J, Way D: Correlation of DNA content and histology in prognosis of astrocytomas. **Am J Clin Pathol** 90:289–293, 1988.
6. Eyre H, Crowley J, Townsend J, *et al.:* A randomized trial of radiotherapy versus radiotherapy plus CCNU for incompletely resected low-grade gliomas: A Southwest Oncology Group study. **J Neurosurg** 78:909–914, 1993.
7. Fazekas J: Treatment of grades I and II brain astrocytomas: The role of radiation therapy. **Int J Radiat Oncol Biol Phys** 2:661–666, 1977.
8. Fujimoto M, Fults D, Thomas G, *et al.:* Loss of heterozygosity on chromosome 10 in human glioblastoma multiforme. **Genomics** 4:210–214, 1989.
9. Fults D, Brockmeyer D, Tullos M, *et al.:* p53 mutation of loss of heterozygosity on chromosomes 17 and 10 during human astrocytoma progression. **Cancer Res** 52:674–679, 1992.
10. Glass J, Hochberg F, Gruber M, *et al.:* The treatment of oligodendrogliomas and mixed oligodendroglioma-astrocytoma with PCV chemotherapy. **J Neurosurg** 76:741–745, 1992.
11. Ito S, Chandler K, Prados M, *et al.:* Proliferative potential and prognostic evaluation of low-grade astrocytomas. **J Neurooncol** 19:1–9, 1994.
12. Jacoby L: Clonal origin of nervous system tumors, in: *Molecular Genetics of Nervous System Tumors.* New York,Wiley-Liss, 1993, pp 209–216.
13. James C, Collins P: Glial tumors, in: *Molecular Genetics of Nervous System Tumors.* New York, Wiley-Liss, 1993, pp 241–248.
14. James C, He J, Carlbom E, *et al.:* Chromosome 9 deletion mapping reveals interferon alpha and interferon beta-1 gene deletions in human glial tumors. **Cancer Res** 51:1684–1688, 1991.
15. Janny P, Cure H, Mohr M, *et al.:* Low grade supratentorial astrocytomas: Management and prognostic factors. **Cancer** 73:1937–1945, 1994.
16. Jenkins R, Kimmel D, Moertel C, *et al.:* A cytogenetic study of 53 human gliomas. **Cancer Genet Cytogenet** 39:253–279, 1989.
17. Kepes J, Rubenstein L, Eng L: Pleomorphic xanthoastrocytoma: A distinctive

meningocerebral glioma of young subjects with relatively favorable prognosis. **Cancer** 44:1839–1852, 1979.

18. Kikuchi T, Van Meir E, de Tribolet N: p53 expression in low-grade astrocytomas. Proceedings of the American Association of Neurological Surgeons, 1993 Annual Meeting, p 487.

19. Kimmel D, O'Fallon J, Scheithauer B, *et al.:* Prognostic value of cytogenetic analysis in human cerebral astrocytomas. **Ann Neurol** 31:534–542, 1992.

20. Kondziolka D, Lunsford D, Martinez J: Unreliability of contemporary neurodiagnostic imaging in evaluating suspected adult supratentorial (low-grade) astrocytoma. **J Neurosurg** 79:533–536, 1993.

21. Kros J, Pieterman H, van Eden C, *et al.:* Oligodendroglioma: The Rotterdam-Dijkzigt experience. **Neurosurgery** 34:959–966, 1994.

22. Lang F, Miller D, Kaslow M, *et al.:* Pathways leading to glioblastoma multiforme: A molecular analysis of genetic alterations in 65 astrocytic tumors. **J Neurosurg** 81:427–436, 1994.

23. Laws E, Taylor W, Clifton M, *et al.:* Neurosurgical management of low-grade astrocytoma of the cerebral hemispheres. **J Neurosurg** 61:665–673, 1984.

24. Leibel S, Sheline G, Wara W, *et al.:* The role of radiation therapy in the treatment of astrocytomas. **Cancer** 35:1551–1557, 1975.

25. Libermann T, Nusbaum H, Razon N, *et al.:* Amplification, enhanced expression and possible rearrangement of EGF receptor gene in primary human brain tumors of glial origin. **Nature** (Lond) 313:144–147, 1985.

26. McCormack B, Miller D, Budzilovich G, *et al.:* Treatment and survival of low-grade astrocytomas in adults 1977–1988. **Neurosurgery** 31:636–642, 1992.

27. Medberry C, Straus K, Steinberg S, *et al.:* Low-grade astrocytomas: Treatment results and prognostic variables. **Int J Radiat Oncol Biol Phys** 15:837–841, 1988.

28. Mizuno M, Yoshida J, Sugita K, *et al.:* Growth inhibition of glioma cells transfected with the human beta-interferon gene by liposomed coupled with a monoclonal antibody. **Cancer Res** 50:7826–7829, 1990.

29. Müller W, Afra D, Schroder R: Supratentorial recurrences of gliomas: Morphological studies in relation to time intervals with astrocytomas. **Acta Neurochir** 37:75–91, 1977.

30. Nowell P: The clonal evolution of tumor cell populations. **Science** 194:23–28, 1976.

31. Perry M, Levine A: The cell cycle, in: *Molecular Genetics of Nervous System Tumors.* New York, Wiley-Liss, 1993, pp 83–88.

32. Piepmeier J: Observations on the current treatment of low-grade astrocytic tumors of the cerebral hemispheres. **J Neurosurg** 67:177–181, 1987.

33. Piepmeier J: Research strategies for evaluating the biological diversity of low-grade astrocytomas. **Perspect Neurosurg** 4:1–20, 1994.

34. Piepmeier J, Fried I, Makuch R: Low-grade astrocytomas may arise from different astrocyte lineages. **Neurosurgery** 33:627–632, 1993.

35. Recht L, Lew R, Smith T: Suspected low-grade glioma: Is deferring treatment safe? **Ann Neurol** 31:431–436, 1992.

36. Rey J, Bello J, de Campos J, *et al.:* Chromosomal composition of a series of 22 human low-grade gliomas. **Cancer Genet Cytogenet** 29:223–237, 1987.

37. Rubenstein L: *Tumors of the Central Nervous System* Washington, D.C., Armed Forces Institute of Pathology, 1972, pp 19–40.

38. Scoffietti R, Chio A, Giordana M, *et al.:* Prognostic factors in well-differentiated cerebral astrocytomas in the adult. **Neurosurgery** 24:686–692, 1989.

39. Shaw E, Daumas-Duport C, Scheithauer B, *et al.:* Radiation therapy in the man-

agement of low-grade supratentorial astrocytomas. **J Neurosurg** 70:853–861, 1989.

40. Shaw E, Scheithauer B, Gilbertson D, *et al.:* Postoperative radiotherapy of supratentorial low-grade gliomas. **Int J Radiat Oncol Biol Phys** 16:663–668, 1989.
41. Shaw E, Scheithauer B, O'Fallon J, *et al.:* Mixed oligoastrocytomas: A survival and prognostic factor analysis. **Neurosurgery** 34:577–582, 1994.
42. Sidransky D, Mikkelsen T, Schwechheimer K, *et al.:* Clonal expansion of p53 mutant cells is associated with brain tumor progression. **Nature** 355:846–847, 1992.
43. Steiger H, Markwalder R, Seiler R, *et al.:* Early prognosis of supratentorial astrocytomas in adult patients after resection or stereotactic biopsy. **Acta Neurochir** 106:99–105, 1990.
44. Terasima R, Tomalch T: X-ray sensitivity and DNA synthesis in synchronous populations of HeLa cells. **Science** 140:490–492, 1963.
45. Venter D, Bevan K, Ludwig R, *et al.:* Retinoblastoma gene deletions in human glioblastomas. **Oncogene** 6:445–448, 1991.
46. Venter D, Thomas D: Multiple sequential abnormalities in the evolution of human gliomas. **Br J Cancer** 63:753–757, 1991.
47. Vertosick F, Selker R, Arena V: Survival of patients with well-differentiated astrocytomas diagnosed in the era of computed tomography. **Neurosurgery** 28:496–501, 1991.
48. Von-Deimling A, Louis C, von-Ammon K, *et al.:* Evidence for a tumor suppressor gene on chromosome 19q associated with human astrocytomas, oligodendrogliomas and mixed gliomas. **Cancer Res** 52:5277–5279, 1992.
49. Wacker M, Hoshino T, Ahn D, *et al.:* The prognostic implications of histologic classification and bromodeoxyuridine labeling index of mixed gliomas. **J Neurooncol** 19:113–122, 1994.
50. Watanabe K, Nagai M, Wakai S, *et al.:* Loss of constitutional heterozygosity on chromosome 10 in human glioblastoma. **Acta Neuropatholo** 80:251–254, 1990.
51. Westergaard L, Gjerris F, Klinken L: Prognostic parameters in benign astrocytomas. **Acta Neurochir** 123:1–7, 1993.
52. Weir B, Grace M: The relative significance of factors affecting postoperative survival in astrocytomas, grades one and two. **Can J Neurol Sci** 3:47–50, 1976.
53. Yoshida D, Piepmeier J, Weinstein M: Estramustine sensitizes human glioblastoma cells to irradiation. **Cancer Res** 54:1415–1417, 1994.

V

General Scientific
Session V

32

Interactive Audience Participation

MARK N. HADLEY, M.D.

The annual meeting organizers of the Congress of Neurological Surgeons have experimented with the use of an interactive audience participation system during the scientific sessions of the 1993 and 1994 annual meetings. The following is a compilation of the responses of the neurosurgeons in attendance at the 1994 annual CNS meeting in Chicago, IL, to questions posed by a variety of speakers.

This interesting information is worthy of several comments. The concept of audience participation allowing "real-time" interaction with topic presenters, is fascinating and represents a potentially powerful and useful tool to sample contemporary opinions, practice patterns, even biases, of active neurological surgeons. While the "answers" derived are by no means binding or even necessarily "correct," they do represent what the responding audience "knows" (or thinks they know) about a given topic. At its best, this "point in time" polling technique could be used to assess important information about current neurosurgical practice, training, continuing education, medicolegal issues, *etc.,* potentially representing the concerns and mentality of mainstream neurosurgery. It also might be used to test or assess our knowledge about specific topics to better direct our future training and education.

Interpretation of this carefully collected data could improve the ability of the leadership of our professional organizations to meet our speciality's specific needs and concerns, organize our annual meetings, and improve the way neurosurgeons are trained and are offered continuing medical education. The *valid* interpretation of the answers provided by the audience is directly related to the quality of the questions posed, the ease of providing an accurate response to those questions (proper question design), and the number of respondents willing to participate.

At our 1994 annual meeting in Chicago, CNS meeting organizers provided 500 IRIS electronic response terminals for the audiences of the major scientific sessions. For the most part, neurosurgeons in the audience were reluctant to participate. Only rarely were there more than 100 to 150 responses to a given question even when the auditorium was full.

The following is a review of the questions posed and the responses recorded from the audience. The number of respondents is listed for each question. Without deciding a "right" or "wrong" answer for any question, the opinions expressed by the small audience are interesting. The potential of this type of information transfer is real, but has yet to be fully realized, either by those posing the questions or by those responding.

HEALTH CARE ISSUES/REFORM*

1. What is your age? (126 respondents)

25–35 years:	13.5%
36–45 years:	26.2%
46–55 years:	24.6%
56–65 years:	15.9%
>65 years:	5.6%

2. Which best describes your practice? (96 respondents)

Resident:	6.3%
Private:	68.8%
Academic:	14.6%
Other:	1.0%
Retired, not practicing:	2.1%
Not neurosurgery:	6.3%

3. Where are you from? (88 respondents)

Northeast:	26.1%
Northwest:	14.8%
Southeast	17.0%
Southwest:	29.5%
Canada:	0.0%
Other:	10.2%

4. Should a Federal health care reform law require all health plans to contract with "any willing" neurosurgeon? (85 respondents)

Yes:	65.9%
No:	23.5%
Not sure:	3.5%

5. Should the Federal government adopt a plan to reduce nonprimary training positions?

Yes:	53.8%
No:	40.4%
Not sure:	1.9%

---

*Percentages may not total 100% for a given question due to respondent error, that is, keying an electronic response for which there is no answer option.

6. If the Federal government requires reductions in nonprimary care residence positions, what do you believe would be the appropriate percentage of reduction? (203 respondents)

More than 50%:	14.4%
41–50%:	13.4%
33–40%	12.4%
20–32%:	26.8%
10–19%	20.6%
1–9%:	3.1%
None:	8.2%

7. What is the major reason policymakers are concerned about what you do? (120 respondents)

Too expensive:	32.0%
Power:	7.4%
Quality of care:	9.9%
They need a job:	4.9%

8. What is a reasonable amount to spend to achieve an additional year of life? (47 respondents)

$100:	6.4%
$10,000:	21.3%
$50,000:	57.4%
$1 million:	8.5%
$5 million:	6.4%

9. Has health care reform had an impact on your practice income in the past year? (89 respondents)

>25% reduction:	32.2%
1–25% reduction:	26.7%
No or unsure:	33.3%
1–25% increase:	5.6%
>25% increase:	1.1%

10. Has health care reform had an impact on your surgical case volume in the past year? (91 respondents)

>25% reduction:	13.0%
1–25% reduction:	23.9%
No or unsure:	45.7%
1–25% increase:	14.1%
>25% increase:	2.2%

11. Has health care reform had an impact on your nonsurgical case volume in the past year? (93 respondents)

>25% reduction:	4.3%
1–25% reduction:	16.0%
No change:	52.1%
1–25% increase:	24.5%
>25% increase:	0.0%

12. Has health care reform had an impact on your administrative burden in the past year? (87 respondents)

>25% reduction:	4.6%
1–25% reduction:	4.6%
No change:	9.2%
1–25% increase:	37.9%
>25% increase:	41.4%

13. Has health care reform had an impact on patients' access to your services in the past year? (87 respondents)

Substantially worse:	41.1%
Somewhat worse:	43.2%
No or uncertain:	9.5%
Somewhat improved:	1.1%
Substantially improved:	3.2%

14. Has health care reform had an effect on the quality of care you delivered in the past year? (89 respondents)

Substantially worse:	16.9%
Somewhat worse:	42.7%
No or uncertain:	32.6%
Somewhat improved:	2.2%
Substantially improved:	4.5%

15. The percentage of the total population enrolled in managed care products (health maintenance organizations (HMOs) and preferred provider organizations (PPOs)) in my local market is: (166 respondents)

0–10%:	10.7%
11–25%:	21.0%
26–50%:	17.3%
Over 50%:	12.8%
Don't know:	6.6%

CLINICAL TRIALS

1. Have you participated in clinical trial? (73 respondents)
   Yes: 25.0%
   No: 75.0%

2. Would you enroll your patients in a prospective clinical trial that is randomized? (26 respondents)
   Yes: 73%
   No: 23%

3. Would you enroll your patients in a prospective clinical trial that is nonrandomized? (27 respondents)
   Yes: 55.6%
   No: 37.0%

SPINE

1. Rheumatoid involvement of the craniovertebral area occurs: (77 respondents)
   Early in the disease: 25.3%
   Well into the disease: 34.2%
   Late in the disease: 38.0%

2. In rheumatoid cranial settling there is: (76 respondents)
   Instability: 2.5%
   Destruction: 3.8%
   Pannus: 3.8%
   Invagination: 1.3%
   All of the above: 84.8%

3. Rheumatoid atlanto-axial dislocation occurs in what percentage of patients with rheumatoid arthritis? (78 respondents)
   10%:   55.0%
   20–25%:   33.8%
   50%:   8.8%

4. A transoral approach should never be used for intradural lesions because of the risk of a cerebrospinal fluid (CSF) leak. (35 respondents)
   True: 20%
   False: 80%

5. Compared with transoral exposure, the transmandibular-translingual approach: (53 respondents)
   Decreases the operating distance: 17.1%
   Provides greater superior exposure: 17.1%
   None of the above: 7.1%
   All of the above: 34.3%

6. If spinal instability is present after transoral odontoid resection, a posterior fusion should be done between: (32 respondents)

C1 and occiput:	9.4%
C1 and C2:	25.0%
Occiput and C2:	65.6%

7. How often do you perform a craniocervical fusion procedure? (92 respondents)

Often:	19.6%
Infrequently:	22.4%
Rarely:	29.0%
Never:	15.0%

8. Of those who perform these procedures, do you perform them in conjunction with an orthopaedic surgeon? (68 respondents)

Yes:	10.3%
No:	89.7%

9. If you perform these procedures, do you use: (61 respondents)

Autograft bone:	91.8%
Allograft bone:	6.6%
Neither:	1.6%

10. If you perform these procedures, do you utilize: (70 respondents)

Fixation hardware:	42.9%
Rigid orthosis (halo):	12.9%
Both:	44.3%
Neither:	0.0%

11. The most common symptom in the patient with degenerative spondylolithesis is: (79 respondents)

Back pain:	65.9%
Radicular pain:	14.6%
Claudication:	9.8%
Bladder dysfunction:	6.1%

12. Factors that may influence the decision to fuse include: (63 respondents)

Back pain:	4.5%
Level of slip:	18.2%
Physiologic age:	20.5%
Load bearing:	6.8%
All of the above:	26.1%
None of the above:	6.8%

13. Which of the following is not true of mechanical low back pain? (61 respondents)

The pain is deep, not superficial:	12.0%
The pain is agonizing:	7.6%
The pain is worsened by bed rest:	31.5%
The pain is worsened by activity (loading):	15.2%

TUMOR

1. A 44-year-old woman presents with mild facial numbness. Magnetic resonance imaging (MRI) shows a 2-cm × 3-cm enhancing lesion within the cavernous sinus consistent with meningioma. The intracavernous carotid artery (ICA) is deviated but not constricted. How would you manage this patient? (209 respondents)

Observation with sequential MRI:	25.4%
Conventional radiation only:	2.9%
Biopsy/debulking + radiation:	16.3%
Total resection:	23.4%
Stereo radiosurgery:	17.7%

2. If you attempted to resect this lesion, how would you manage the carotid artery? (226 respondents)

Avoid at all costs:	19.5%
Skeletonize but leave patent:	64.2%
Resect:	0.9%
Resect if tolerated test occlusion:	9.3%
Resect and reconstruct:	4.9%

3. How would you treat a small meningioma in the cavernous sinus? (167 respondents)

Radical resection	12.0%
Conservative resection (or biopsy) and conventional radiation	3.0%
Conservative resection and stereotactic radiosurgery	21.0%
No treatment until tumor extends outside cavernous sinus	62.3%

4. How would you treat a medial sphenoid-ridge meningioma with cavernous sinus invasion in a 45-year-old patient? (225 respondents)

Radical resection:	26.2%
Conservative resection (or biopsy) and conventional radiation:	12.9%
Conservative resection and stereotactic radiosurgery:	60.9%

5. How would you treat a medial sphenoid ridge meningioma with cavernous sinus invasion in a 60-year-old patient? (226 respondents)

Radical resection:	11.1%
Conservative resection and conventional radiation:	17.7%
Conservative resection and stereotactic radiosurgery:	71.2%

6. Would you observe (clinically and radiographically follow) a 45-year-old patient with the same pathology? (212 respondents)

Yes:	51.4%
No:	46.7%

7. Would you observe (clinically and radigraphically follow) a 60-year-old patient with the same pathology? (229 respondents)

Yes:	60.7%
No:	38.0%

8. How would you treat a malignant tumor involving the anterior fossa, orbit, and frontal sinus in a 55-year-old patient? (231 respondents)

Radical resection	35.9%
Conservative resection and conventional radiation:	37.2%
Conservative resection and stereotactic radiosurgery:	17.3%
Radiation alone:	8.2%

9. How would you treat a meningioma encasing the petrous or cavernous carotid artery (failed test occlusion)? (206 respondents)

Radical resection with carotid grafting:	11.7%
Radical resection after bypass to the middle cerebral artery (MCA):	19.9%
Subtotal resection with carotid preservation:	39.3%

VASCULAR

1. Asymptomatic cavernous segment ICA aneurysm. Treatment you would recommend: (162 respondents)

Observation:	34.6%
Proximal occlusion of the ICA (no bypass):	4.3%
Proximal occlusion/trapping of aneurysm with vascular bypass:	11.1%
Endovascular coil occlusion of aneurysm:	11.7%
Endovascular balloon occlusion of aneurysm:	6.8%
Direct dissection and clipping of aneurysm:	27.2%

2. Symptomatic cavernous segment ICA aneurysm. Treatment you
   would recommend: (72 respondents)

Observation:	8.3%
Proximal occlusion of the ICA (no bypass):	9.7%
Proximal occlusion/trapping of aneurysm with vascular bypass:	25.0%
Endovascular coil occlusion of aneurysm:	20.8%
Endovascular balloon occlusion of aneurysm:	9.7%
Direct dissection and clipping of aneurysm:	22.2%

3. Asymptomatic giant basilar tip aneurysm. Treatment options you
   would recommend: (151 respondents)

Observation with no intervention:	6.6%
Direct exposure and clipping of the aneurysm:	19.2%
Exposure and clipping under hypothermic-circulatory arrest:	64.2%
Endovascular coil occlusion of aneurysm:	9.3%
Endovascular balloon occlusion of aneurysm:	0.0%

4. Asymtomatic giant MCA aneurysm. Treatment options you would
   recommend: (153 respondents)

Observation with no intervention:	2.6%
Direct exposure and clipping of the aneurysm:	74.5%
Exposure and clipping under hypothermic-circulatory arrest:	20.3%
Endovascular coil occlusion of aneurysm:	1.3%
Endovascular balloon occlusion of aneurysm:	0.0%

5. Asymptomatic small left frontal arteriovenous malformation
   (AVM). Treatment options you would recommend: (82 respondents)

Observation with no intervention:	15.9%
Endovascular embolization:	2.4%
Stereotactic radiosurgery:	19.5%
Direct surgical resection:	43.9%
Combination of embolization and resection:	12.2%

6. Ruptured 4-cm right temporal lobe AVM. Treatment options you
   would recommend: (60 respondents)

Observation with no intervention:	5.0%
Endovascular embolization:	5.0%
Stereotactic radiosurgery:	1.7%
Direct surgical resection:	36.7%
Combination of embolization and resection:	50.0%

7. Giant posterior left frontal AVM. Treatment options you would recommend: (59 respondents)

Observation with no intervention:	47.5%
Endovascular embolization:	10.2%
Stereotactic radiosurgery:	8.5%
Direct surgical resection:	5.1%
Combination of embolization and resection:	25.4%

8. Asymptomatic small left frontal AVM. Treatment options you would recommend: (60 respondents)

Observation with no intervention:	8.3%
Endovascular embolization:	1.7%
Stereotactic radiosurgery:	15.0%
Direct surgical resection:	68.3%
Combination of embolization and resection:	6.7%

9. Giant posterior left frontal AVM. Treatment options you would recommend: (60 respondents)

Observation with no intervention:	69.8%
Endovascular embolization:	7.9%
Stereotactic radiosurgery:	0.0%
Direct surgical resection:	0.0%
Combination of embolization and resection:	19.0%

Index

Page numbers in italics denote figures; those followed by a "t" denotes tables

AANS. *See* American Association of Neurological Surgeons

Abducens nerve (cranial nerve VI), intra-operative monitoring, 189

Abducens palsy, 127, *128*

Accessory nerve (cranial nerve XI), intra-operative monitoring, 200

Acetate polymer, cellulose, 284–285

Acoustic neuromas
  removal, 208–212, *209, 211*
    auditory nerve monitoring during, 198–199, 199t, 210–212, *211*
    facial nerve monitoring during, 193–194, 195t
    translabyrinthine approach to, 194, 195t
  tumor size, facial nerve function according to, 195, 196t

Adhesive, liquid polymeric, 283–284

Age, factor in decision making, 350

American Association of Neurological Surgeons (AANS), 9, 10

American College of Surgeons, 40

American health care
  employer pressure, 5–6
  financial evolution of, 1–6
  government cost containment, 4–5
  government involvement, 3–4

American Medical Association, 18

Aneurysms
  alternative techniques, 259–260
  bilobed, 277, *277*
  debulking, 261
  endovascular techniques for, 267–268, *268*
  giant cavernous, 127, *129*, 228–231, 239
    indications for treatment, 235–237
    skull bypass I for, 127, *128, 129, 130*
  giant intracranial, 214–244, 239
    definition of, 245
    endovascular management, 267–293
    surgical management of, 245–266
  giant intradural, 226–228, 238–239
    indications for treatment, 231–237
  recanalization or regrowth after coil occlusion, 277, *278*
  skull base approaches to, 256–257

Angiofibroma, transfacial approach to, 60, *60*

Angiographically occult vascular malforma-tions, 344–345

Angiographic thrombosis rates, 329–331

Anterior communicating artery, giant aneurysm of, 222, *223*

Anterior cranial fossa
  sinus carcinoma growing into, 93
  transfrontal approach, 44t, *45*, 50
  transfrontal-nasal approach, 44t, *46*, 50–53
  transfrontal-nasal-orbital approach, 44t, *47, 52*, 53–54

Anterior skull base tumors, 71–98
  ICA sacrifice for, 63–67
    clinical materials and methods, 63
    results, 63
  meningiomas, radiosurgery for
    clinical status after, 103–104, 105t
    tumor control and neurologic status after, 106t, 106–107
    tumor imaging changes after, 103, 103t
  metastatic, stereotactic radiosurgery for, 115–116
  radical resection of, 43–70
  stereotactic radiosurgery for, 99–118, 100t
  surgery for, 73–74
  that can be exposed by transfacial routes, 43–44, *44*
  transfacial approach, 43–62
    case report, 60, *60*
    clinical experience, 58–59
    general treatment techniques, 56–58
    lesion types, 58, 59t
    levels, 43–44, *44*
    transfrontal (level I), 44t, *45*, 50
    transfrontal-nasal (level II), 44t, *46*, 50–53
    transfrontal-nasal-orbital (level III), 44t, *47, 52*, 53–54
    transmaxillary (level V), 44t, *49, 52*, 55–56
    transnasomaxillary (level IV), 44t, *48*, 55
    transpalatal (level VI), 44t, *51–52*, 56
  treatment of, 73–79

Anticoagulant therapy, for giant aneurysms, 235, *236*

Antiplatelet therapy, for giant aneurysms, 235, *236*

Any willing provider laws, 17

AOVMs. *See* Angiographically occult
vascular malformations
Arrest, hypothermic circulatory, 258–259
Arteriovenous malformations
angiographic cure, 335, 337, *338*
angiographic failure, 335, 337
cavernous, 344–345
cerebral, decision making, 348–351, 364–365
death during follow-up, 336, 339
decision analysis, 294–312, 348–351, 364–365
age vs Spetzler grade, *302*, 302–303, *304*
alternate grading system, 299–300, 300t
ASA grades, 303, 303t
baseline values, 297–300, *298*, 299t
model failure, 303–306
results, 300–303, 301t, *301*
summary, 303, 305t, 306
technique (methods), 295–297
decision tree, 300–301, *301*
embolization and gamma knife
radiosurgery for
case, 323, *325*
follow-up results, 318
embolization and radiosurgery for, 342–344, *343–344*
embolization and resection for, cases, 319–323, *321*, *322*, *324*
embolization of, 313–327, 314–315, 315t
bleeding rates, 317
cases, 318–323, *320*
complications of, 317
cost effectiveness, 323–326, 325t
Martin gradings, 315–316, 316t
materials, 313–314
in modern era, 301t, 301–302
nidus volume changes, 316–317, *317*
obliteration rates, 315–316, 316t
outcomes, 318, 318t
results, 315–318
Spetzler gradings, 315–316, 316t
treatment methods, 313–315
volume reduction, 315–317
gamma knife radiosurgery costs, 323–326, 325t, 326t
initial treatment indications, 314
intracerebral hemorrhage risk, 358
intracranial
decision making, 348–351
surgical treatment for, 348–369
indications, 348–351
large, sensitivity analysis of age vs Spetzler grade for, *302*, 302–303, *304*
life expectancy, 361, 362t
locations, 350
lost to follow-up, 336, 339
mortality rates, 358–359
MRI suggestive of cure, 336, 339
MRI suggestive of failure, 336, 339
multimodality treatment, 342–344
natural history, 351–352
patients refusing follow-up, 336, 339
radiosurgery for, 328–347
angiographic thrombosis rates, 329–331
complications, 331–333, 341–342
follow-up, 335
outcome analysis, 336–339, 337t
outcome categories, 335–336
outcome endpoint summary, 339–340, 341t
patient population, 333t, 333–335, 334t
radiation-induced complications, 332–333
University of Florida experience, 333–342
resection costs, 323–326, 325t, 326t
retreatment, 336, 337–339, *340*
sizes, 350
small
sensitivity analysis of age vs Spetzler grade for, *302*, 302–303, *304*
SRNS for, 303–306, *307–308*
treatment analysis, 362, 363t
surgical treatment of
complications, 352–356
cost effectiveness, 356–364
cost estimates, 359t, 359–360
decision analysis
model overview, 357–358
utilities, 360
methodology, 356–360
results, 352–356, 353t, 360t, 360–362, 361t, 362t
therapeutic choices, 294, *295*
treatment costs, 323–326, 325t, 326t, 361–362, 362t
treatment of, 313–314, 314t
Astrocytomas
associated with intractable seizures, 453–454, *454*, *455*
brain, 464–479
cerebral
surgical mortality rates, 375–476, 476t

survival rates, 473, 474t
clinical features, 467–468, 468t
CT-defined characteristics, 467–468, 468t
cytoreductive surgery for, 465–466
definition of, 464–465
diffuse fibrillary
  survival curves, 489–491, *490, 491*
  survival rates, 488–489, 489t
fibrillary, 392
malignant, 465
neurodiagnostic technique for, 467–469
nonpilocytic, 426–427
ordinary, 392
pilocytic, 391–392, 404, *404*, 407, *408*
  management of, 421–423, *422*
  survival rates, 488–489, 489t
protoplasmic, 404
radiation therapy for, 466–467
stereotactic biopsy and fractionated
    radiation therapy for, 467–473
  clinical response, 469–471, *470*
  imaging-defined response, *471*, 471–473,
    472
  Karnofsky performance rating, 469–471,
    470t
  medial survival, 473, 474t
  survival curves, 473, *473*
  survival rates, 473, 473t
  survival statistics, 473, 473t
stereotactic biopsy vs resection of, 473–476
surgical debulking, 467–473
Audience participation
  interactive, 508–517
  IRIS electronic response system, 508–509
Auditory canal, internal, posterior wall
    drilling, 210–211, *211*
Auditory evoked responses. *See also* Evoked
    potentials
  intra-operative monitoring, 210
Auditory nerve (cranial nerve VIII),
    monitoring, 196–199, *197*, 210–212,
    211
AVMs. See Arteriovenous malformations
Awake cortical mapping, 442–443, *443*

BAEP. *See* Brainstem auditory evoked
    potentials
Balloon occlusion, of giant aneurysms, 272–
    273
Balloons, detachable silicone, *272*, 272–273
Balloon test occlusion, 136–137, 158

patients that clinically fail, 143–144
studies, 137t, 137–138
Barrow Neurological Institute, surgical
    management of giant intracranial
    aneurysms at, 245–266
Basilar artery, giant aneurysm of, 233, *233*,
    235, *236*
Biopsy
  stereotactic, of astrocytomas, 473–476
  stereotactic serial, 409
    studies in low-grade gliomas, 400–402,
      401, 402–403
Bleeding rates, after embolization of AVMs,
    317
Blue Cross and Blue Shield plans, 2–3, 4
Brain, stimulation mapping of functional
    areas, 440–448
Brain astrocytomas, 464–479. *See also*
    Astrocytomas
Brain compression, from giant aneurysms,
    222–225
Brain necrosis, with fractionated stereotactic
    proton therapy, 77–78
Brainstem auditory evoked potentials, 181.
    See also Evoked potentials
  intra-operative monitoring, 186, *197*, 197–
    198
Brainstem compression, from giant
    aneurysms, 222–225, *224*
Brain tissue, handling of, rules of
    perioperative care, 205–206
Brain tumor gene therapy
  with *CYP2B1* gene, experimental, *376*,
    376–379, *377–378*, 379t
  in mice, 370–382
  viral vectors for, 372–373, 373t
Broca's area, stimulation parameters, 445,
    446
BTO. *See* Balloon test occlusion
Bystander effect, in gene therapy, 375

Cancer, metastatic, stereotactic radiosurgery
    for, 115–116
Capitation, 24
CAPs. See Compound action potentials
Carcinomas, 156
  sinus, growing into anterior fossa, 93
Carotid bypass
  Fukushima (cavernous), 119, 120t, 125–
    127, *126*
  Fukushima skull base bypass I, 125–127, *126, 132*

Fukushima skull base bypass II, 127–130, *131*, *132*
Fukushima skull base bypass III, 130–132, *132*
occipital artery to middle cerebral artery, 142
superficial temporal artery to middle cerebral artery, 141, 141t, 142, 160
Carotid-cavernous fistulas, 221, 229–231
Cavernous carotid artery
aneurysms of, 228–231
asymptomatic, 228–229, *230*
compressive symptoms, 231
giant, 127, *129*
indications for treatment, 235–237
skull bypass I for, 127, *128*, *129*, *130*
vascular symptoms, 229–231
preservation, 154–170
Cavernous carotid bypass, 119, 120t, 125–127, *126*
Cavernous hemangioma, direct surgery for, 119, 120t
Cavernous malformations, 344–345
Cavernous sinus
anterolateral triangle, 125
anteromedial triangle, 122
last no man's land, 119
lateralmost triangle, 125
lateral triangle, 123
medial triangle, 122–123
microsurgical anatomy, *121*, 121–125
posteroinferior triangle, 123
posterolateral triangle, 123
posteromedial triangle, 123
postmeatal triangle, 124
premeatal triangle, 123–124
superior triangle, 123
triangles, 122, *122*
Cavernous sinus tumors, 71–98, 155–156
benign, 155
direct surgery for, 119, 120t
meningiomas, 88–90
management of, 88–89
recurrent petroclival, skull bypass I technique for, 127, *130*
results, 89t, 89–90
volume changes after radiosurgery, 103, *104*
surgery for, 73–74
treatment of, 73–79
Cellulose acetate polymer, 284–285

Cerebral arteriovenous malformations, decision making for, 348–351, 364–365
Cerebral artery, middle
common carotid artery vein graft to, 160
external carotid artery vein graft to, 141, 141t, 160
giant aneurysm of, 222–225, *225*
long cervical artery vein grafts to, 142
occipital artery carotid bypass to, 142
superficial temporal artery carotid bypass to, 141, 141t, 142, 160
superficial temporal artery vein graft to, 160
Cerebral astrocytomas. *See also* Astrocytomas
surgical mortality rates, 475–476, 476t
survival rates, 473, 475t
Cerebral blood flow
low, patients that show, 144
measurement of, 136–137, 158
patients who have no asymmetry of, 144
Cerebral hemispheres, diffuse gliomas of, 392–393
Cerebral protection, intra-operative, 258
Cerebral revascularization, 260–261
Cerebral ventricles, fourth, recording electrical potentials from lateral recess of, 198
Cervical artery to middle cerebral artery vein graft, 142
Chemodectoma, infratemporal, 130, 131
Children, gangliogliomas in, 409, 409–410
Chondroma, direct surgery for, 119, 120t
Chondrosarcomas, 90–91, 156
management of, 90–91
radiotherapy for, 91, 91t
results, 91, 91t
stereotactic radiosurgery for, 111–113
neurologic status after, 111, 112t
tumor imaging changes after, 111, 111t
Chordomas, 91–92, 156
direct surgery for, 119, 120t
management of, 91–92
radiotherapy for, 92, 92t
results, 92, 92t
stereotactic radiosurgery for, 111–113
neurologic status after, 111, 112t
tumor imaging changes after, 111, 111t
tumor volume changes after, 111, *112*
Cingulate gyrus, 443

Circulatory arrest, hypothermic, 258–259
Clinical condition, factor in decision making, 350
Clinical trials, 1994 CNS audience responses, 512
Clinoidal meningiomas, 85–88
  tumor growth arrest after radiosurgery, 103, *105*
Clinton bill. *See* Health Security Act of 1994
Clipping, direct, 257–258
Clivus
  transfrontal-nasal approach, 44t, *46*, 50–53
  transfrontal-nasal-orbital approach, 44t, *47*, *52*, 53–54
  transmaxillary approach, 44t, *49*, *52*, 55–56
  transnasomaxillary approach, 44t, *48*, 55
  transpalatal approach, 44t, *51–52*, 56
CN. *See* Cranial nerve
CNS. *See* Congress of Neurological Surgeons
CNS/AANS Computer Task Force, 10
Coil occlusion, of giant aneurysms, 273–279
Coils
  electrically detachable, 275–279
  fibered, 274, *274*
  flower petal design, 271, 274
  platinum, 273–275
Common carotid artery to middle cerebral artery vein grafts, 160
Communicating artery, anterior, giant aneurysm of, 222, *223*
Communication, challenges for, 10
COMPASS stereotactic frame (Stereotactic Medical Systems, Inc.), 413, 414
Competition, managed, 8
Compound action potentials (CAPs), 172
Compression
  from cavernous segment aneurysms, 231
  from giant aneurysms, 222–225, *224*
  from intracavernous aneurysms, 231
Computational Diagnostics Inc., NEURONET monitoring system, 181
Computed tomography
  astrocytoma characteristics, 467–468, 468t
  of low-grade gliomas, histologic correlations, 403–406
  Xenon
    CBF measurement, 137, 158
    moderate-risk patients treated by, 144
Computer-assisted stereotactic volumetric resection
  of deep-seated tumors, 418, *419*
  of low-grade gliomas, 412–413
    database acquisition, 413
    methods, 413–418
    results, 418–427
    surgical planning, 414
    surgical procedures, 414–417
    technical aspects, 417–418
Congressional Budget Office, 21
Congress of Neurological Surgeons (CNS), 9
  COSIN (Clinical Outcomes Studies in Neurosurgery) office, 10
Cortical mapping, awake, 442–443, *443*
Cost containment, government, 4–5
Cost effectiveness
  embolization of AVMs, 323–326, 325t
  of neurophysiologic monitoring during cranial base surgery, 200
  surgical treatment of AVMs, 356–364
Costs
  acute hemorrhage, 359t, 359–360
  AVM treatment, 323–326, 325t, 326t, 361–362, 362t
  endovascular management of giant aneurysms, 285–287, *287*
  gamma knife radiosurgery, 323–326, 325t, 326t
  giant intracranial aneurysm treatment, 237–238
  Guglielmi detachable coil system, 285–287, *286*
  health care, 1–6, 24
  health care reform, 16
  inpatient rehabilitation, 359t, 359–360
  nursing home care, 359t, 359–360
  resection, 323–326, 325t, 326t
  surgical treatment of AVMs, 359t, 359–360
CPA. *See* Cyclophosphamide
CPT codes. *See* Current Procedural Terminology codes
Cranial base, anterior
  radiation damage to, 78
  tumors, 71–98
    ICA sacrifice for, 64–66
    radical resection of, 43–70
    stereotactic radiosurgery for, 99–118, 100t
Cranial base surgery
  cranial nerve monitoring during, 187–200
  neurologic deficits after
    and intraoperative SSEP changes, 185, 186t
    pathogenesis of, 180–181

neurophysiologic monitoring during, 180–
202
BAEP, 186
cost effectiveness, 200
EEG, 182, *183*, *184*
motor evoked potentials, 186
SSEP, 182–186, 185t, 186t, *187–192*
techniques, 181–200
Cranial fossa, anterior
sinus carcinoma growing into, 93
transfrontal approach, 44t, *45*, 50
transfrontal-nasal approach, 44t, *46*, 50–53
transfrontal-nasal-orbital approach, 44t,
47, *52*, 53–54
Cranial nerve(s). *See also specific nerve*
monitoring, 181, 187–200
stimulation, 181
Cranial nerve I. *See* Olfactory nerve
Cranial nerve II. *See* Optic nerve
Cranial nerve III. *See* Oculomotor nerve
Cranial nerve V. *See* Trigeminal nerve
Cranial nerve VI. *See* Abducens nerve
Cranial nerve VII. *See* Facial nerve
Cranial nerve VIII. *See* Auditory nerve
Cranial nerve X. *See* Vagus nerve
Cranial nerve XI. *See* Accessory nerve
Cranial nerve XII. *See* Hypoglossal nerve
Cranial neuropathy, from giant aneurysms,
222, *223*
Craniectomy, left-sided suboccipital, 207, *207*
Craniopharyngiomas, stereotactic
radiosurgery for, 113–115
neurologic status after, 114, 114t
tumor imaging changes after, 113t, 113–
114
Craniotomy, cost estimates, 359t, 359–360
Credentialing, economic, 7
Cribriform plate, preservation of, *53*, *54*, 54–
55
CT. *See* Computed tomography
Current Procedural Terminology (CPT)
codes, 4, 40
Cyclophosphamide
bioactivation pathway, 370–371, *371*
characteristics of, 370–371, *372*
sensitivity to, 371, *372*
Cylindrical retractor, stereotactic, 416, 416–
417
CYP2B1 gene, experimental brain tumor
therapy with, *376*, 376–379, *377–378*, 379t
Cystic tumors, stereotactic resection of, 417, *418*

Cysts, direct surgery for, 119, 120t
Cytochrome P450-2B1 enzyme, immunocytochemical analysis, *376*, 376–377
Cytoreductive surgery, for astrocytomas,
465–466
Cytotoxicity, in tumor cell death after
transfer of drug-sensitivity genes,
375–376

Data, meaningful, 12–13
DATA software (TreeAge), 296
Debulking
of aneurysms, 261
of astrocytomas, 467–473
Decision analysis, 295
for AVMs, 294–312
age vs Spetzler grade, *302*, 302–303, *304*
alternate grading system, 299–300, 300t
ASA grades, 303, 303t
baseline values, 297–300, *298*, 299t
model failure, 303–306
results, 300–303, 301t, *301*
summary, 303, 305t, 306
technique (methods), 295–297
for cerebral AVMs, 348–351, 364–365
ethical considerations, 351
example, *310*, 310–312, *311*
factors, 349–351
for glial tumors, 406, *407*
for intracranial AVMs, 348–351
Decision tree, 295
for AVMs, 300–301, 301
constructed, 295–297
sample, 296, *296*
Dermoid cysts, direct surgery for, 119, 120t
Diagnosis-Related Groups (DRGs), 4
Direct auditory nerve action potential, 198
DNEs. *See* Dysembryoplastic
neuroepitheliomas
DNETs. *See* Dysembryoplastic
neuroepithelial tumors
DRGs. *See* Diagnosis-Related Groups
Drug-sensitivity genes, cytotoxic mecha-
nisms of tumor cell death after
transfer, 375–376
Dysembryoplastic neuroepithelial tumors,
455
Dysembryoplastic neuroepitheliomas, 409–410
ECOG. *See* Electrocochleography
ECoG. *See* Electrocorticography
Economic credentialing, 7

Edema/necrosis, radiation, 342
Education, graduate medical, 18–19
EEG. *See* Electroencephalography
Electrically detachable coils, 275–279
Electrical potentials, from lateral recess of fourth ventricle, recording, 198
Electrocardiography, intra-operative, 203
Electrocochleography, 198
Electrocorticography
  indications for, 459–461
  pre- and postresection, 448–449, *449*
  resection of low-grade gliomas without, 453–463
Electroencephalography, 181
  intra-operative, 182, *183, 184*
Electromyography
  cranial nerve monitoring with, 189
  potentials, 174
Elekta Instruments
  Gamma Knife, 100
  Leksell Model G stereotactic frame, 100
Embolization, of AVMs, 313–327
  bleeding rate, 317
  cases, 318–323, *320*
  complications of, 317
  cost effectiveness, 323–326, 325t
  with gamma knife radiosurgery, 318, 323, *325*
  materials, 313–315
  methods, 315
  in modern era, 301t, 301–302
  nidus volume changes after, 316–317, *317*
  obliteration rates, 315–316, 316t
  outcomes, 318, 318t
  with radiosurgery, 342–344, *343–344*
  with resection, 319–323, *321, 322, 324*
  results, 315–318
  role, 314–315, 315t
  treatment methods, 313–315
  volume reduction by, 315–317
EMG. *See* Electromyography
Employers, pressure from, 5–6
Endocrine deficiency, after fractionated stereotactic proton therapy, 78
Endovascular management, of giant aneurysms, 261, 267–293
  cost analysis, 285–287, *287*
  endovascular approach, 272–279
  experimental techniques, 282–285
  techniques, 267–268, *268*
Enzymes, CYP2B1, *376*, 376–377

Ependymomas, low-grade, 423–426
Epidermoid cysts, direct surgery for, 119, 120t
Epidermoid tumors, 94–95
Epilepsy
  intractable, with low-grade gliomas, 448–449
  surgically remediable syndromes of, 453
Epileptogenesis, local and remote, 458–459
Epileptogenic foci, 456
Epileptogenic zones, 456
Epistaxis, 221, 231
Equipment
  coils
    electrically detachable, 275–279
    fibered, 274, *274*
    flower petal design, 271, 274
    platinum, 273–275
  detachable silicone balloons, *272*, 272–273
  for intra-operative neurophysiologic monitoring, 204–205, *205*, 206
  self-retaining retractors, 205, *206*, 207–208, *208*
Esthesioneuroblastoma, 92–93
Ethernet, 101
Ethics, considerations for decision making, 351
Evoked facial nerve discharge, 191–193, *194*
Evoked potentials, 174
  intra-operative monitoring, 180, 186, 187–189, *204*, 204–205, 210
    equipment for, 204–205, *206*
  somatosensory, 181
    intra-operative monitoring, 182–186, *187–192*, 203–204
      classification of changes, 185, 185t
      correlation with postoperative neurologic deficits, 185, 186t
External carotid artery to middle cerebral artery vein grafts, 141, 141t, 160

Facial nerve (cranial nerve VII)
  evoked discharge, 191–193, *194*
  function according to tumor size, 195, 196t
  intra-operative monitoring, 189–196, *194*, 209, *209*
    bursts, 191
    dissection, 191
    non-repetitive discharges, 191
    postoperative facial nerve function, 193–194, 195t

repetitive discharges, 191
trains, 191
outcome after translabyrinthine approach
to acoustic neuroma, 194, 195t
stimulation of, 210
Fibered coils, 274, *274*
Field effect, tumorigenic, 483
Financing. *See also* Costs
American health care, 1–6
health care reform, 16
health care spending, 23–24
Fistulas, carotid-cavernous, 221, 229–231
Floor of frontal fossa meningiomas, 84
Flower petal coils, 271, 274
Focal seizures, from giant aneurysms, 226
Fourth ventricle, recording electrical
potentials from lateral recess of, 198
Fractionated external-beam radiation
therapy, for astrocytomas, 467–473
Fractionated photon radiotherapy
for anterior cranial base neoplasms, 71–73
for cavernous sinus meningiomas, 89t, 89–
90
for cavernous sinus neoplasms, 71–73
for medial sphenoid wing meningiomas,
87–88, 88t
for olfactory groove meningioma, 80, 81t
for tuberculum sellae meningioma, 83, 83t
Fractionated stereotactic proton radiotherapy, 74–79
for anterior cranial base neoplasms, 71–73
background, 74
for cavernous sinus meningiomas, 89t, 89–
90
for cavernous sinus neoplasms, 71–73
for chondrosarcoma, 90–91, 91t
for chordoma, 92, 92t
complications of, 76–78
for medial sphenoid wing meningiomas,
87–88, 88t
medical therapy with, 78
MGH program, 75
observation, 78–79
for olfactory groove meningioma, 80, 81t
treatment planning, 75
treatment program, 75–76
for tuberculum sellae meningioma, 83, 83t
Frontal fossa floor meningiomas, 84
Frontal skull anatomy, *53*
Fukushima bypass, 119, 125–127, *126*
skull base I, 125–127, *128, 129, 130, 132*

skull base II, 127–130, *131, 132*
skull base III, 130–132, 132
Functional areas, stimulation mapping of,
440–448
Functional mapping, guided resection of low-
grade gliomas with, 437–452

Gamma Knife (Elekta Instruments), 100
Gamma knife radiosurgery, for AVMs
costs, 323–326, 325t, 326t
after embolization
case, 323, *325*
follow-up result, 318
Gangliogliomas, 391, 404, 409, *409*
management of, 423–426
in young patients, *409*, 409–410
Gangliomas, giant, 425, *425*
Garfield, Sidney, 2
GDC system. *See* Guglielmi detachable coil
system
Geisel, Theodore, 11, 13
Genes
drug-sensitivity, cytotoxic mechanisms of
tumor cell death after transfer, 375–
376
therapeutic, 372, 373t
Gene therapy, 370, 371–372
bystander effect in, 375
experimental, with *CYP2B1* gene, *376*,
376–379, *377–378*, 379t
vectors for gene transfer *in vivo*, 372–375
Giant aneurysms
debulking, 261
of internal carotid artery, 233, 233
intracavernous, 127, *129*, 239
skull bypass I for, 127, *128, 129, 130*
treatment of
goals, 237
indications for, 235–237
options, 237
intracranial, 214–244
age and gender of patients, 215–216, *216*
alternative techniques, 259–260
of anterior communicating artery, 222, *223*
balloon occlusion of, 272–273
classification of, 269, *270*
clinical presentation, 217–226, *223, 224*
coil occlusion of, 273–279
definition of, 245
diagnostic evaluation, 247
direct clipping, 257–258

endovascular approach, 272–279
endovascular management, 267–293
  cost analysis, 285–287
  experimental techniques, 282–285
  hemodynamic considerations, 269–272
endovascular therapy for, 261
epidemiology, 215–216
flow within, 269, *270*
growth of, 222–225
hemorrhage, 219–221
Hunt-Hess grade, *153*, 252, *252*
incidence of, 215, 215t
location, 217, 218t, 219t
mass effect, *221*, 221–225
multiplicity, 217
natural history, 226–231
parent artery occlusion, 279–282
pathogenesis, 214
patient population, 245
patient presentation, 246
postoperative management, 261–262
pre-operative management, 247–248
skull base approaches, 256–257
surgical management of, 245–266
  clinical materials and methods, 245–251
  Glasgow outcome scores, 252–253, 254t
  intra-operative cerebral protection, 258
  mortality rate, 252, 253
  operative approach and exposure, 255–
    257
  outcomes, 251–254, *252*, *253*, 254t, 255t
  techniques, 248t, 248–249, 249t
  therapeutic options, 232–235, *233*, *235*,
    236
  treatment, 248–251
  treatment costs, 237–238
  treatment techniques, 257–261
intradural, 238–239
treatment of
  goals, 232
  indications for, 231–237
  options, 232–235, *233*, *235*, *236*
midbasilar, 233, *233*
of middle cerebral artery, 222–225, *225*
of proximal basilar artery, 235, *236*
of vertebral artery, 222, *224*
Giant gangliomas, 425, *425*
Giant subependymomas, 423–426, *424*
Glasgow outcome scores, after surgical
    management of giant intracranial
    aneurysms, 252–253, 254t

Gliomas
  associated with intractable seizures, 453–
    456
  diffuse, of cerebral hemispheres, 392–393
  high-grade
    internal decompression, 411
    surgical microanatomy, 400
  infiltrating, 426
  mixed, 392
  pre-operative diagnosis, 481–482
  radical resection of, 480–487
    alternatives to, 485–486
    arguments against, 483, 484t
    arguments for, 482t, 482–483
    methods, 484
    results, 484–485
  variants, 391–392
Gliomas, low-grade
  associated with seizures, 461
    extent of resection for, 456–457
  biologic markers, 498–499
  classification of, 497, 498
  clinical markers, 497–498
  computer-assisted stereotactic volumetric
      resection of, 412–413
    database acquisition, 413
    methods, 413–418
    results, 418–427
    surgical planning, 414
    surgical procedures, 414–417
  CT/histologic correlations, 403–406
  delayed radiotherapy strategy, 502–503
  delayed surgery for, 391–398, 395t
    benefits and risks, 393–397
    indications for, 393, 393t, 396–397, 397t
  early radiotherapy for, 488–494
    supporting evidence, 488–493
  early surgery for, 383–390
    extent of resection, 388–389
    indications for, 393, 393t
  functional mapping-guided resection of,
      437–452
  glial tumor spatial types in, 404–406
  grading systems, 429
  histologic circumscription, 411
  hypothetical data sheet, 504t, 504–505
  infiltrated parenchyma, 402–403
  intractable epilepsy associated with, 448–
    449
  labeling indices, 429–430
  local and remote epileptogenesis, 458–459

misdiagnosis, 394–395, 395t
morbidity, 491–493
natural history, 488–489
pathology, 488–489
prognostic factors, 395–396, 396t, 496t,
    496–500
  biologic, 498–499
  clinical, 497–498
  therapeutic, 499–500
proliferative potential, 386–388, 387t
radiographic diagnosis, 384–386
radiotherapy for, 433
  adjuvant vs at recurrence, 500–502, *501,*
    503
  delayed strategy, 502–503
  early, 488–494
  efficacy of, 489–491
  at recurrence, 495–496, 500–502, *501,*
    503, 504–505
  strategy for, 501–502
  toxicity of, 491–493
recurrence
  effects of volume on, 438t, 438–440, 439t
  radiotherapy at, 495–496, 500–502, *501,*
    503, 504–505
resectability, 411
resection of
  benefits of, 428
  electrocorticography before and after, 448–
    449, *449*
  extent influencing outcome, 438–440
  outcome based on language mapping,
    447–448, *448*
  risk:benefit ratio, 399–400
  stereotactic volumetric, 420t, 433–434
  technical aspects, 417–418
  without electrocorticography, 453–463
spatial types, *404,* 404–406, *405, 406*
stereotactic serial biopsy studies, 400–402,
    401, 402–403
supratentorial
  surgical complications, 393–394, 394t
  surgical issues, 399–436
  survival curves, 489, *490*
surgery for, 431–433
  early, 383–390
  planning and case selection, 406–411, *409,*
    410
  procedures, 411–412
surgical decision making for, 406, *407*
survival rates, 488–489, 489t

therapeutic markers, 499–500
treatment benefits, 430–431
tumor tissue, 402, 402t
volume, effects on recurrence, 438t, 438–
    440, 439t
Global budgeting, 24
Governmental regulations, 10
Graduate medical education, 18–19
Graduate Medical Education National
    Advisory Council, 35
Granulomas, direct surgery for, 119, 120t
Group Health Cooperative of Puget Sound,
    19
Guglielmi detachable coil (GDC) system,
    275, 276, *276,* 277, 279
  cost analysis, 285–287, *286*

Harvard Cyclotron, 75
HCFA. *See* Health Care Financing
    Administration
Health, factor in decision making, 350
Health care
  costs of, 24
  financial evolution of, 1–6
  inflation rate, 34
  managed, 6–8
Health Care Financing Administration
    (HCFA), 5
Health care reform, 1–14, 27–29, 30–36
  agenda, 19–21
  1994 CNS audience responses, 509–511
  financing, 16
  fundamental issue, 25
  immediate future, 33–35
  implications for neurologic surgeons, 25–26
  Magnum Opus, 21–22
  national, 8–9
  and neurosurgery, 35–36
  paradigm shift, 23–25
  politics of, 15–22
  reasons for optimism, 29
  strategies for change, 23–29
  surgeons' response to, 37–42
Health care spending, 23–24. *See also* Costs
Health insurance
  any willing providers, 16, 17
  benefits, 16–18
  first physician-directed prepaid plans, 2
  industry, 2–3
  primary payers, 17
  providers, 16–18

Health insurance purchasing cooperatives
(HIPCs), 20
Health Security Act of 1994, 30–32
Health states, 310, *310*
Hearing preservation, with auditory nerve
monitoring, 198–199, 199t, 210–212,
211
Hemangiomas, 205
cavernous, direct surgery for, 119, 120t
Hemorrhage, 219–221, 331–332
acute, cost estimates, 359t, 359–360
intracerebral, 220, *220*
risk with AVMs, 358
with radiosurgery for AVMs, 341–342
subarachnoid, 219, 229
Hemostasis, intraoperative, 213
Hill-Burton Act, 3
HIPCs. *See* Health insurance purchasing
cooperatives
HMOs, 6, 7–8, 19
Hospital networks, 27
Hospital Survey and Construction Act, 3
House Resolution 4527. *See* Patient
Protection Act
Hunt-Hess grading, of giant intracranial
aneurysms, 252, *252*
Hypoglossal nerve (cranial nerve XII),
monitoring of, 200
Hypothermic circulatory arrest, 258–259

ICA. *See* Internal carotid artery
Incentives for physicians, corrected, 11–12
Independent practice associations (IPAs), 7,
26–27
Infiltrated parenchyma, in low-grade
gliomas, 402–403
Infiltrating gliomas, 426
Infratemporal chemodectoma, 130, *131*
Injury, optic pathway, with fractionated
stereotactic proton therapy, 76–77
Injury potentials, 191
Innovation, 13
Inpatient rehabilitation, cost estimates,
359t, 359–360
Interactive audience participation, 508–517
clinical trials responses, 512
health care issues/reform responses, 509–
511
spine responses, 512–514
tumor responses, 514–515
vascular responses, 515–517

Internal auditory canal, posterior wall
drilling, 210–211, *211*
Internal carotid artery
cavernous
aneurysms of, 228–231
asymptomatic, 228–229, *230*
compressive symptoms, 231
giant, 127, *128*, *129*, *130*, 235–237
vascular symptoms, 229–231
preservation, 154–170
giant aneurysm of, 233, *233*
ligation, preoperative testing, 136–138
BTO studies, 137, 137t
case studies, 138–141, *139*, *140*
preservation of, 165–168
reconstruction or revascularization, 66–67,
119–134, *156*, 156–162, *159*
case studies, *145*, 145–146, *147*
choice of, 143–145
clinical material for, 120–124
Fukushima bypass, 119, 120t, 125–127,
126
high-risk patients, 143–144
indications for, 135
low-risk patients, 144
moderate-risk patients treated by Xe CT,
144
operative results, 132
operative technique, 125–132
options for, 141–146
risks of, 146–151
skull base bypass I, *124*, 125–127, *126*,
132
skull base bypass II, 127–130, *131*, *132*
skull base bypass III, 130–132, *132*
technique pros and cons, 141, 141t
resection, oncologic effects, *156*, 162–165,
163, *164*, *165*, *166*
sacrifice, 63–67
for benign skull base tumors, 64–66
clinical materials and methods, 63
for malignant skull base tumors, 66
on one side, 135–141
results, 64
segments and nomenclature, *121*, 121–122
vein graft occlusion
case study, 149–151, *150*
management of, 148–149
Internal carotid artery to internal carotid
artery vein grafts, 141, 141t, 142–
143, 160

Intracavernous aneurysms, 228–231
  asymptomatic, 228–229, *230*
  compressive symptoms, 231
  giant, 127, *129*, 239
    indications for treatment, 235–237
    skull bypass I for, 127, *128*, *129*, *130*
  vascular symptoms, 229–231
Intracerebral hemorrhage, 220, *220*
  risk with AVMs, 358
Intracranial aneurysms, giant, 214–244, 239
  definition of, 245
  endovascular management, 267–293
  surgical management of, 245–266
Intracranial arteriovenous malformations,
    surgical treatment of, 348–369
Intradural aneurysms, giant, 238–239
  indications for treatment, 231–237
Intra-operative cerebral protection, for
    aneurysm patients, 258
Intra-operative neurophysiologic monitoring,
    171–179, 203–213
  advantages, 174
  basis, 172–173
  benefits
    for patient, 173
    for surgeon, 173–174
  during cranial base surgery, 180–202
  equipment, 204–205, *205*, *206*, 207–208,
    208
  implementation, 174–177
  medicoeconomic aspects, 177–179
  medicolegal aspects, 177–179
Intravascular stents, 282–283
IPAs. *See* Independent practice associations
IRIS electronic response audience participa-
    tion system, 508–509
Ischemia, distal, from giant aneurysms,
    225–226

Joint Managed Care Task Force, 9

Kaiser, Henry, 2
Kaiser Permanente Health Plan, 2
Kaiser Portland, 19
Karnofsky Performance Scale (KPS), rating
    with stereotactic biopsy and
    irradiation of astrocytomas, 469–471,
    470t
Key Person Program, 10
KPS. *See* Karnofsky Performance Scale

Labeling indices, for low-grade gliomas, 429–
    430
Laminectomy, for spinal cord tumors, 212–
    213
Language mapping
  penumbras, 447–448
  postoperative outcome based on, 447–448,
    448
  stimulation parameters, 445–448, *447*
  supplementary penumbra, 448
  suprasylvian essential site, 446–447, *447*
Leadership, needs for, 26–27
Left abducens palsy, 127, *128*
Left-sided suboccipital craniectomy, with
    removal of mastoid, 207, *207*
Legislation. *See also specific acts*
  any willing provider laws, 17
Leksell Model G stereotactic frame (Elekta
    Instruments), 100
Lesionectomy, stereotactic, 456
Lesions. *See also* Tumors
  deep-seated, stereotactic resection of, *416*,
    416–417
  superficial, management of, 423–426
  well-circumscribed, management of, 423–
    426
LGGs. *See* Gliomas, low-grade
Lifestyle, factor in decision making, 350
Liquid polymeric adhesive, 283–284
Literature review, radiosurgery for AVMs,
    329–333

Magnetic resonance imaging (MRI), of AVMs
  suggestive of cure, 336, 339
  suggestive of failure, 336, 339
Magnum Opus, 21–22
Managed care, 6–8
Managed competition, 8
Mapping
  awake cortical, 442–443, *443*
  stimulation
    of functional areas, 440–448
    language parameters, 445–448, *447*
    motor parameters, 441–445
    sensory parameters, 441–445
Marker balls, radiographically opaque, 417,
    418
Markov cycling, 297
  decision analysis model for AVMs, 357–358
  example, *310*, 310–312, *311*
Martin grading, of AVMs, 315–316, 316t

Massachusetts General Hospital, fractionated proton program, 75
Mastoid process, removal of, 207, *207*
Materials, for embolization of AVMs, 313–314
Mayfield's law, 205
Medial sphenoid wing meningiomas, 85–88
  management of, 85–86
  radiotherapy for, 87–88, 88t
  results, 87–88
  surgery for, 87, 87t
  tumor growth arrest after radiosurgery, 103, *105*
Medicaid
  cost containment, 4–5
  waivers, 34–35
Medical education, graduate, 18–19
Medical therapy, with fractionated stereotactic proton therapy, 78
Medicare, 3, 36
  cost containment, 4–5
  intermediaries for, 3–4
Medicare Prospective Payment System, 4
Medicare Volume Performance Standard, 41
Meningiomas, 155, *156*, *158*
  anterior skull base, radiosurgery for
  clinical status after, 103–104, 105t
  tumor control and neurologic status after, 106t, 106–107
  tumor imaging changes after, 103, 103t
  cavernous sinus, 88–90
  recurrent petroclival, skull bypass I technique for, 127, *130*
  volume changes after radiosurgery, 103, *104*
  direct surgery for, 119, 120t
  floor of frontal fossa, 84
  medial sphenoid wing (clinoidal), 85–88
  tumor growth arrest after radiosurgery, 103, *105*
  olfactory groove, 79–80
  optic sheath, 84–85
  stereotactic radiosurgery for, 101–107
  tuberculum sellae, 81–83
Metastatic cancer, stereotactic radiosurgery for, 115–116
Mice, brain tumor gene therapy in, 370–382
Microtechnique, 205
Middle cerebral artery
  common carotid artery vein graft to, 160
  external carotid artery vein graft to, 141,

  141t, 160
  giant aneurysm of, 222–225, 225
  long cervical artery vein grafts to, 142
  occipital artery carotid bypass to, 142
  superficial temporal artery carotid bypass to, 141, 141t, 142, 160
  superficial temporal artery vein graft to, 160
Middle fossa rhomboid complex, 124, *124*
Monitoring
  cranial nerve, 187–200
  intra-operative neurophysiologic, 171–179, 203–213
  during cranial base surgery, 180–202
  equipment, 204–205, *205*, *206*, 207–208, *208*
Moniz, Egas, 267
Morbidity, acute, with radiosurgery for AVMs, 341
Mortality rates
  with AVMs, 358–359
  after surgical management of giant intracranial aneurysms, 252, *253*
Motor cortex, supplementary, tumor infiltrating, 443, *444*
Motor deficits, postoperative, 443
Motor evoked potentials. *See also* Evoked potentials
  during cranial base surgery, 186
Motor mapping, stimulation parameters for, 441–445
Motor pathways, subcortical, preservation of, 443–445, *444*

Nasomaxillary osteotomy, 44t, *48*, 55
Nasopharynx
  transfrontal-nasal approach, 44t, *46*, 50–53
  transfrontal-nasal-orbital approach, 44t, *47*, *52*, 53–54
  transmaxillary approach, 44t, *49*, 55–56
  transnasomaxillary approach, 44t, *48*, 55
National health care reform, 8–9
National Institutes of Health, 3
Natwest Securities Corporation, 15
Necrosis
  brain, with fractionated stereotactic proton therapy, 77–78
  radiation, 342
Neoplasms. *See* Tumors
Neurinoma, direct surgery for, 119, 120t
Neuroblastoma, olfactory, 92–93

Neurocytomas, 423–426
Neuro-endovascular therapy. *See* Endovascular management
Neuroepitheliomas, dysembryoplastic, 409–410, 455
Neurologic deficits, after cranial base surgery
and intraoperative SSEP changes, 185, 186t
pathogenesis of, 180–181
Neuromas
acoustic
removal, 208–212, *209, 211*
auditory nerve monitoring, 198–199, 199t, 210–212, *211*
facial nerve monitoring, 193–194, 195t
translabyrinthine approach to, 194, 195t
tumor size, facial nerve function according to, 195, 196t
trigeminal, 94
NEURONET monitoring system (Computational Diagnostics Inc.), 181
Neuropathy, cranial, 222
Neurophysiologic monitoring, intra-operative, 171–179, 203–213
cost effectiveness, 200
during cranial base surgery, 180–202
equipment, 204–205, *205, 206,* 207–208, *208*
techniques, 181–200
Neurosurgeons
implications of health care reform for, 25–26
leadership needs, 26–27
response to health care reform, 28–29, 37–42
role of, 10–13
Neurosurgery
challenges for, 9–13
educational role, 9–10
health care reform and, 35–36
Nursing home care, cost estimates, 359t, 359–360

Occipital artery to middle cerebral artery bypass, 142
Occlusion
alternative techniques, 259–260
balloon, 272–273
balloon test, 136–137, 158
patients that clinically fail, 143–144
studies, 137t, 137–138
coil, 273–279
parent artery, 279–282
Occupation, factor in decision making, 350
Oculomotor nerve (cranial nerve III), intra-operative monitoring, 189
Oculomotor nerve palsy, 127, *128, 129*
Oh, The Places You'll Go! (Seuss), 11, 13
Olfactory groove meningioma, 79–80
management, 79
radiotherapy for, 80, 81t
results, 79–80
surgery for, 79–80, 80t
Olfactory neuroblastoma, 92–93
Oligo-astrocytomas, 410, *410*
management of, 427
survival curves, 489–491, *490, 491*
survival rates, 488–489, 489t
Oligodendrogliomas, 392, 404, *405*
management of, 427
survival rates, 488–489, 489t
very low-grade, 409–410
Ophthalmoplegia, due to recurrent petroclival-cavernous sinus meningioma, 127, *130*
Optic nerve (cranial nerve II), monitoring, 187–189
Optic pathways, injury with fractionated stereotactic proton therapy, 76–77
Optic sheath meningiomas, 84–85
management of, 84
results, 84–85
surgery for, 84–85, 85t
Optimism, reasons for, 29
Osteonecrosis, after fractionated stereotactic proton therapy, 78
Osteotomy
anterior, *53,* 54–55
circumferential cribriform plate, *53, 54,* 54–55
nasomaxillary, 44t, *48,* 55
parasagittal, *53,* 54–55

Palsy
left abducens, 127, *128*
oculomotor nerve, 127, *128, 129*
right oculomotor nerve, 127, *128*
Parenchyma, infiltrated, 402–403
Parent artery occlusion, for giant aneurysms, 279–282
Patient Access to Specialty Care Coalition, 10

Patient age, factor in decision making, 349
Patient health and clinical condition, factor in decision making, 349–350
Patient occupation and lifestyle, factor in decision making, 350
Patient Protection Act (HR4527), 10
Petroclival cavernous sinus meningioma, recurrent, skull bypass I technique for, 127, *130*
PHOs. *See* Physician-hospital organizations
Photon radiotherapy, fractionated
  for anterior cranial base and cavernous sinus neoplasms, 71–73
  for cavernous sinus meningiomas, 89t, 89–90
  for medial sphenoid wing meningiomas, 87–88, 88t
  for olfactory groove meningioma, 80, 81t
  for tuberculum sellae meningioma, 83, 83t
Physician-hospital organizations (PHOs), 27
Physician organizations, 26–27, 28–29
Physician Payment Review Commission, 6
Physicians
  corrected incentives for, 11–12
  in-network, 17
  out-of-network, 17
Pilocytic astrocytomas, 391–392, 404, *404*, 407, *408*
  management of, 421–423, *422*
  survival rates, 488–489, 489t
Pituitary tumors
  direct surgery for, 119, 120t
  stereotactic radiosurgery for, 107–110
    ACTH levels after, 107–108, *109*
    endocrine function after, 107–108, 108t
    neurologic status after, 108–109, 109t
    tumor imaging changes after, 107t, 107–108
    tumor volume changes after, 107–108, *108*
Platinum coils, 273–275
Pleomorphic xanthoastrocytoma, 391
Politics, of health care reform, 15–22
Polymer
  cellulose acetate, 284–285
  liquid adhesive, 283–284
PPOs, 6, 7
Proton radiotherapy, fractionated stereotactic, 74–79
  for anterior cranial base neoplasms, 71–73
  for cavernous sinus meningiomas, 89t, 89–90

  for cavernous sinus neoplasms, 71–73
  for chondrosarcoma, 90–91, 91t
  for chordoma, 92, 92t
  for medial sphenoid wing meningiomas, 87–88, 88t
  for olfactory groove meningioma, 80, 81t
  for tuberculum sellae meningioma, 83, 83t
Protoplasmic astrocytomas, 404
Proximal basilar artery, giant aneurysm of, 235, *236*

Quality objectives, clinical, 25

Radiation injury
  complications of radiosurgery for AVMs, 332–333
  edema/necrosis, 342
  optic pathway, 76–77
  skull base damage, 78
Radiographically opaque marker balls, 417, *418*
Radiography, diagnostic, of low-grade glioma, 384–386
Radioneurosurgery, stereotactic, for small AVMs, 303–306, *307–308*
Radiosurgery
  for AVMs, 328–347
    angiographic thrombosis rates, 329–331
    complications, 331–333
    cost estimates, 359t, 359–360
    literature review, 329–333
    radiation-induced complications, 332–333
    University of Florida experience, 333–342
  and embolization, for AVMs, 342–344, *343–344*
  gamma knife
    for AVMs, costs, 323–326, 325t, 326t
    and embolization, for AVMs
      case, 323, *325*
      follow-up result, 318
    general paradigm, 328–329
  stereotactic
    for anterior skull base tumors, 99–118, 100t
    for small AVMs, 303–306, *307–308*
Radiotherapy
  adjuvant, for low-grade gliomas, 500–502, *501, 503*
  for astrocytomas, 466–467
  controversy, 466–467
  efficacy of, 489–491

fractionated external-beam, stereotactic
biopsy and, 467–473
fractionated photon
for anterior cranial base neoplasms, 71–73
for cavernous sinus meningiomas, 89t, 89–
90
for cavernous sinus neoplasms, 71–73
for medial sphenoid wing meningiomas,
87–88, 88t
for olfactory groove meningioma, 80, 81t
for tuberculum sellae meningioma, 83, 83t
fractionated stereotactic proton, 74–79
for anterior cranial base and cavernous
sinus neoplasms, 71–73
for cavernous sinus meningiomas, 89t, 89–
90
for chondrosarcoma, 90–91, 91t
for chordoma, 92, 92t
for medial sphenoid wing meningiomas,
87–88, 88t
for olfactory groove meningioma, 80, 81t
for tuberculum sellae meningioma, 83, 83t
for low-grade gliomas, 433
efficacy, 489–491
at recurrence, 495–496, 500–502, *501,
503*, 504–505
toxicity, 491–493
RBRVS. *See* Resource-Based Relative Value
System
Reference balls, steel, 417, *418*
Rehabilitation, inpatient, cost estimates,
359t, 359–360
Relative value unit (RVU), 4–5
Resection
of astrocytomas, vs stereotactic biopsy, 473–
476
of AVMs
costs, 323–326, 325t, 326t
after embolization, 319–323, *321, 322, 324*
computer-assisted stereotactic volumetric
of cystic tumors, 417, *418*
of deep-seated tumors, *416*, 416–417, 418,
419
of low-grade gliomas, 412–413
database acquisition, 413
methods, 413–418
results, 418–427
surgical planning, 414
surgical procedures, 414–417
technical aspects, 417–418
of superficial tumors, *415*, 415–416

early, of low-grade gliomas, 388–389
electrocorticography before and after, 448–
449, *449*
and embolization, of AVMs, 319–323, *321,
322, 324*
extent influencing outcome, 438–440
functional mapping-guided, of low-grade
gliomas, 437–452
of gliomas, radical, 480–487
internal carotid artery, oncologic effects,
156, 162–165, *163, 164, 165, 166*
of low-grade gliomas
benefits of, 428
early, 388–389
extent influencing outcome, 388–389,
438–440
functional mapping-guided, 437–452
outcome based on language mapping,
447–448, *448*
risk:benefit ratio, 399–400
technical aspects, 417–418
without electrocorticography, 453–463
of low-grade gliomas associated with
seizures, extent of, 456–457
radical
of anterior skull base tumors, 43–70
of gliomas, 480–487
alternatives to, 485–486
arguments against, 483, 484t
arguments for, 482t, 482–483
methods, 484
results, 484–485
stereotactic volumetric, of low-grade
gliomas, 420t, 433–434
without electrocorticography, of low-grade
gliomas, 453–463
Resource-based Relative Value System
(RBRVS), 4, 5
Retractors
self-retaining, 205, *206*, 207–208, *208*
stereotactic cylindrical, *416*, 416–417
Revascularization, cerebral, 260–261
Right oculomotor nerve palsy, 127, *128*
RU486, 78
RVU. *See* Relative value unit

Seizures
focal, from giant aneurysms, 226
intractable
gliomas associated with, 453–456
low-grade astrocytomas associated with,

453–454, *454*, *455*
low-grade gliomas associated with, 461
Self-retaining retractors, 205, *206*, 207–208, *208*
Sensitivity, CPA, 371, *372*
Sensitivity analysis, of AVMs
  age vs Spetzler grade, *302*, 302–303, *304*
  summary, 303, 305t
Sensory mapping, stimulation parameters for, 441–445
Sensory pathways, subcortical, preservation of, 443–445, *444*
Seuss, Dr., 11, 13
Silicone balloons, detachable, *272*, 272–273
Single photon emission computed tomography
  CBF measurement, 137
  patients that show low CBF on, 144
  patients who have no asymmetry of CBF by, 144
Sinus carcinoma, growing into anterior fossa, 93
Skull, frontal anatomy, 53
Skull base, anterior
  radiation damage to, 78
  tumors, 71–98
    ICA sacrifice for, 64–66
    meningiomas, radiosurgery for, 103t, 103–104, 105t, 106t, 106–107
    metastatic, stereotactic radiosurgery for, 115–116
    radical resection of, 43–70
    stereotactic radiosurgery for, 99–118, 100t
Skull base bypass I, 125–127, *128*, *129*, *130*, *132*
Skull base bypass II, 127–130, *131*, *132*
Skull base bypass III, 130–132, *132*
Skull base surgery
  approaches to aneurysms, 256–257
  cranial nerve monitoring during, 187–200
  neurologic deficits after
    and intraoperative SSEP changes, 185, 186t
    pathogenesis of, 180–181
  neurophysiologic monitoring during, 180–202
    BAEP, 186
    cost effectiveness, 200
    EEG, 182, *183*, *184*
    motor evoked potentials, 186
    SSEP, 182–186, 185t, 186t, *187–192*

techniques, 181–200
Software, DATA (TreeAge), 296
Somatosensory evoked potentials, 181
  intra-operative monitoring, 182–186, *187–192*, 203–204
    classification of changes, 185, 185t
    correlation with postoperative neurologic deficits, 185, 186t
SPECT. *See* Single photon emission computed tomography
Speech arrest, 445, *446*
Spetzler grading, of AVMs
  pre- and postembolization, 315–316, 316t
  sensitivity analysis of, *302*, 302–303, *304*
Sphenoid wing, medial, meningiomas of, 85–88
Spinal cord tumors, laminectomy for, 212–213
Spine, 1994 CNS audience responses, 512–514
SRNS. *See* Stereotactic radioneurosurgery
SSEP. *See* Somatosensory evoked potentials
Steel reference balls, 417, *418*
Stents, intravascular, 282–283
Stereotactic biopsy
  for astrocytomas, 467–473, 473–476
  and fractionated external-beam radiation therapy, for astrocytomas, 467–473
  serial, 409
    of low-grade gliomas
      results, 402–403
      studies, 400–402, *401*
Stereotactic cylindrical retractors, *416*, 416–417
Stereotactic fractionated proton radio-therapy, 74–79
  for anterior cranial base neoplasms, 71–73
  for cavernous sinus meningiomas, 89t, 89–90
  for cavernous sinus neoplasms, 71–73
  for chondrosarcoma, 90–91, 91t
  for chordoma, 92, 92t
  for medial sphenoid wing meningiomas, 87–88, 88t
  for olfactory groove meningioma, 80, 81t
  for tuberculum sellae meningioma, 83, 83t
Stereotactic frames
  COMPASS, 413, 414
  Leksell Model G, 100
Stereotactic lesionectomy, 456
Stereotactic Medical Systems, Inc.,

COMPASS stereotactic frame, 413,
414
Stereotactic radioneurosurgery, for small
AVMs, 303–306, *307–308*
Stereotactic radiosurgery
for anterior skull base tumors, 99–118, 100t
results, 101–116
technique, 100–101, *102*
Stereotactic volumetric resection
computer-assisted
of cystic tumors, 417, *418*
of deep-seated lesions, *416*, 416–417
of deep-seated tumors, 418, *419*
of low-grade gliomas, 412–413
methods, 413–418
results, 418–427
of superficial tumors, *415*, 415–416
of low-grade gliomas, 420t, 433–434
Stereotaxis, volumetric, purpose of, 418
Stimulation mapping, of functional areas,
440–448
Subarachnoid hemorrhage, 219, 229
Subcortical pathways, preservation of, 443–
445, *444*
Subependymomas, management of, 423–426
Suboccipital craniectomy, left-sided, 207, *207*
Superficial temporal artery to middle
cerebral artery bypass, 141, 141t,
142, 160
Superficial temporal artery to middle
cerebral artery vein graft, 160
Superficial tumors
management of, 423–426
stereotactic resection method for, *415*, 415–
416
Supratentorial astrocytomas, diffuse
fibrillary, survival curves, 489–491,
490, 491
Supratentorial gliomas, low-grade
surgical complications, 393–394, 394t
surgical issues, 399–436
survival curves, 489, *490*
Surgeon experience, factor in decision
making, 350
Surgeons. *See* Neurosurgeons
Surgery. *See also* Radiosurgery
for anterior cranial base neoplasms, 71–73,
73–74
for cavernous sinus tumors, 71–73, 73–74
direct, 119, 120t
conservative

definition of, 71
factors favoring, 72
cranial base
neurologic deficits after, 180–181
neurophysiologic monitoring during, 180–
202
cytoreductive, for astrocytomas, 465–466
for giant aneurysms, 245–266
cost analysis, 285–287, *286*
techniques, 248t, 248–249, 249t
for low-grade gliomas, 431–433
decision making, 406, *407*
delayed, 391–398, 395t
early, 383–390
indications for, 393, 393t
for medial sphenoid wing (clinoidal)
meningiomas, 87, 87t
for olfactory groove meningiomas, 79–80,
80t
for optic sheath meningiomas, 84–85, 85t
for tuberculum sellae meningiomas, 82t,
82–83
Surgical debulking, of astrocytomas, 467–
473
Surgically remediable syndromes, of
epilepsy, 453

Temporal artery, superficial
bypass to middle cerebral artery, 141, 141t,
142, 160
vein graft to middle cerebral artery, 160
Temporal lobectomy, 457, 461
Thrombo-embolism, 231
Thrombosis, angiographic rates, 329–331
Toxicity, of radiation therapy, 491–493
Tracker microcatheter, with fibered coil, 274,
274
Transfacial approach, to anterior skull base
tumors, 43–62
case report, 60, *60*
classification of, 44t, 44–50
clinical experience, 58–59
general treatment techniques, 56–58
lesion types, 58, 59t
levels, 43–44, *44*
transfrontal (level I), 44t, 45, 50
transfrontal-nasal (level II), 44t, *46*, 50–53
transfrontal-nasal-orbital (level III), 44t,
47, 52, 53–54
transmaxillary (level V), 44t, *49, 52*, 55–56
transnasomaxillary (level IV), 44t, *48*, 55

transpalatal (level VI), 44t, *51–52*, 56
Transfrontal approach, to anterior skull
  base tumors, 44t, *45*, 50
Transfrontal-nasal approach, to anterior
  skull base tumors, 44t, *46*, 50–53
Transfrontal-nasal-orbital approach, to
  anterior skull base tumors, 44t, *47*,
  52, 53–54
Translabyrinthine approach, to acoustic
  neuromas, facial nerve outcome with,
  194, 195t
Transmaxillary approach, to anterior skull
  base tumors, 44t, *49*, *52*, 55–56
Transnasomaxillary approach, to anterior
  skull base tumors, 44t, *48*, 55
Transpalatal approach, to anterior skull
  base tumors, 44t, *51–52*, 56
TreeAge, DATA software, 296
Trigeminal nerve (cranial nerve V), intra-
  operative monitoring, 189
Trigeminal neuroma, 94
Tuberculum sellae meningioma, 81–83
  management of, 81–82
  radiotherapy for, 83, 83t
  results, 82–83
  surgery for, 82t, 82–83
Tumor cell death, after transfer of drug-
  sensitivity genes, 375–376
Tumorigenesis, field effect, 483
Tumors. *See also specific types*
  anterior skull base, 71–98
    ICA sacrifice for, 63–67
    radical resection of, 43–70
    stereotactic radiosurgery for, 99–118, 100t
    transfacial approach to, 43–60
  benign
    of cavernous sinus, 155
    skull base, ICA sacrifice for, 64–66
  brain, gene therapy for, in mice, 370–382
  cavernous sinus, 71–98, 155–156
    benign, 155
    direct surgery for, 119, 120t
    1994 CNS audience responses, 514–515
  cystic, stereotactic resection of, 417, *418*
  deep-seated, stereotactic resection of, *416*,
    416–417, 418, *419*
  dysembryoplastic neuroepithelial, 409–410,
    455
  epidermoid, 94–95
  glial
    spatial types, 404–406

  surgical decision making for, 406, *407*
    infiltrating supplementary motor cortex,
      443, *444*
  malignant
    direct surgery for, 119, 120t
    skull base, ICA sacrifice for, 66
  metastatic, stereotactic radiosurgery for,
    115–116
  pituitary, stereotactic radiosurgery for, 107–
    110
  recurrence, volume effects on, 438t, 438–
    440, 439t
  skull base, ICA sacrifice for, 66
  spinal cord, laminectomy for, 212–213
  superficial
    management of, 423–426
    stereotactic resection method for, *415*,
      415–416
  volume, effects on recurrence, 438t, 438–
    440, 439t
  well-circumscribed, management of, 423–
    426

United States
  health care reform, 8–9
  health care system, 23
Universal coverage, 12
University of Florida, radiosurgery for AVMs
  at, 333–342

Vagus nerve (cranial nerve X), monitoring of,
  200
Vascular malformations
  angiographically occult, 344–345
  1994 CNS audience responses, 515–517
Vectors, viral, for brain tumor gene therapy,
  372–373, 373t
Vein grafts
  common carotid artery to middle cerebral
    artery, 160
  external carotid artery to middle cerebral
    artery, 141, 141t, 160
  internal carotid artery to internal carotid
    artery, 141, 141t, 160
  long, from cervical arteries to middle
    cerebral artery, 142
  occlusion of, 148–149
  petrous ICA to supraclinoid ICA, 142–143
  superficial temporal artery to middle
    cerebral artery, 160
VERs. *See* Visual evoked responses

Vertebral artery, giant aneurysm of, 222, *224*
Vestibulocochlear nerve (cranial nerve VIII).
	See Auditory nerve
Viral vectors, for brain tumor gene therapy,
	372–373, 373t
Visual evoked responses. *See also* Evoked
	potentials
 intra-operative monitoring, 187–189, *204,*
	204–205
Volumetric stereotactic resection
 computer-assisted
  of deep-seated tumors, 418, *419*
  of low-grade gliomas, 412–413
   methods, 413–418
   results, 418–427
   surgical planning, 414
   surgical procedures, 414–417
 of low-grade gliomas, 420t, 433–434
Volumetric stereotaxis

database acquisition, 413
 purpose of, 418

WADA tests, 440
Waivers, Medicaid, 34–35
Washington Committee, 10
Water-hammer effect, 273
Wilcoson rank-sum test, 194, 195t

Xanthoastrocytomas, 404
 management of, 423–426
 pleomorphic, 391
Xenon computed tomography (Xe CT)
 CBF measurement, 137, 158
 moderate-risk patients treated by, 144

Young patients, gangliogliomas in, *409,* 409–
	410